CANCER
RISK
ASSESSMENT

BASIC AND CLINICAL ONCOLOGY

Editor

Bruce D. Cheson, M.D.

National Cancer Institute
National Institutes of Health
Bethesda, Maryland

ADDITIONAL VOLUMES IN PREPARATION

CANCER RISK ASSESSMENT

edited by

PETER G. SHIELDS

Georgetown University Medical Center
Washington, D.C., U.S.A.

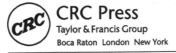

CRC Press
Taylor & Francis Group
Boca Raton London New York

CRC Press is an imprint of the
Taylor & Francis Group, an **Informa** business

A TAYLOR & FRANCIS BOOK

Published in 2005 by
Taylor & Francis Group
6000 Broken Sound Parkway NW, Suite 300
Boca Raton, FL 33487-2742

© 2005 by Taylor & Francis Group, LLC
CRC Press is an imprint of Taylor & Francis Group, an Informa business

First issued in paperback 2019

No claim to original U.S. Government works

ISBN 13: 978-0-367-45414-2 (pbk)
ISBN 13: 978-0-8247-2984-4 (hbk)

Library of Congress Cataloging-in-Publication Data

Catalog record is available from the Library of Congress

**Visit the Taylor & Francis Web site at
http://www.taylorandfrancis.com**

**and the CRC Press Web site at
http://www.crcpress.com**

Contents

Preface

Humans are continuously exposed to carcinogens from environmental, occupational, and endogenous sources. Health professionals, regulatory agencies, and cancer researchers are frequently challenged to identify the causes of cancer, to predict risks, and to develop methods to prevent cancer. The assessment of cancer risk in individuals or the population is a complex process that reflects both actual science and scientific intuition. There is an exploding amount of information—in many cases conflicting information—and a confusing array of sources to consider about the applicability and use of biomarkers. New data from the Human Genome Project, the latest technologies in molecular genetics (e.g., proteomics, microarrays, high-throughput assay methods), are rapidly being incorporated into risk assessment and epidemiological studies, and there are many challenges to the interpretation of the resulting data. Clearly, the use of biomarkers and genetic susceptibility analysis is improving our ability to predict risk in the population and the individual, but it is a rapidly evolving and complicated area of research. Students of molecular epidemiology and people outside of the field need guidance to use and interpret biomarker data, and a context from to evaluate whether the data improve the risk assessment process.

This book is intended for health professionals, public health specialists, persons within regulatory agencies, and cancer researchers who need more than a summary of recent data. It provides a practical approach to conducting risk assessment for the population and the individual in the context of biomarkers and genetic susceptibilities, especially within a broader perspective of background cancer risk and an individual's exposures within a complex environment. While the risk assessment process usually focuses on a single particular exposure, people are constantly exposed to a multitude of known and potential human carcinogens—from the air, their diet and lifestyle, etc. When setting public health priorities or evaluating a person with cancer, this broader context makes the risk assessment process much more challenging. This text helps the reader place cancer risk within such a context, and understand the relative risks from different exposures and how biomarkers and genetic susceptibilities help in the risk assessment process.

Biomarkers are tests conducted on any biological tissue or fluid, including air. Assays to assess an individual's risk through specific genes, thereby assessing genetic susceptibilities, also are a type of biomarker. However, the term *biomarker* usually refers to an assay of exposure, biologically effective dose, or some effect of exposure. The term *genetic susceptibility* refers to an individual's heritable capacity to respond to exposures, which would therefore result in modifying cancer risk. Biomarkers can be used as intermediate markers of cancer risk, reflecting a mechanistic pathway to cancer. Genetic susceptibilities would therefore affect the level of biomarkers, reflecting a gene–environment interaction. Therefore, the term *gene–environment interaction* refers to an effect of exposure that is increased or decreased by genetic susceptibilities; it is used generically and there are formal statistical methods to assess interactions. Most cancers are considered to be caused by carcinogenic exposures, although with most cancers and therefore in most people, the causes have not been identified. Although the body has the capacity to repair much of the damage from gene–environment interactions, it is the sheer number of gene–environment interactions that actually contribute to the carcinogenic process. Biomarkers now are enhancing our understanding about the causes of cancer, and in some cases are helping identify what specifically caused a cancer in a particular person.

The use of biomarkers is not new and has been around for more than 50 years. But the last 20 years have seen rapidly developing technologies, which recently have greatly accelerated. These newer methods bring analytical and bioinformatic challenges but nonetheless show great promise for enhancing our risk assessment processes further.

Frequently the public and individuals with cancer make conclusions about the causes of cancer that are not founded upon sound data or based on appropriate assessment methodologies. The public health community is obligated to understand and communicate the latest scientific data in the context of the risk assessment process for the general population, persons at high risk, and individuals within the general population. This text provides the reader with the tools to assess cancer causation with specific methodologies, rather than relying on intuition and speculation.

Cancer is a multistage process that is triggered by multiple steps through many pathways. There are many repair and protective mechanisms in the human body to prevent most DNA damage that would otherwise lead to cancer. Typically, the determination of a cancer risk factor requires the examination of a potential etiological agent against a background of many real etiological agents. Many new laboratory and epidemiological findings are impacting how we think about cancer risk, while many principles used in the assessment of causation remain conceptually important. This book presents recent data that impact cancer risk for the general population and individual, and reviews data for some known and potential human carcinogens. It reviews the methods for determining what causes cancer and what does not. Practical approaches to the determination of cancer risk in individuals and the population are offered, including counseling of individuals, groups of exposed persons, and society as a whole.

This text is organized to provide the most current information in two ways. The first approaches risk assessment from a methodological perspective. The reader is provided information about carcinogenesis in general and then specifically for chemical, radiation, viral, occupational, and familial cancers. While there is overlap in some of these mechanisms (e.g., chemical and occupational carcinogenesis), there are different mechanistic approaches to consider depending on the perspective. One particular focus includes recent data for tobacco, alcohol, and hormonal mechanisms in cancer risk, as these are among the major known human carcinogens and carcinogenic mechanisms. Additionally, how people are exposed to known and suspected carcinogens is identified, with particulars on how to measure this in the workplace using industrial hygiene methods. Information about differences in cancer risk among various ethnic and racial populations in the context of different exposures and mechanistic etiologies are also discussed.

The second methodology includes basic epidemiological approaches as they apply to molecular epidemiology, including both the use of biomarkers and genetics within an epidemiological framework. Detailed approaches in the use of genetic testing for cancer risk, using both markers in cancers and then measures of genetic damage in persons without cancer, are given. The actual approach to risk assessment is highlighted in detail in three separate chapters. The readers are provided with the distinct approaches to population and individual risk assessment, and also with information about how regulatory agencies determine what is a carcinogen. The chapter on individual risk assessment is particularly unique as the reader is provided with a framework for evaluating an individual who has cancer, or is thought to be at risk for cancer.

The second half of the text provides the reader with cancer risk information by organ system for major cancers. It uses the principals established in the first part of the text, which provided the reader with the tools to evaluate risk, and applies them to single organ sites. While this text provides a summary of the latest data for biomarkers and genetic susceptibilities within the risk assessment process, it cannot provide a critique of all available data. However, it will equip the reader to explore and assess further data.

The production of this text required the hard work of many people, and I would like to thank my co-authors and contributors specifically for their patience and multiple iterations to produce what are outstanding chapters. I also will like to thank Sandi Crawford and Regina Jackson for the expert organizational assistance, without which this book would never have been completed.

Peter G. Shields

Contributors

Christine B. Ambrosone   Department of Epidemiology, Roswell Park Cancer Institute, Buffalo, New York, U.S.A.

Melissa L. Bondy Department of Epidemiology, M. D. Anderson Cancer Center, University of Texas, Houston, Texas, U.S.A.

Anne-Lise Børresen-Dale Department of Genetics, Institute for Cancer Research, University Clinic of the Norwegian Radium Hospital, Oslo, Norway

Diane L. Carlisle Department of Pharmacology, University of Pittsburgh, Pittsburgh, Pennsylvania, U.S.A.

James R. Cerhan   Health Sciences Research, Mayo Clinic College of Medicine, Rochester, New York, U.S.A.

Susan S. Devesa Division of Cancer Epidemiology and Genetics, National Cancer Institute, Bethesda, Maryland, U.S.A.

Mustafa Dosemeci   Occupational and Environmental Epidemiology Branch, Division of Cancer Epidemiology and Genetics, National Cancer Institute, Rockville, Maryland, U.S.A.

Randa El-Zein Department of Epidemiology, M. D. Anderson Cancer Center, University of Texas, Houston, Texas, U.S.A.

Heather Spencer Feigelson Department of Epidemiology and Surveillance Research, American Cancer Society, Atlanta, Georgia, U.S.A.

Christina Frank Department of Epidemiology, University of Maryland School of Medicine, Baltimore, Maryland, U.S.A.

Helena Furberg Department of Genetics, University of North Carolina at Chapel Hill, Chapel Hill, North Carolina, U.S.A.

Laura Gunn Division of Environmental Health Sciences, School of Public Health, University of California at Berkeley, Berkeley, California, U.S.A.

Pierre Hainaut International Agency for Research on Cancer, Lyon, France

Aage Haugen Department of Toxicology, National Institute of Occupational Health, Oslo, Norway

Richard B. Hayes Division of Cancer Epidemiology and Genetics, National Cancer Institute, DHHS, Bethesda, Maryland, U.S.A.

Kathy J. Helzlsouer Bloomberg School of Public Health, Johns Hopkins University, Baltimore, Maryland, U.S.A., and Prevention and Research Center, Mercy Medical Center, Baltimore, Maryland, U.S.A.

Michie Hisada Viral Epidemiology Branch, Division of Cancer Epidemiology and Genetics, National Cancer Institute, Bethesda, Maryland, U.S.A.

Carrie P. Hunter North Potomac, Martland, U.S.A.

Alan M. Jeffrey Department of Pathology, New York Medical College, Valhalla, New York, U.S.A.

Charles E. Land Radiation Epidemiology Branch, Division of Cancer Epidemiology and Genetics, National Cancer Institute, Bethesda, Maryland, U.S.A.

Loïc Le Marchand Cancer Research Center of Hawaii, University of Hawaii, Honolulu, Hawaii, U.S.A.

Martha S. Linet Division of Cancer Epidemiology and Genetics, National Cancer Institute, Bethesda, Maryland, U.S.A.

Christopher Loffredo Cancer Genetics and Epidemiology Program, Department of Oncology, Georgetown University School of Medicine, Washington, D.C., U.S.A.

Ragnhild A. Lothe   Department of Genetics, Institute for Cancer Research, University Clinic of the Norwegian Radium Hospital, Oslo, Norway

Robert J. McCunney   Department of Biological Engineering, Massachusetts Institute of Technology, Pulmonary Division, Massachusetts General Hospital, Boston, Massachusetts, U.S.A.

Roberta McKean-Cowdin   Norris Comprehensive Cancer Center, Keck School of Medicine, Los Angeles, California, U.S.A.

Yuri Minn   Department of Epidemiology, M. D. Anderson Cancer Center, University of Texas, Houston, Texas, U.S.A.

Ruggero Montesano   International Agency for Research on Cancer, Lyon, France

Gareth J. Morgan   Department of Hematology, Institute of Pathology, University of Leeds, Leeds, U.K.

Kirsten B. Moysich   Department of Epidemiology, Roswell Park Cancer Institute, Buffalo, New York, U.S.A.

Lee Okurowski   Department of Orthopedics, Occupational Health, New England Baptist Hospital, Boston, Massachusetts, U.S.A.

Steven R. Patierno   Department of Pharmacology, George Washington University, Washington, D.C., U.S.A.

Charles S. Rabkin   Viral Epidemiology Branch, Division of Cancer Epidemiology and Genetics, National Cancer Institute, Bethesda, Maryland, U.S.A.

Jerry M. Rice   Department of Oncology, Lombardi Comprehensive Cancer Center, Georgetown University, Washington, D.C., U.S.A.

Hongbing Shen   Department of Epidemiology, M. D. Anderson Cancer Center, University of Texas, Houston, Texas, U.S.A.

Peter G. Shields   Cancer Genetics and Epidemiology Program, Department of Medicine and Oncology, Lombardi Comprehensive Cancer Center, Georgetown University Medical Center, Washington, U.S.A.

Martyn T. Smith   Division of Environmental Health Sciences, School of Public Health, University of California at Berkeley, Berkeley, California, U.S.A.

Margaret R. Spitz   Department of Epidemiology, M. D. Anderson Cancer Center, University of Texas, Houston, Texas, U.S.A.

Erich M. Sturgis   Department of Head and Neck Surgery, M. D. Anderson Cancer Center, University of Texas, Houston, Texas, U.S.A.

Haruhiko Sugimura   Department of Pathology, Hamamatsu University School of Medicine, Hamamatsu, Shizuoka, Japan

Philippe Tanière   International Agency for Research on Cancer, Lyon, France

Paolo Vineis   Unit of Cancer Epidemiology and Chair of Biostatistics, Dipartimento di Scienze Biomediche e Oncologia Umana, University of Turim, Turim, Italy

Kala Visvanathan   Bloomberg School of Public Health, Johns Hopkins University, Baltimore, Maryland, U.S.A.

Elizabeth Ward   Industrywide Studies Branch Division of Surveillance, Hazard Evaluations and Field Studies, National Institute for Occupational Safety and Health, Cincinnati, Ohio, U.S.A.

Qingyi Wei   Department of Epidemiology, M. D. Anderson Cancer Center, University of Texas, Houston, Texas, U.S.A.

John Whysner   Washington Occupational Health Associates, Washington, D.C., U.S.A.

Gary M. Williams   Department of Pathology, New York Medical College, Valhalla, New York, U.S.A.

Margaret Wrensch   Department of Epidemiology, M. D. Anderson Cancer Center, University of Texas, Houston, Texas, U.S.A.

Luoping Zhang   Division of Environmental Health Sciences, School of Public Health, University of California at Berkeley, Berkeley, California, U.S.A.

1

Carcinogenesis and Molecular Genetics

Diane L. Carlisle

Department of Pharmacology, University of Pittsburgh, Pittsburgh, Pennsylvania, U.S.A.

Steven R. Patierno

Department of Pharmacology, George Washington University, Washington, D.C., U.S.A.

1. INTRODUCTION

All tissues have a rate at which cells naturally die, while other cells divide to take their place. The skin, for example, consists of large numbers of cells that are dying or dead and are constantly sloughed off, while new layers of skin regenerate by cell division beneath the cell surface. Maintaining the homeostatic balance of cell loss and cell gain is crucial to the health and survival of the tissue and organism, and so the balance is tightly regulated in all tissues throughout the body. Disturbing this balance of cell loss and cell proliferation can lead to disease. Tumor formation occurs when cell division exceeds cell death. This happens in one of two ways: either cell proliferation is increased so that it occurs faster than cell death or cell death is prevented or slowed so that it no longer keeps up with cell division. The progression of cellular changes leading to this excess growth and formation of a malignant tumor is the process known as multistage carcinogenesis. Most, if not all, of the morphological and biochemical characteristics of malignant cells have as their source either genetical or epigenetical alterations in gene expression. Therefore, the controls that usually tightly regulate the cell growth and death processes on a molecular level must be examined and manipulated in order to fully understand multistage

1

carcinogenesis. Many factors can contribute to carcinogenesis, including viruses, chemicals, radiation, diet, hormones, and genetical predisposition.

Currently, there is much attention ascribed to cancer genes that can increase or decrease an individual's chance of getting cancer and influence a person's prognosis after the diagnosis of cancer has been made. In addition to providing risk assessment information, knowledge of why these genes are important and how they work may yield important clues to the molecular causes of cancer. Genes that are important in cancer come in two general types, operationally defined as oncogenes and tumor suppressor genes (1).

Oncogenes are genes which act to stimulate cell division or increase cell survival, when expressed in a biochemically abnormal environment which is permissive for their growth stimulatory effects. When overexpressed or expressed aberrantly, they may disrupt the division–death ratio. Tumor suppressor genes have an equally important role in tissues, but in preventing in tumor formation. Normally, they protect cells from abnormal growth in several ways and, in cancers, are often found to be mutated so that their function is either altered or lost entirely. The complex interplay between oncogenes and tumor suppressor genes can be exemplified using the *ras* oncogene which becomes oncogenic by expressing altered function after a single base change, and the *bcl-2* gene, which codes for a mitochondrial protein that helps prevent apoptotic cell death. Overexpression of a mutant *ras* oncogene is actually lethal to normal cells, but in the context of a cell which has lost expression of *bcl-2,* mutant *ras* becomes promitogenic (2).

2. STEPS IN CARCINOGENESIS

The carcinogenic process is complex and involves many genetical changes. For example, mutation of the *brca1* or *brca2* gene, which has been implicated in familial breast cancer (3,4), leads only to an *increased risk* of breast cancer; it does not mean that there is a 100% certainty of any particular woman having breast cancer during her lifetime. In fact, the penetrance of *brca1* mutation, i.e., the chance that a woman with a *brca1* mutation will be diagnosed with breast cancer by age 70, has been shown to be anywhere from 37% to 90%, depending on the population studied (5). In order to study carcinogenesis, the process has been historically and conceptually divided operationally into three steps: initiation, promotion, and progression. These divisions are a helpful starting point, but as we learn more about the molecular genetics and epigenetics of cancer, the distinctions between these divisions become less and less clear.

The first step in carcinogenesis, historically referred to as initiation, is one that produces an altered cell that has some selectable growth advantage over other cells. This step can be facilitated by genetical predisposition, and caused by exposure to chemicals, radiation, viruses, or other permanent cellular changes. These changes reduce the stringency of the regulation of cell growth and death. Initiation is always a permanent event and may occur at any time during a person's lifetime, but usually many years before cancer is diagnosed. Historically, the initiation event was thought to be nearly synonymous with mutation after genotoxic insult. Recently, however, this notion has been challenged. More and more evidence is accumulating, linking cancer initiation with epigenetical alterations in transcriptional patterning, perhaps invoked as a cellular response to genotoxic insult and other forms of cellular stress (6,7).

The next operationally defined stage in the development of cancer is promotion. Promotion is not a permanent event, but a transient process that promotes cell growth. However, because initiation is permanent, promotion can occur at any time, either at the same time as initiation, or many years after initiation takes place (Fig. 1). The role of promotion is to stimulate an initiated cell to divide, and then to stimulate the net accumulation of initiated cells by either stimulating cell division or inhibiting cell death (8). Promotion may have indirect effects as well. For example, the stimulation of cell division increases the possibility that a mistake in the fidelity of DNA replication may occur, leading to mutation. This situation could be especially dangerous if the cell being provoked to divide has already incurred alterations in the function of genes required for DNA repair or for governing the cell cycle. For example, the *p53* gene, often referred to as the guardian of the genome, functions to inhibit the cell from entering the DNA synthesis (S) phase of the cell cycle, in the presence of unrepaired DNA damage (9). Forcing a cell with defective *p53* to enter the S phase with unrepaired DNA damage may increase the frequency of mutation and lead to genomic instability and development of the mutator phenotype (see below).

While some agents are strictly initiating agents, and others strictly promoting agents, many of the most potent carcinogens are both initiators and promoters. Cigarette smoke is one such example (10). Many of the chemicals in cigarette smoke are both genotoxic and toxic, cause mutations and gene expression changes, as well as cell death. The events associated with the genotoxic insult may be initiating events, creating populations of abnormal cells. Cigarette smoke also serves as a promoter, for example, by stimulating proliferation of genetically damaged cells following cytotoxicity and loss of neighboring cells.

The final stage of carcinogenesis is historically defined as progression. Progression occurs when an initiated cell undergoes promotion, and that promotion leads to cellular changes that deregulate the cell growth controls. This stage of carcinogenesis is self-sustaining, but occurs in part by chance. Cells that are growing without the normal controls will, by chance, gain mutations. If a mutation occurs in a tumor suppressor gene such as a DNA repair gene, this will allow that cell to acquire mutations at an even higher rate. A cell which has this type of mutation is said to have a mutator

79. Welcsh PL, Schubert EL, King MC. Inherited breast cancer: an emerging picture. Clin Genet 1998; 54:447.
80. Meyn MS. Ataxia-telangiectasia, cancer and the pathobiology of the ATM gene. Clin Genet 1999; 55:289.
81. Skomedal H, Helland A, Kristensen GB, Holm R, Borresen-Dale AL. Allelic imbalance at chromosome region 11q23 in cervical carcinomas. Eur J Cancer 1999; 35:659.
82. Starostik P, Manshouri T, O'Brien S, Freireich E, Kantarjian H, Haidar M, Lerner S, Keating M, Albitar M. Deficiency of the ATM protein expression defines an aggressive subgroup of B-cell chronic lymphocytic leukemia. Cancer Res 1998; 58:4552.
83. Bullrich F, Rasio D, Kitada S, Starostik P, Kipps T, Keating M, Albitar M, Reed JC, Croce CM. ATM mutations in B-cell chronic lymphocytic leukemia. Cancer Res 1999; 59:24.
84. Friedman LS, Ostermeyer EA, Szabo CI, Dowd P, Lynch ED, Rowell SE, King MC. Confirmation of BRCA1 by analysis of germline mutations linked to breast and ovarian cancer in ten families. Nat Genet 1994; 8:399.
85. Castilla LH, Couch FJ, Erdos MR, Hoskins KF, Calzone K, Garber JE, Boyd J, Lubin MB, Deshano ML, Brody LC, et al. Mutations in the BRCA1 gene in families with early-onset breast and ovarian cancer. Nat Genet 1994; 8:387.
86. Steichen-Gersdorf E, Gallion HH, Ford D, Girodet C, Easton DF, DiCioccio RA, Evans G, Ponder MA, Pye C, Mazoyer S, et al. Familial site-specific ovarian cancer is linked to BRCA1 on 17q12-21. Am J Hum Genet 1994; 55:870.
87. Gao X, Zacharek A, Salkowski A, Grignon DJ, Sakr W, Porter AT, Honn KV. Loss of heterozygosity of the BRCA1 and other loci on chromosome 17q in human prostate cancer. Cancer Res 1995; 55:1002.
88. Yu JJ, Mu C, Lee KB, Okamoto A, Reed EL, Bostick-Bruton F, Mitchell KC, Reed E. A nucleotide polymorphism in ERCC1 in human ovarian cancer cell lines and tumor tissues. Mutat Res 1997; 382:13.
89. Liang BC, Ross DA, Reed E. Genomic copy number changes of DNA repair genes ERCC1 and ERCC2 in human gliomas. J Neurooncol 1995; 26:17.
90. Benachenhou N, Guiral S, Gorska-Flipot I, Labuda D, Sinnett D. Frequent loss of heterozygosity at the DNA mismatch-repair loci hMLH1 and hMSH3 in sporadic breast cancer. Br J Cancer 1999; 79:1012.
91. Bapat BV, Madlensky L, Temple LK, Hiruki T, Redston M, Baron DL, Xia L, Marcus VA, Soravia C, Mitri A, Shen W, Gryfe R, Berk T, Chodirker BN, Cohen Z, Gallinger S. Family history characteristics, tumor microsatellite instability and germline MSH2 and MLH1 mutations in hereditary colorectal cancer. Hum Genet 1999; 104:167.
92. Simpkins SB, Bocker T, Swisher EM, Mutch DG, Gersell DJ, Kovatich AJ, Palazzo JP, Fishel R, Goodfellow PJ. MLH1 promoter methylation and gene silencing is the primary cause of microsatellite instability in sporadic endometrial cancers. Hum Mol Genet 1999; 8:661.
93. Strathdee G, MacKean MJ, Illand M, Brown R. A role for methylation of the hMLH1 promoter in loss of hMLH1 expression and drug resistance in ovarian cancer. Oncogene 1999; 18:2335.

94. Risinger JI, Umar A, Boyd J, Berchuck A, Kunkel TA, Barrett JC. Mutation of MSH3 in endometrial cancer and evidence for its functional role in heteroduplex repair. Nat Genet 1996; 14:102.
95. Hosoya N, Hangaishi A, Ogawa S, Miyagawa K, Mitani K, Yazaki Y, Hirai H. Frameshift mutations of the hMSH6 gene in human leukemia cell lines. Jpn J Cancer Res 1998; 89:33.
96. Nicolaides NC, Papadopoulos N, Liu B, Wei YF, Carter KC, Ruben SM, Rosen CA, Haseltine WA, Fleischmann RD, Fraser CM, et al. Mutations of two PMS homologues in hereditary nonpolyposis colon cancer. Nature 1994; 371:75.
97. Kondoh M, Ueda M, Nakagawa K, Ichihashi M. Siblings with xeroderma pigmentosum complementation group A with different skin cancer development: importance of sun protection at an early age. J Am Acad Dermatol 1994; 31:993.
98. Baylin SB, Herman JG, Graff JR, Vertino PM, Issa JP. Alterations in DNA methylation: a fundamental aspect of neoplasia. Adv Cancer Res 1998; 72:141.
99. Belinsky SA, Nikula KJ, Palmisano WA, et al. Aberrant methylation of p16(INK4a) is an early event in lung cancer and a potential biomarker for early diagnosis. Proc Natl Acad Sci USA 1998; 95:11891.

2

Epidemiological Approaches to Studying Cancer I: Study Design, Confounding Variables, Misclassification, and Cancer Clusters

Elizabeth Ward

Industrywide Studies Branch Division of Surveillance, Hazard Evaluations and Field Studies, National Institute for Occupational Safety and Health, Cincinnati, Ohio, U.S.A.

1. INTRODUCTION

In recent years, several authors have advocated the use of epidemiological data, if available, in developing cancer risk assessments (1–5). Epidemiological data may be used in a variety of ways in risk assessment, principally in hazard identification and exposure–response analysis (4). This chapter will review basic concepts in the design and interpretation of epidemiological studies, focusing on their application in risk assessment.

Two major epidemiological study designs have contributed substantially to understanding the etiology of human cancer. *Cohort studies* are studies in which a defined group of people are followed for a period of time. They can be either retrospective studies, in which the group is defined at a point or period in the past and followed to the present, or prospective, in which the group is defined in the present and followed into the future. The cohorts can be derived from the general population, to study the effects of common exposures such as smoking and diet, or selected on the basis of a particular exposure. Outcomes measured may be intermediate markers, incident disease, or death. Cohort studies can detect the effect of a rare exposure because by design a relatively large number of exposed subjects can be assembled and studied; cohort studies often focus on a single exposure and multiple outcomes. *Case–control studies* are studies in which risk factors for disease are compared between individuals with the disease and those without. Case–control studies may be community based or nested within cohorts. In community based case–control studies, information about risk factors is generally obtained directly from study subjects, but in some cases, additional measurements are made of biological tissues or environmental exposures, or supplementary information is gained from medical or other records. Case–control studies are particularly useful for studying rare diseases; they examine the relationship between a single outcome and multiple exposures. General aspects of the design and analysis of both types of studies are covered in textbooks of epidemiology (6,7).

Cohort studies of occupational groups or populations with environmental exposure to radiological or chemical hazards have been the primary source of information for a number of important risk assessments to date (e.g., asbestos, arsenic, benzene, and radon daughters) (1). The use of case–control studies in risk assessment has been more limited, with some noteworthy exceptions, such as environmental tobacco smoke and lung cancer (8,9) and residential radon exposure and lung Cancer (10).

Epidemiological studies may be hypothesis testing or hypothesis generating. Ecological studies, in which correlations are made at a group level (i.e., comparing fat consumption and breast cancer incidence by country) are often used to generate hypotheses about exposure–disease associations and typically cannot do more than that. Cohort and case–control studies may be hypothesis generating when the basis for a priori hypotheses is limited, but they are often designed to test hypotheses about disease causation. A causal association between an exposure and disease is rarely established by the results of a single epidemiological study. A number of investigators have proposed criteria for defining causality based on epidemiological study results (6). Some of the most important criteria include temporal sequence (the cause must precede the effect), strength of the association, dose–response relationship, replication of the findings, and biological plausibility (6). Table 1 defines some important terms used in epidemiological studies.

2. COHORT STUDIES

Occupational cohort studies have played a central role in the understanding of radiation-induced and chemically related cancer, because occupational exposures are often orders of magnitude higher than exposures in the general population, making exposure effects easier to observe in relatively small populations. As early as the 1950s, occupational cohort studies documented

Table 1 Definitions of Some Important Terms Used in Epidemiological Studies

Term	Definition
Incidence	The number of new cases of a disease that occur in a specified period of time divided by the number of people in the population at risk of developing the disease
Prevalence	The number of cases of a disease present in a population at a specified time divided by the number of persons at that point in time
Period prevalence	How many people have had the disease at any time during a certain period
Mortality rate	The number of deaths in the population divided by the number of persons in the population at midyear
Proportionate mortality ratio (PMR)	The number of deaths from a particular cause divided by the total number of deaths
Standardized mortality ratio (SMR)	Observed number of deaths per year divided by expected number of deaths; expected number of deaths based on age, calendar time, gender- and race-specific death rates in the referent population
Standardized incidence ratio (SIR)	Observed number of new cases per year divided by expected number of new cases; expected number of new cases based on age, calendar time, gender- and race-specific incidence rates in the referent population
Relative risk (RR)	Disease risk (incidence rate) in an exposed population divided by disease risk (incidence rate) in an unexposed population
Odds ratio	Estimate of association calculated in a case-control study; approximates relative risk when the risk of disease is low (see Section 3 for how to calculate)
Attributable risk	The amount or proportion of disease incidence (or disease risk) that can be attributed to a specific exposure

Source: Adapted from Refs. 6, 7, 63, 64.

the risk of cancer associated with occupational exposure to aromatic amines (beta-naphthylamine, benzidine) (11) and asbestos (12). Many occupational cohort studies have used duration of employment in the occupation or industry under study as an index of cumulative exposure. However, as methods were developed and utilized to measure air concentrations of chemicals in the workplace, studies began to incorporate quantitative estimates of exposure, enabling researchers to associate level of exposure with level of risk (13). In some studies, exposure estimates are generated for multiple agents in a single population, with the goal of evaluating which agents are associated with observed cancer excesses. For example, in a study of the synthetic rubber industry, quantitative estimates of exposure to 1,3-butadiene, styrene, and benzene were developed to evaluate exposure–response relationships with leukemia (14).

Occupational cohort studies include all individuals entering and leaving a workforce during a defined time period (for example, from January 1, 1940, to January 1, 1979) and observe the number of incident cases or deaths during the time interval of study per number of person-years of observation (15). Most commonly, occupational cohort studies use mortality as the outcome, ascertaining deaths from national vital registry data. Use of mortality as the outcome has the advantage that it is possible to achieve nearly 100% ascertainment of deaths, at least in the United States. There is, however, a significant possibility of misclassification of cancer site on death certificates (16) and histologic type is often unspecified. Occupational cohort studies may be analyzed using life table methods, in which person-years-at-risk (PYAR) are accumulated for each individual from the time they enter the cohort until death, loss to follow-up, or end of study. Person-years-at-risk may be stratified by age, calendar time, race, time since first employment, duration of employment, and other occupational exposure characteristics. The number of expected deaths is calculated by multiplying age, calendar time, and race-specific PYAR by the relevant referent rates in the general population, such as national mortality or state-based cancer registry data. Life table analysis yields standardized mortality ratios (SMRs) or standardized incidence ratios (SIRs), which compare the number of observed and expected deaths, based on indirect standardization to control for age, calendar time, and race. Life table analysis programs are available from several sources (17–19). Analysis of cohort studies using external referents suffers from the problem that the external referent population may not be comparable to the study population in attributes other than the one under study. For example, it is common to find that occupational cohorts have substantially lower mortality than the general population due to selection of healthy individuals into the workforce and the survival of healthier individuals, which permits long-term employment (this has been called the "healthy worker effect") (13). This effect is strongest for cardiovascular disease and is less apparent for cancer (13). Use of internal referents, i.e., members of the cohort with no or minimal exposure, may circumvent this problem. Internal comparisons within cohort studies require additional analytical methods, such as direct standardization or Mantel–Haenzel techniques, to adjust for age and other factors that may differ between subcohorts. Poisson regression analysis can be utilized to to examine the effect of all the study variables on the disease incidence or mortality rate simultaneously (6,20).

There are a number of important issues to be considered in the design of cohort studies intended to assess the carcinogenicity of chemical or physical exposures. Often chemical studies are triggered by new, positive animal bioassay results. The first step in designing a cohort study is to determine in what occupations and industries the chemical is used, the numbers of workers exposed, and a selection of those industries or occupations that provide the best opportunity for study. Important factors in choosing the occupation or industry to study include the level of exposure to the chemical and the presence of potential confounding exposures. Once an industry or occupational group has been selected, factors considered in choosing the actual study sites include length of operation, numbers of workers, and quality of personnel, production, and exposure records (21). Great care must be taken to ensure that the entire targeted study population is identified, because nonrandom losses, such as failing to identify records of retirees or other subgroups, may seriously bias the study results.

Exposure assessment in occupational cohort studies should include, at a minimum, a complete history of plant operations, including major products, starting materials, by-products, and potential contaminants present in all major departments or process areas and review of existing environmental or personal monitoring data. Such data can be used to classify workers (through their department and job codes) as exposed or unexposed to the chemical of interest, as well as potential confounders, and to establish the date at which exposure began and its duration. Once preliminary data have been collected for a retrospective study, a decision is made about whether it is feasible to reconstruct historical exposures and conduct an exposure–response assessment. Factors in this decision include whether there is sufficient detail in the personnel records to determine the detailed job history of individuals (i.e., department, operation, starting and ending dates) and whether there are sufficient monitoring data available to generate meaningful exposure estimates. Often these conditions are not met, but a decision is made to proceed with a study because it is the best available population or because there is interest in the health effects in a specific population although it does not have sufficient information to characterize exposure–response.

Issues in the reconstruction of historical exposures for occupational cohort studies have recently been reviewed (22,23). Stewart et al. (22) define several steps in developing quantitative retrospective exposure estimates for epidemiological studies: (1) identification of appropriate agents of exposure, including consideration of physical states and routes of exposure; (2) development of "exposure groups," defined as groups of persons whose exposures are similar enough so that monitoring of any worker in the group provides data useful for predicting the exposure of the remaining workers; (3) evaluation of availability and representativeness of existing sampling data; development of procedures for generating quantitative estimates by exposure group, including methods of extrapolation or interpolation for time periods and exposure groups where data are sparse or nonexistent. Often there are no exposure measurements for early decades of plant operation. Assumptions made in deriving exposure estimates for these time periods may lead to considerable variation in the estimates (24,25) and the resulting risk assessments (26,27).

Cohort studies also have been conducted among individuals in the general population who have one-time (or short term) exposure to chemical or physical agents as a result of accidental or intentional releases. One of the earliest such studies was initiated in 1946 among atomic bomb survivors in Hiroshima and Nagasaki (28). Prospective study cohorts (or registries) have been established for individuals exposed to 2,3,7,8-tetradichlorodibenzo dioxin (TCDD) after an accidental release in Seveso, Italy, in 1976 (29) and individuals exposed to radioactive isotopes after a nuclear reactor malfunctioned in Chernobyl, USSR, in 1986 (30). Cox regression may be used to analyze clinical trials or cohort study in which the event times are observed (17). When the relationship between predictor variables and disease outcome are modeled using Cox regression, the partial regression coefficients of the model are the natural logarithms of the respective rate ratios (6).

Prospective study cohorts may also be established to study chronic rather than one-time exposures. In the United States, a large prospective cohort has been established of registered pesticide applicators in two states; the cohort will be followed periodically to ascertain pesticide exposure and health status (31). Because of the high cost and great effort required by researchers, a prospective study should be launched only for high-priority topics for which retrospective studies cannot provide adequate data, for example, when retrospective exposure assessment is difficult due to substitution of products over time and varied use over workers in similar job categories (31).

Cohorts may also be assembled from the general population without regard to a specific exposure, and subsequently exposure groups can be identified (e.g., smokers). Population-based cohort studies, such as the Framingham study, have been invaluable in understanding the etiology of cardiovascular disease (33), and have contributed to the understanding of cancer etiology as well (34). Prospective studies of the general population may be geographically based, including a sample or the total of a defined population, or defined by other criteria, such as membership in a health maintenance organization (35). For example, a prospective mortality study [Cancer Prevention II Study (CPS II)] of about 1.2 million U.S. men and women was begun by the American Cancer Society in 1982. Participants were identified and enrolled in by more than 77,000 ACS volunteers in all 50 states, the District of Columbia, and Puerto Rico. Data collected at baseline included personal identifiers, demographic characteristics, personal and family history of cancer and other diseases, reproductive history, and various behavioral, environmental, occupational, and dietary exposures. This study has yielded information on health effects of occupational exposure to diesel exhaust (36), aspirin use, and reduced risk of gastrointestinal tract cancers (37) and the relationship between exposure to environmental tobacco smoke and lung cancer (38). Other recent findings from population-based cohort studies relate to the relationship between aflatoxin exposure, hepatitis B infection, and hepatocellular carcinoma (39,40) the effects of hepatitis B and hepatitis C infection on the development of hepatocellular carcinoma (41), and the relationship between alcohol consumption and breast cancer in women (42). While some population-based studies have involved measurement of risk factors at baseline and follow-up for mortality as the outcome, prospective studies may involve multiple measurements of risk factors in individuals over time, intermediate outcomes, and incident disease. Studies in which there are repeated measures of exposure and outcome over time, and whose focus is to examine individual heterogeneity, time-dependent changes, rates of change, or natural history of complex disease states have been termed "longitudinal" cohort studies (43). Such studies may play an important role in understanding gene–environment interaction, and the interplay of multiple risk factors, in cancer and other diseases.

3. CASE–CONTROL STUDIES

The case–control design has played an important role in the understanding of lifestyle, infections, and familial risk factors for cancer, and in generating and testing hypotheses about environmental and occupational causes. For example, the first evidence for a strong association between cigarette smoking and lung cancer was derived from two case–control studies, published in 1950 (44,45). Much of our current knowledge of the contribution of alcohol consumption and cigarette smoking to esophageal cancer (46,47) and hepatitis B and C infection to liver cancer (48) has been derived from case–control studies, to give just two of numerous examples.

Unlike cohort studies, which measure rates of disease and relative risks, case–control studies compare probabilities (or odds ratios) of exposure and disease between cases and controls. Case–control studies are often community based, where both cases and controls are drawn from the general population. A second type of case–control study is nested within a retrospective cohort study; this design is often used in occupational studies when the cost of obtaining detailed exposure information for every cohort member is high. The nested case–control design is also an integral part of many prospective studies. For example, in a large prospective study of pesticide applicators in the United States (known as the Agricultural Health Study), nested case–control studies will be conducted to examine the association between specific cancers and pesticide exposures (31). In the EPIC project, a prospective study of nutritional and other risk factors for cancer, blood samples have been collected from approximately 400,000 men and women; plasma, serum, white blood cells, and erythrocytes have been banked for future analyses on cancer cases and matched healthy controls (49). The emergence of new technologies for gene sequencing, identifying genetic polymorphisms, and determining their functional significance (50,51) will make this and similar studies particularly powerful tools in the assessment of gene–environment interactions.

Methods for the design and analysis of case–control studies are available from many sources (6,7,52). Case definition for cancer studies is facilitated by highly standardized methods for classification and coding of neoplasms (53); cases may be selected from hospital records or from geographically based cancer registries. In some instances, cases may be further restricted by age or other factors. For example, in designing a study of the relationship between oral contraceptives, which began being marketed in the United States in the 1960s, and breast cancer, cases were restricted to women under 45 years who had opportunity for exposure throughout their entire reproductive years (54).

Perhaps the most difficult and critical issue in case–control studies is appropriate control selection. Issues in control selection are best understood in the conceptual context that every case-control study takes place within some hypothetical cohort (55). Cases and controls should be "representative of the same base experience" or members of the same underlying cohort or source population (55). In order to meet this condition when hospital controls are utilized, care must be taken that the catchment area and referral patterns for the disease under study and diseases included in the control group are similar (56). A second important feature in selecting hospitalized controls is that diseases or conditions thought to be related to the exposure of interest should be excluded (56). Population controls are an appropriate choice when there is a high degree of case ascertainment from the base population (56). Population controls have been identified by a variety of methods, including random digit dialing, selection from neighborhood rosters or Department of Motor Vehicle records, and selection from case-nominated friends or relatives (56,57). In all of these methods, procedures must be carefully evaluated to ensure as much as possible that the control group is representative of the base population (or that a random sample of eligible subjects is obtained). For example, in the use of random digit dialing to identify controls, factors such as incomplete phone coverage, residences that can be reached by more than one telephone number, more than one person in the house who is eligible to be a control, and nonresponse bias among selected individuals can lead to possible selection bias (56).

Another important issue in the design of case-control studies is whether individual matching will be employed in the selection of controls. Matching is often done to improve efficiency in the estimation of the effect of exposure by protecting against the situation where the distributions of a confounder (a factor that is related to both the exposure and the disease under study, but not in the causal pathway between the exposure and the disease of interest) are substantially different in cases and controls (58). Other reasons to match are to control unmeasured confounders and to ensure time comparability for exposures that vary over time (58). On the other hand, there is a danger of overmatching, where reducing the variability of potential confounding variables may also reduce variability in exposures of interest (58). The latter are critical to observe differences in disease rate by exposure level. In studies where individual matching is employed, analysis methods must be used that take the matching into account.

The data layout for an unmatched case–control study with a bivariate risk factor is shown below:

Exposure status	Cases	Controls
Yes	a	b
No	c	d

The odds ratio is the ratio ad/bc and is interpretable as the ratio of incidence rates for disease among exposed vs. unexposed members of the population (59). The data layout for a matched study, with one control per case, is shown below:

	Control exposed	Control not exposed
Case exposed	a	b
Control exposed	c	d

For an analysis that incorporates control only for the matching variables, the odds ratio is calculated as b/c (59). Multivariate methods for the analysis of case–control studies are covered in textbooks of epidemiology (6,7) and other sources (59). The goals of such analyses are: (1) to determine whether there is a statistically significant association between the exposure and the disease of interest after accounting for the possibly confounding variables; (2) to determine whether there is evidence for effect modification (heterogeneity in the association under study across the strata); and (3) to provide an estimate of the overall odds ratio and confidence limits (6). Unmatched case–control studies may be analyzed using multiple logistic regression, in which the partial regression coefficients are estimates of the natural logarithms of the adjusted odds ratios contrasting exposed (coded as 1) with unexposed (coded as 0) persons (6). Matched case–control studies are analyzed using conditional logistical regression (6).

One of the frequently cited concerns about the case–control study design relates to the reliability and validity of the (necessarily retrospective) exposure data (60). Correa et al. (60) reviewed exposure measurement methods in 223 reports of population-based case–control studies conducted in 34 countries and published in 25 journals during 1992; 143 of these studies had cancer as the outcome. Most of these studies relied on a questionnaire as the primary source of exposure data; relatively few employed biological monitoring or other types of information (60). Recent methodological refinements increase the potential for case–control data to generate semiquantitative or even quantitative information on occupational and environmental exposures. These methods include expert review of detailed occupational history data to identify potential exposures and estimate the level, frequency, and mode of exposure (61) and use of computer assisted interviews with job-specific modules that ask detailed questions relevant to exposure assessment for that particular job (62).

4. ISSUES IN INTERPRETING EPIDEMIOLOGICAL STUDY RESULTS

4.1. Statistical Power

Statistical power is the ability of a study to demonstrate an association if one exists. The power of a study is determined by several factors, including the frequency of the condition under study, the magnitude of the effect, the study design, and the sample size (63).

4.2. Bias

Bias has been defined as "any systematic error in the design, conduct, or analysis of a study that results in a mistaken estimate of an exposure's effect on the risk of disease" (63). Some important potential biases in epidemiological studies are:

Selection bias: Error due to systematic differences in characteristics between members of the source or base population who are selected for study and those who are not (63).

Ascertainment bias: Error due to systematic failure to represent equally all classes of cases or persons supposed to be represented in a sample. Ascertainment bias may arise from the nature of the sources from which the persons come (63).

Response (or participation) bias: Error due to systematic differences in characteristics between those who choose to volunteer to take part in a study and those who do not (63).

Information (or observational) bias: A flaw in measuring exposure or outcome data that results in differences in the quality (accuracy) of information between comparison groups (63).

Recall bias: Systematic error due to differences in accuracy or completeness of recall to memory of past events or experiences (63). For example, a mother whose child has leukemia is more likely than the mother of a healthy child to remember details of past experiences such as the use of x-ray services when the child was in utero.

Surveillance bias: Systematic error due to differences in monitoring between the groups under study: for example, better detection of cases of thrombophlebitis among patients taking oral contraceptives than among those who are not (64).

Interviewer bias: Systematic error due to interviewers' subconscious or conscious gathering of selective data (63), for example, more extensive probing when interviewing cases compared to controls.

Minimizing the potential for such biases is important in the design of epidemiological studies. Interviewer bias may be avoided if it is possible to blind interviewers to case or control status. Other biases, such as recall bias, may be unavoidable, but measures may be taken to evaluate or control for them. For example, recall bias may be evaluated by asking questions about exposures thought not to be plausibly related to the disease under study, and comparing the responses of cases and controls. Some reported exposures, such as in utero x-rays, may be subject to validation from record sources, thus minimizing the impact of recall bias.

4.3. Confounding and Interaction

Confounding refers to a distortion in the apparent effect of the exposure of interest due to an extraneous factor. Confounding is of particular concern in epidemiological studies because if it is not recognized, study results may be interpreted as suggesting a causal relationship between the risk factor and the disease of interest, when in fact there is none. An example of confounding that is easy to understand is provided in Rothman and Greenland (7). In this example, an investigator wishes to examine the relationship between alcohol consumption and oral cancer. Even in the absence of any causal association, alcohol drinkers will have a higher incidence of oral cancer than nondrinkers because consumers of alcoholic beverages are more likely to be smokers, and smoking is associated with oral cancer. In order to understand whether alcohol consumption itself is associated with oral cancer, one would have to analyze this relationship separately in smokers and nonsmokers. A stratified analysis of this sort, with a subsequent calculation of a single relative risk (a weighted average across strata), is what is meant by "adjusting for" or "controlling for" smoking. In order to be a confounder, the extraneous variable must be associated with both the exposure under study and the disease.

Factors that are on the causal pathway between exposure and disease should not be considered confounders. Determining whether a factor is likely to be on the causal pathway requires integration of clinical, epidemiological, and mechanistic data, and the answer may not be clear-cut (7).

Controlling for a factor that is on the causal pathway may lead to underestimation of the relationship between the exposure and the disease.

Many epidemiological studies, particularly case–control studies, examine the relationship between multiple risk factors and disease outcome. For example, in the study of oral cancer discussed above, the investigator might be interested in the independent effects of alcohol and smoking, and also their effects in combination. The concept of interaction in the simplest sense means that the effect of factor A differs depending on the level of factor B. Such would be the case, for example, if after examining the effects of alcohol consumption and smoking, one found that among nonsmokers, alcohol consumption was not associated with oral cancer, but among smokers, it was highly associated. In practice, the definition of interaction depends on whether an expected relationship under conditions of no interaction is defined to be additive or multiplicative. For example, if there is a fivefold risk of oral cancer associated with smoking and a threefold risk associated with alcohol consumption, a multiplicative model would predict a 15-fold risk among those with both exposures, while an additive model would predict an eightfold risk. While there has been considerable debate in the epidemiological literature on the statistical and conceptual meaning of interaction, a pragmatic approach is to evaluate whether an additive or a multiplicative model provides the best fit to the data (65).

In occupational cancer studies, concerns about confounding often relate to a higher prevalence of adverse lifestyle factors, such as smoking, in the study population than in the referent population, and also to the presence of potential confounding exposures in the work environment. Siemiatycki et al. (66) have shown, however, that even for lung cancer, differences in smoking habits between an occupational group and the general population from which referent rates are derived are unlikely to result in a relative risk or SMR greater than 1.2–1.4. Although there are rarely any data on smoking status available for all members of an occupational cohort, smoking data may be available for a subset of the cohort, which are used to estimate the magnitude of the predicted smoking related effect (67). With regard to the potential confounding effect of concomitant chemical exposures in the work environment, a preliminary assessment may be made from the toxicological and epidemiological literature of whether the chemicals present are likely to be carcinogenic. Depending on the distribution of the exposures and hypothesized target organs, it may or may not be possible to control for potential confounding. For example, in a study of bladder cancer incidence related to occupational exposure to *o*-toluidine and aniline, the presence of vinyl chloride at the study plant was considered unlikely to be a confounding exposure, because the bladder is not a target organ for vinyl chloride. In addition, potential confounding by vinyl chloride could be assessed in the analysis because exposure to aromatic amines and vinyl chloride took place in separate areas of the plant. However, it was not possible to separate the effects of *o*-toluidine and aniline because these exposures occurred in the same area and both chemicals were likely to have the bladder as a target organ (68).

4.4. Measurement Error and Misclassification

Exposure measurement error is an inherent part of epidemiological studies because of the way information is obtained. Table 2 summarizes the sources of information for epidemiological studies and their advantages and limitations. No source of information can be considered absolutely accurate; even "objective" measurements such as levels of a contaminant in the environment or in biological fluids may be affected by sampling method, biological variability, or laboratory error (69). The terms "measurement error" and "misclassification" both refer to any discrepancy between the true value of a variable x and its measured value z, although the term misclassification is more often used with categorical variables and measurement error with continuous variables (69). Errors may be systematic or random; systematic errors refer to errors that are not distributed randomly around the true value (69). Both systematic and random errors may be "differential" or "nondifferential" with respect to disease status. In nondifferential misclassification, the probability and/or direction of misclassification differs between those with disease and those without, as might occur, for example, if an interviewer who knew the health status of the subjects and the study hypotheses probed more intensely when asking about these exposures in case compared to control interviews. Nondifferential misclassification can introduce serious bias in the study results, but can often be avoided by a good study design, i.e., blinded assessment of the study variables (69). Prior to the late 1980s, it was thought that nondifferential exposure measurement error or misclassification would bias studies toward the null (i.e., in the direction of finding no effect), but it is now recognized that there are exceptions to this rule (71).

Where possible, epidemiologic studies try to minimize measurement error and also to estimate its magnitude. For example, in classifying subjects with respect to current smoking status, self-reported data may be compared to the serum cotinine level; for self-reported exposures, data reported at two different times may be evaluated for consistency; in studies where laboratory analyses are done, blinded split sample analysis and spiked samples with known standard compounds may be used to estimate laboratory error.

5. OTHER STUDY DESIGNS

In reviewing the epidemiological literature on cancer, there are a number of other epidemiological study designs that the reader should be familiar with. All of the study designs are covered in detail in epidemiology textbooks (6,7,64).

Table 2   Commonly Used Assessments for Exposures in Epidemiological Studies

Source of exposure data	Advantages/limitations
Measurement of substance in biological samples	Good methods available for measuring recent exposures (i.e., cotinine and current smoking status) or retrospective exposure to chemical or physical agents with long half-lives (i.e., organochlorines such as DDT) Time period of interest in cancer studies is often 20–30 years prior to onset of disease; some shorter half-lived exposures can be detected in stored sera or urine, if available Accessible samples in living individuals (blood, urine, buccal cells, etc.) may not reflect exposure at the target tissue of interest (i.e., asbestos in lung tissue) Studying intermediate markers such as hemoglobin or urothelial cell adducts may yield information about biologically effective dose (84)
Interview data	Able to gain information about a wide range of risk factors throughout life, which is generally not possible with any single record source Interview data are dependent on the accuracy and completeness of participant recall, may lack detail on specific exposures, such as chemicals or medications, and may be influenced by recall bias
Medical records	May be an excellent source for confirming self-reported medically related exposures; medical records are especially valuable for identifying cohorts for follow-up of medical exposures, i.e., children exposed to diethylstilbestrol during pregnancy Location and retrieval of medical records may be difficult in retrospective studies; investigator may need patient's permission to access medical records
Work history records	Generally a good source to identify individuals for cohort studies, provided that they are complete; may or may not contain detailed information about jobs held, which is needed

(Continued)

Table 2 Commonly Used Assessments for Exposures in Epidemiological Studies (*Continued*)

Source of exposure data	Advantages/limitations
	to provide a more detailed assessment of exposure
Industrial hygiene monitoring data	Only in rare instances, such as film badge data available for radiation workers, is it possible to reconstruct exposure data for individuals based on their own measured exposures
	Exposure reconstruction in cohort studies is based on industrial hygiene samples to characterize exposures by work area, rather than on sampling results for individuals; sampling data are often incomplete and may not cover specific jobs or time periods; assumptions are made to extrapolate data to these periods; often there are no air sampling results available for early decades of operation
	Exposure reconstruction for case-control studies is usually based on information provided by the study subject combined with

(*Continued*)

Ecological studies: There are enormous variations in the incidence of some cancers worldwide; correlations between site-specific cancer incidence and dietary and other risk factors may lead to potential clues about cancer etiology. Studies looking at such correlations on a population level are termed ecological studies; the unit of observation is a group and not an individual.

Cross-sectional (or prevalence) studies: These studies examine risk factors and the presence of disease or disease markers simultaneously. In the area of cancer risk assessment, cross-sectional studies may provide valuable information on exposure, including biological indicators such as levels of DNA adducts.

Proportionate mortality ratio (PMR) studies: In some instances, it is not possible to enumerate the entire population at risk for a cohort study, but it is possible to identify deaths that have occurred, for example, from a union-based pension plan. Proportionate mortality ratio studies compare the proportion of deaths by cause in the study and the referent populations, with appropriate control for age, calendar time, gender and race.

Case–cohort studies: A variant of the nested case–control study design, in which cases occurring in a study cohort are compared to a sample of the whole cohort (which may include some cases).

6. METHODS FOR COMBINING THE RESULTS OF EPIDEMIOLOGICAL STUDIES

There are two main methods for combining the results of epidemiological studies: meta-analysis and pooled analysis. These methods are important for the application of epidemiological study results to risk assessment, as they may provide an overall summary of effect across all studies.

Meta-analysis: A meta-analysis is a statistical analysis of a collection of studies with the aim of identifying consistent patterns and sources of disagreement among the results. Meta-analysis generally relies on study results provided in the published literature (72).

Pooled analysis: In a pooled analysis, the investigator conducts a combined analysis of a collection of studies, after standardization of the studies to allow exposure variables to be combined. Unlike in meta-analysis, in pooled analysis the investigator uses the primary data (73). A recent article compared the results of a meta-analysis and a pooled analysis of studies of sinonasal cancer among wood workers and proposed criteria for whether a pooled analysis of raw data or a meta-analysis should be carried out (74).

7. CANCER CLUSTERS

A cluster refers to an unusual aggregation of health events that are grouped together in time and space. Although clusters may come to light through surveillance systems, more often they are reported to public health agencies by concerned citizens or groups. Responses to inquiries about perceived clusters may consume substantial resources on the part of public health agencies, yet rarely lead to the identification of etiological agents (75–78). Those clusters that have led to important etiological findings have often been clusters of new or rare diseases, and/or clusters of disease in very highly defined populations. For example, the well-known association between vinyl chloride and angiosarcoma of the liver was first recognized through a cluster of cases at a single company (79).

Many observations of apparent clusters since the early part of this century have involved leukemia (80), childhood leukemia in particular (81). There is currently little understanding of the causes of leukemia, which is the most common childhood cancer. There has been considerable interest in the possibility that childhood leukemia has an infectious etiology, although in recent years, residence near nuclear facilities, contaminated water, and electromagnetic fields have been studied (81). A systematic investigation of spatial clustering of 13,351 cases of childhood leukemia in 17 European countries between 1980 and 1989 found evidence of clustering of total childhood leukemia within small census areas, but the magnitude of the clustering was small (81). No specific cell type, age group, or etiology was highlighted.

Although the study of cancer clusters has not had direct applicability to regulatory risk assessment to date, knowledge and perspective on this topic are of considerable value to the public health and medical practitioner. The U.S. Centers for Disease Control and Prevention has provided recommendations for local and state health departments in the management and investigation of cancer and other disease clusters reported by the public (82). A scientific publication of the International Agency for Research on Cancer provides information on choices of statistical methods for investigating localized clustering of disease (83).

REFERENCES

1. Stayner LT, Smith RJ. Methodologic issues in using epidemiologic studies of occupational cohorts for cancer risk assessment. Epidemiol Prev 1992; 14: 32–39.
2. Samet JM, Schnatter R, Gibb H. Invited commentary: epidemiology and risk assessment. Am J Epidemiol 1998; 148:929–936.
3. Shore RE. Editorial: epidemiologic data in risk assessment—imperfect but valuable. Am J Public Health 1995; 85:474–475.
4. Hertz-Piccioto I. Epidemiology and quantitative risk assessment: a bridge from science to policy. Am J Public Health 1995; 85:484–491.
5. Wartenberg D, Simon R. Comment: integrating epidemiologic data into risk assessment. Am J Public Health XXXX; 85:491–493.
6. MacMahon B, Trichopoulos D. Epidemiology: Principles and Methods. 2nd ed. New York: Little, Brown and Company, 1996.
7. Rothman KJ, Greenland S . Modern Epidemiology. 2nd ed. Philadelphia: Lippincott-Raven, 1998.
8. Fontham ETH, Correa P, Reynolds P, Wu-Williams A, Buffler PA, Greenberg RS, Chen VW, Alterman T, Boyd P, Austin DF, Liff J. Environmental tobacco smoke and lung cancer in nonsmoking women: a multi center study. J Am Med Assoc 1994; 271:1752–1759.
9. Occupational Safety and Health Administration, Department of Labor. Notice of proposed rulemaking; notice of informal public hearing. 29 CFR Parts 1910, 1915, 1926, 1928. Federal Register 59, No. 65: 1994; 15968–16039.
10. Lubin JH, Boice JD Jr. Lung cancer risk from residential studies: meta analysis of eight epidemiologic studies. J Natl Cancer Inst 1997; 89:49–57.
11. Case RA, Hosker ME, McDonald DB, Pearson JT. Tumors of the urinary bladder in workmen engaged in the manufacture and use of certain dyestuff intermediates in the British Chemical Industry. Part I: the role of aniline, benzidine, alpha-naphthylamine and beta-naphthylamine. Br J Ind Med 1993; 50:389–411. (1954, classical article).

12. Doll R. Morality from lung cancer in asbestos workers. Br J Ind Med 1993; 50:485–490. (1955 classical article).

13. Checkoway H, Eisen EA. Developments in occupational cohort studies. Epidemiol Rev 1998; 20:100–111.

14. Macaluso M, Larson R, Delzell E, Sathiakumar N, Hovinga M, Julian J, Muir D, Cole P. Leukemia and cumulative exposure to butadiene, styrene and benzene among workers in the synthetic rubber industry. Toxicology 1996; 113:190–202.

15. Monson RR. Occupational Epidemiology. 2nd ed. Boca Raton, FL: CRC Press, 1990.

16. Percy C, Stanck E III, Gloeckler L. Accuracy of cancer death certificates and its effect on cancer mortality statistics. Am J Public Health 1981; 71:242–250.

17. Marsh GM, Youk AO, Stone RA, Sefeik S, Alcorn C. OCMAP-Plus: a program for the comprehensive analysis of occupational cohort data. J Occup Environ Med 1998; 40:351–362.

18. Steenland K, Beaumont J, Spaeth S, Brown D, Okun A, Jurcenko L, Ryan B, Phillips S, Roscoe R, Stayner L, Morris J. New developments in the life table analysis system of the National Institute for Occupational Safety and Health. J Occup Med 1990; 32:1091–1098.

19. Steenland K, Spaeth S, Cassinelli R II, Laber P, Chang L, Koch K. NIOSH life table program for personal computers. Am J Ind Med 1998; 34:517–518.

20. Thomas D. New techniques for the analysis of cohort studies. Epidemiol Rev 1998; 20:122–133.

21. Steenland K, Stayner L, Greife A. Assessing the feasibility of retrospective cohort studies. Am J Ind Med 1987; 12:419–430.

22. Stewart PA, Lees PSJ, Francis M. Quantification of historical exposures in occupational cohort studies. Scand J Work Environ Health 1996; 22:405–414.

23. Seixas NS, Checkoway H. Exposure assessment in industry specific retrospective occupational epidemiology studies. Occup Environ Med 1995; 52:625–633.

24. Paustenbach DJ, Price PS, Ollison W, Blank C, Jernigan JD, Bass RD, Petersen HD. Reevaluation of benzene exposure for the Pliofilm (rubberworker) cohort (1936–1976). J Toxicol Environ Health 1992; 36:177–231.

25. Utterback DF, Rinsky RA. Benzene exposure assessment in rubber hydrochloride workers: a critical evaluation of previous estimates. Am J Ind Med 1995; 27:661–676.

26. Rinsky RA, Smith AB, Hornung R, Filloon TG, Young RJ, Okun AH, Landrigan PJ. Benzene and leukemia: an epidemiologic risk assessment. New Engl J Med 1987; 316:1044–1050.

27. Crump KS. Risk of benzene-induced leukemia predicted from the Pliofilm cohort. Environ Health Perspect 1996; 104(suppl 6):1437–1441.

28. Pierce DA, Shimizu Y, Preston DL, Vaeth M, Mabuchi K. Studies of the mortality of atomic bomb survivors. Report 12, Part I. Cancer: 1950–1990. Radiat Res 1996; 146:1–27.

29. Bertazzi PA, Zocchetti C, Guercilena S, Consonni D, Tironi A, Landi MT, Pesatori AC. Dioxin exposure and cancer risk: a 15-year mortality study after the "Seveso accident". Epidemiology 1997; 8:646–652.

30. Buzunov VA, Strapko NP, Pirogova EA, Krasnikova LI, Bugayev VN, Korol NA, Treskunova TV, Ledoschuk BA, Gudzenko NA, Bomko EI, Bobyleva OA, Kartushin GI. Epidemiological survey of the medical consequences of the Chernobyl accident in Ukraine. World Health Stat Q 1996; 49:4–6.
31. Alavanja MC, Sandler DP, McMaster SB, Zahm SH, McDonnell CJ, Lynch CF, Pennybacker M, Rothman N, Dosemeci M, Bond AE, Blair A. The Agricultural Health Study. Environ Health Perspect 1996; 104:362–369.
32. Blair A, Hayes RB, Stewart PA, Zahm SH. Occupational epidemiologic study design and application. Occup Med State Art Rev 1996; 11:403–417.
33. Sytkowski PA, D'Agostino RB, Belanger AJ, Kannel WB. Secular trends in long-term sustained hypertension, long-term treatment and cardiovascular mortality. The Framingham Heart Study 1950 to 1990. Circulation 1996; 93: 697–703.
34. Zhang Y, Kiel DP, Kreger BE, Cupples LA, Ellison RC, Dorgan JF, Schatzkin A, Levy D, Felson DT. Bone mass and risk of breast cancer among postmenopausal women. N Engl J Med 1997; 336:611–617.
35. Szklo M. Population-based cohort studies. Epidemiol Rev 1998; 20:81–90.
36. Boffetta P, Stellman SD, Garfinkel L. Diesel exhaust exposure and mortality among males in the American Cancer Society prospective study. Am J Ind Med 1988; 14:403–415.
37. Thun MJ, Heath CW Jr. Aspirin use and reduced risk of gastrointestinal tract cancers in the American Cancer Society prospective studies. Prev Med 1995; 24:116–118.
38. Cardenas VM, Thun MJ, Austin H, Lally CA, Clark WS, Greenberg RS, Heath CW Jr. Environmental tobacco smoke and lung cancer mortality in the American Cancer Society's Cancer Prevention Study II. Cancer Causes Control 1997; 8:57–64.
39. Sun Z, Lu P, Gail MH, Pell D, Zhang Q, Ming L, Wang J, Wu Y, Liu G, Wu Y, Zhu Y. Increased risk of hepatocellular carcinoma in male hepatitis B surface antigen carriers with chronic hepatitis who have detectable urinary aflatoxin metabolite M1. Hepatology 1999; 30:379–383.
40. Ross RK, Yuan JM, Yu MC, Wogan GN, Qian GS, Tu JT, Groopman JD, Gao YT, Henderson BE. Urinary aflatoxin biomarkers and risk of hepatocellular carcinoma. Lancet 1992; 339:943–946.
41. Tsai JF, Jeng JE, Ho MS, Chang WY, Hseih MY, Lin ZY, Tsai JH. Effect of hepatitis C and B virus infection on risk of hepatocellular carcinoma: a prospective study. Br J Cancer 1997; 76:968–974.
42. Garland M, Hunter DJ, Colditz GA, Spiegelman DL, Manson JE, Stampfer MJ, Willet WC. Alcohol consumption in relation to breast cancer risk in a cohort of United States women 25–42 years of age. Cancer Epidemiol Biomarkers Prev 1999; 8:1017–1021.
43. Tager IB. Outcomes in cohort studies. Epidemiol Rev 1998; 20:15–28.
44. Levin ML, Goldstein H, Gerhardt PR. Cancer and tobacco smoking: a preliminary report. J Am Med Assoc 1950; 143:336–338.
45. Wynder EL, Graham EA. Tobacco smoking as a possible etiologic factor in bronchogenic carcinoma: a study of 684 proved cases. J Am Med Assoc 1950; 143:329–336.

46. Launoy G, Milan CH, Faivre J, Pienkowski P, Milan CI, Gignoux M. Alcohol, tobacco and oesophageal cancer: effects of the duration of consumption, mean intake, and current and former consumption. Br J Cancer 1997; 75: 1389–1396.
47. Valsecchi MG. Modeling the relative risk of esophageal cancer in a case-control study. J Clin Epidemiol 1992; 45:347–355.
48. Donato F, Bofetta P, Puoti M. A meta-analysis of epidemiologic studies on the combined effect of hepatitis B and C virus infections in causing hepatocellular carcinoma. Int J Cancer 1998; 75:347–354.
49. Riboli E, Kaaks R. The EPIC project: rationale and study design. Int J Epidemiol 1997; 26:S6–S14.
50. Ishibe N, Kelsey KT. Genetic susceptibility to environmental and occupational cancers. Cancer Causes and Control 1997; 8:504–513.
51. Guengerich FP. The environmental genome project: functional analysis of polymorphisms. Environ Health Perspect 1998; 106:365–368.
52. Epidemiologic Reviews. Vol. 16. Case–Control Studies, 1994.
53. Muir CS, Percy C. Cancer registration: principles and methods. Classification and coding of neoplasms. IARC Sci Publ 1991; 95:64–81.
54. Brinton LA, Daling JR, Liff JM, Schoenberg JB, Malone KE, Stanford JL, Coates RJ, Gammon MD, Hanson x L, Hoover RN. Oral contraceptives and breast cancer risk among younger women. J Natl Cancer Inst 1995; 87:827–835.
55. Wacholder S, McLaughlin JK, Silverman DT, Mandel JS. Selection of controls in case-control studies: I. Principles. Am J Epidemiol 1992; 135: 1019–1028.
56. Wacholder S, Silverman DT, McLaughlin JK, Mandel JS. Selection of controls in case-control studies: II. Types of controls. Am J Epidemiol 1992; 135: 1029–1041.
57. Lasky T, Stolley PD. Selection of cases and controls. Epidemiol Rev 1994; 16:6–17.
58. Thompson WD. Statistical analysis of case–control studies. Epidemiol Rev 1994; 16:33–50.
59. Correa A, Stewart WF, Yeh H-C, Santos-Burgoa C. Exposure measurement in case-control studies: reported methods and recommendations. Epidemiol Rev 1994; 16:18–32.
60. Gerin M, Siemiatycki J, Kemper H, Begin D. Obtaining occupational exposure histories in epidemiologic case–control studies. J Occup Med 1985; 27: 420–446.
61. Stewart PA, Stewart WF, Heineman EF, Dosemeci M, Linet M, Inskip PD. A novel approach to data collection in a case–control study of cancer and occupational exposures. Int J Epidemiol 1996; 25:744–752.
62. Last JM, ed. A Dictionary of Epidemiology. 3rd ed. New York: Oxford University Press, 1995.
63. Gordis L. Epidemiology. Philadelphia: W.B. Saunders Company, 1996.
64. Steenland K. Age specific interactions between smoking and radon among United States uranium miners. Occup Environ Med 1994; 51:192–194.

65. Siemiatycki J, Wacholder S, Dewar R, Cardis E, Greenwood C, Richardson L. Degree of confounding bias related to smoking, ethnic group, and socioeconomic status in estimates of the associations between occupation and cancer. J Occup Med 1988; 30:617–625.
66. Axelson O, Steenland K. Indirect methods of assessing the effects of tobacco use in occupational studies. Am J Ind Med 1988; 13:105–118.
67. Ward E, Carpenter A, Markowitz S, Roberts D, Halperin W. Excess number of bladder cancers in workers exposed to ortho-toluidine and aniline. J Natl Cancer Inst 1991; 83:501–506.
68. Thomas D, Stram D, Dwyer J. Exposure measurement error: influence of exposure disease relationships and methods for correction. Annu Rev Public Health 1993; 14:69–93.
69. Steenland K, Deddens JA. Design and analysis of studies in environmental epidemiology. In: Steenland K, Savitz DA, eds. Topics in Environmental Epidemiology. New York, Oxford: Oxford Press, 1997:9–27.
70. Flegal KM, Keyl PM, Nieto FJ. Differential misclassification arising from non-differential errors in exposure measurement. Am J Epidemiol 1991; 134:1233–1244.
71. Normand S. Meta-analysis: formulating, evaluating, combining, and reporting. Stat Med 1999; 18:321–359.
72. Friedenreich CM. Methods for pooled analyses of epidemiologic studies. Epidemiology 1993; 4:295–302.
73. Gordon I, Boffetta P, Demers PA. A case study comparing meta-analysis and a pooled analysis of studies of sinonasal cancer among wood workers. Epidemiology 1998; 9:518–524.
74. Schulte PA, Ehrenberg RL, Singal M. Investigation of occupational cancer clusters: theory and practise. Am J Public Health 1987; 77:52–56.
75. Caldwell GG. Twenty-two years of cancer cluster investigations at the Centers for Disease Control. Am J Epidemiol 1990; 132:S43–S47.
76. Bender AP, Williams AN, Johnson RA, Jagger HG. Appropriate public health responses to clusters: the art of being responsibly responsive. Am J Epidemiol 1990; 132:S48–S52.
77. King WD, Darlington GA, Krieger N, Fehringer G. Response of a cancer registry to reports of disease clusters. Eur J Cancer 1993; 29A:1414–1418.
78. Creech JL Jr, Johnson MN. Angiosarcoma of the liver in the manufacture of poylvinyl chloride. J Occup Med 1974; 16:150–151.
79. Boyle P, Walker AM, Alexander FE. Historical aspects of leukemia clusters. In: Alexander FE, Boyle P, eds. Methods for Investigating Localized Clusters of Disease. IARC Scientific Publications No. 135. Lyon: International Agency for Research on Cancer, 1996:1–20.
80. Alexander FE, Boyle P, Carli P-M, Coebergh JW, Draper GJ, Ekbom A, Levi F, McKinney PA, McWhirter W, Michaelis J, Peris-Bonet R, Pertidou E, Pompe-Kirn V, Plisko I, Pukkala E, Rahu M, Storm H, Terracini B, Vatten L, Wray N. Spatial clustering of childhood leukemia: summary results from the EUROCLUS project. Br J Cancer 1998; 77:818–824.
81. Centers for Disease Control and Prevention. Guidelines for Investigating Clusters of Health Events. MMWR XXXX; 39:1–22.

82. Alexander FE, Boyle P, eds. Methods for Investigating Localized Clusters of Disease. IARC Scientific Publications No. 135. Lyon: International Agency for Research on Cancer, 1996.
83. Farmer PB. Studies using specific biomarkers for human exposure assessment for exogenous and endogenous chemical agents. Mutat Res 1999; 16:69–81.

3

Epidemiological Approaches to Studying Cancer II: Molecular Epidemiology

Loïc Le Marchand

Cancer Research Center of Hawaii, University of Hawaii, Honolulu, Hawaii, U.S.A.

1. INTRODUCTION

It is thought that most cancers result from the combined effects of environmental factors and inherited susceptibilities and that only few cancers (5–10%) are due to purely genetic or endogenous factors (1,2). Thus substantial prevention opportunities should result from the identification of key environmental risk factors (i.e., lifestyle factors, environmental pollutants, drugs, radiation, and infectious agents) and the characterization of genetic susceptibilities involved in the process. Epidemiology has already played a crucial role in identifying important causes of cancer in populations, such as smoking in lung cancer, hepatitis B virus in liver cancer, and UV radiation in skin cancer. However, the traditional epidemiologic approach, relying mainly on record and questionnaire information, has had difficulty detecting weak or attenuated associations. Studies have often been inconsistent when the relative risk associated with exposure has been smaller than 2.0. For example, despite 20 years of intense effort, only few specific dietary components have been convincingly demonstrated to be risk factors for cancer (3). Difficulty in measuring exposure accurately and the inability to distinguish susceptible from resistant individuals have been major impediments to the study of cancer risk.

The field of epidemiology has dramatically changed in the past 10 years and, as a result, is poised to make new major contributions to our understanding of cancer etiology, risk assessment and prevention. Taking advantage of new advances in laboratory methods, epidemiologists and laboratory scientists have worked toward refining measurement of study variables through the use of biomarkers. The widespread incorporation of biological measurements at the cellular and molecular levels into large-scale studies has given rise to the term *molecular epidemiology*, which characterizes more an evolutionary step than the birth of a new discipline. In this regard, an analogy can be drawn with the effects of the computer revolution in the 1980s and the 1990s on the field of epidemiology. Enhanced computational power has made possible the application of sophisticated statistical techniques (e.g., logistic regression, proportional hazards regression, generalized estimating equation) aimed at identifying new risk factors from an intricate web of causal factors, confounders, and effect modifiers. These methods have allowed the investigation of inter-related exposures (e.g., lifestyle factors) in the etiology of complex diseases, such as cancer and coronary heart disease. The sequencing of the human genome and the genomics/proteomics revolution that is currently unfolding, and other technical advances, such as in analytical chemistry, are providing epidemiologists with the capability for an even greater methodological leap based on increasingly sensitive and accurate measurements of susceptibility, exposure, and disease. With some of these scientific advances, however, come social and ethical issues that need to be addressed before the potential benefits can be fully realized.

This chapter provides an overview of the opportunities offered by the use of biomarkers in cancer epidemiology and risk assessment, as well as summarizes the main categories of biomarkers and the issues related to their application. For further exploration of these topics, we refer the reader to recent textbooks on molecular epidemiology (4–6).

2. APPLICATIONS OF BIOMARKERS

Although biomarkers have limitations of their own (see secs. 4 and 5), their use offers new opportunities in cancer epidemiology. At the least, the use of biomarkers can provide independent confirmation of results obtained with exposure information collected through questionnaire or external monitoring. More importantly, it can also help to identify new associations or refine risk estimates for exposures that have been difficult to assess or quantify by conventional means. It also offers the possibility of delineating mechanistic pathways between exposures and disease, and identifying milestones along these pathways that could not be tested or recognized before. Thus, molecular epidemiology has the potential for contributing greatly to our further understanding of cancer biology, as well as to early detection and risk assessment. The current paradigm guiding molecular epidemiology and risk assessment is illustrated in Figure 1.

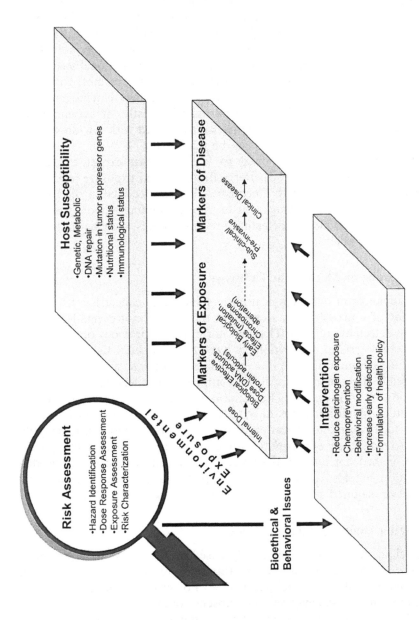

Figure 1 Current paradigm for molecular epidemiology and risk assessment. *Source:* Modified from Refs. 7, 8.

2.1. Assessing Health Effects of Small Doses and Past Exposures

Powerful analytical techniques have markedly lowered the detection limits of many biological measurements, making possible the study of the health effects associated with low-dose exposures, such as those typically experienced by the general population. Most health regulations for suspected or established carcinogens have been derived from data obtained in individuals exposed to moderate or high doses; for example, in occupational settings or in the aftermath of an environmental disaster. Because, in most cases, the marked reduction or complete elimination of a known carcinogen from the environment is socially and economically costly, it is important to determine with greater certainty the risk associated with low-dose exposures and whether such exposures can be tolerated.

Biomarkers can also be used to integrate past exposure over an extended period of time; thus, better reflecting usual exposure [e.g., trace elements in toenails (9)], or to "reconstruct" doses received in the past by estimating body burden through, for example, sampling adipose tissue for lipid soluble compounds or detecting protein adducts, somatic mutations, or chromosome aberrations (7).

2.2. Focusing on Mechanistic Pathways

Recent advances in our biological understanding of cancer has led to the unraveling of some of the many steps in the sequence of events leading to clinically detectable tumors. This new information provides opportunities for epidemiologists to refine etiologic hypotheses, identify the most appropriate study design, examine more specific forms of exposure, and consider new possible effect modifiers. All these improvements lead to a more effective testing of an hypothesis. Epidemiologists now have the capability of contributing significantly not only to the identification of cancer causes but also to the further clarification of the mechanisms involved, potentially leading to major new opportunities for prevention. Information can potentially be gained not only on the specific nature and extent of the needed intervention but also on its most appropriate target groups, defined by inherited or acquired susceptibility and/or preclinical events (7).

2.3. Better Defining Disease Entities

Tumor characterization is increasingly based on the use of molecular markers. They help to define disease variants that are unrecognizable through traditional clinical and pathological tools. For example, molecular assays applied to tumor tissue may reveal an absence of expression, or overexpression, of a particular protein (e.g., through immunohistochemistry), or the presence of a localized or genome-wide genetic defect (e.g., chromosome translocation or microsatellite instability due a DNA mismatch repair deficiency). These defects may point to a specific disease pathway or help to identify a subgroup of patients that may differ in their prognosis or respond differently to treatment.

Recent progress in the development of DNA microarrays and in bioinformatics have also made possible the classification of tumors based on their genome-wide patterns of gene expression. Through these techniques, the expression of thousands of genes can be assessed in a semiquantitative fashion and clustering algorithms are used to identify tumor expression profiles. These expression patterns can then be statistically associated with different exposures or clinical outcomes (10).

2.4. Assessing Host Susceptibility

The fact that not all similarly exposed individuals (e.g., smokers) get the same disease (e.g., lung cancer, coronary heart disease), or any disease at all, is central to assessing risk at the individual level. However, health and regulatory policies have historically been based on the working assumption that all individuals in a population have the same biological response to a specified dose of carcinogens (10). Molecular epidemiology techniques have allowed for major advances in our ability to define the role of host factors, particularly genetic factors, in accounting for the interindividual variation in response.

The discoveries of a number of familial cancer genes (e.g., *BRCA1, BRCA2*) have received a great deal of attention from the public in recent years because an inherited mutation in one of these genes confers a dramatic increase in cancer risk. However, these highly penetrant mutations are rare and explain only a small percentage of cancer cases in the population. More common and, thus, potentially more important to public heath, are a number of inherited sequence variations (polymorphisms) in genes regulating key physiological processes (e.g., carcinogen metabolism, growth factors, cell signaling, cell cycle regulation, angiogenesis, oxidative stress, inflammation, DNA synthesis and repair) or health-related behaviors (e.g., nicotine addiction), which may affect cancer risk. Because their effects on cancer risk are usually small to moderate, these genetic polymorphisms are unlikely to be useful for predictive genetic testing in individuals. However, these associations may provide a basis for defining population groups with an increased susceptibility to a specific exposure, for example, based on ethnic origin, which could be the focus of special interventions (11). At the least, associations of functional genetic variants with disease are helpful in establishing the relevance of the mechanistic pathway under study.

2.5. Improving Early Detection

In the past 10 years, there has only been limited progress in the application of biomarkers to the early detection of cancer. Only the prostate-specific antigen (PSA) test has been widely adopted in clinical practice to screen for prostate cancer. Elevated and, especially, rising PSA indicates cell proliferation in prostatic tissue and, thus, is a marker of disease progression. Similarly, a decrease in the level of this marker can be used as an endpoint for interventions. Unfortunately, no comparable markers have been identified for other common cancers.

Molecular genetics may provide new sensitive detection methods in the coming years. Recent studies have shown that circulating tumor DNA ("cell-free DNA") can be isolated in peripheral blood and used to detect selected mutations that, individually or as a group, can be highly specific of the solid tumor from which the DNA originated (12). Tumor DNA with signature mutations have also been detected in sputum, breast fluid, and feces. However, it is still unclear how early in the disease process these tests could be used. Another emerging approach, namely proteomics, allows for the screening of hundreds or thousands of proteins in peripheral blood to detect patterns that may be highly specific for certain diseases, including cancers (13).

2.6. Improving Risk Assessment

More homogeneous disease groupings, improved measurement of study variables, and accounting for effect modification due to genetic or acquired susceptibility result in reduced misclassification in epidemiological studies, allowing for risk estimates that are more precise and that pertain to more refined subgroups of the population. Since epidemiological data are used in risk assessment to formulate individual risk functions, molecular epidemiologic studies can increase the validity and specificity of these functions.

3. CATEGORIES OF BIOMARKERS

Biomarkers used in epidemiological studies have been classified into markers of internal dose, markers of biologically effective dose, markers of susceptibility, and markers of early biological effects. These categories of biomarkers are better suited to some study designs than others, as described below.

3.1. Markers of Internal Dose

Biomarkers of internal dose typically measure a compound in biological specimens to assess the subjects' exposure to biological, nutritional, occupational, medical, or environmental agents, or to levels of endogenously produced compounds, such as hormones (7). Examples of markers of internal dose are given in Table 1. The utility of this type of biomarkers depends upon the half-life of the agent in the body and the pattern of the exposure it is measuring (e.g., daily vs. episodic). If the compound measured is rapidly

Table 1 Examples of Markers of Internal Dose

Biomarkers	Specimens	Exposure	Half-life	Target organ	Reference
Aflatoxin B1 and metabolites	Urine	Aflatoxin in diet		Liver	14
Arsenic	Urine	Copper smelting	1 week	Lung	15
Cotinine	Urine	Tobacco	3 days	Lung	16
DDE	Serum	DDT	Several months/years	Breast	17
Ascorbic acid	Plasma	Dietary vit. C	Few hours	All	18
Folate	Red blood cell	Dietary folate	120 days	All	19
Selenium	Toe nails	Dietary selenium	>1 year	Prostate	20
Estradiol	Plasma	Endogenous estrogens		Breast	

Source: Modified from Refs. 8 and 21.

eliminated or if the exposure is episodic, multiple measurements may be required in order to reduce the ratio of within- to between-individual variance (see Sec. 4) and estimate a "usual" level. Biomarkers of internal dose are particularly useful in prospective studies because the problem of reverse causality (i.e., disease status affecting the level of the biomarker) that can plague case–control studies is minimized or eliminated. However, markers of internal dose can sometimes be used in case–control studies when it is unlikely that either the exposure or the markers have been affected by the disease process or treatment (i.e., when studying a precursor lesion or early disease stage), or when the marker reflects past (presumably, prediagnostic) exposure (e.g., DDT metabolites in adipose tissue) and is not affected by disease status.

3.2. Markers of Biologically Effective Dose

In contrast to markers of internal dose, which measure the internal level of a compound or its metabolites, markers of biologically effective dose assess the amount of this compound that interacts with critical subcellular or cellular targets. Thus, these markers have the advantage of integrating the effects of both exposure and host susceptibility. For example, certain chemicals can bind covalently to proteins in the cell to form an adduct (Table 2). DNA adduct formation often occurs after metabolic activation of a carcinogen and can be followed by DNA repair. Thus, measurement of adducts can assess both exposure to a specific carcinogen and the individual's capacity to activate this carcinogen and repair DNA, as well as other possible host factors. Since formation of chemical–DNA adducts are thought to be important in carcinogenesis, individuals with the highest levels of DNA adducts are expected to be at greater cancer risk. A frequent limitation of adduct studies is that samples of target tissues are often not available and that surrogate tissue needs to be used. DNA adducts have limited applications in case–control studies due to the relatively short life of most adducts evaluated to date. However, protein adducts (hemoglobin or albumin adducts) have a longer half-life and, thus, their use may be possible in retrospective studies of early-stage cancers.

3.3. Markers of Susceptibility/Resistance

Cancer families have been noted for centuries. Linkage studies followed by positional cloning have allowed the identification of the genes responsible for a number of familial cancer syndromes, such as retinoblastoma, Wilm's tumor, Li–Fraumeni syndrome, Von Hipple–Lindau disease, familial adenomatous polyposis (FAP), hereditary nonpolyposis colorectal cancer (HNPCC), and familial breast–ovary cancers (44). These mutations are typically rare in populations but carry a high disease risk (high penetrance).

Table 2 Examples of Markers of Biologically Effective Dose

Adducts[a]	Exposure	Biospecimen[b]	Population	Reference
Alkylated Hb	Propylene oxide	RBC	Workers	22
4-Aminobiphenyl–Hb	Cigarette smoking	RBC	Smokers	23
AFB_1–guanine	Diet	Urine	Chinese	24
AFB_1–DNA	Diet	Liver tissue	Taiwanese	25
PAH–DNA	PAH in cigarette smoke/ environment	WBC	Lung cancer patients, smokers, workers	26
NNK–Hb	Cigarette smoke	RBC	Smokers	27

[a]AFB_1, aflatoxin B_1; PAH, polycyclic aromatic hydrocarbon; NNK, 4-(methylnitrosamino)-1-(3-pyridyl)-1-butanone.
[b]RBC, red blood cells; WBC, white blood cells.
Source: Modified from Ref. 8.

They can be used for predictive genetic testing in situations where preventive interventions are possible.

Potentially more relevant to public health are low-penetrance but common susceptibility genes, such as those listed in Table 3. Examples include genetic polymorphisms associated with interindividual differences in the metabolism of xenobiotics, DNA repair, or metabolism of hormones or key nutrients. Markers of susceptibility to behavioral exposures include genetic polymorphisms controlling metabolic processes affecting one's adoption of healthy or unhealthy lifestyle habits (e.g., toxic reaction to alcohol curtailing ethanol consumption; biological basis for susceptibility to nicotine or ethanol addiction).

Measuring enzymes or hormones that are thought to be the basis for the susceptibility, directly by assessing their levels in plasma or tissue, or

Table 3   Examples of Low Penetrance Susceptibilty Genes

Mechanism	Gene examples	Cancer	Reference
Dominant oncogene	*ras, myc*	Lung	28
Tumor suppressor genes	*p53, rb*	Lung, bladder	29
Carcinogen activation	*CYP1A1*	Lung	30
	CYP1A2	Bladder, colon	31
	CYP2E1	Lung, NPC	30, 32, 33
	NAT2	Colon	31
Carcinogen detoxification	*GSTM1*	Lung, bladder	34
	NAT2	Bladder	35
Hormone metabolism	*CYP17*	Breast	36
Hormone receptor	Androgen receptor	Prostate	37
Vitamin metabolism	Vitamin D receptor	Prostate	38
	MTHFR	Colon	39
Alcohol metabolism	*ADH, ALDH*	Oral	40
Addiction	Dopamine receptors	Smoking related cancers	41
DNA repair	*XP, AT hOGGI*	Skin, Burkitt lymphoma, lung	43

Source: Modified from Ref. 44.

indirectly by using a pharmacological probe (e.g., caffeine for NAT2 or CYP1A2 activity, chlorzoxazone for CYP2E1), is often possible in order to characterize the phenotype of interest. Such phenotyping assays are often difficult to use in case–control studies as the disease or its treatment may affect these measurements. In contrast, genotyping using genomic DNA has often been favored in case–control studies since the genotype of an individual is determined at birth and remains unaffected by disease or treatment. However, even with genotyping, the prospective design remains optimal when studying rapidly lethal diseases because of biases resulting from potential differential survival (e.g., due to differences in response to therapy by genotypes (45)) that may plague case–control studies. Moreover, the genes studied may convey an increased or decreased risk only in individuals who have been exposed (gene–environment interaction); hence, the importance of carefully assessing exposure. Compared to case–control studies, prospective studies offer the advantage of generating exposure data that are devoid of recall bias since this information is collected before the disease develops.

3.4. Markers of Early Biological Effects

Markers of early biological effects represent processes that are intermediate on the etiological pathway between exposure and clinically detectable disease. Examples of such markers are given in Table 4. These markers may help identify a mechanistic link between exposure and disease. They may also be used as disease surrogates for intervention studies or as screening tools for primary

Table 4 Examples of Markers of Early Biological Effect

Marker	Exposure	Biospecimen	Reference
Sister chromatid exchange	Industrial, radiation	WBC	46
Micronuclei	Cigarette smoke	WBC	47
	Betal quid	Buccal cells	48
Chromosomal aberrations	Industrial, radiation	WBC	49
Mutations in tumor suppressor genes			
Codon 249^{ser} *p53*	Dietary AFB1	Liver cells	50
p53 hot spot mutations at codons 157, 248 and 273	Benzo[α]pyrene	Bronchial epithelial cells	51
CC to *TT* mutation in p53	UV	Skin	52

and secondary prevention. For example, somatic mutations may be identified in target genes (e.g., p53), providing evidence of irreversible genetic damage. In some cases, specific mutations in the gene may indicate exposure to specific agents (DNA fingerprints) or may point to specific mechanisms. They may also be used clinically as prognostic factors or as endpoints in intervention studies evaluating genetic responses to various exposures.

Chromosomal aberrations are less specific markers but they are also thought to be intermediate in the etiological pathway to cancer. They have been used as markers of exposure or to evaluate individual sensitivity to mutagens or carcinogens.

4. DEVELOPMENT OF A BIOMARKER

A model for the development and validation of a biomarker is illustrated in Figure 2. Biomarkers are selected on their biological relevance to the question under study and on their practicality and validity. The biological relevance of a biomarker is usually established in animal studies and other experimental systems. It is based on specific knowledge about metabolism, product formation, and general mechanism of action. The development of a biomarker in the laboratory also includes the optimization of the specificity, sensitivity, and reproducibility of the assay used in its measurement, as well as the determination of the most appropriate biospecimen for the measurement (serum, plasma, red blood cells, spot urine, overnight urine, 24-h urine, etc.). In addition, optimal conditions are established for collecting, processing, and storing the samples in which the assay will be performed.

Whether a biomarker appears promising for use in large-scale studies rests on its validity, reliability, and practicality, which need to be assessed in preliminary field studies. A biomarker is considered valid if it measures well what it is supposed to measure. Although the concept is straightforward, validity is often difficult to establish as it requires a comparison to a gold standard that is rarely available. In contrast, reliability measures the extent to which a marker provides consistent results across repeated measurements. Although high validity implies high precision and reliability, high reliability can be obtained with a highly biased measure. Validity and reliability are, thus, two different attributes that are important in assessing the potential value of a biomarker (54). Considerations about the feasibility of using a biomarker in the field include the amount and type of biological specimen needed, the time required for the assay, and its cost.

When the potential value of a biomarker has been established, information on the extent and sources of its variability needs to be collected in order to adequately design studies that will use the biomarker. An estimate of the variation in the biomarker measurement in the population under study is required in order to carry out power estimations. Information on

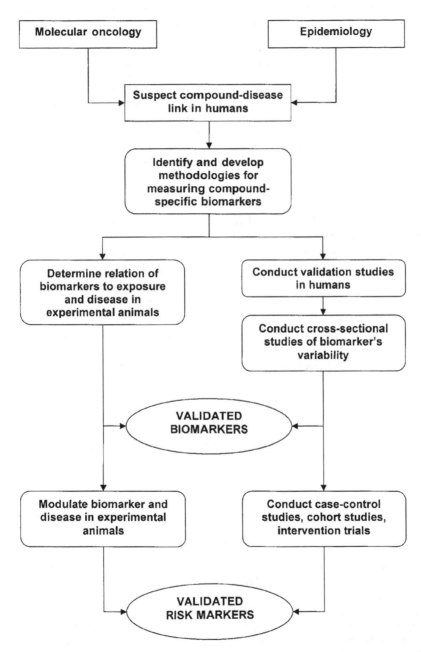

Figure 2   Model for the development of a biomarker. *Source*: Modified from Ref. 59.

Table 5 Determinants of Variability in Laboratory Results

Relative degree of variability	Comparison	Assessment
Minimal	Same analytical run	Duplicate samples
	Different analytical runs	Duplicate samples of known concentration
	Different laboratories	Exchange of samples
Maximal	Different methods	Split samples

Source: Modified from Ref. 54.

sources of variability is needed in order to identify potential confounders and effect modifiers that will need to be assessed as covariates.

The variation in a biomarker measurement is made up of two components, the intra- and interindividual variations. The intraindividual variability represents the extent to which the biomarker changes when measured several times on the same individual. Intraindividual variability is itself composed of laboratory variation (due to technical variation in the laboratory), sampling variation (variation resulting from a change in the way the sample was collected, processed, or stored), and intrasubject variation (true variation in the marker over a certain period of time). The components of laboratory variability are described in Table 5, along with the types of quality control samples required to assess them. Sources of sampling variability due to differences in biospecimen collection, processing, and storage are listed in Table 6. The true interindividual variability is the extent to which the level of the marker differs among individuals (due to exposure, host characteristics, etc.). The intraindividual variability can be considered as

Table 6 Sources of Variability in Sample Collection, Processing, and Storage

Collection	Processing	Storage
Donor (e.g., fasting vs. nonfasting; sitting vs. supine)	Time since collection	Temperature (−20°C, −70°C, −150°C, −196°C)
Time of venipuncture	Refrigeration	
Type of collection tube/additives	Exposure to light (carotenoids)	Thawing history
Duration of collection (e.g., spot vs. 12 hr urine)	Speed of centrifugation	Evaporation
Hemolysis	Contamination	Duration

noise and the interindividual variability as the signal of interest. Biomarkers that have a high interindividual variability compared to its intraindividual variability (i.e., a high signal-to-noise ratio) are particularly useful and will require a smaller sample size to test an hypothesis.

When the inter- vs. intraindividual variability of a biomarker has been described, additional investigations need to be conducted to characterize the main sources for this variability. These studies will help to identify potential confounders or effect modifiers that should be considered in hypothesis-testing studies using the biomarker. These preliminary studies typically use a cross-sectional design to assess the level of the marker by subject characteristics, such as age, sex, ethnic group, and other known risk factors for the disease of interest (e.g., dietary factors, smoking, and genotypes). They may also be small intervention studies assessing the effects of important modifiable variables (e.g., diet, smoking) on the level of a marker.

5. METHODOLOGICAL ISSUES

Although the use of biomarkers may increase the amount of useful information gained from epidemiological studies, the validity of the results, as in traditional epidemiology, rests on the adherence of these studies to time-tested epidemiologic principles. Of primary importance are the concepts of selection bias, random and systematic errors, confounding, and effect-modification. As primarily an observational science, molecular epidemiology is subject to the same biases and limitations as traditional epidemiology and should be practiced and evaluated with the same rigor.

It has been construed that molecular epidemiologic studies, because they deal with biological measurements, are less affected by selection bias or confounding. This view is untenable and should be rejected. In biology, cause and effect relationships rarely occur in isolation. They are often impacted upon by multiple host or extraneous factors that, themselves, may correlate with subject selection factors (resulting in selection bias) or other risk factors (resulting in confounding).

Although the justification for using biomarkers in an epidemiological study is that they will yield better measurements of study variables than conventional methods, minimizing measurement error and avoiding systematic error is even more a priority in molecular epidemiology than in traditional epidemiology. This is because inferences in traditional epidemiology are typically made based on relative differences using categorical exposures (e.g., quartiles), whereas the interpretation of biomarker data emphasizes more absolute levels and individual results. Strict quality standards are required in the laboratory and in the field to maximize the accuracy of the results and minimize measurement error due to laboratory and sampling variability. Particularly problematic is the systematic error that may occur if samples of cases and controls (or "exposed" and "nonexposed" subjects in prospective studies) are collected, processed, stored, or analyzed under different conditions. As a rule, samples for cases and controls (or "exposed" and "nonexposed" subjects) should be matched on collection conditions and storage duration, and the matched samples analyzed together in the same batch. Also, laboratory personnel analyzing the samples should remain blind to the case–control status of the samples. Duplicate samples should be used to monitor both intra- and inter-run laboratory variability throughout the study and those data should be published with the study findings.

Also of particular relevance to molecular epidemiological studies is the need for adequate statistical power in order to accept or reject the null hypothesis with confidence. Because molecular epidemiological studies are often expensive and logistically complex to carry out, many studies have been small and, as the result, inconclusive. Since studies with positive findings, even if they are inadequately small, are more likely to be published than negative studies, the influence on the field of these small studies tends to be excessive. Furthermore, when studying complex diseases, such as cancer, using a molecular epidemiology approach to home in on a specific step of a particular biological pathway, effect size is expected to be smaller than when studying a complex exposure that acts through multiple pathways (e.g., smoking, specific dietary components or patterns, hormones). Thus, it is an imperative for null studies to report their statistical power to detect weak effects. Finally, sample size requirements are especially taxing when interactions are tested, as very large sample sizes (sometimes in the thousands) are typically needed (55).

Because molecular epidemiological studies often attempt to identify individual susceptibility factors, the relationships observed are often found to be limited to, or stronger for, subgroups of the study population (56). Sometimes even opposite effects are expected for different study subgroups (57). Exploration of these interactions must be part of an a priori, biology-based hypothesis since the testing of an association in multiple subgroups increases the likelihood of a chance finding. A related problem is the testing of multiple hypotheses in the same study, a common practice to increase cost-efficiency. This practice also increases the probability that a chance association emerges as statistically significant. Thus, the knowledge of the number of hypotheses tested in a study is useful in interpreting the results. Similarly, findings that were not part of the initial study hypotheses should clearly be identified as such, as they need to be reproduced in other studies before being given much credence.

6. ETHICAL ISSUES

The use of biomarkers may present ethical issues that do not manifest themselves as acutely in traditional epidemiological studies. Biomarker studies may generate particularly sensitive information on exposure, early biological effects, or susceptibility to cancer about individual research participants. This information may be misused, for example, as the basis for denying insurance coverage or employment. In order to protect the participants from any kind of stigmatization or discrimination, as well as to assure their privacy in general, strict confidentiality measures are required. Access to physical and electronic files must be severely restricted. This includes the use of encryption, fire walls, and passwords to protect electronic datafiles. In addition, in the United States, when the information to be collected is particularly sensitive, investigators may apply, at the start of the study, for a "Certificate of Confidentiality," which would prevent the researcher from having to release data to a third party, even if required as part of a legal proceeding (58). There remains differences in opinion as to whether research participants should be told of test results obtained in a research setting. This is particularly relevant to those biomarkers that have a high predictive value. In addition to the risks involved in participating in the study, the type of tests conducted and the significance and limitations of the test results should be explained to the subjects as part of the study informed consent process. The decision to report results to the subjects should be limited to preventable conditions and should be based on the degree of clinical usefulness and the reliability of the information provided by the biomarker. Positive results may require repeat testing, counseling, and diagnostic evaluation.

7. CONCLUSION

Historically, epidemiologists have investigated the distributions of diseases by person, time, and place in order to make inferences about their causes. Over the years, methodological tools have been introduced in order to better characterize each of these three key elements. For example, laboratory assays have been used to monitor the ambient environment (air, food, soil, water, etc.) or to detect present or past exposure to an infectious agent. The recent interest in the development of exquisitely sensitive and specific biomarkers offers much promise for the continued contributions of epidemiology to our knowledge of cancer etiology, risk assessment, and prevention. The purpose of this chapter was to summarize the applications of biomarkers, as well as the methodological aspects of their use. It should be stressed that, although the current technology permits the detection of changes at the cellular and molecular levels, and of very low doses of exposure, at these levels inherited and acquired host factors can be strong sources of variability and confounding. Thus, more than ever, the soundness of the epidemiological approach remains critical to the quality of the data.

REFERENCES

1. Doll R, Peto R. The Causes of Human Cancer: Quantitative Estimates of Avoidable Risk of Cancer in the United States Today. New York: Oxford University Press, 1981.
2. Higginson J, Muir CS. The role of epidemiology in elucidating the importance of environmental factors in human cancer. Cancer Detect Prev 1976; 1:79–105.
3. World Cancer Research Fund/American Institute for Cancer Research. Food, Nutrition and the Prevention of Cancer: a Global Perspective. Washington: American Institute for Cancer Research, 1997.
4. Hulka BS, Wilcosky TC, Griffith JD, eds. Biological Markers in Epidemiology. New York: Oxford University Press, 1990.
5. Shulte PA, Perera FP, eds. Molecular Epidemiology: Principles and Practices. San Diego: Academic Press, 1993.
6. Toniolo P, Boffetta P, Shuker DEG, Rothman N, Hulka B, Pearce N. Applications of Biomarkers in Cancer Epidemiology. Lyon: International Agency for Research on Cancer IARC Scientific Publications No. 142, 1997.
7. Shulte PA. A conceptual and historical framework for molecular epidemiology. In: Shulte PA, Perera FP, eds. Molecular Epidemiology: Principles and Practices. San Diego: Academic Press, 1993:3–44.
8. Perera FP, Santella R. Carcinogenesis. In: Shulte PA, Perera FP, eds. Molecular Epidemiology: Principles and Practices. San Diego: Academic Press, 1993:277–300.
9. Longnecker MP, Stram DO, Taylor PR, Levander OA, Howe M, Veillon C, McAdam PA, Patterson KY, Holden JM, Morris JS, Swanson CA, Willett WC. Use of selenium concentration in whole blood, serum, toenails, or urine as a surrogatemeasure of selenium intake. Epidemiology 1996; 7:384–390.
10. Shipp MA, Ross KN, Tamayo P, Weng AP, Kutok JL, Aguiar RC, Gaasenbeek M, Angelo M, Reich M, Pinkus GS, Ray TS, Koval MA, Last KW, Norton A, Lister TA, Mesirov J, Neuberg DS, Lander ES, Aster JC, Golub TR. Diffuse large B-cell lymphoma outcome prediction by gene-expression profiling and supervised machine learning. Nat Med 2002; 8:68–74.
11. Perera FP. Environment and cancer: who are susceptible? Science 1997; 278:1068–1073.
12. Kirk GD, Camus-Randon AM, Mendy M, Goedert JJ, Merle P, Trepo C, Brechot C, Hainaut P, Montesano R. Ser-249 p53 mutations in plasma DNA of patients with hepatocellular carcinoma from The Gambia. J Natl Cancer Inst 2000; 92:148–153.
13. Petricoin EF, Ardekani AM, Hitt BA, Levine PJ, Fusaro VA, Steinberg SM, Mills GB, Simone C, Fishman DA, Kohn EC, Liotta LA. Use of proteomic patterns in serum to identify ovarian cancer. Lancet 2002; 359:572–577.
14. Ross RK, Yuan JM, Yu MC, Wogan GN, Qiao GS, Tu JT, Groopman JD, Gao YT, Henderson BE. Urinary aflatoxin biomarkers and risk of hepatocellular carcinoma. Lancet 1992; 339:943–946.
15. Enterline PE, Marsh GM. Cancer among workers exposed to arsenic and other substances in a copper smelter. Am J Epidemiol 1982; 116:895–911.
16. de Waard F, Kemmeren JM, van Ginkel LA, Stolker AA. Urinary cotinine and lung cancer risk in a female cohort. Br J Cancer 1995; 72:784–787.

17. Wolf MS, Toniolo PG, Lee EW, Rivera M, Dubin N. Blood levels of organo-chlorine residues and risk of breast cancer. J Natl Cancer Inst 1993; 85:648–652.
18. Sinha R, Block G, Taylor PR. Determinants of plasma ascorbic acid in a healthy male population. Cancer Epidemiol Biomarkers 1992; 1:297–302.
19. Wild J, Seller MJ, Schorah CJ, Smithells RW. Investigation of folate intake and metabolism in women who have had two pregnancies complicated by neural tubal defects. Br J Obstet Gynecol 1994; 101:197–202.
20. Swanson CA, Longnecker MP, Veillon C, Howe SM, Levander OA, Taylor PR, McAdam PA, Brown CC, Stampfer MJ, Willett WC. Selenium intake, age, gender, and smoking in relation to indices of selenium status of adults residing in seleniferous area. Am J Clin Nutr 1990; 52:856–862.
21. Coggon D, Friesen MD. Markers of internal dose: chemical agents. In: Toniolo P, Boffetta P, Shuker DEG, Rothman N, Hulka B, Pearce N, eds. Applications of Biomarkers in Cancer, Epidemiology. Lyon: International Agency for Research on Cancer, IARC Scientific Publications No.142, 1997:95–101.
22. Osterman-Golkar S, Bailey E, Farmer PB, Gorf SM, Lamb JH. Monitoring exposure to propylene oxide through the determination of hemoglobin alkylation. Scand J Work Environ Health 1984; 10:99–102.
23. Bryant MS, Skipper PL, Tannenbaum SR. Hemoglobin adducts of 4-aminobiphenyl in smokers and nonsmokers. Cancer Res 1987; 47:602–608.
24. Groopman JD, Donahue PR, Zhu J, Chen J, Wogan GN. Aflatoxin metabolism and nucleic acid adducts in urine by affinity chromatography. Proc Natl Acad Sci USA 1985; 82:6492–6496.
25. Zhang Y-J, Chen C-J, Lee C-S, Haghighi B, Yang G-Y, Wang L-W, Feitelson M, Santella R. Aflatoxin B-DNA adducts and hepatitis B virus antigens in hepatocellular carcinoma and non-tumerous tissue. Carcinogenesis 1991; 12:2247–2252.
26. Santella RM. Application of new techniques for the detection of carcinogen adducts to human population monitoring. Mutat Res 1988; 205:271–282.
27. Carmella SG, Kagan SS, Kagan M, Foiles PG, Palladino G, Quart AM, Quart E, Hecht SS. Mass spectrometric analysis of tobacco-specific nitrosamine hemoglobin adducts in snuff dippers, smokers, and nonsmokers. Cancer Res 1990; 50:5438–5445.
28. Tamai S, Sugimura H, Caporaso NE, Reseau JH, Trump BF, Weston A, Harris CC. Restriction fragment length polymorphism analysis of the L-myc gene locus in a case-control study of lung cancer. Int J Cancer 1990; 41:411–415.
29. Wu W-J, Kakehi Y, Habuchi T, Kinoshita H, Ogawa O, Terachi T, Huang C-H, Chiang CP, Yoshida O. Allelic frequency of p53 gene codon 72 polymorphism in urologic cancers. Jpn J Cancer Res 1995; 86:730–736.
30. Le Marchand L, Sivaraman L, Pierce L, Seifried A, Lum A, Wilkens LR, Lau AF. Associations of CYP1A1, GSTM1, and CYP2E1 polymorphisms with lung cancer suggest cell type specificities to tobacco carcinogens. Cancer Res 1988; 58:4858–4863.
31. Lang NP, Butler MA, Massengill J, Lawson M, Stotts RC, Hauer-Jensen M, Kadlubar FF. Rapid metabolic phenotypes for acetyltransferase and cyto-chrome P4501A2 and putative exposure to food-borne heterocyclic amines increase the risk of colorectal cancer and polyps. Cancer Epidemiol Prev Biomarkers 1994; 3:657–682.

32. Uematsu F, Kikuchi H, Motomiya M, Abe T, Sagami I, Ohmachi T, Wakui A, Kanamaru R, Watanabe M. Association between restriction fragment length polymorphism of the human cytochrome P450IIE1 gene and susceptibility to lung cancer. Jpn J Cancer Res 1991; 82:254–256.

33. Hildesheim A, Chen CJ, Caporaso NE, Cheng YJ, Hoover RN, Hsu MM, Levine PH, Chen LH, Chen JY, Yang CS, Daly AK, Idle JR. Cytochrome P4502E1 genetic polymorphisms and risk of nasopharyngeal carcinoma: results from a case–control study conducted in Taiwan. Cancer Epidemiol Biomarkers Prev 1995; 4:607–610.

34. Bell DA, Taylor JA, Paulson DF, Robertson CN, Mohler JL, Lucier GW. Genetic risk and carcinogen exposure: common inherited defect of the carcinogen-metabolism gene glutathione S-transferase M1 (GSTM1) that increases susceptibility to bladder cancer. J Natl Cancer Inst 1993; 85:1159–1164.

35. Cartwright RA, Glashan RW, Rogers HJ, Ahmad RA, Barham-Hall D, Higgins E, Kahn MA. Role of N-acetyltransferase phenotypes in bladder carcinogenesis: a pharmacogenetic epidemiological approach to bladder cancer. Lancet 1982; 2:842–845.

36. Feigelson HS, Coetzee GA, Kolonel LN, Ross RK, Henderson BE. A polymorphism in the CYP17 gene increases the risk of breast cancer. Cancer Res 1997; 57:1063–1065.

37. Irvine RA, Yu MC, Ross RK, Coetzee GA. The CAG and GGC microsatellites of the androgen receptor gene are in linkage disequilibrium in men with prostate cancer. Cancer Res 1995; 55:1937–1940.

38. Taylor JA, Hirvonen A, Watson M, Pittman G, Mohler JL, Bell DA. Association of prostate cancer with vitamin D receptor gene polymorphism. Cancer Res 1996; 56:4108–4110.

39. Chen J, Giovannucci E, Kelsey K, Rimm EB, Stampfer MJ, Colditz GA, Spiegelman D, Willett WC, Hunter DJ. A methylenetetrahydrofolate reductase polymorphism and the risk of colorectal cancer. Cancer Res 1996; 56:4862–4864.

40. Harty LC, Caporaso NE, Hayes RB, Winn DM, Bravo-Otero E, Blot WJ, Kleinman DV, Brown LM, Armenian HK, Fraumeni JF Jr, Shields PG. Alcohol dehydrogenase 3 genotype and risk of oral cavity and pharyngeal cancers. J Natl Cancer Inst 1997; 89:1698–1705.

41. Comings DE, Muhleman D, Ahn C, Gysin R, Flanagan SD. The dopamine D2 receptor gene: a genetic risk factor for substance abuse. Drug Alcohol Depend 1994; 34:175–180.

42. Hanawalt PC. Role of transcription-coupled DNA repair in susceptibility to environmental carcinogenesis. Environ Health Perspect 1996; 104(Suppl 3):547–551.

43. Le Marchand L, Donlon T, Lum-Jones A, Seifried A, Wilkens LR. Association of the hOGG1 Ser326Cys polymorphism with lung cancer risk. Cancer Epidemiol Biomarkers Prev 2002; 11:409–412.

44. Caporaso N, Goldstein A. Issues involving biomarkers in the study of the genetics of human cancer. In: Toniolo P, Boffetta P, Shuker DEG, Rothman N, Hulka B, Pearce N, eds. Applications of Biomarkers in Cancer Epidemiology. Lyon: International Agency for Research on Cancer, IARC Scientific Publications No. 142, 1997:237–250.

45. Kelsey KT, Hankinson SE, Colditz GA, Springer K, Garcia-Closas M, Spiegelman D, Manson JE, Garland M, Stampfer MJ, Willett WC, Speitzer FE, Hunter DJ. Glutathione S-transferase class mu deletion polymorphism and breast cancer: results from prevalent versus incident cases. Cancer Epidemiol Biomarkers Prev 1997; 6:511–515.

46. Wilcosky TC, Rynard SM. Sister chromatic exchanges. In: Hulka B, Wilcosky TC, Griffith JD, eds. "Biological Markers in Epidemiology". New York: Oxford University Press, 1990:28–55.

47. Hogstedt B, Akesson B, Axell K, Gullberg B, Mitelman F, Pero RW, Skerving S, Welinder H. Increased frequency of lymphocyte micronuclei in workers producing reinforced polyester resin with low exposure to styrene. Scand J Work Environ Health 1983; 49:271–276.

48. Stich HF, Dunn BP. DNA adducts, micronuclei, and leukoplakias as intermediate endpoints in intervention trials. IARC Sci Publ 1988; 89:137–145.

49. Perera FP, Hemminki K, Gryzbowska E, Motykiewicz G, Michalska J, Santella RM, Young T, Dickey C, Brandt-Rauf P, DeVivo I, Blaner W, Tsai W, Chorazi M. Molecular and genetic damage in humans from environmental pollution in Poland. Nature 1992; 360:256–258.

50. Hsu IC, Metcalf R, Sun T, Welsh JA, Wang NJ, Harris CC. Mutational hotspot in the p53 gene in human hepatocellular carcinomas. Nature 1991; 350: 427–428.

51. Denissenko MF, Pao A, Tang M-S, Pfeifer GP. Preferential formation of benzo[a]pyrene adducts at lung cancer mutational hotspots in p53. Science 1996; 274:430–432.

52. Brash DE, Rudolph JA, Simon JA, Lin A, McKenna GJ, Baden HP, Halperin AJ, Ponten J. A role for sunlight in skin cancer: UV-induced p53 mutation in squamous cell carcinoma. Proc Natl Acad Sci USA 1991; 88:10124–10128.

53. Hussain SP, Harris CC. Molecular epidemiology of human cancer: contribution of mutation spectra studies of tumor suppressor genes. Cancer Res 1988; 58:4023–4037.

54. Vineis P, Schulte PA, Vogt RF Jr. Technical variability in laboratory data. In: Shulte PA, Perera FP, eds. Molecular Epidemiology: Principles and Practices. San Diego: Academic Press, 1993:109–135.

55. Garcia-Closas M, Rothman N, Lubin J. Misclassification in case-control studies of gene-environment interactions: assessment of bias and sample size. Cancer Epidemiol Biomarkers Prev 1999; 8:1043–1050.

56. Garte S. Metabolic susceptibility genes as cancer risk factors: time for a reassessment? Cancer Epidemiol Biomarkers Prev 2001; 10:1233–1237.

57. Thompson PA, Shields PG, Freudenheim JL, Stone A, Vena JE, Marshall JR, Graham S, Laughlin R, Nemoto T, Kadlubar FF, Ambrosone CB. Genetic polymorphisms in catechol-O-methyltransferase, menopausal status, and breast cancer risk. Cancer Res 1998; 58:2107–2110.

58. Earley CL, Strong LC. Certificate of confidentiality: a valuable tool for protecting genetic data. Am J Hum Genet 1995; 57:727–731.

59. Groopman JD, Kensler TW. The light at the end of the tunnel for chemical-specific biomarkers: daylight or headlight? Carcinogenesis 1999; 20:1–11.

4

Methods for Genetic Testing I: Assessing Mutations in Cancers

Haruhiko Sugimura

Department of Pathology, Hamamatsu University School of Medicine, Hamamatsu, Shizuoka, Japan

Peter G. Shields

Cancer Genetics and Epidemiology Program, Department of Medicine and Oncology, Lombardi Cancer Center, Georgetown University Medical Center, Washington, D.C., U.S.A.

1. INTRODUCTION

There are over 100,000 human genes located on 46 chromosomes. Genes are composed of deoxyribonucleic acid (DNA) in two strands joined by nucleotide base pairing. The DNA sequence provides a written language of three base codons that are transcribed to mRNA, which then are translated to proteins. These expressed proteins then govern cellular function. The codons code for specific amino acids. Not all of a gene, however, and not all of a chromosome, codes for amino acids. The nucleotides are organized together into either exons, which are transcribed, and introns, which are not. There also are promoter regions within introns that decide when and how much a gene is transcribed. Among people, most of the genetical sequence is the same, but there are important differences too, which affect such things as hair color, height, and facial characteristics. This diversity is controlled through variations in DNA sequence. Any variation that occurs in more than 1% of the population is considered a polymorphism (a single-base polymorphism also is known as an SNP). It is estimated that genetical polymorphisms occur approximately every 500 bases. But other polymorphisms include more than one base insertion or deletion (and there can be variable numbers in different people—variable nucleotide tandem repeats). In some cases, whole exons or large parts of genes can be inserted or deleted.

Familial cancers involving highly penetrant mutations of single genes account for less than 5–10% of human cancers (1,2). The identification of these cancers is not difficult with an adequate level of curiosity and knowledge. But to do this, it is essential that clinicians make a thorough record of clinical information, including the onset of symptoms, other sites of malignancy, family history, the ages of both affected and unaffected family members, lifestyle information, occupations, ethnicity, and consanguity. This information is confirmed or supplemented with mutational analysis. But, molecular techniques for detecting inherited mutations cannot compensate for a lack of clinical data.

Human tumors occur through an accumulation of multiple mutations and genetical changes (3–5). They affect gene function and the coding of proteins, which allows cancer to develop. The study of mutations provides insights into tumorigenesis and forecasting of clinical behavior. The significance of mutations also provide etiological clues for associations with individual and population cancer risks. Genetical changes that are acquired and seen in tumors include point mutations, base deletions, base insertions, loss of heterozygosity (LOH) (gene deletion), chromosomal loss, amplifications, microsatellite instability, rearrangements, translocation, and chromosomal instability.

Mutations affect genetical function as they alter the genetical code in an exon, splice-site region or promoter region. Thus, mutations can be nonsense (change into stop codon), frame-shift (three bases plus one or two bases insertion or deletion change a reading frame or possibly generate a premature stop codon), or missense (amino acid substitution) mutations. Mutations also can be silent (no amino acid change). Nonsense and frame-shift mutations have potentially drastic effects on the gene product by causing a truncated protein. Amino acid substitutions may or may not be associated with a change in protein function, polarity, or pK_a.

In this chapter, possible interpretations of the mutations in tumors and how they are identified are addressed from the standpoint of individual cancer risk. The assessment of mutations in cancer must always be done from the viewpoint of its primary role in initial tumorigenesis.

2. MUTATED GENES IN HUMAN CANCERS

Mutations in the early stages of cancer and precancerous lesions are among the most informative for providing information about the carcinogenic process. These mutations can be directly involved in augmenting carcinogenesis. However, some mutations occur without consequence and result from an abnormal cellular process (6). These mutations are also called "passenger" mutations, the sequels of the genetical instability during the tumorigenesis, and are probably not the cause of the tumor development, although, it is still possible that these "passenger" mutations may confer some peculiar characteristics to the biological behavior of the tumors. When studying cancer risk and the resulting mutations, lesions in genes affecting early stages probably represent early exposures.

We can categorize cancer genes as oncogenes (including signal transduction molecules, receptor and nonreceptor kinases and phosphatases) and suppressor genes (nuclear transcription factors, cell cycle dependent genes, and cell adhesion molecules). The former are genes that augment cell proliferation and tumorigenesis by increasing gene expression. The latter augments cell proliferation and tumorigenesis when function is lost due to a mutation. Oncogenes and tumor suppressor genes are mutated in essentially every human tumor. Interestingly, only a few genes play a role in cancers from multiple organs, but most appear to be specific to some tumors.

Cancer-related genes also can be categorized into gatekeeper, caretaker, and landscaper genes (7). Caretaker genes are responsible for maintaining cell integrity (i.e., DNA repair). Mutations in gatekeeper genes are nearly always found in early precursor lesions and their (in) activation is essential for initiation of specific neoplasms. These genes include BRCa1, p53, and others. Inactivation of gatekeeper genes may be necessary for passing the genetical "threshhold" of the neoplastic process. Gatekeepers control cell proliferation in each tissue and include APC (8–10), beta-catenin (11–14); NF1 (15), patched (16), and others. Generally speaking, once inactivation occurs (for example, in the case of ret) in a gatekeeper gene, clonal expansion is more likely to occur followed by the accumulation of multiple genetical events.

An individual's risk for cancer is a function of their genetical predisposition (preinherited mutations found in the germline) and environmental exposures. This is then added to by acquired mutations that occur as a result of those gene–environment interactions, such as a mutation in a caretaker gene. We believe that mutations are nonrandom profiles of what caused a particular cancer. Nonrandomness of the mutations of certain genes (p53, ATM, Brca1, APC, and others) help us understand what causes cancer, especially when studied in animal and in vitro cell culture models. This so-called "carcinogen fingerprint," as methodologies are further developed, is considered among the best ways of determining carcinogenic etiologies.

3. GENETICAL ASSAYS

In this chapter, the practical aspects of mutation assessment are reviewed. Physicians, surgeons, diagnostic pathologists, laboratory technologists, nurses, epidemiologists, and other health workers need to be prepared for research studies and clinical decision making (17,18). Health professionals working in developing countries also are encouraged to participate in this field (19). Every cancer patient, whether suspected as representing a familial cancer syndrome or not, should be considered unique and their tissues irreplaceable. Biopsy and other surgical specimens must be properly handled, and different simultaneous pathological processing procedures should be used to allow for different types of assays. More and more, tissues collected in community hospitals, otherwise not involved in research, are serving as a valuable resource in large studies. So, staff members must prevent autolysis. It is helpful to use different fixations because these provide different DNA yields. As described later, a success rate for DNA recovery from the paraffin blocks depends on appropriate fixation. For example, long immersion of resected tissues in formalin fixatives damages tissues for further molecular investigations. Frozen tissue is essential for many genetical assays, but is not sufficient for RNA analysis or cell culture without special processing. Quick fixation is required for electron microscopy, but not for DNA extraction.

Good pathological examination using standard techniques is required to ensure success at subsequent analysis. The histological type of cancer should be confirmed when planning to assay DNA, then microdisection is needed so tumor cells are separated from other cells. This is best done from fixed tissues.

Every step in the process of tumor collection, fixation, and storage affects the ability to perform subsequent genetical assays because they can affect DNA quality and quantity. The most commonly used fixative is formaldehyde (so-called 1/10, which is 3.6%). Many laboratories recommend neutral buffered formalin. Some institutes use AMEX fixation, which has been asserted to be one of the best ways to keep the tissues as a possible good source of DNA, RNA, and protein (20,21). This procedure takes some extra steps in the routine histopathological laboratory and at least one person knowledgable in that procedure is needed. The time between resection and fixation should be short and the fixation time should be short. An alternate fixative is ethanol, which is better for subsequent DNA studies. And more laboratories are using OCT with rapid freezing with success.

Other variables that affect DNA quality and quantity occur during DNA extraction, such as insufficient time for dewaxing with xylene, detergent (SDS or tween-20) or insufficient time for proteinase K digestion. Greater quantities of the paraffin embedded tissue are not necessarily better for DNA assays, because this allows for greater amounts of inhibitors from the blocks. Several agents are available for extracting DNA from fixed tissues that are thought to reduce these inhibitors, e.g., Chelex-100 (22).

Table 1 lists the biomarker assays used for risk assessment and diagnosis. Basic and additional protocols are available elsewhere (23–26).

There are many types of genetical assays in use today. Some of these will be described below. The majority of molecular genetic tests used today begin with the polymerase chain reaction (PCR). There are emerging

Table 1   Biomarkers of Cancer Risk and Diagnosis

Biomarkers for disease risk
Markers of inherited susceptibility
    Genetical variation causing impaired metabolic activation or excretion of
        toxins
    Genetical variation causing defects in the repair of DNA, cell cycle control, or
        programmed cell death
Markers of acquired susceptibility
    Formation of DNA adducts
    Integration of viral DNA
    Mutations in critical genes
    Mutations in noncritical genes
    Hypermethylation of gene promoter region
    Altered gene expression
    Clastogenic abnormalities
    Antibodies to DNA adducts
    Altered protein or mRNA expression patterns

Biomarkers for preclinical disease
Markers of cellular alteration
    Altered morphology of cells
    Altered phenotypic expression of cells
    Clonal proliferation of cells
    Altered gene expression
    Antibodies to gene products
    Altered protein or mRNA expression patterns

Biomarkers for clinical disease
Markers of cellular alteration
    Altered morphology of cells
    Altered phenotypic expression of cells
    Immunohistochemical staining
    Clonal proliferation of cells
    Altered gene expression
    Antibodies to gene products
    Altered protein or mRNA expression patterns
Markers of prognosis
    Pathological diagnosis
    Immunohistochemical staining
    Altered gene expression
    Cytogenetic abnormalities
    Altered protein or mRNA expression patterns

technologies that will eliminate this need, but none have been sufficiently validated for use in the clinical setting. Polymerase chain reaction, in fact, is among the most important recent advances in molecular genetics. The reaction is the amplification of small amounts of DNA to make lots of DNA, which are then available for subsequent analyses. Polymerase chain reaction is facile and inexpensive. It has been used in forensic medicine for DNA fingerprinting from a single hair follicle or blood stain (27); mutation detection in single sperm cells to assess teratogenicity rates (28); and amplification of DNA from paraffin embedded tissue blocks (29), serum (30) or ancient DNA (31). It also forms the basis for microarray technology (32,33). Polymerase chain reaction relies upon a temperature stable enzyme (*Taq* polymerase) that can replicate DNA when using gene- and site-specific primers that begin the reaction. While PCR is generally used for DNA amplification, it also can be used for RNA amplification using a different enzyme (reverse transcriptase) (34). The major limitations of PCR lie in its sensitivity that allows for contamination by unwanted DNA from other sources. It also is critical to choose primers carefully to ensure specificity and prevent amplifying the wrong gene.

There are many applications for PCR. It is being used directly without other techniques for diagnosing viral infections (e.g., HIV in lymphocytes (35), hepatitis B virus in liver and serum (36), and papilloma virus in uterine cervix (37)). It can be used to amplify mutated and structurally altered regions of a given gene (e.g., translocation of chromosomes by determining the breakpoint cluster region for the *bcr-abl* oncogene for the diagnosis of chronic myelogenous leukemia (38). Other applications involve the identification of single-base mutations or genetical polymorphisms by designing primers that anneal only if matched to the unique sequence (e.g., oligo-specific PCR for the identification of polymorphisms in the *N*-acetyl transferase gene predictive of cancer risk in workers exposed to aromatic amines (39). Polymerase chain reaction also is combined with other techniques whereby PCR amplification products can be subjected to restriction enzyme digestion to identify genetical polymorphisms or mutations [e.g., restriction fragment length polymorphism (RFLP) analysis for cytochrome P450 genetical polymorphisms (40)] or used for hybridization with mutation-specific probes (e.g., oligonucleotide hybridization for the detection of *Ras* mutations (41). Another important application is the use of PCR to amplify sufficient quantities of DNA fragments for nucleotide sequencing. This method allows for the determination of specific sequences from unknown genes or for the detection of mutations (42).

3.1. Genotyping

Genotyping to determine genetical variation (e.g., color of hair, metabolic activity, DNA repair) can be done by using different types of detection methods following PCR. This genetical variation can happen via SNPs, or multiple-base pair insertions or deletions. A common way is to utilize RFLP analysis. Restriction fragment length polymorphism enzymes identify short, specific DNA sequences, cutting the DNA at those sequences into uniquely sized fragments that can be separated electrophoretically. Restriction enzymes recognize palindromic sites where the sequence on each strand is identical with each other (when read in 5′ to 3′ direction). Restriction fragment length polymorphism enzymes are only useful when a palindromic site exists. In other cases, the variant may be determined using single-strand conformational polymorphism (SSCP) analysis. If the variant results in the insertion or deletion of a base or bases, then electrophoretic methods that separate fragments based on size can be used. The fortunate property of DNA, where each strand is complementary and annealed by nucleic acid base-pairing (guanine to cytosine and adenine to thymine), can be taken advantage of to identify specific genetical sequences. Under experimental conditions the two complementary DNA strands can be separated and reannealed. Single-stranded probes of short DNA fragments can be used to identify a specific genetical sequence by exposing DNA to the probe. Using oligo-specific hybridization, a radioactive or fluorescently labeled probe marker will bind to the matched DNA. Two probes are used in tandem that are matched to one variant or the other. This unique property allows for Southern blot analysis of DNA (43), which subjects DNA to restriction enzyme digestion, separation of the resulting fragments by electrophoresis, and then probing the fragments for the genetical sequence and measuring the lengths of the fragments. The method also is used for northern blot analysis of messenger RNA (mRNA) (44), which is almost identical with Southern blot analysis except that RNA is used instead of DNA.

Several new methodologies exist for high through-put genotyping. These include microarrays that can determine 2000 SNPs following 24 different PCR assays, real-time PCR that allows for detection of SNPs without gel electrophoresis, matrix-assisted laser desorbtion/ionization time of flight (Maldi-TOF) mass spectroscopy (45), denatured high-performance liquid chromatography (46), capillary gel electrophoresis, and flourescence detection (47) and pyrosequencing (48).

3.2. Sequencing

DNA sequencing can be used to determine the actual genetical code. This may be used for identifying an inherited code (i.e., sequence of entire gene or SNPs) or mutations in tumors. The dideoxy-mediated chain termination method was among the first established and allows for the determination of the nucleic acid sequence of a gene (49). For example, a PCR fragment is amplified and four dideoxy reactions are carried out for each of the four nucleotides. The amplified product, radiolabeled nucleotides, 2,3′- dideoxynucleotides, and a polymerase are mixed so that the 2,3′-dideoxynucleotide is randomly incorporated into the DNA. Based on the location of the dideoxynucleotide incorporation, the DNA sequence can be determined after electrophoretic separation. More recent high-throughput methods rely on microarray technology following PCR (32) or capillary electrophoresis.

Because sequencing can be labor intensive, some investigators use methods to screen for mutations. The SSCP analysis was originally developed by Orita et al. (50) as such a screening method. Here, DNA is denatured into single strands and analyzed by gel electrophoresis. If there are base changes, then the migratory distance on the gel changes. The basis for this technique is still empirical, thus the sensitivity of the detection of mutation depends on which product you like to screen (51). The electrophoresis conditions including the glycerol content and gel temperature determine the specifity and sensitivity of the procedures, but there is no general principle about which condition is the best. For some fragments, only 12.5% glycerol can identify the migrationdifferences while at other times electrophoresis at 4°C is needed.

3.3. Gene Loss and Loss of Heterozygosity

Assessing for loss at heterozygosity (LOH) is a major way for determining gene deletions. Using PCR and SNP analysis, we examine tumors in people who are heterozygous for the loci (germline polymorphisms where each allele is different) and determine if both or only one allele is present in the tumor. This only works in persons who have inherited different sequences on the allele from each parent, but then in the tumor only one of those alleles is seen. Southern blotting is the classical technique for LOH, named after the inventor. In this procedure, extracted DNA is enzymatically digested with restriction enzymes and the digested products are transferred to a membrane. The membrane with the products is then hybridized to a "probe." The probe is a labeled marker matching the gene of interest. The procedure usually takes 3 days or more including electrophoresis, transferring, hybridization, washing, and exposure to the film. The required DNA amounts are greater than in other procedures described in the following sections. This method requires that the DNA is of good quality. Previously a few years ago, Southern blotting has essentially been replaced by PCR amplification of several genes assessment for loss of heterozygosity, using the SNP analysis. This allows for greater odds for informative cases, especially if the loci is a minisatellite (tandem repeats of 20–30 DNA bases).

Several methods are available to analyze the gross structure of chromosomes in metaphase and prophase of mitosis. Chromosome aberrations can be observed by identifying each of the 23 chromosomal pairs for completeness and number (52). Common uses of such analyses include the detection of trisomy 21, which is diagnostic for Down's syndrome, and the detection of a translocation between chromosomes 9 and 21, which is diagnostic for chronic myelogenous leukemia and the Philadelphia chromosome. The availability of specific chromosomal markers now makes this method more specific. Another gross chromosomal change detectable in human cells includes the sister chromatid exchange (53). In this case, sister chromatids of one chromosome are switched, which can be counted using nonspecific markers and correlated with exposures to tobacco and certain chemicals. A method of detecting DNA damage that does not require cell culture and examination of chromosomes during mitosis is the detection of micronuclei (54). Small chromosomal fragments are sometimes found to exist outside the nucleus.

3.4. Microsatellite Instability

The assessment of microsatellite instability is a marker for altered DNA repair. Analysis of tumors indicates that there are increased numbers of repeat DNA sequences that are not present in the patient's nontumor tissues. Thus, there were errors during DNA replication. Mono-, di-, tri-, quadra-, and pentanucleotide repeats are ubiquitous in human genomes, probably due to replication errors through evolution, but then in tumors, these loci are possible sites for more slippage during replication. Microsatellite instability is one of the common genetical alterations in human tumors where the repeats might be more or less. They are caused by somatic changes, and also occur in people with genetical mismatch repair deficiencies in hereditary nonpolyposis colorectal cancer. The germline mutations of MLH1 and MSH2 (PMS1, PMS2, MSH6) have been most commonly documented in some, not all, families with high rates of colon cancer (55,56) . Target molecules can be surrogate markers for microsatellite instability (replication error type). These include TGF beta II receptor, MSH3, MSH6, IGF II receptor, and *Bax* gene (57). The alterations in repetitive sequences in the coding exon of these genes can be predictive of progress.

3.5. Immunohistochemistry

Overexpression of genes relating to DNA damage can be detected with immunohistochemistry. Using tumor tissues fixed on slides, antibodies raised against specific proteins can be labeled and used to bind to the protein on the slide. The more the binding, the more the overexpression. This method, though, can have pitfalls like false positives (the antibody is not specific for the protein of interest) and negatives (the antibody is not good enough to stay bound to the protein during binding). In addition to the quality of the antibody, these can occur because of poor slide preparation, denatured antibodies, or high background.

3.6. Carcinogen–DNA Adducts

There are many types of DNA damage that can be detected using molecular genetical methods, such as carcinogen–DNA adduct detection. Chemicals or their reactive metabolites can bind to DNA, resulting in promutagenic lesions. The combination of the chemical and the nucleotide is an adduct. The measurement of DNA adducts allows for the distinction between the measurement of chemicals in the environment and exposures inside the body and in target organs, because the former is not always indicative of the latter. DNA adducts reflect the biologically effective dose of an exposure, resulting from the competition of exposure, absorption, activation, detoxification, and DNA repair. Thus, the measurement of DNA adducts reflects both exposure and inherited susceptibilities. Elevated levels of DNA adducts have been correlated with cigarette use (58), occupational exposures to polycyclic aromatic hydrocarbons (59), and air pollution (60).

Several methods are currently available for the measurement of DNA adducts, although all remain research tools. These include the ^{32}P-postlabeling assay that uses hydrolytic enzymes to reduce DNA to individual nucleotides and then uses another enzyme to radiolabel the nucleotides (61). Any adducts that are present are then resolved chromatographically and quantitated by measuring the radioactivity incorporated into the nucleotide. This assay can be used as a screening method to detect unknown adducts (61) or can be combined with purification techniques to identify specific compounds such as adducts formed from polycyclic aromatic hydrocarbons (62) and N-nitrosamines (63). Several important immunological methods are available for the detection of DNA adducts. Using procedures such as enzyme-linked immunoadsorbant assays (ELISA) or radioimmunoassays, adducts for polycyclic aromatic hydrocarbons can be measured (64–66). More recent methods utilize improved mass spectroscopy methods (67) and flourescence detection.

4. CONCLUSIONS

Advances in technology will improve accuracy, cost, and speed of genetical testing. Further studies will elucidate the mechanistic relationships of genetics to disease, while epidemiology will assist in the identification of relevant assays for human risk. Ultimately, the institution of any clinical test depends on its reliability, sensitivity, specificity, predictive value, and cost. Quality control and quality insurance are critical parts of genetical testing (68). The evaluation of research findings requires an understanding and evaluation of the research tools that produce the findings. New assays should be evaluated against proven assays, and methods should be shown to measure what they purport to measure. The technological advances happening today are coming more rapidly then ever before.

REFERENCES

1. Cohen MM Jr. Some neoplasms and some hamartomatous syndromes: genetic considerations. Int J Oral Maxillofac Surg 1998; 27:363–369.

2. Hussain SP, Harris CC. Molecular epidemiology of human cancer: contribution of mutation spectra studies of tumor suppressor genes. Cancer Res 1998; 58:4023–4037.

3. Kinzler KW, Vogelstein B. Lessons from hereditary colorectal cancer. Cell 1996; 87:159–170.

4. Knudson AG. Hereditary predisposition to cancer. Ann N Y Acad Sci 1997; 833:58–67.

5. Sugimura T, Terada M, Yokota J, Hirohashi S, Wakabayashi K. Multiple genetic alterations in human carcinogenesis. Environ Health Perspect 1992; 98:5–12.

6. O'Brien C. Cancer genome anatomy project launched. Mol Med Today 1997; 3:94.

7. Kinzler KW, Vogelstein B. Gatekeepers and caretakers. Nature 1997; 386:761–763.

8. Spirio LN, Samowitz W, Robertson J, Robertson M, Burt RW, Leppert M, White R. Alleles of APC modulate the frequency and classes of mutations that lead to colon polyps. Nat Genet 1998; 20:385–388.

9. O'Sullivan MJ, McCarthy TV, Doyle CT. Familial adenomatous polyposis: from bedside to benchside. Am J Clin Pathol 1998; 109:521–526.

10. Mulkens J, Poncin J, Arends JW, De Goeij AF. APC mutations in human colorectal adenomas: analysis of the mutation cluster region with temperature gradient gel electrophoresis and clinicopathological features. J Pathol 1998; 185: 360–365.

11. Polakis P. The oncogenic activation of beta-catenin. Curr Opin Genet Dev 1999; 9:15–21.

12. Rimm DL, Caca K, Hu G, Harrison FB, Fearon ER. Frequent nuclear/ cytoplasmic localization of beta-catenin without exon 3 mutations in malignant melanoma. Am J Pathol 1999; 154:325–329.

13. Koch A, Denkhaus D, Albrecht S, Leuschner I, von Schweinitz D, Pietsch T. Childhood hepatoblastomas frequently carry a mutated degradation targeting box of the beta-catenin gene. Cancer Res 1999; 59:269–273.

14. Fukuchi T, Sakamoto M, Tsuda H, Maruyama K, Nozawa S, Hirohashi S. Beta-catenin mutation in carcinoma of the uterine endometrium. Cancer Res 1998; 58:3526–3528.

15. Garicochea B, Giorgi R, Odone VF, Dorlhiac-Llacer PE, Bendit I. Mutational analysis of N-RAS and GAP-related domain of the neurofibromatosis type 1 gene in chronic myelogenous leukemia. Leuk Res 1998; 22:1003–1007.

16. Sidransky D. Is human patched the gatekeeper of common skin cancers? Nat Genet 1996; 14:7–8.

17. Rieger PT. Overview of cancer and genetics: implications for nurse practitioners. Nurse Pract Forum 1998; 9:122–133.

18. Roberts R, Ryan TJ. Task force 3: clinical research in a molecular era and the need to expand its ethical imperatives. J Am Coll Cardiol 1998; 31:942–949.

19. Erasmus RT, Murthy DP, Ogunbanjo BO. Basics of molecular biology and its applications: I Molecular biology in medicine: basic concepts. P N G Med J 1996; 39:56–66.

20. Sato Y, Mukai K, Matsuno Y, Furuya S, Kagami Y, Miwa M, Shimosato Y. The AMeX method: a multipurpose tissue-processing and paraffin-embedding

method. II. Extraction of spooled DNA and its application to Southern blot hybridization analysis. Am J Pathol 1990; 136:267–271.

21. Sato Y, Mukai K, Furuya S, Shimosato Y. The AMeX method: a multipurpose tissue-processing and paraffin-embedding method. III. Extraction and purification of RNA and application to slot-blot hybridization analysis. J Pathol 1991; 163:81–85.

22. Yoshimi N, Suzuki M, Wang A, Kojima T, Mori H. One step procedure of PCR-DNA extraction from paraffin-embedded materials by Chelex-100. Acta Pathol Jpn 1993; 43:790–791.

23. Innis M, Gelfand D, Sninsky JJ. PCR Protocols: A Guide to Methods and Applications. San Diego: Academic Press, Inc, 1990.

24. Sambrook J, Russel DW. Molecular Cloning, A Laboratory Manual. 2nd ed. New York: Cold Spring Harbor Laboratory Press, 1989.

25. Diffebach CW, Dveksler GS. PCR Primer, A Laboratory Manual. New York: Cold Spring Harbor Laboratory Press, 1995.

26. Birren B, Green ED, Klapholz S, Myers RM, Roskams J. Analyzing DNA. In: Birren B, Green ED, Klapholz S, Myers RM, Hieter P, eds. Genome Analysis: A Laboratory Manual. Vol. 1. New York: Cold Spring Harbor Laboratory Press, 1997:1.

27. Sambrook J, Russel DW. PCR Technology: Principles and Applications for DNA Amplification. New York: W. H. Freeman and Co., 1991.

28. Zhang L, Cui X, Schmitt K, Hubert R, Navidi W, Arnheim N. Whole genome amplification from a single cell: implications for genetic analysis. Proc Natl Acad Sci USA 1992; 89:5847–5851.

29. Vahakangas KH, Samet JM, Metcalf RA, Welsh JA, Bennett WP, Lane DP, Harris CC. Mutations of p53 and ras genes in radon-associated lung cancer from uranium miners. Lancet 1992; 339:576–580.

30. Martin M, Carrington M, Mann D. A method for using serum or plasma as a source of DNA for HLA typing. Hum Immunol 1992; 33:108–113.

31. Paabo S. Amplifying ancient DNA. In: Innis MA, Gelfand DH, Sninsky JJ, White TJ, eds. PCR Protocols: A Guide to Methods and Applications. San Diego: Academic Press, 1990:159–166.

32. Ahrendt SA, Halachmi S, Chow JT, Wu L, Halachmi N, Yang SC, Wehage S, Jen J, Sidransky D. Rapid p53 sequence analysis in primary lung cancer using an oligonucleotide probe array. Proc Natl Acad Sci USA 1999; 96: 7382–7387.

33. Ramaswamy S, Golub TR. DNA microarrays in clinical oncology. J Clin Oncol 2002; 20:1932–1941.

34. Kawasaki ES, Clark SS, Coyne MY, Smith SD, Champlin R, Witte ON, McCormick FP. Diagnosis of chronic myeloid and acute lymphocytic leukemias by detection of leukemia-specific mRNA sequences amplified in vitro. Proc Natl Acad Sci USA 1988; 85:5698–5702.

35. Hewlett IK, Laurian Y, Epstein J, Hawthorne CA, Ruta M, Allain JP. Assessment by gene amplification and serological markers of transmission of HIV-1 from hemophiliacs to their sexual partners and secondarily to their children. J Acquir Immune Defic Syndr 1990; 3:714–720.

36. Kato N, Yokosuka O, Omata M, Hosoda K, Ohto M. Detection of hepatitis C virus ribonucleic acid in the serum by amplification with polymerase chain reaction. J Clin Invest 1990; 86:1764–1767.

37. Manos MM, Ting Y, Wright DK, Lewis AJ, Broker TR, Wolinsky SM. Cancer cells: Molecular diagnostics of human cancer. In: Furth M, Greaves M, eds. Cancer Cells: Molecular Diagnostics of Human Cancer. 7th ed. New York: Cold Spring Harbor Press, 1989:209–214.

38. Kurzrock R, Shtalrid M, Gutterman JU, Talpaz M. Molecular diagnostics of chronic myelogenous leukemia and Philadelphia-positive acute leukemia. In: Furth M, Greaves M, eds. Cancer Cells: Molecular Diagnostics of Human Cancer. 7th ed. New York: Cold Spring Harbor Laboratory, 1989:9–13.

39. Blum M, Demierre A, Grant DM, Heim M, Meyer UA. Molecular mechanism of slow acetylation of drugs and carcinogens in humans. Proc Natl Acad Sci USA 1991; 88:5237–5241.

40. Kawajiri K, Nakachi K, Imai K, Yoshii A, Shinoda N, Watanabe J. Identification of genetically high risk individuals to lung cancer by DNA polymorphisms of the cytochrome P450IA1 gene. FEBS Lett 1990; 263:131–133.

41. Rodenhuis S, Van de Wetering ML, Mooi WJ, Evers SG, van Zandwijk N, Bos JL. Mutational activation of the K-ras oncogene A possible pathogenetic factor in adenocarcinoma of the lung. N Engl J Med 1987; 317:929–935.

42. Pawson T, Olivier P, Rozakis-Adcock M, McGlade J, Henkemeyer M. Proteins with SH2 and SH3 domains couple receptor tyrosine kinases to intracellular signalling pathways. Philos Trans R Soc Lond B Biol Sci 1993; 340:279–285.

43. Southern EM. Detection of specific sequences among DNA fragments separated by gel electrophoresis. J Mol Biol 1975; 98:503–517.

44. Maniatis T, Fritsch EF, Sambrook J. Molecular Cloning: A Laboratory Manual. New York: Cold Spring Harbor Press, 1982.

45. Bray MS, Boerwinkle E, Doris PA. High-throughput multiplex SNP genotyping with MALDI-TOF mass spectrometry: practice, problems and promise. Hum Mutat 2001; 17:296–304.

46. Matyas G, De Paepe A, Halliday D, Boileau C, Pals G, Steinmann B. Evaluation and application of denaturing HPLC for mutation detection in Marfan syndrome: identification of 20 novel mutations and two novel polymorphisms in the FBN1 gene. Hum Mutat 2002; 19:443–456.

47. Moretti TR, Baumstark AL, Defenbaugh DA, Keys KM, Brown AL, Budowle B. Validation of STR typing by capillary electrophoresis. J Forensic Sci 2001; 46:661–676.

48. Fakhrai-Rad H, Pourmand N, Ronaghi M. Pyrosequencingtrade mark: an accurate detection platform for single nucleotide polymorphisms. Hum Mutat 2002; 19:479–485.

49. Sanger F, Nicklen S, Coulson AR. DNA sequencing with chain-terminating inhibitors. Proc Natl Acad Sci U.S.A. 1977; 74:5463–5467.

50. Orita M, Iwahana H, Kanazawa H, Hayashi K, Sekiya T. Detection of polymorphisms of human DNA by gel electrophoresis as single-strand conformation polymorphisms. Proc Natl Acad Sci USA. 1989; 86:2766–2770.

51. Hayashi K, Yandell DW. How sensitive is PCR-SSCP? Hum Mutat 1993; 2:338–346.

52. Bender MA, Awa AA, Brooks AL, Evans HJ, Groer PG, Littlefield LG, Pereira C, Preston RJ, Wachholz BW. Current status of cytogenetic procedures to detect and quantify previous exposures to radiation. Mutat Res 1988; 196:103–159.

53. Latt SA. Microfluorometric detection of deoxyribonucleic acid replication in human metaphase chromosomes. Proc Natl Acad Sci USA. 1973; 70: 3395–3399.

54. Heddle JA, Hite M, Kirkhart B, Mavournin K, MacGregor JT, Newell GW, Salamone MF. The induction of micronuclei as a measure of genotoxicity A report of the US Environmental Protection Agency Gene-Tox Program. Mutat. Res 1983; 123:61–118.

55. de la CA, Peltomaki P. The genetics of hereditary common cancers. Curr Opin Genet Dev 1998; 8:298–303.

56. Akiyama Y, Sato H, Yamada T, Nagasaki H, Tsuchiya A, Abe R, Yuasa Y. Germ-line mutation of the hMSH6/GTBP gene in an atypical hereditary non-polyposis colorectal cancer kindred. Cancer Res 1997; 57:3920–3923.

57. Souza RF, Appel R, Yin J, Wang S, Smolinski KN, Abraham JM, Zou TT, Shi YQ, Lei J, Cottrell J, Cymes K, Biden K, Simms L, Leggett B, Lynch PM, Frazier M, Powell SM, Harpaz N, Sugimura H, Young J, Meltzer SJ. Microsatellite instability in the insulin-like growth factor II receptor gene in gastrointestinal tumours. Published erratum appears in Nat Genet 1996; 14(4):488. Nat Genet 1996; 14:255–257.

58. Phillips DH, Hewer A, Martin CN, Garner RC, King MM. Correlation of DNA adduct levels in human lung with cigarette smoking. Nature 1988; 336:790–792.

59. Savela K, Hemminki K, Hewer A, Phillips DH, Putman KL, Randerath K. Interlaboratory comparison of the 32P-postlabelling assay for aromatic DNA adducts in white blood cells of iron foundry workers. Mutat Res 1989; 224:485–492.

60. Perera FP, Hemminki K, Gryzbowska E, Motkiewicz G, Michalska J, Santella RM, Young TL, Dickey C, Brandt-Rauf P, DeVivo I, Blaner W, Tsai WY, Chorazy M. Molecular and genetic damage in humans from environmental pollution in Poland. Nature 1992; 360:256–258.

61. Randerath E, Agrawal HP, Weaver JA, Bordelon CB, Randerath K. ^{32}P-postlabeling analysis of DNA adducts persisting for up to 42 weeks in the skin, epidermis, and dermis of mice treated topically with 7,12-dimethylbenz[a]-anthracene. Carcinogenesis 1985; 6:1117–1126.

62. Shields PG, Bowman ED, Harrington AM, Doan VT, Weston A. Polycyclic aromatic hydrocarbon-DNA adducts in human lung and cancer susceptibility genes. Cancer Res 1993; 53:3486–3492.

63. Shields PG, Povey AC, Wilson VL, Weston A, Harris CC. Combined high performance liquid chromatography/^{32}P-postlabeling assay of N7-methyldeoxyguanosine. Cancer Res 1990; 50:6580–6584.

64. Van Schooten FJ, Hillebrand MJ, Van Leeuwen FE, Lutgerink JT, van Zandwijk N, Jansen HM, Kriek E. Polycyclic aromatic hydrocarbon-DNA adducts in lung tissue from lung cancer patients. Carcinogenesis 1990; 11:1677–1681.

65. Perera F, Mayer J, Jaretzki A, Hearne S, Brenner D, Young TL, Fischman HK, Grimes M, Grantham S, Tang MX. Comparison of DNA adducts and sister chromatid exchange in lung cancer cases and controls. Cancer Res 1989; 49:4446–4451.
66. Perera FP, Hemminki K, Young TL, Brenner D, Kelly G, Santella RM. Detection of polycyclic aromatic hydrocarbon-DNA adducts in white blood cells of foundry workers. Cancer Res 1988; 48:2288–2291.
67. Goldman R. Quantitation of benzo[alpha]pyrene-DNA adducts by postlabeling with 14C-acetic anhydride and accelerator mass spectrometry. Chem Biol Interact 2000; 126:171–183.
68. Blomeke B, Shields PG. Chapter 13. Laboratory methods for the determination of genetic polymorphisms in humans. IARC Sci Publ 1999; 148:133–147.

5

Methods for Genetic Testing II: New Methods for Assessing Acquired DNA Damage in Humans Without Cancer

Laura Gunn, Luoping Zhang, and Martyn T. Smith

Division of Environmental Health Sciences, School of Public Health, University of California at Berkeley, Berkeley, California, U.S.A.

1. INTRODUCTION

Cancer is an abnormal genetic phenomenon, involving multiple steps of somatic mutation (1,2). Genetic damage can occur at the level of the gene (e.g., point mutations and deletions) or the chromosome (e.g., aneuploidy, translocations). During the last two decades, a wide spectrum of biomarkers of genetic damage have been developed to detect early mutational and chromosomal effects of carcinogenic exposure in humans (3). Historically, biomarkers have tended to measure mutations in surrogate genes, including hypoxanthine phosphoribosyltransferase (*HPRT*) and glycophorin A (*GPA*) (4), or use cytogenetics to assess overall changes in chromosome structure and number, such as classical and banded chromosomal aberrations (CAS), sister chromatid exchanges (SCEs), and micronucleus formation (MN) (5–7). These biomarkers have been shown to be associated with a wide range of carcinogenic exposures, but they are not truly biomarkers of early effect as they are not on the causal pathway of disease.

Identification of early causal genetic events in cancer has been the key to the recent development of novel biomarkers of early effect in high-risk populations. These novel biomarkers measure changes frequently observed among cancer patients, including point mutations in genes such as *p53* and *RAS*, altered gene methylation, aneuploidy (chromosome loss or gain) including monosomy 7 and trisomy 8, and specific chromosome rearrangements such as translocations. Application of these biomarkers to study individuals who may be at risk, but who do not yet have cancer, will result in improved early detection, as well as better understanding of carcinogenesis itself.

The development of valid biomarkers of early effect in individuals without cancer depends on the ability to detect infrequent mutational events at critical loci in a large background of normal DNA. Therefore, detection of these novel biomarkers employs cutting edge technologies, such as real-time quantitative polymerase chain reaction (PCR), fluorescence in situ hybridization (FISH) analysis, and genotypic selection methods which introduce new levels of sensitivity and specificity. Such biomarkers will be useful in epidemiological studies of environmentally induced cancers which have long latency periods as well as provide early detection for those individuals at risk. This chapter outlines a number of these new methods and examines their potential application in detecting novel biomarkers of early effect.

2. ROLE OF DIFFERENT TYPES OF GENETIC DAMAGE IN CANCER

Carcinogenesis is a complex, multistage process which involves the accumulation of a variety of mutations within a particular cell and its progeny (1). Although carcinogenesis depends on a number of factors including exposure, genetics, and target tissue, certain general characteristics of cancers are known. The role of particular genes in cancer has opened a new avenue of research over the past two decades. Oncogenes and tumor suppressor genes have taken center stage with their respective roles in cancer. Alterations in these genes ranging from small insertions, deletions, point mutations, and aberrant methylation, to gross chromosomal aberrations, like translocations, and gene amplification either enhance or inactivate the normal function of the gene and lead to abnormal proliferation, lack of cell cycle control, genomical instability, and eventually cancer. Mutations in these genes provide telltale signs of genetical changes or damage and possible cancer risk, often long before the onset of cancer. Particular genes, chromosomal regions, or entire chromosomes are vulnerable to mutation at variable points in carcinogenesis (1). This suggests that certain mutations play a specific role in the ability of a cell to survive and continue to the next step of this multistep process, as well as potentially determining what the next mutation will be. These mutations, particularly early events, may provide markers, which are indicative of genetical damage and potential cancer risk.

Thus far, few cancers have been well characterized in terms of which mutations occur at what point in the multistep process. Because much of cancer research depends on backtracking from tumor tissue, it is virtually impossible to assess the point at which one mutation arose relative to another and how that mutation may encourage future hits. However, a few models exist which have provided valuable information about the clonal evolution of cancer. Possibly the best known model that exists is the Vogelstein and Kinzler (1) model of colon cancer (Fig. 1A). This model provides a unique opportunity to observe morphological changes resulting from each mutation acquired in a stepwise progression. From normal tissue, the cells acquire one mutation after another, beginning with the loss of a key gene involved in cell proliferation (*APC*), aberrant methylation, further mutation of oncogenes (*RAS*), and finally, loss of the *DCC* and *p53* genes, which pushes the cell over the cancer threshold. Although the order of mutation may vary slightly in the later stages, the pattern is strikingly similar in approximately 50% of colorectal cancers. For example, late events such as the loss of *p53* and *DCC* are only observed in late adenomas, whereas loss of *APC* is observed even in benign polyps. This suggests that each type of mutation plays a unique, key role in the clonal evolution, without which the cells might not transform to malignancy.

Since the original model of colon cancer, a few other models have emerged demonstrating similar patterns of mutation accumulation. Figure 1 shows three hypothetical models for three different cancer types. It is important to observe the differences in mutation pattern in each cancer type; for example, *p53* mutations are believed to be early events in astrocytoma, in contrast to *p53* mutations in colon cancer, which are later events. However, although the specific mutation varies among different cancers, the pattern of accumulation of mutation and the progressive impact of each mutation on cell proliferation and morphology are similar in each.

3. MEASURING POINT MUTATIONS IN CANCER-RELATED GENES

Conventional methods used to detect point mutations such as single-stranded conformation polymorphism (SSCP) and sequencing, are labor intensive and require the use of radionucleotides. Recently, a number of assays, most of which employ PCR, have been developed which do not require radioactivity, are relatively quick, and are much more sensitive than conventional methods.

The use of PCR technology has vastly improved detection and identification of mutations in cancers. Increased sensitivity and reproducibility have provided the possibility of utilizing these mutation assays as biomarkers of early effect, and for detection of minimal residual disease or precursors to relapse. Because of the low frequency of many of these mutations in the normal population, the normal background levels and variability have not yet been established. Recently, a number of assays have been developed

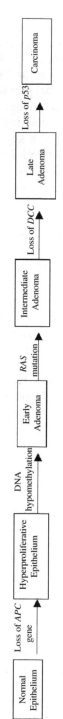

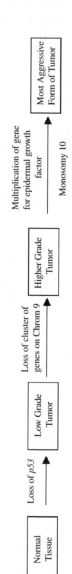

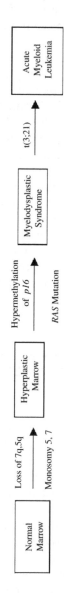

Figure 1 Three multistep models of carcinogenesis. (A) Vogelstein and Kinzler model of mutation pattern in colon cancer. (B) Cavanee and White model (1) of astrocytoma. (C) Theoretical model of therapy-induced leukemia.

which improve sensitivity orders of magnitude over previously used methods. Many of these assays employ methods to selectively amplify the relative number of mutants in a large pool of wild type in order to increase the sensitivity of detecting rare mutant alleles, a method referred to as genotypic selection.

3.1. Measurement of Point Mutations in *RAS*

One recently published assay used genotype selection for the detection of mutations in the *H-RAS* gene. By combining two previously published methods (8,9), the MutEx + allele-specific competitive blocker PCR (ACB-PCR) technique (10) is one of the most sensitive methods of genotypic selection. This assay begins with the denaturation of a heterogenous sample of mutant and wild-type double-stranded DNA. When reannealing, mutant DNA forms heteroduplex DNA with normal strands, while normal DNA strands form homoduplexes. Mut S, a thermostable protein, is added which binds to the mispaired sequence of the heteroduplex which protects the short sequence of mutant DNA from digestion from 3′–5′ exonuclease activity of T7 DNA polymerase, whereas the wild-type DNA is digested. This Mut-Ex step results in a 1000-fold enrichment of mutant alleles relative to wild type. To further increase sensitivity, the next step utilizes an additional selection technique, ACB-PCR. This genotypic selection method is based on preferential amplification by allele-specific primers. The first primer has more mismatches to wild type than mutant, resulting in preferential amplification of mutant DNA. The second primer is blocker primer, which preferentially anneals to the wild-type sequence, but is modified with a 3′-dideoxyguanosine residue, which prevents extension. The ACB-PCR method therefore results in preferential amplification of mutant with a sensitivity of as few as 10 mutant alleles detected in the presence of 10^8 copies of the wild-type allele.

As one of the most sensitive methods available for mutation detection, the MutEx+ ACB-PCR technique has many potential applications for mutation detection. This method is based on increasing the ratio of mutant DNA relative to wild type and is therefore a sensitive method for the detection of rare mutations. However, this method is not appropriate for unknown mutations, as the sequence of the mutated region is necessary for the design of ACB-PCR primers.

3.2. Measurement of Point Mutations in *p53*

Genotypic selection methods have also been applied to *p53* mutation detection. Sites which are commonly mutated in the *p53* gene, referred to as mutational hotspots, have been targeted as potential biomarkers of early effect. Assays utilizing allele-specific PCR have been designed to detect and preferentially amplify mutations in these hotspots. These assays either used alone or in combination with SSCP and sequencing result in a considerable improvement in sensitivity over conventional methods of mutation detection. For example, an allele-specific PCR method developed by Wada et al. (11) has been shown to be more sensitive than SSCP alone. Allele-specific PCR resulted in the detection of mutated cells accounting for 0.01–1% of cells, in comparison to SSCP alone which has a detection limit of approximately 10% mutant cells. This method has been successfully applied to *p53* hotspots to detect rare point mutations in acute myeloid leukemia (AML) and acute lymphocytic leukemia (ALL) relapse cases (12). Behn and Schuermann (13) developed a similar method called *p53*-mutant enriched PCR-SSCP which also targets mutational hotspots in the *p53* gene. This method combines PCR-SSCP with sequence specific-clamping by peptide nucleic acids (PNAs). Peptide nucleic acids are designed to preferentially bind to wild-type DNA, and do not extend, thereby blocking amplification of wild-type DNA. This results in a mutant enriched sample. Mutations are then detected by SSCP and identified by sequencing. This combination of PCR with PNAs and SSCP improves sensitivity 10–50-fold higher than conventional PCR-SSCP.

As in Mut-EX + ACB-PCR, these methods are only appropriate for certain applications. Because they target mutational hotspots of *p53*, they do not account for mutations outside this region, and are therefore not applicable to mutation spectrum analysis. In general, genotypic selection methods offer higher specificity and sensitivity than traditional methods. Although they are not appropriate for all applications, they are vast improvements over conventional methods previously used for these applications, including SSCP analysis.

4. MEASURING GENETIC DAMAGE AT THE CHROMOSOME LEVEL

Genetic damage at the chromosome level has been shown to be involved in the development of cancer. For example, leukemias and lymphomas are characterized by clonal chromosomal aberrations that appear to have a central role in tumorigenesis (14,15). Chromosome aberrations encompass all types of changes in chromosome structure and number. The most common numerical changes called aneuploidy are the loss (monosomy) or gain (trisomy) of one chromosome; less frequent types include the loss of both copies or the gain of more than one copy of a chromosome. Structural changes include translocations, inversions, breaks, and deletions. Generally, chromosome loss can lead to the loss of tumor suppressor genes, while chromosome gain can lead to increased oncogene expression. Further, chromosome translocations or other types of chromosome rearrangements may lead to the formation of fusion genes that are oncogenic.

4.1. Conventional Cytogenetics

Classical chromosome aberrations are the only cytogenetical end point that have been shown to have predictive value for risk of cancer (6,16), particularly for hematologic malignancies (17). Therefore, classical chromosome aberrations appear to be a particularly promising early-effect biomarker of carcinogen exposure. However, classical aberrations are a measure of overall chromosome damage, not of specific events on the causal pathways of particular diseases. In order to understand the mechanisms of exposure-related diseases, we need to measure specific events on the causal pathways of those diseases. Since these specific events are relatively rare among non-diseased populations, it is important to screen levels among much larger populations or examine much greater quantities of cells from each subject in order to attain sufficient statistical power.

In myeloid leukemia, loss of part or all of chromosomes 5 and 7 is a common event, along with trisomy of chromosome 8 and various specific translocations and inversions including inv(16), t(8;21), t(9;22), t(15;17), and t(11q23) (18). These rearrangements are associated with particular types of myeloid leukemia (Fig. 2). In ALL,particularly in childhood ALL, translocation t(12;21) is common (~25%) and in non-Hodgkin lymphomas the translocation t(14;18) is found in follicular lymphoma (14). Therefore, the

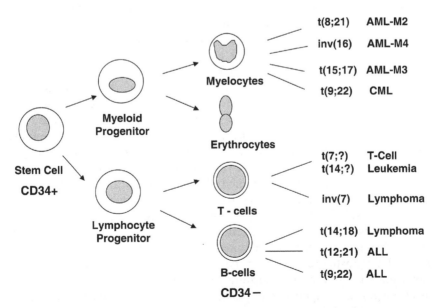

Figure 2 Chromosome rearrangements in leukemias and lymphomas. AML = acute myeloid leukemia; CML = chronic myeloid leukemia, ALL = acute lymphocytic leukemia.

detection of these changes at the chromosomal level could be very important in predicting risk of these diseases.

Many specific chromosome aberrations have been recognized using classic karyotyping among patients with clinical syndromes. For example, an extra copy of chromosome 21 is routinely detected among children born with Down syndrome. As a result, classic karyotyping has become a widely used tool of clinical diagnosis for many diseases, including leukemia. However, classic cytogenetical techniques have several drawbacks for the detection of chromosome-specific aneusomy and rearrangements. For example, the cells must be cultured to make metaphase spreads, a limited number (25–100) of scorable cells can be examined, and recognition of specific chromosomes is problematic. In addition, certain rearrangements, such as t(12;21), cannot be detected by classic banding assays because the rearranged fragments barely affect the morphology of the involved chromosomes. These problems can be now overcome by using FISH to measure aberrations in specific chromosomes in large numbers of interphase cells and metaphase spreads (19,20).

4.2. Measurement of Specific Chromosome Aberrations by Molecular Cytogenetics

Fluorescence in situ hybridization has several advantages over conventional cytogenetics, including selectivity of specific DNA probes, multiple color labeling, sensitivity of detection, and speed of microscopic analysis. Interphase FISH, in particular, offers several advantages over classical cytogenetics (21). First, interphase FISH allows analysis of non-dividing cells. Second, a much larger number of cells, at least 1000 or more, may be analyzed. Third, the detection of aneuploidy is facilitated by simply counting the number of labeled regions representing a particular chromosome of interest within the isolated interphase nucleus. By contrast, metaphase FISH can readily detect structural rearrangements in addition to aneuploidy. Furthermore, because metaphase FISH, like classical cytogenetics, analyzes dividing cells, the results from these two methods may be directly compared. A number of studies have determined that FISH is both more sensitive and convenient than classical cytogenetics (22–24). Therefore, FISH appears to be the more suitable method for large-scale population biomonitoring

Fluorescence in situ hybridization is now a widely used tool in the analysis of chromosomal changes in human cancers, including leukemias, and in prenatal diagnostics (20,25). It has been extensively used to analyze chromosomal damage induced by exposure to ionizing radiation (26,27) and has also been gradually applied to populations exposed to chemicals and various carcinogens (28–30).

One example of a specialized FISH assay primarily employed in radiation research is that developed by Tucker and coworkers (31,32). This assay uses single-color FISH by painting the chromosome pairs 1, 2, and 4 (or 3, 5, and 6) the same color, which allows for the detection of (1) numerical and structural chromosome aberrations among these painted chromosomes and (2) structural rearrangements between these and other untargeted chromosomes. This assay has been applied in vitro and in vivo in both animal and human studies (31–33). Since radiation is thought to cause equal levels of damage across all chromosomes (34), and chromosomes 1 through 6 (the largest chromosomes) make up 40% of the genome (35), it is hypothesized that measurement of damage in these large chromosomes can be extrapolated to the whole genome (31). This may not be true for chemical exposures as certain chemicals may have selective or preferential effects on certain chromosomes (36). For example, we showed that epoxide metabolites of 1,3-butadiene had more effect on some chromosomes than on others (37). Indeed, the hypothesis of equal levels of damage across the genome may not hold true even for low doses of radiation, as inversion of chromosome 10 has been shown to be highly sensitive to low-intensity radiation exposure (38). Interestingly, inv(10) rearranges the *RET* gene and is associated with thyroid cancer, potentially caused by linear energy transfer (LET) radiation.

Our laboratory is currently employing FISH to examine the cytogenetical changes in human blood cells caused by exposure to the established leukemogen, benzene. Our plan is to examine all 22 autosomes and to particularly examine for chromosome changes associated with the development of leukemia. This study is being performed along with Drs. Rothman and Hayes of the National Cancer Institute (NCI), Drs. Li and Yin at the Chinese Academy of Preventive Medicine in Beijing, and others at the Shanghai Anti-Epidemic Center as well as other institutions in the United States. We have applied various FISH techniques in this collaborative study of 43 Chinese workers highly exposed to benzene (median exposure level = 31 ppm, 8 h. time-weighted average) and 44 frequency-matched controls. To date, five chromosomes (1, 5, 7, 8, and 21) have been examined by metaphase FISH in these highly exposed Chinese workers and their matched controls. Frequencies of monosomy 5, 7, and 8, but not 1 or 21, increased with elevated exposure levels, whereas a significant trend was observed for trisomy of all five chromosomes (36,39). The most striking dose-dependent increases were found in monosomy 7 and trisomy 7, 8 and 21. The most common structural changes detected among chromosomes 1, 5, 7, 8, and 21 were t(8;21), t(8;?) (translocation between chromosome 8 and another unidentified chromosome), breakage of chromosome 8, and deletions of the long (q) arms of chromosomes 5 and 7. A significant trend was observed for all these changes (36,39). The loss and long arm deletion of chromosomes 5 and 7, two of the most common cytogenetical changes in therapy- and chemical-related leukemia, were significantly increased in benzene-exposed workers over controls (36).

Since the development and popularization of FISH, other novel cytogenetical methods, such as comparative genome hybridization (CGH), spectral karyotyping (SKY), and color banding, have been developed. Comparative genome hybridization involves the comparison of total DNA extracted from normal and cancerous cells in order to look for specific gains or losses in genetical material associated with cancer (27). The SKY method involves painting each of the 24 different chromosomes a different color using four or five fluorophores with combined binary ratio labeling, which allows the entire karyotype to be screened for chromosome aberrations (40). Since the human eye cannot effectively distinguish the 24 colors, this method requires the use of an automated imaging system. In color banding, which is based on traditional banding techniques, each chromosome is labeled by subregional DNA probes in different colors, resulting in a unique "chromosome bar code" (41). This method allows the rapid identification of chromosomes and chromosome rearrangements. These techniques, however, are at present relatively new and have not been employed as widely or as extensively as FISH.

4.3. Limitations of FISH

While FISH can be used to measure both structural and numerical chromosome aberrations and is a powerful tool in molecular epidemiology, its sensitivity is limited to 1 in 10^{3-4} cells and it is relatively expensive because of the high cost of probes. This makes it difficult to use FISH to detect rare translocations between multiple chromosomes, such as t(21q22) and t(11q23). The PCR technique allows much more sensitive detection of these types of changes and is also less expensive in comparison with FISH.

5. MEASUREMENT OF CHROMOSOME REARRANGEMENTS BY PCR

Chromosome translocations produce novel fusion genes or products that can be detected at the DNA or RNA level by PCR or reverse-transcriptase PCR (RT-PCR) as well as by FISH. Polymerase chain reaction holds a number of advantages over FISH, including: (1) the ability to detect very rare events (1 copy/10^{6-7} cells vs. $1/10^{3-4}$ cells by FISH) and (2) the ability to study large numbers of people easily and at low cost. These potent advantages are accompanied, however, by two disadvantages. First, the high sensitivity of PCR makes it prone to false-positive results caused by sample contamination. However, contamination artifacts can be overcome with extremely rigorous laboratory procedures (42) as well as the use of dUTP and uracil glycosylase in PCR reactions to prevent carryover contamination. Second, until recently, quantitation was difficult, especially for RT-PCR. Quantitation has also become feasible through recent advances in exonuclease-dependent real-time PCR. This quantitative PCR assay, now generally called real-time PCR, allows for an absolute number of novel sequences to be quantified in a cell population without the need for gel electrophoresis. In addition, real-time PCR is more sensitive than conventional PCR, where a sensitivity of 1 in 10^7 can be reached if a stochastic multitube approach is taken (43,44). This technology has therefore paved the way for a new generation of biomarkers to be developed. While no methods yet exist which employ PCR to measure rare aneuploidies or genome-wide structural damage, real-time and conventional PCR techniques which measure specific chromosome rearrangements, such as translocations and inversions, and the methylation status of genes have become available.

5.1. Conventional PCR Detection of Chromosome Rearrangements

Reverse-transcriptase PCR and PCR have previously been used to detect a number of translocations including t(14;18), t(8;21), t(9;22) and t(4;11). Using these techniques, t(9;22) and t(14;18) have been detected in unexposed individuals of different ages and in smokers (45–47). Both translocations were found to increase with age and the t(14;18) translocation was increased in cigarette smokers (48). Studies from our laboratory showing detectable t(8;21) by RT-PCR in an otherwise healthy benzene exposed worker (39) clearly demonstrate the potential of RT-PCR for monitoring specific aberrations in populations exposed to suspected or established leukemogens. Because many of these translocations have multiple breakpoints or translocation partners, multiplex assays have also been developed to detect multiple or unknown rearrangements. Despite recent improvements in sensitivity and applicability, conventional PCR methods remain semiquantitative. However, with the recent advent of real-time PCR, quantitation is no longer an obstacle. Now that quantitation problems can be overcome, a whole new avenue of biological monitoring for early detection of cancer has been opened. Polymerase chain reaction-based procedures therefore hold further promise for detecting specific chromosome aberrations, especially when used in combination with FISH.

5.2. The Development of Quantitative Real-Time PCR Methods for Chromosome Rearrangements

Real-time PCR is comparable to conventional PCR in that it uses sense and antisense primers to amplify a targeted sequence of DNA. However, real-time PCR employs an additional, nonextendable oligonucleotide probe, which is positioned between the two primers during the annealing phase of amplification (Fig. 3) (49). The oligonucleotide probe is labeled with a fluorescent reporter dye [such as FAM 6-carboxy-fluorescein] at the 5' end and a quencher fluorescent dye [such as TAMRA 6-carboxy-tetramethyl-

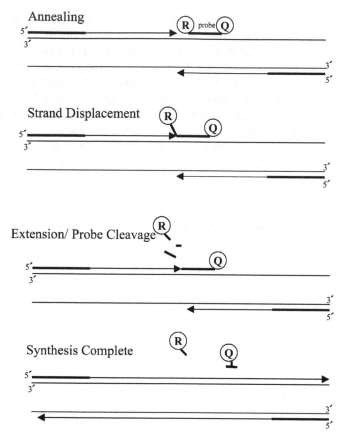

Figure 3 Diagram of TaqMan technology in quantitative PCR R, reporter dye; Q, quencher dye. *Source*: Adapted from PCR Applications (49), 1999.

rhodamine] at the 3′ end. When the probe is intact, fluorescence resonance energy transfer to TAMRA quenches the FAM emission. During the extension phase of amplification, the *Taq* polymerase extends the primer to the region of the probe, at which point the 5′ exonuclease property of *Taq* cleaves the reporter dye from the probe. This results in an increase in fluorescent signal that is proportional to the amount of amplification product. The increase in reporter molecules is measured in real time by the ABI Prism 5700 or 7700 Sequence Detection Systems (PE Applied Biosystems). After each cycle fluorescence signal is measured resulting in an amplification plot, in which the point at which the fluorescence crosses a defined threshold, C_t, is proportional to the starting copy number. C_ts of positive control samples are used to generate a standard curve. From this standard curve, it is possible to calculate the copy number of unknown samples. Methods for the quantitative detection of translocations using the above TaqMan technology have recently been reported. For example, methods for the analysis of t(14;18), t(8;21), t(9;22), and other translocations have been presented or published (43,50–53).

5.3. Measurement of t(14;18) Found in Lymphocytic Leukemia and Lymphoma

The structural rearrangements observed in lymphocytic leukemia and lymphoma may be caused by mistakes made by the V(D)J recombinase enzyme complex while it is generating new immunoglobulin and T-cell receptor gene rearrangements (54). Illegitimate V(D)J recombinase activity could therefore be centrally involved in the development of these blood cancers and could result from mistakes brought on by chemical exposure.

The t(14;18) translocation is thought to arise by illegitimate V(D)J recombination in pre-B cells as a result of aberrant immoglobulin gene rearrangement. Liu et al. (45) first described the fact that this translocation was found at low levels in normal, healthy individuals. They subsequently showed that the incidence of t(14;18) increased with age and was higher in the blood of smokers (48). Recently, two groups have described novel quantitative PCR procedures that measure very low levels of t(14;18) (43,44). Luthra et al. (43) detected rearrangements at the bcl-2 mbr in 36% of lymphoma cases and found a 98% concordance between real-time PCR and conventional PCR (43). In addition, using serial dilution they demonstrated that real-time PCR was 100-fold more sensitive than conventional PCR. BCL-$2/JH$ fusion sequences were consistently detected when diluted 10^5 fold with normal genomic DNA. Doelken et al. (44) confirmed the sensitivity of this assay and concluded that the detection of single-genome copies is possible if a stochastic multiple tube approach is taken.

5.4. Measurement of t(8;21) Associated with Acute Myeloid Leukemia and Myelodysplasia

The t(8;21) translocation results in the fusion of the *ETO* gene, at 8q22, with the *AML1* gene at chromosome 21q22. This translocation is one of the most frequent karyotypic abnormalities observed in acute myeloid leukemia. The presence of t(8;21) is associated with a high complete remission rate and a high survival rate (55), suggesting that the levels of the translocation may be predictive of relapse. On the basis of potential prognostic value of the t(8;21), Marcucci et al. (56) developed a real-time reverse-transcriptase PCR method to detect *AML1/ETO* fusion transcript in patients with AML. Each patient showed 10^3 copies of *AML1/ETO* transcript at diagnosis and each showed a 2–4-log decrease in copy number following successful induction chemotherapy. The sixth patient had a high copy number immediately following successful remission induction chemotherapy, which continued to increase during early remission, and was followed by relapse.

These results suggest that t(8;21) translocation is detectable at low levels and may be a valuable biomarker of early effect or potential relapse.

5.5. Measurement of t(9;22) Associated with Leukemia

A real-time RT-PCR method has also been developed for the detection of the t(9;22) translocation (57), which is common in CML (chronic myelogenous leukemia). This translocation results in the fusion of the *ABL* gene, an oncogene, with the *BCR* gene (58). Under the regulation of the *BCR* promoter, a fusion gene product is expressed in malignant cells. By performing serial dilutions of a positive control diluted in wild-type RNA, a sensitivity of 10^{-5} was achieved, which is comparable to conventional PCR methods.

6. OTHER POTENTIAL APPLICATIONS OF REAL-TIME PCR
6.1. Measurement of Aberrant Gene Methylation

In addition to the wide range of genetical damage involved in carcinogenesis, epigenetic mechanisms, such as DNA methylation, have gained attention as potential key players in certain cancer types. Aberrant methylation, which may be induced by environmental exposures, may result in altered carcinogen metabolism, cell cycle regulation, and DNA repair. For example, in leukemia and lymphoma translocations cause the formation of novel fusion genes that produce excessive growth (14,15), and other genes undergo transcriptional silencing by methylation, which causes aberrant cell cycle control (59). Aberrant methylation and transcriptional silencing appear to be early events in both solid tumors, including lung (60), colon (61), hepatocellular (62), and bladder (63), as well as hematological malignancies (59). A number of different methods have been developed to detect aberrant methylation of genes, including the use of methylation sensitive restriction enzymes, bisulfite sequencing, and methylation-specific PCR (MSP).

Perhaps one of the most interesting targets of aberrant methylation is the tumor suppressor gene $p16^{INK4a}$, which is a key component in the G1/S cell cycle check point and has been shown to be involved in colon cancer, leukemia, and lung cancer. Recently, a real-time methylation specific PCR protocol has been developed by Lo et al. (64) and applied to bone marrow samples of patients with multiple myeloma as well as cell lines with known methylation status. The authors demonstrated that the real-time method had very high concordance with the conventional method, but with the added sensitivity and specificity of the real-time technology. In addition, the authors correlated methylation status with p16 mRNA expression and observed that transcription was inversely correlated with methylation status. As with other real-time methods, this application shows great potential for future studies involving methylation of key genes in carcinogenesis as well as other biological processes.

6.2. Multiplex Real-Time PCR with Molecular Beacons

Yet another novel application of real-time PCR technology is the multiplex amplification of DNA by Vet et al. (65). Using molecular beacons (MB) rather than TaqMan probes, the authors successfully performed multiplex PCR reactions which were monitored in real time. Although similar to Taq-Man probes, molecular beacons do not require the 5' exonuclease properties of *Taq* polymerase. Instead, when unbound, the fluorescent moiety is kept in physical proximity to the quencher in a loop conformation. When the probe anneals to a target sequence, the loop is linearized and the reporter and quencher are separated in space, and the reporter emits fluorescence. In a multiplex reaction, different colored fluorescent moieties are used for each amplicon. The potential applications of this assay are very promising. Unfortunately, research potential is often limited by the amount of material available for analysis. The possibility of real-time multiplex PCR provides the opportunity to examine multiple points of interest simultaneously with the same amount of material previously required for one point.

6.3. Digital PCR

Another recent contribution to this spectrum of novel methods combines the process of genotypic selection with the sensitive new molecular beacon-based PCR methodologies. Digital PCR, developed by Vogelstein and Kinzler (66) is an assay designed to quantitatively measure the proportion of mutant sequences within a DNA sample. Single molecules of DNA are isolated and amplified by PCR in a multiple-well plate, resulting in completely mutant or completely wild-type products. After amplification, asymmetric PCR is used to generate a single-stranded product to which the molecular beacons could anneal. Two molecular beacons (red and green) are added, one which recognizes only wild-type sequence and one which is common to all PCR products. Using mutations in the *RAS* gene, the authors designed the wild-type beacon which would react better with the wild type than any mutant sequence within the target sequence. In other words, any mutations in the region complementary to the molecular beacon sequence would inhibit wild-type beacon binding. This was possible due to the fact that *RAS* has proximal mutational hotspots within codons 12, 13 which are within the range of the probe sequence. This assay, however, in most cases, would require molecular beacons for the expected mutational sequences, as well as wild-type beacons. Each well is then analyzed separately for the presence (or absence) of mutation by the fluorescent probes. The ratio of red/green is determined and normalized against known controls. Those wells containing mutant sequences are then analyzed by sequencing to determine the nature of the mutation. Although the authors chose to add the molecular beacons after amplification, the beacons may also be used during the amplification process and monitored in real time.

Digital PCR is only appropriate for predefined mutations. As with genotypic selection methods, the specific area or mutational hotspot must be known in order to design primers and beacon sequences. In addition, unless the molecular beacons are added prior to amplification, the amplification will not be monitored in real time. Like many other PCR methods, this method assumes 100% efficient PCR and that both wild type and mutant will amplify with equal efficiencies. Because the results are based on the ratio of the red/green signal, any discrepancies in amplification efficiencies may affect this ratio. Finally, it is important to understand that this method is only a quantitative measure of the proportion of mutant sequences within a sample, but is not a measure of the starting number of mutant and wild-type copies.

7. CONCLUSIONS

A new generation of biomarkers of early effect in carcinogenesis are now available and widely employed. These methods utilize the latest advances in molecular cytogenetics and PCR allowing for mutations to be detected and measured in cancer-related genes and in specific regions of chromosomes that are rearranged, lost, or amplified in carcinogenesis. Measurement of aberrant gene methylation and loss of heterozygosity is also possible. These new early-effect biomarkers are on the causal pathway to disease and, as such, should be predictive markers of future cancer risk. In addition, the high sensitivity of these assays will allow the detection of genetical damage in normal, healthy individuals, which is a key to the validation of these potential biomarkers. However, their true value can only be tested in prospective epidemiological studies. It is important that epidemiologists begin to collect biological samples from large cohorts of people being followed for disease onset and process them in a sophisticated manner so that large quantities of RNA and DNA are available for analysis as the studies progress. In this manner development and validation can proceed hand in hand.

ACKNOWLEDGMENTS

This work was supported by grants from the National Institute for Environmental Health Sciences RO1 ES06721, P42 ES04705, and P30 ES01896 and the National Foundation for Cancer Research.

REFERENCES

1. Vogelstein B, Kinzler KW. The multistep nature of cancer. Trends Genet 1993; 9(4):138–141.
2. Lengauer C, Kinzler KW, Vogelstein B. Genetic instabilities in human cancers. Nature (Lond) 1998; 396(6712):643–649.

3. Toniolo P, Boffetta, P, Shuker DEG, Rothman N, Hulka B, Pearce N, eds. Application of Biomarkers in Cancer Epidemiology. Vol. 142. Lyon France: International Agency for Research on Cancer Scientific Publications, 1997: 1–18.

4. Albertini RJ, Hayes RB. Somatic cell mutations in cancer epidemiology. IARC Sci Publ 1997; 6(142):159–184.

5. Sorsa M, Wilbourn J, Vainio H. Human cytogenetic damage as a predictor of cancer risk. IARC Sci Publ 1992; 18(116):543–554.

6. Hagmar L, Brogger A, Hansteen I-L, Heim S, Hogstedt B, Knudsen L, Lambert B, Linnainmaa K, Mitelman F. Cancer risk in humans predicted by increased levels of chromosomal aberrations in lymphocytes: Nordic Study Group on the Health Risk of Chromosome Damage. Cancer Res 1994; 54(11):2919–2922.

7. Hagmar L, Bonassi S, Stromberg U, Mikoczy Z, Lando C, Hansteen I-L, Montagud AH, Knudsen L, Norppa H, Reuterwall C, Tinnerberg H, Brogger A, Forni A, Hogstedt B, Lambert B, Mitelman F, Nordenson I, Salomaa S, Skerfving S. Cancer predictive value of cytogenetic markers used in occupational health surveillance programs: a report from an ongoing study by the European Study Group on cytogenetic biomarkers and health. Mutat Res 1998; 405(2):171–178.

8. Parsons BL, Heflich RH. Evaluation of MutS as a tool for direct measurement of point mutations in genomic DNA. Mutat Res 1997; 374(2):277–285.

9. Parsons BL, Heflich RH. Detection of a mouse H-ras codon 61 mutation using a modified allele-specific competitive blocker PCR genotypic selection method. Mutagenesis 1998; 13(6):581–588.

10. Parsons BL, Heflich RH. Detection of basepair substitution mutation at a frequency of $1 \times 10\text{-}7$ by combining two genotypic selection methods, MutEx enrichment and allele-specific competitive blocker PCR. Environ Mol Mutagen 1998; 32(3): 200–211.

11. Wada H, Asada M, Nakazawa S, Itoh H, Kobayashi Y, Inoue T, Fukumuro K, Chan LC, Sugita K, Hanada R, Akuta N, Kobayashi N, Mizutani N. Clonal expansion of p53 mutant cells in leukemia progression in vitro. Leukemia (Basingstoke) 1994; 8(1):53–59.

12. Zhu YM, Foroni L, McQuaker IG, Papaioannou M, Haynes A, Russell HH. Mechanisms of relapse in acute leukaemia: involvement of p53 mutated subclones in disease progression in acute lymphoblastic leukaemia. Br J Cancer 1999; 79(7–8):1151–1157.

13. Behn M, Schuermann M. Sensitive detection of p53 gene mutations by a 'mutant enriched' pCR-SSCP technique. Nucleic Acids Res 1998; 26(5): 1356–1358.

14. Ong ST, Beau MML. Chromosomal abnormalities and molecular genetics of non-Hodgkin's lymphoma. Semin Oncol 1998; 25(4):447–460.

15. Rowley JD. The critical role of chromosome translocations in human leukemias. Ann Rev Genet 1998:495–519.

16. Hagmar L, Bonassi S, Stromberg U, Brogger A, Knudsen LE, Norppa H, Reuterwall C. ESGOCBA Health. Chromosomal aberrations in lymphocytes

predict human cancer: a report from the European Study Group on cytogenetic biomarkers and health (ESCH). Cancer Res 1998; 58(18):4117–4121.

17. Bonassi S, Abbondandolo A, Cumurri L, Dal Pra L, De Ferrari M, Degrassi F, Forni A, Lamberti L, Lando C, Padovani P, Sbrana I, Vecchio D, Puntoni R. Are chromosome aberrations in circulating lymphocytes predictive of future cancer onset in humans?: preliminary results of an Italian cohort study. Cancer Genet Cytogenet 1995; 79(2):133–135.

18. Pedersen-Bjergaard J, Pedersen M, Roulston D, Philip P. Different genetic pathways in leukemogenesis for patients presenting with therapy-related myelo-dysplasia and therapy-related acute myeloid leukemia. Blood 1995; 86(9): 3542–3552.

19. Eastmond DA, Pinkel D. Detection of aneuploidy and aneuploidy-inducing agents in human lymphocytes using fluorescence in situ hybridization with chromosome-specific DNA probes. Mutat Res 1990; 234(5):303–318.

20. Gray JW, Pinkel D. Molecular cytogenetics in human cancer diagnosis. Cancer 1992; 69(suppl 6):1536–1542.

21. Eastmond DA, Schuler M, Rupa DS. Advantages and limitations of using fluorescence in situ hybridization for the detection of aneuploidy in interphase human cells. Mutat Res 1995; 348(4):153–162.

22. Kadam P, Umerani A, Srivastava A, Masterson M, Lampkin B, Raza A. Combination of classical and interphase cytogenetics to investigate the biology of myeloid disorders: detection of masked monosomy 7 in AML. Leuk Res 1993; 17(4):365–374.

23. Kibbelaar RE, Mulder JWR, Dreef EJ, Van Kamp H, Fibbe WE, Wessels JW, Beverstock GC, Haak HL, Kluin PM. Detection of monosomy 7 and trisomy 8 in myeloid neoplasia: a comparison of banding and fluorescence in situ hybridization. Blood 1993; 82(3):904–913.

24. Poddighe PJ, Moesker O, Smeets D, Awwad BH, Ramaekers FC, Hopman AH. Interphase cytogenetics of hematological cancer: comparison of classical karyo-typing and in situ hybridization using a panel of eleven chromosome-specific DNA probes. Cancer Res 1991; 51(7):1959–1967.

25. Cohen MM, Rosenblum-Vos LS, Prabhakar G. Human cytogenetics: a current overview. Am J Dis Child 1993; 147(11):1159–1166.

26. Tucker JD, Senft JR. Analysis of naturally occurring and radiation-induced breakpoint locations in human chromosomes 1, 2 and 4. Radiat Res 1994; 140(1):31–36.

27. Gray JE, Pinkel D, Brown JM. Fluorescence in situ hybridization in cancer and radiation biology. Radiat Res 1994; 137(3):275–289.

28. Dulout FN, Grillo CA, Seoane AI, Maderna CR, Nilsson R, Vahter M, Darroudi F, Natarajan AT. Chromosomal aberrations in peripheral blood lymphocytes from native Andean women and children from north-western Argentina exposed to arsenic in drinking water. Mutat Res 1996; 370(3–4):151–158.

29. Rupa DS, Hasegawa L, Eastmond DA. Detection of chromosomal breakage in the 1cen-1q12 region of interphase human lymphocytes using multicolor fluorescence in situ hybridization with tandem DNA probes. Cancer Res 1995; 55(3):640–645.

30. Zhang L, Rothman N, Wang Y, Hayes RB, Bechtold W, Venkatesh P, Yin Y, Wang Y, Dosemeci M, Li G, Lu W, Smith MT. Interphase cytogenetics of workers exposed to benzene. Environ Health Perspect 1996; 104(suppl 6): 1325–1329.

31. Matsumoto K, Ramsey MJ, Nelson DO, Tucker JD. Persistence of radiation-induced translocations in human peripheral blood determined by chromosome painting. Radiat Res 1998; 149(6):602–613.

32. Tucker JD, Tawn EJ, Holdsworth D, Morris S, Langlois R, Ramsey MJ, Kato P, Boice JD, Tarone RE, Jensen RH. Biological dosimetry of radiation workers at the Sellafield nuclear facility. Radiat Res 1997; 148(3):216–226.

33. Tucker JD, Breneman JW, Briner JF, Eveleth CG, Langlois RG, Moore DHI. Persistence of radiation-induced translocations in rat peripheral blood determined by chromosome painting. Environ Mol Mutagen 1997; 30(3): 264–272.

34. Sachs RK, Chen AM, Brenner DJ. Review: proximity effects in the production of chromosome aberrations by ionizing radiation. Int J Radiat Biol 1997; 71(1):1–19.

35. Morton NE. Parameters of the human genome. Proc Natl Acad Sci USA 1991; 88(17):7474–7476.

36. Zhang L, Rothman N, Wang Y, Hayes RB, Li G, Dosemeci M, Yin S, Kolachana P, Titenko-Holland N, Smith MT. Increased aneusomy and long arm deletion of chromosomes 5 and 7 in the lymphocytes of Chinese workers exposed to benzene. Carcinogenesis 1998; 19(11):1955–1961.

37. Xi L, Zhang L, Wang Y, Smith MT. Induction of chromosome-specific aneuploidy and micronuclei in human lymphocytes by metabolites of 1,3-butadiene. Carcinogenesis (Oxford) 1997; 18(9):1687–1693.

38. Scarpato R, Lori A, Panasiuk G, Barale R. FISH analysis of translocations in lymphocytes of children exposed to the Chernobyl fallout: preferential involvement of chromosome 10. Cytogenet Cell Genet 1997; 79(1–2):153–156.

39. Smith MT, Zhang L, Wang Y, Hayes RB, Li G, Wiemels J, Dosemeci M, Titenko-Holland N, Xi L, Kolachana P, Yin S, Rothman N. Increased translocations and aneusomy in chromosomes 8 and 21 among workers exposed to benzene. Cancer Res 1998; 58(10):2176–2181.

40. Schröck E, du Manoir S, Veldman T, Schoell B, Wienberg J, Ferguson-Smith MA, Ning Y, Ledbetter DH, Bar-Am I, Soenksen D, Garini Y, Ried T. Multicolor spectral karyotyping of human chromosomes. Science 1996; 273(5274): 494–497.

41. Müller S, Rocchi M, Ferguson-Smith MA, Wienberg J. Toward a multicolor chromosome bar code for the entire human karyotype by fluorescence in situ hybridization. Hum Genet 1997; 100(2):271–278.

42. Kwok S, Higuchi R. Avoiding false positives with PCR. (Published erratum appears in Nature 1989; 339(6224):490.) Nature 1989; 339(6221):237–238.

43. Luthra R, McBride JA, Cabanillas F, Sarris A. Novel 5′ exonuclease-based real-time PCR assay for the detection of t(14;18)(q32;q21) in patients with follicular lymphoma. Am J Pathol 1998; 153(1):63–68.

44. Doelken L, Schueler F, Doelken G. Quantitative detection of t(14;18)-positive cells by real-time quantitative PCR using fluorogenic probes. Biotechniques 1998; 25(6):1058–1064.
45. Liu Y, Hernandez AM, Shibata D, Cortopassi GA. BCL2 translocation frequency rises with age in humans. Proc Nat Acad Sci USA 1994; 91(19):8910–8914.
46. Biernaux C, Loos M, Sels A, Huez G, Stryckmans P. Detection of major bcr-abl gene expression at a very low level in blood cells of some healthy individuals. Blood 1995; 86(8):3118–3122.
47. Fuscoe JC, Setzer RW, Collard DD, Moore MM. Quantification of t(14;18) in the lymphocytes of healthy adult humans as a possible biomarker for environmental exposures to carcinogens. Carcinogenesis (Oxford) 1996; 17(5): 1013–1020.
48. Bell DA, Liu Y, Cortopassi GA. Occurrence of bcl-2 oncogene translocation with increased frequency in the peripheral blood of heavy smokers. J Natl Cancer Institute (Bethesda) 1995; 87(3):223–224.
49. Innis M, Gelfand DH, Sninsky JJ, eds. PCR Applications: Protocols for Functional Genomics. San Diego: Academic Press, 1999.
50. Bories D, Dumont V, Belhadj K, Bernaudin F, Raffi H, Kuentz M, Cordonnier C, Tulliez M. Real-time quantitative RT-PCR monitoring of chronic myelogenous leukemia. Blood 1998; 92(10 suppl 1, parts 1–2):73A.
51. Krauter J, Wattjes M, Nagel S, Heidenreich O, Bunjes D, Bergmann L, Heil G, Ganser A. AML1/MTG8 real-time RT-PCR for the detection of minimal residual disease in patients with T[8;21] positive AML. Blood 1998; 92(10 suppl 1, parts 1–2):74A–75A.
52. Preudhomme C, Merlat A, Roumier C, Duflos-Gardel N, Jouet JP, Cosson A, Fenaux P. Detection of BCR-ABL transcripts in chronic myeloid leukemia (CML) using a novel "real time" quantitative RT-PCR assay: a report on 15 patients. Blood 1998; 92(10 suppl 1, parts 1–2):93.
53. Saal RJ, Gill DS, Cobcroft RG, Marlton P. Quantitation of AML-ETO transcripts using real-time PCR on the ABI7700 sequence detection system. Blood 1998; 92(10 suppl 1, parts, 1–2):74A.
54. Cayuela J-M, Gardie B, Sigaux F. Disruption of the multiple tumor suppressor gene MTS1/p16-INK4a/CDKN2 by illegitimate V(D)J recombinase activity in T-cell acute lymphoblastic leukemias. Blood 1997; 90(9):3720–3726.
55. Satake N, Maseki N, Kozu T, Sakashita A, Kobayashi H, Sakurai M, Ohki M, Kaneko Y. Disappearance of AML1-MTG8(ETO) fusion transcript in acute myeloid leukaemia patients with t(8;21) in long-term remission. Br J Haematol 1995; 91(4):892–898.
56. Marcucci G, Livak KJ, Bi W, Strout MP, Bloomfield CD, Caligiuri MA. Detection of minimal residual disease in patients with AML1/ETO-associated acute myeloid leukemia using a novel quantitative reverse transcription polymerase chain reaction assay. Leukemia (Basingstoke) 1998; 12(9):1482–1489.
57. Mensink E, van de Locht A, Schattenberg A, Linders E, Schaap N, Geurts van Kessel A, De Witte T. Quantitation of minimal residual disease in Philadelphia chromosome positive chronic myeloid leukaemia patients using real-time quantitative RT-PCR. Br J Haematol 1998; 102(3):768–774.

58. Heisterkamp N, Stephenson JR, Groffen J, Hansen PF, de Klein A, Bartram CR, Grosveld G. Localization of the c-abl oncogene adjacent to a translocation break point in chronic myelocytic leukaemia. Nature 1983; 306(5940): 239–242.

59. Issa JP, Baylin SB, Herman JG. DNA methylation changes in hematologic malignancies: biologic and clinical implications. Leukemia (Basingstoke) 1997; 11(suppl 1):S7–S11.

60. Belinsky SA, Nikula KJ, Palmisano WA, Michels R, Saccomanno G, Gabrielson E, Baylin SB, Herman JG. Aberrant methylation of p16INK4a is an early event in lung cancer and a potential biomarker for early diagnosis. Proc Natl Acad Sci U S A 1998; 95(20):11891–11896.

61. Hsieh C-J, Klump B, Holzmann K, Borchard F, Gregor M, Porschen R. Hypermethylation of the p16INK4a promoter in colectomy specimens of patients with long-standing and extensive ulcerative colitis. Cancer Res 1998; 58(17):3942–3945.

62. Kanai Y, Ushijima S, Tsuda H, Sakamoto M, Sugimura T, Hirohashi S. Aberrant DNA methylation on chromosome 16 is an early event in hepatocarcinogenesis. Jpn J Cancer Res 1996; 87(12):1210–1217.

63. Jones PA, Gonzalgo ML, Tsutsumi M, Bender CM. DNA methylation in bladder cancer. Eur Urol 1998; 33(suppl 4):7–8.

64. Lo YMD, Wong IHN, Zhang J, Tein MSC, Ng MHL, Hjelm NM. Quantitative analysis of aberrant p16 methylation using real-time quantitative methylation-specific polymerase chain reaction. Cancer Res 1999; 59(16):3899–3903.

65. Vet JAM, Majithia AR, Marras SAE, Tyagi S, Dube S, Poiesz BJ, Kramer FR. Multiplex detection of four pathogenic retroviruses using molecular beacons. Proc Natl Acad Sci U S A 1999; 96(11):6394–6399.

66. Vogelstein B, Kinzler KW. Digital PCR. Proc Natl Acad Sci U S A 1999; 96(16):9236–9241.

6

Quantitative Cancer Risk Assessment

John Whysner
Washington Occupational Health Associates, Washington, D.C., U.S.A.

1. INTRODUCTION

Risk assessment provides a quantitative approach to toxicology and chemical carcinogenesis. Before the development of risk assessment methods, there was no established method to determine the probability of disease due to measured exposure levels. The Food Additives Amendment of 1958 included the Delaney Clause, which required that no chemical determined to be carcinogenic in either humans or animals be allowed as a food additive by the Food and Drug Administration (FDA). As a consequence, food additives were regulated without risk assessment determinations. Later, in the case of residues of animal drugs in foods, acceptable levels were determined by the FDA based upon calculated risks of cancer. However, these risk estimates developed by the FDA were not derived using a particular model of carcinogenesis, but were calculated based upon probabilities of differences in sensitivities of individuals within a population.

During the 1970s, risk assessment methods were developed by the U.S. Environmental Protection Agency (EPA) and the U.S. Occupational Health and Safety Administration (OSHA). It was largely assumed that all carcinogens were DNA reactive, and that such interactions requiring only one event could be additive to ongoing, spontaneous gene mutation. The Armitage and Doll multistage model of cancer (1) proposed that the carcinogenic agent caused several irreversible steps of genetic change. Cancer policy and statistical methods for high- to low-dose extrapolations were developed using this model, which included an assumption of the lack of a threshold for chemicals producing neoplastic development. However, it is now known that carcinogens may act by mechanisms that may exhibit a threshold due to the role of target organ toxicity in the carcinogenic process.

In 1983, the National Academy of Sciences (NAS) published a study of how risk assessment should be conducted in the Federal government (2). The NAS established a framework to guide future risk assessment by Federal agencies, which included the use of default assumptions where gaps were present in general knowledge or available data for a particular chemical. As defined by the NAS and is now generally recognized, risk assessment consists of the following four steps:

1. Hazard identification
2. Dose–response assessment
3. Exposure assessment
4. Risk characterization

Hazard identification is the review of relevant biological and medical information to determine whether or not particular substances may cause adverse health effects. Dose–response assessment defines the relationships between the exposure or dose of an agent and the magnitude of the health response. This includes a quantitative estimate of the possible impact of a health effect for a range of doses. Exposure assessment produces an estimate of the extent of exposure to the populations of interest. Risk characterization integrates the hazard identification, dose–response assessment, and exposure assessment, in order to describe the nature and the magnitude of health risk. The risk characterization includes presentation of uncertainties and provides a framework to help judge the significance of the risks.

2. HAZARD IDENTIFICATION FOR CARCINOGENS

Carcinogen risk assessment begins with an evaluation of whether a chemical has been shown to cause increased rates of specific neoplasms in either humans or animals. Various types of information are available for determining the carcinogenic potential of a compound. Useful data for hazard identification comes from epidemiological studies, controlled human experiments, in vivo and in vitro toxicological tests, and analysis of physical/chemical properties, structure–activity relationships, and pharmacokinetic properties. Epidemiological studies of humans and toxicological studies of experimental animals provide the most important information and are essential in determining the hazardous potential of a compound. The other types of information serve mainly as supporting data to the toxicological and epidemiological studies, although data on cancer mechanisms are being increasingly used to evaluate whether certain rodent tumors are relevant to human cancer risk determination.

The resulting data are evaluated and chemicals have been classified according to the "strength of evidence" for positive responses, and usually with little regard for studies showing no carcinogenic effects. Major default assumptions used by regulatory agencies are that neoplastic responses in rodents are potentially relevant to human cancer and that target organ site concordance in not necessary for extrapolation to humans. However, it is now recognized that these assumptions are naive and that many tumor types are not relevant for human cancer risk assessment.

One source of hazard identification information is the EPA's Integrated Risk Information System (IRIS), which is available on-line (http://www.epa.gov/iris). Another source is the *IARC Monographs on the Evaluation of the Carcinogenic Risks to Humans*, published by the International Agency for Research on Cancer (IARC), which is part of the World Health Organization.

2.1. Carcinogen Classifications

An EPA carcinogen group designation that characterizes the strength of evidence for human cancer risk, has been established for each substance reviewed by the intra-agency work group, which consists of scientists from throughout the EPA. The basis for the classification is included in the IRIS database. In the case of the IARC, the classification is based upon the deliberations by cancer experts from throughout the world at meetings that develop the monographs. The classifications systems for carcinogens vary somewhat among the IARC, other nations and regulatory agencies within the United States.

Traditionally, there has been an alphanumeric system used with Group A (EPA) and Group 1 (IARC) identifying chemicals *known* to produce cancer in humans based upon epidemiology studies. Other groups such as Groups B and C (EPA) or Group 2 (IARC) identify chemicals that are known to produce cancer in animals but not proven in humans. These are termed probable or possible carcinogens based upon the premise that it is prudent for regulatory purposes to act as if they represent a risk to humans. However, this does not imply that a causal relationship has been proven between the agent and human cancer. The EPA classification system for the characterization of the overall weight of evidence (animal, human, and other supportive data) of carcinogenicity of a substance includes the following five groups (3):

1. *Group A: Human carcinogens.* Sufficient evidence from epidemiological studies to support a causal association between exposure to the agents and cancer.
2. *Group B: Probable human carcinogens.* Sufficient evidence of carcinogenicity based on animal studies. This group is divided into two subgroups. Group B1 is reserved for agents for which there

is limited evidence of carcinogenicity from epidemiological studies. Agents for which there is "sufficient" evidence from animal studies and for which there is "inadequate evidence" or "no data" from epidemiological studies would usually be categorized under Group B2.

3. *Group C: Possible human carcinogens.* Limited evidence of carcinogenicity in animals in the absence of human data. This group includes a wide variety of evidence such as (1) a malignant tumor response in a single well-conducted experiment that does not meet conditions for sufficient evidence, (2) tumor responses of marginal statistical significance in studies having inadequate design or reporting, (3) benign, but not malignant tumors with an agent showing no response in a variety of short-term tests for mutagenicity, and (4) responses of marginal statistical significance in a tissue known to have a high or variable background rate.

4. *Group D: Not classifiable as to human carcinogenicity.* Inadequate (or negative) human and animal evidence of carcinogenicity, or no data are available.

5. *Group E: Evidence of noncarcinogenicity for humans.* No evidence for carcinogenicity in at least two adequate animal tests in different species or in both adequate animal tests in different species or in both adequate epidemiological and animal studies.

Groups A and B and, in some cases, C are treated similarly for risk assessment purposes. In general, once a chemical has been shown to produce a particular tumor type in rodents by two independent studies, risk assessment proceeds regardless of whether humans studies are positive, negative or nonexistent.

2.2. Changes in the Carcinogen Classification Systems

Recently, the EPA has begun to move away from alphanumeric systems for classification and instead to integrate additional information into a weight of evidence approach, which includes the mode of action and exposure conditions required to express a neoplastic response (4). One category "known/likely" may approximately replace the designation of known and probable according to proposed new regulations (5). In the case of agents that have data that raise the suspicion of carcinogenicity, but the data is not adequate to convincingly demonstrate a carcinogenic potential, the designation would be "cannot be determined."

In addition, regulatory agencies have been changing hazard identification methodology by using additional information available for the chemicals. For example, they have been incorporating a "weight of evidence" approach, whereby well-conducted negative studies are used in the evaluation process (5). Such negative studies may be used to contradict poorly conducted studies that have reported a positive finding.

It is now recognized that certain chemical-induced neoplastic effects in animals within certain target organs may not be predictors of risks for humans, especially at human exposure levels. Such mechanistic evaluations formed the basis for a monograph published by the International Expert Panel on Carcinogen Risk Assessment (6). In these series of evaluations, evidence whether a chemical produced cancer in animals by a DNA-reactive mechanisms was found to be of primary importance in the assessment of human cancer risk. The designation of a chemical as producing tumors in animals by a non-DNA-reactive mechanism raises the possibility that these chemicals would not produce cancer in humans. Several chemicals have been evaluated and found to be unlikely to cause cancer in humans. These include the food additives D-limonene (7), butylated hydroxyanisole (8), and saccharin (9).

In those cases where a chemical has been shown to produce neoplasms in animals by a mode of action that could not be operative in humans, risk assessment is not performed based upon such neoplasms. In the case of the EPA's proposed descriptors (5), such agents would be designated as "not likely to be carcinogenic in humans." This is the same designation as for chemical that have been shown to be negative in adequate well-conducted rodent testing. The IARC has also begun using cancer mechanism data for risk assessment, and several chemicals including melamine, D-limonene, saccharin, and atrazine were placed in Group 3 (insufficient evidence) based on such considerations (10).

3. DOSE–RESPONSE ASSESSMENT

After a chemical has been identified as a human or experimental carcinogen, the dose–response for the tumor response is assessed. Dose–response assessment for a chemical is the key element in the risk assessment process, because this forms the basis for the quantitative nature of the process. Epidemiological data are preferred over animal data when conducting a dose–response assessment since extrapolation from animals to humans is not required (3). This eliminates the uncertainty associated with interspecies extrapolation. For many known human carcinogens, studies of humans have included exposure information sufficient to determine the dose–response relationship. In most instances, human exposure information comes from industrial hygiene measures in the workplace.

In order to estimate the dose–response, either an upper bound estimate or a maximum likelihood estimate (MLE) is derived, which is the statistically best estimate of the value of a parameter from a given data set. The difference between the upper bound estimate and the MLE is that the upper bound is more conservative in the face of uncertainty due to a lesser amount of data, whereas the MLE is better if there is a significant level of confidence in deriving point estimates of risk. An MLE approach is better to use with large numbers of data points. For most chemicals, the only reliable dose–response information comes from studies in rats or mice. In these cases the upper bound estimate is used, and various mathematical models can be used to fit the data (Fig. 1A).

3.1. Extrapolation to Doses Below the Observed Effects

The relationship between dose and toxicological response of any particular chemical is usually a complex one and may involve sublinear, linear, and supralinear components (Fig. 1). This is also true of neoplastic responses and depends upon the mode of action. When cancer risk assessment was first developed, all carcinogens were believed to act as mutagens producing irreversible changes and acting at one or more steps in a sequence of events leading to neoplasia. It is now known that chemicals may be involved in many steps of a neoplastic process in which they may directly or indirectly produce mutagenic effects, alternatively they may produce other changes that enhance neoplastic conversion or development.

The underlying default assumption for dose–response has been that the low-dose portion of the curve is linear unless proven otherwise. The original justification for this assumption was mathematical and derived from the multistage model of carcinogenesis. Animal tumor data is analyzed by the linearized multistage (LMS) procedure, which provides a first-order cancer potency factor at low dosage levels. The cancer slope factor (q_1^*) is

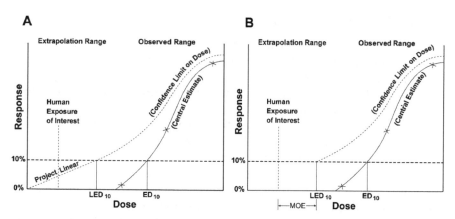

Figure 1 Dose–response extrapolation for carcinogens. Data points represent hypothetical data for tumor response versus dose. (**A**) Dose–response extrapolation using a linear-at-low-dose approach for estimates of human risk. (**B**) Dose response extrapolation using the margin of exposure (MOE) approach. Abbreviations are defined in the text. Note that the "human exposure of interest" is usually much nearer to the zero dose than shown.

the linear extrapolation line of the dose–response data and is expressed in units of risk per dosage $(mg/kg\ b.w./day)^{-1}$. The q_1^* represents the 95% upper confidence limit on that slope.

Since the early 1980s, the FDA has used a somewhat different low-dose extrapolation where linear extrapolation to zero proceeds from the upper confidence limit on the lowest experimental dose (11). In this procedure, a point on the dose–response curve (tumor incidence vs. dose) for a chemical is chosen below which the data no longer appear to be reliable and a straight line is drawn form the upper confidence limit to the origin. The EPA has recently developed a similar method for deriving the relationship between dose and response for low doses (4,5), which uses a straight line extrapolation to the origin from the low-end dose of the observed tumor data, usually the 10% tumor response, which is termed the LED_{10} (Fig. 1A).

Several other procedures have been used for dose–response extrapolation, which lead to widely differing estimates of potency. The model with the most significant departure from the LMS model is the threshold model, which assumes that no significant risk is present below an identified exposure. In this model, a no-observed-adverse effect level (NOAEL) is determined, which serves a point of departure for the development of an acceptable dose. The NOAEL approach has been used extensively along with safety or uncertainty factors for the determination of acceptable doses for toxic effects other than cancer. However, this procedure has also been used by some European nations and on a limited basis in the United States where the chemical is believed to produce neoplasia by a process that involves a threshold (12). The major determinant for the use of a threshold model for a chemical is the lack of DNA reactivity coupled with a plausible explanation, such as chronic toxicity of the target organ, as the basis for the tumorigenic response.

The EPA has recently developed a similar procedure for carcinogens that exhibit a dose–response that either has a lack of demonstrated effect at low doses (threshold dose) or a much lower than expected effect at low doses (sublinear dose–response) (5). In this case a margin of exposure (MOE) is determined, which is the difference between the LED_{10} and the estimated human exposure level (Fig. 1B). This procedure is similar to the use of uncertainty factors with a NOAEL; however, the use of the MOE method does not require the experimental determination of a threshold dose for the neoplastic effect.

3.2. Rodent-to-Human Extrapolation

Although humans have been exposed to many chemicals classified as carcinogens, usually adequate exposure information is lacking from epidemiology studies for use in dose–response development. Also, for most chemicals that have been found to produce tumors in experimental animals, human studies are lacking or have not found increases in cancer that can be quantified. Consequently, the estimation of cancer risks for humans are usually based upon extrapolation from rodents. In addition, animal studies have two primary advantages over epidemiological studies: 1) dose, environmental, and extraneous exposures are strictly controlled, and 2) adverse affects are directly measured through pathological examination and necropsy. The obvious disadvantage is that humans may not respond to chemicals in the same manner as rodents either qualitatively or quantitatively.

For carcinogens, the EPA's default method of extrapolation from animals to humans has been traditionally based upon comparative surface areas, which is related to metabolic rate. The surface area is approximately proportional to the two-third power of body weight. However, based upon empirical data for chemotherapeutic drugs in rodents and humans, the ratio of the three-quarter power of body weight or $(BW_1)^{3/4}/(BW_2)^{3/4}$ is now used both by the EPA and FDA (13). In practice, this means that the cancer slope factor in mg/kg/day for the rat or mouse would be multiplied by a factor of between 5 and 10 for humans.

If data regarding the chemical-specific relative metabolic rates, tissue distributions, or other factors are available for rodents and humans, pharmacologically based pharmacokinetic (PBPK) modeling may be used to extrapolate between species. PBPK modeling is a mathematical method for extrapolating between species that accounts for differences in target organ concentrations of the reactive metabolite(s) due to absorption, biotransformation, distribution and elimination. Difficulty in applying this level of sophistication to the species-to-species extrapolation is usually due to the lack of information in human parameters for many chemicals. Furthermore, individual differences among humans for many of these parameters requires that PBPK modeling use statistical distributions of parameters, and the combinations of distributions may give a result with a large range of values.

Ideally, the route of administration of animal studies used for dose–response data should be the same as the human route of exposure (i.e., inhalation, dermal contact, ingestion). If it is not, an extrapolation from the animal route of administration to the human route of exposure may be possible. The target organ(s) and mechanism(s) of action determine whether route-to-route extrapolation is appropriate. For an agent causing adverse effects at the point of contact (e.g., skin, lung) extrapolation from one route of administration is usually not valid. But for carcinogens with a systemic mode of action, route-to-route extrapolation may be biologically plausible. In order to perform route-to-route extrapolation, pharmacokinetic data for the substance being evaluated are desirable, but not always available, and estimates can be made in the absence of such data. Pharmacokinetic data can also be used in PBPK models to convert the dose to a different route.

4. EXPOSURE ASSESSMENT

In exposure assessment, the amount of a chemical that may contact the human body is determined, but there is also a difference between external exposure and internal exposure, which is the dose, and this depends on the efficiency of absorption. The dosage is summed for all pathways and routes of exposure resulting in an numerical estimate that is usually expressed in units of milligrams per kilogram body weight per day (mg/kg/day).

For pharmaceuticals, food additives, food contaminants, and drinking water contaminants, the only pathway of concern is usually oral ingestion and the amount of the medicine, food, or water can be estimated with some degree of certainty. As a default assumption, the external and internal exposure is often considered to be the same, i.e., there is 100% absorption. For contaminants in food regulated by the FDA, the average total diet of an adult is generally assumed to include 1500 g of solid food and 1500 g of liquid per day. In the absence of a measured distribution of intakes among individuals in a population or a direct measure of the 90th percentile, a two- to three-fold excess is used on the observed average consumption of the medium that contains the contaminant (11).

The exposure assessment process varies in complexity depending upon the conditions under which individuals may contact the agent. For example, dermal exposure usually results in a lower dose to the target organ than an oral dose, and in the dermal exposure scenario, the chemical may be bound to a matrix such as soil, which would be expected to decrease dermal absorption. In other cases, the exposure estimate includes the use of sophisticated mathematical models, and the exposures related to all significant potential pathways are estimated (14). An example of a complicated site-specific exposure assessment is that of a hazardous waste incinerator where air levels are models based upon meteorological data, and deposition of particulates on edible plants and water are estimated. These data are then used to calculate the amount inhaled or ingested from consumption of plants and animals including fish. Route- and chemical-specific absorption factors are then used to translate exposure to doses, which are summed for all exposure pathways. Current EPA risk assessment guidelines promote estimating "high end" and "central tendency" exposures (14). High end exposure scenarios are supposed to result in reasonable but highly conservative estimates of risk that generally represent the degree of exposure to only the most exposed members of the population (2–10%). Central tendency exposure scenarios reflect the degree of exposure of typical or average individuals. Unfortunately, the exposure assessment may also include highly implausible estimates that would include few, if any, of the people with potential exposures.

A detailed description of exposure assessment methods is beyond the scope of this chapter. However, two of the most common and direct risk scenarios will be briefly described: oral ingestion of contaminated drinking water and inhalation of contaminated air. These will provide the reader with some understanding of the estimates made of exposure. More detailed guidance for exposure assessment is available from EPA publications (14–16).

4.1. Drinking Water

Exposure to drinking water is direct and does not require the differentiation between external and internal exposure. A default assumption used is that adults can consume up to 2 L of water per day. Therefore, for a one part per billion (ppb) level of contamination in drinking water, a person may consume the following:

$$\frac{1\,\mu g\ contaminant}{kg\ water} \times \frac{1\,kg\ water}{1\,L\ water} \times \frac{2\,L\ water}{day}$$

$$\times \frac{1}{70\,kg\ b.w.} = 3 \times 10^{-5}\,mg/kg/day$$

4.2. Inhalation and the Inhalation Unit Risk

For breathing contaminants in air, the amount of exposure is usually determined by the breathing volume per day divided by the human body weight. In this case there usually are no adjustments made for the difference between external and internal dose. The calculation of exposure for microgram per cubic meter contaminant level in air is shown below:

$$1\,\mu g/m^3 \times 20\,m^3/per\ day \times 1/70\,kg\ (b.w.)$$

$$\times 10^{-3}\,mg/\mu g = 0.0003\,mg/kg/day$$

For some inhalation exposures, it is a relatively straightforward procedure to translate cancer slope factors into mathematical relationships that are termed unit risk levels, which represent an estimate of the increased cancer risk from a lifetime (70-year) exposure to a concentration of one unit of exposure. Unit risk values incorporate the cancer potency and the amount of air consumed per day. The inhalation unit risk (IUR) is expressed as risk per micrograms per cubic meter.

For radionuclides in air such as uranium-238 and thorium-232, data is published yearly by the EPA in the Health Effects Assessment Summary Tables (HEAST) that estimate risks based upon total lifetime dose in risk/pCi, which is irrespective of body weight. In the case of radionuclides, the IUR can be calculated from the data presented in the HEAST tables as follows:

$$IUR = \frac{risk}{pCi} \times \frac{20\,m^3}{day} \times \frac{25,550\,days}{lifetime} = Risk(pCi/m^3)^{-1}$$

5. RISK CHARACTERIZATION

In risk characterization, exposure assessment is coupled with the dose–response information. By this method risks can be estimated based upon various exposure scenarios. Along with quantitative estimates of risk, risk characterization should identify the key assumptions, their rationale, and the effect of reasonable alternative assumptions on the conclusions and estimates. Second, the risk characterization identifies any important uncertainties in the assessment.

In order to calculate risk, the dose determined by exposure assessment is multiplied by the cancer slope factor, which in this example is 0.1 risk $(mg/kg/day)^{-1}$, as in the following example:

$$3 \times 10^{-5} \, mg/kg \ b.w./day \times 0.1 \ risk \ (mg/kg/day)^{-1}$$
$$= 3 \times 10^{-6} \ risk$$

In site-specific risk assessment, all significant exposure routes are determined related to contaminant levels in a specific situation such as a Superfund site. Based upon exposure assessment calculations, a risk is determined. Alternatively, the calculation can be performed in reverse order to develop regulatory levels for chemicals in air, water, soil, or food based upon specified risk levels.

The risk assessment of chemical mixtures results in an estimation of the total risk for all chemicals to which an individual is exposed from a particular source. In the case of carcinogens, the risks are assumed to be additive, since most risks are calculated assuming a linear risk–dose relationship, and the risks calculated are incremental risks.

5.1. Individual vs. Population Risks

Maximum individual lifetime risk (MIR) is commonly used to express individual risks. MIR is defined as the hypothetical probability of cancer following exposure to an agent at the maximum modeled long-term exposures assuming a 70-year (lifetime) duration of exposure. Estimates of MIR are usually expressed as a probability represented in scientific notation as a negative exponent of 10, which may be indicated in the tables by "e." For example, 5e-8 is the same as 5×10^{-8}, which is 0.00000005.

Population risk descriptors are intended to estimate the extent of risk for the population as a whole. This typically represents the sum total of individual risks within the exposed population. Two important population risk descriptors are usually estimated and presented (14):

- the probabilistic number of health effect cases estimated in the population of interest over a specified time period; and
- the percentage of the population, or the number of persons, above a specified level of risk or range of health benchmark levels.

5.2. Sensitive Subpopulations

Individual risk descriptors are intended to estimate the risk borne by individuals within a specified population or subpopulation. These descriptors are used to answer questions concerning the affected population, the risk levels of various groups within the population, and the maximum risk for individuals within the population. The "high end" risk descriptor is intended to estimate the risk that is expected to occur in a small but definable segment of the population. The intent is to convey an estimate of risk in the upper range of the distribution, but to avoid estimates which are beyond the true distribution. Conceptually, high end risk means risk above the 90th percentile of the population distribution, but not higher than the individual in the population who has the highest risk (14).

Certain groups within a population may be more sensitive to environmental exposure than other groups. However, EPA considers the linear default assumption for low-dose extrapolation to be health protective to the extent that human variability of response would be taken into account (5). Concerns regarding exposures to children have been given special attention. However, for carcinogens and most noncarcinogens, the particular sensitivity of children has not been characterized. In risk assessment calculations involving contaminated soil that could be ingested by children, the young child's exposure is calculated separately due to the possibility of children ingesting soil directly. Contamination of food sources are also calculated separately for children due to the greater consumption of certain foods per body weight compared to adults.

5.3. Uncertainty Analysis

EPA guidance calls for a full characterization of risk, not just the single point estimate, which has become synonymous with risk characterization. Critical to full characterization of risk is a discussion of the uncertainty in the overall assessment and in each of its components. Uncertainty in risk assessment can be classified into three broad categories according to EPA (14):

1. Uncertainty regarding missing or incomplete information needed to fully define the exposure and dose (scenario uncertainty)
2. Uncertainty regarding some parameter (parameter uncertainty)
3. Uncertainty regarding gaps in scientific theory required to make predictions on the basis of causal inferences (model uncertainty)

Uncertainty can be introduced into a health risk assessment at many steps in the process. It occurs because risk assessment is a complex process, requiring the integration of many items. The fate and transport of substances in a variable environment that require complex models with uncertain assumptions. The potential for adverse health effects in humans may require uncertain extrapolations from animal bioassays; and the probability of adverse effects in a human population may be variable genetically, in age, in activity level, and in lifestyle.

Even using the most accurate data with the most sophisticated models, uncertainty is inherent in the process. In order to account for uncertainty, risk assessment generally uses assumptions that overestimate the risks so that the risks are likely to be less, rather than greater, than those predicted.

6. RISK MANAGEMENT CONSIDERATIONS

Risk management has been described as the process of evaluating alternative regulatory actions and selecting among them. This selection process necessarily requires the use of value judgements on such issues as the acceptability of risk (2). Risk levels that have been deemed "acceptable" range from one per thousand (10^{-3}) lifetimes to less than one per million (10^{-6}). Differences in acceptable risk depend upon judgments that are based on societal values. Risk assessment has been used by the OSHA to regulate cancer risks resulting in air levels that have associated risks of one per thousand (10^{-3}) lifetimes or less. The use of risk assessment by OSHA balances the reduction of risk with practical concerns in the workplace. The resulting unit dose is called the permissible exposure limit (PEL), which is based upon exposures over a working lifetime, 8 hr per day, 5 days per week.

For the general public, air levels have also been developed by air toxics programs of the states. In the case of the general public, risks of one per one-hundred thousand (10^{-5}) or one per million (10^{-6}) are generally used as a starting point. The 10^{-6} risk level has been chosen historically in an arbitrary manner as a basis for regulation (17), and the EPA has regulated chemicals involving exposures to large populations at about this risk level. For decisions where the population risk is a fraction of a cancer case per year for the entire population, a 10^{-5} risk level seems to be in the range of what EPA might consider to be an insignificant average individual lifetime risk (18). A review of policies by Travis et al. (19) has found that EPA does not consider individual risks of less than 10^{-4} in small geographic areas to necessarily require regulation. The legislation that created superfund clean-up standards has indicated that a range of 10^{-4}–10^{-6} risk level is generally acceptable. At these specified hypothetical risk levels, the actual risk to an individual is usually negligible due to the many health protective assumptions that are incorporated into the risk assessment process.

7. DISCUSSION AND FUTURE DIRECTIONS

The risk assessment methodology has now been used extensively in a wide variety of circumstances, and due to the quality of the database the results have ranged from reasonable estimates of cancer probability for known human carcinogens to controversial risk speculations that are seemingly improbable. Consequently, it is important to understand that quality and validity of the data regarding a particular chemical greatly affects the reliability of the risk estimate. Even where the data are technically sound but the extrapolation of risk to humans is unclear, the relevance to human risks may be questionable. It is likely that many chemicals pose no cancer risk to humans at any realistic exposure level although risks can be calculated.

Risk assessment does not determine real probabilities of an individual or a population developing cancer from a particular agent. Calculated risks are intended to provide upper-bound estimates, and one must understand that the real risks may be much lower or zero (3). In other words, one cannot deduce the true probability of cancer causation by doing a risk assessment calculation since there are usually several health protective assumptions that inflate the risk. An excellent argument has been made that a MOE-type approach (Fig. 1) be used for assessment of all toxic effects including cancer, since the toxicological information generally available does not warrant numerical estimates of risk at low levels of human exposure (20).

Risk assessment does provide a framework for decreasing the probability of harm from chemical exposures. Consequently, it is useful for regulatory purposes. The coincidence of real probability and risk assessment calculations will be greater for those agents that have been shown to cause cancer in epidemiology studies, which can be used for dose-response assessment and in which the exposure levels are close to or within the range of observation. However, for those agents that are positive in animal studies but are negative or untested in epidemiology studies, extrapolation is always problematic.

The mode of action by which an agent causes cancer in animals is of primary importance for extrapolation to humans. The induction of neoplasia through a mechanism that is likely to operate both in humans and rodents, such as DNA adduct formation leading to mutation, tends to increase the validity of risk assessment. In contrast, many chemical-related cancer mechanisms are now known to be either unique to the rodent or are suspected to only occur in the rodent at very high exposure levels. In such cases, risk assessment would unrealistically calculate risks to humans.

One of the most important developments in risk assessment is the identification of species-specific modes of actions for some carcinogenic effects in rodents. As a consequence, the EPA has determined that tumors formed in the male rat related to $\alpha_{2\mu}$-globulin nephropathy are not relevant to humans (21). Also, the IARC has determined that chemicals producing tumors by this mode of action do not pose a risk to humans (22). In addition, IARC has found that other agents producing bladder tumors involving calcium phosphate-containing precipitate formation, such as saccharin and certain chemicals producing thyroid follicular-cell neoplasms, do not pose a risk to humans.

The future of risk assessment lies in the development of better epidemiology data and the diversification of rodent to human extrapolation methods based upon sound scientific data regarding mode of action. Consequently, more and more emphasis is being placed on the generation of data regarding cancer mechanisms for use in quantitative risk assessment. As additional data becomes available, the use of chemical-specific information that replaces the traditional default assumptions will provide a enhanced scientific certainty in the risk assessment process.

REFERENCES

1. Armitage P, Doll R. The age distribution of cancer and multistage theory of carcinogenesis. Br J Cancer 1954; 8:1–12.
2. National Research Council. Risk Assessment in the Federal Government: Managing the Process. Washington, DC: National Academy Press, 1983.
3. US Environmental Protection Agency. Guidelines for carcinogen risk assessment. Fed Reg 1986; 41:33992–34005.
4. Wiltse J, Dellarco VL. US Environmental Protection Agency guidelines for carcinogen risk assessment: past and future. Mutat Res 1996; 365:3–15.
5. US Environmental Protection Agency. Proposed guidelines for carcinogen risk assessment. Fed Reg 1996; 61:17960–18011.
6. International Expert Panel on Carcinogen Risk Assessment. The use of mechanistic data in the risk assessments of ten chemicals: an introduction to the chemical-specific reviews. Pharmacol Ther 1996; 71:1–5.
7. Whysner J, Williams GM. D-Limonene mechanistic data and risk assessment: absolute species-specific cytotoxicity, enhanced cell proliferation and tumor promotion. Pharmacol Ther 1996; 71:137–151.
8. Whysner J, Williams GM. Butylated hydroxyanisole mechanistic data and risk assessment: conditional specific-specific cytotoxicity, enhanced cell proliferation and tumor promotion. Pharmacol Ther 1996; 71:137–151.
9. Whysner J, Williams GM. Saccharin mechanistic data and risk assessment: urine composition, enhanced cell proliferation and tumor promotion. Pharmacol Ther 1996; 71:225–252.
10. International Agency for Research on Cancer. IARC Monographs on the Evaluation of the Carcinogenic Risks to Humans, Monograph 73, 2000.
11. Gaylor DW, Axelrad JA, Brown RP, Cavagnaro JA, Cyr WH, Hulebak KL, Lorentzen RJ, Miller MA, Mulligan LT, Schwetz BA. Health risk assessment practices in the US Food and Drug Administration. Regul Toxicol Pharmacol 1997; 26:307–321.
12. Whysner J, Williams GM. International cancer risk assessment: the impact of biologic mechanisms. Regul Toxicol Pharmacol 1992; 15:41–50.
13. Travis CC, White RK. Interspecific scaling of toxicity data. Risk Anal 1988; 8:119–125.
14. US Environmental Protection Agency. Guidelines for exposure assessment. Fed Reg 1992; 57:22888–22938.

15. Environmental Protection Agency. Risk Assessment Guidance for Superfund. Vol. 1. Human Health Evaluation Manual. Part A. EPA/540/1-89/002, 1989.
16. US Environmental Protection Agency. A Descriptive Guide to Risk Assessment Methodologies for Toxic Air Pollutants. EPA-453/R-93-038, Office of Air Quality, 1993.
17. Food Safety Council. Quantitative risk assessment. Fd Cosmet Toxicol 1980; 18:711-734.
18. Rodricks JV, Brett SM, Wrenn GC. Significant risk decisions in Federal regulatory agencies. Regul Toxicol Pharmacol 1987; 7:307-320.
19. Travis CC, Crouch EAC, Wilson R, Klema ED. Cancer risk management: a review of 132 regulatory decisions. Environ Sci Technol 1987; 21:415-420.
20. Gaylor DW, Kodell RL, Chen JJ, Krewski D. A unified approach to risk assessment for cancer and noncancer endpoints based on benchmark doses and uncertainty/safety factors. Regul Toxicol Pharmacol 1999; 29:151-157.
21. Baetcke KP, Hard GC, Rodgers IS, McGaughy RE, Tahan LM . Alpha$_{2u}$-Globulin: Association with Chemically Induced Renal Toxicity and Neoplasia in the Male Rat. Washington, DC: Risk Assessment Forum, US Environmental Protection Agency, 1991.
22. Capen C, Dybing E, Rice J, Wilbourn J, eds. Species Differences in Thyroid, Kidney and Urinary Bladder Carcinogenesis, IARC Scientific Publications No. 147. Lyon, France: IARC, 1998.

7

Cancer Risk Assessment I: How Regulatory Agencies Determine What Is a Carcinogen

Jerry M. Rice*

Department of Oncology, Lombardi Comprehensive Cancer Center, Georgetown University, Washington, D.C., U.S.A.

1. INTRODUCTION

The first stage in cancer risk assessment is the process known as carcinogenic hazard identification. This is the qualitative determination that a substance, complex mixture, agent, or exposure is capable of causing cancer in humans, that is, it is a carcinogen.

An agent is a carcinogen if exposure to it causes an increased incidence of malignant neoplasms at one or more anatomic sites in humans, experimental animals, or both. In experimental animal studies, carcinogenicity may also be indicated by increased multiplicity or accelerated appearance of neoplasms. Known human carcinogens include certain infectious agents; all forms of ionizing radiation; and a wide variety of chemical agents and mixtures, some of which occur naturally and some of which are produced by human activities. Carcinogens rarely increase the frequency of tumors at all organ sites, in either humans or experimental animals. Most carcinogens cause tumors at a single site or at a limited number of sites, which in the

*Chief (Emeritus), IARC Monographs Programme, International Agency for Research on Cancer, Lyon, France.

case of chemicals is largely determined by pathways of metabolism and by the routes of exposure, which affect the dose of active carcinogen delivered to various tissues. Inorganic arsenic, for example, causes human skin cancer when taken in medicinals by ingestion; lung cancer when inhaled under occupational circumstances such as smelting of metal-containing ores; and both of the above plus cancers of the urinary tract and certain other internal organs when present at high concentrations in drinking water (1).

Essentially, all neoplasms occur at some "natural" or "background" frequency. Some human neoplasms are so regularly associated with exposure to a specific agent that diagnosis of a case automatically raises the suspicion that the patient was exposed to a known carcinogen (e.g., mesothelioma suggests previous exposure to asbestos; clear-cell carcinoma of the female reproductive tract suggests prenatal exposure to diethylstilbestrol), but these are exceptions. For most kinds of tumors, at nearly all anatomic sites, it is rarely possible, on the basis of either morphological or molecular characteristics of an individual neoplasm that has been caused by a specific agent, to distinguish it reliably from other cancers of the same kind that may occur naturally or as a result of concurrent exposure to some other carcinogen. This applies to both humans and experimental animals. Accordingly, conclusions regarding causality are almost always based on statistical analyses of tumor frequencies in exposed vs. nonexposed populations. Genetical, molecular, or morphological markers of exposure to a specific carcinogen may sometimes indicate that a specific case of cancer has resulted from exposure to a specific agent (e.g., base-pair-specific mutation of the tumor suppressor gene $TP53$ can implicate exposure to aflatoxin B_1 in human hepatocellular carcinoma). At present, for chemicals and chemical mixtures this situation is the exception rather than the rule.

For suspect agents that are already present in the environment, data that are relevant for carcinogenic hazard identification may be available in the international scientific literature. These may include epidemiological studies of health effects, including cancer experience, in exposed human populations. When such studies exist, they are of primary interest for assessing possible carcinogenic hazard. In the case of widely studied agents or exposures (e.g., ionizing radiation, human papillomaviruses, tobacco use) the database for carcinogenic hazard identification may be extremely robust, and is often strengthened by the existence of studies from several different laboratories or study groups. This allows assessment of the consistency of findings among different studies. Consistently positive findings from several independent studies are strong evidence that a carcinogenic hazard truly exists. However, even for many agents whose existence in the environment has been recognized for decades, epidemiological studies that are adequate to establish whether a given substance is or probably is not a human carcinogen do not exist. Those studies that do exist often are limited by the fact that most environmental exposures are not "pure" exposures to a single substance (e.g., 1-nitropyrene), but rather to multiple suspect substances or to complex mixtures of substances (e.g., to many different nitro-polynuclear aromatic hydrocarbons and other substances that occur together in diesel engine exhaust). In such cases additional data are needed to decide whether a specific substance is in fact a carcinogen.

Carcinogenicity, like most other forms of toxicity, increases in severity with increasing duration and intensity of exposure. However, the relative potencies of various carcinogens are highly variable. Low levels of exposure, especially to weak carcinogens, may not be detectable, either by epidemiological methods in human populations or by increased tumor frequency in bioassays in experimental animals. For this reason, negative epidemiological and experimental findings must be treated with caution when there are strong reasons to suspect that an agent may be carcinogenic, as when a substance is markedly similar in chemical structure to known carcinogens, or if it possesses biological properties that are often associated with carcinogenicity, such as mutagenicity in mammalian or nonmammalian cells and organisms. The most convincing data for establishing carcinogenicity are those that show a statistically significant increasing trend in tumor incidence with increasing intensity and duration of exposure, as well as statistically significantly increased incidences of tumors in populations that have been exposed to doses above the minimum level of detection.

A broadly based data set on which carcinogenic hazard identification can be based includes:

- Epidemiological studies
- Carcinogenicity bioassays in laboratory animals (where appropriate)
- Studies of genetical and related effects in laboratory animals and in human cells, or even in exposed humans
- Studies of mode(s) of carcinogenic action of the agent.

Commonly, however, decisions on whether to treat a substance as a carcinogen must be taken on the basis of incomplete data sets, which lack data from one or more of these categories. For example, for truly novel substances, such as new agricultural chemicals (e.g., herbicides or insecticides) or new drugs, there is no epidemiology. The basis for carcinogenic hazard identification then consists of carcinogenicity studies in experimental animals, generally rats and conventional and/or genetically engineered mice, together with studies on the metabolism of the agent, its genetical and related effects in experimental animals in vivo and in microorganisms, animal cells, and often human cells in vitro. There may also be studies on the mode of action of the agent as a carcinogen in animals. Such studies will usually have been conducted, or contracted for, by a single commercial entity for purposes of compliance with regulatory requirements. Results of such studies that are submitted to regulatory agencies are often unpublished and are usually regarded by the sponsor as proprietary information, i.e., trade secrets, that may never be published in a scientific journal. The database for evaluation of new chemicals as possible carcinogens may therefore be much more limited, and previous scientific peer review much less vigorous, than for environmental agents that have been studied more widely.

Agencies that have responsibilities for carcinogenic hazard identification exist in several international organizations, including the Commission of the European Union and the World Health Organization (WHO). Such agencies also exist in many individual countries, at the national level and sometimes also within the governments of constituent geopolitical units, such as individual states of the United states of America (e.g., California). Generally, all such agencies work from the same basic kinds of data, but they differ fundamentally in whether they evaluate:

- Agents and exposures that already exist in the human environment or
- Novel substances proposed for introduction into that environment.

Within the WHO, an internationally recognized carcinogen identification program is conducted by the International Agency for Research on Cancer (IARC). The *IARC Monographs on the Evaluation of Carcinogenic Risks to Humans* is an international, interdisciplinary approach to carcinogenic hazard identification. *Monographs* evaluations are assessments of the strength of the published scientific evidence for the existence of an environmental carcinogenic hazard to humans, but they are qualitative rather than quantitative in nature and do not address issues of relative carcinogenic potency. Also, the *Monographs* are confined to published scientific data, and therefore do not evaluate novel agents about which only proprietary data exist. The *Monographs* are published as a basis for cancer prevention initiatives, which are not limited to regulation. The IARC is not a regulatory agency, and the *Monographs* explicitly avoid any recommendation regarding regulation or legislation. The *Monographs* are widely consulted by regulatory agencies worldwide, however, and the series can serve as a model for how regulatory agencies determine what is a carcinogen, and how different kinds of data are used to make carcinogenic hazard identifications. The criteria applied, and some examples of overall evaluations based on those criteria, are summarized in the following pages.

2. *IARC MONOGRAPHS* IDENTIFICATIONS OF CARCINOGENIC HAZARD

During the period 1972–2002 a total of 888 agents and exposure circumstances have been reviewed by the IARC Monographs Programme in Volumes 1–84 of the series. Many have been evaluated more than once as new data have become available in the scientific literature. Because the nature and the strength of published evidence for carcinogenicity vary greatly from one agent or exposure circumstance to another, in most cases it is not possible to conclude definitively whether a given agent or exposure is either definitely a human carcinogen or is probably not one. Of these 888 agents and exposure circumstances, only 89 are currently classified as definitely carcinogenic to humans. In 1987 a classification system was introduced (2) which stratifies agents according to the strength of the total evidence for carcinogenicity to humans. This evidence may include epidemiological studies of cancer risk in humans; bioassays for carcinogenicity in experimental animals; and other relevant data of various kinds that may modify the conclusions that would be drawn on the basis of epidemiology and/or bioassays alone.

2.1. Epidemiological Studies

Epidemiological Studies to assess the possibly increased risks of cancer in exposed humans are critically reviewed, and the strength of that evidence is evaluated according to the criteria listed in Table 1. The *IARC Monographs* criteria require specific, critical consideration of the possibility that the results of each published study may be affected by chance, bias or confounding.

The strength of an association between an exposure and a disease outcome, and the possible role of chance are estimated by standard statistical methods. These methods commonly report the strength of an association as an odds ratio, relative risk, standardized mortality ratio, or other measurement that presents the observed incidence of disease in a study population relative to that in an unexposed control population. For example,

Table 1 IARC Criteria for Strength of Evidence for Increased Cancer Risk in Exposed Humans

---

Sufficient—a positive relationship has been established between exposure to the agent and increased risk of cancer in humans, in which chance, bias, and confounding can be ruled out with reasonable confidence.

Limited—a positive relationship has been observed between exposure to the agent and human cancer for which a causal association is credible, but chance, bias, and confounding cannot be ruled out with reasonable confidence.

Inadequate—available studies are of insufficient quality, consistency, or statistical power to permit a conclusion regarding presence or absence of a causal association (or no data are available).

Evidence suggesting lack of carcinogenicity—several adequate studies covering the full range of exposures encountered by humans are mutually consistent in showing no positive association between exposure to the agent and human cancer, at any observed level of exposure.

---

a ratio of 5.0 indicates that there were five times as many cases of the disease in question among members of the study population as among controls. Whether this ratio is consistent with simple chance association or not is indicated by the calculated confidence interval surrounding the point estimate; in this hypothetical case, a 95% confidence interval of 2.8–7.7 would strongly support a significant association. On the other hand, a confidence interval of 0.3–15 for the same ratio would indicate that the ratio is not statistically significant and is likely due to chance. Any confidence interval that includes unity indicates lack of statistical significance at the level specified.

In epidemiology, *bias* refers to "systematic errors in the way subjects are selected or followed up, or in the way information was obtained from them. *Confounding* occurs when an estimate of the association between an exposure [e.g., occupational exposure to mineral dusts containing crystalline silica] and an outcome [e.g., lung cancer] is mixed up with the real effect of another exposure [e.g., cigarette smoking] on the same outcome, the two exposures being correlated" (3).

In general, the criteria for causality in epidemiological studies are those articulated by Hill (4) (Table 2). A comment is in order, however, on the criterion of biological plausibility. What is considered biologically plausible at any given point in time depends on the state of knowledge at that time. Observations of increased cancer rates in certain populations have often been made before the cause was understood. A striking example is that of lung

Table 2   Hill Criteria for Causality

Temporal relationship: for an exposure to be the cause of a disease, it has to precede its biological onset.
Biological plausibility: the association is more likely to be causal if it is consistent with other biological knowledge.
Consistency: the association is more likely to be causal if similar results have been found in different populations (however, a lack of consistency does not exclude a causal association).
Strength: the stronger the association—the greater the relative measure of effect—the more likely it is to reflect a true causal association.
Exposure–response relationship: further evidence is provided if increasing levels of exposure are associated with increasing incidence of disease.
Specificity: if a particular exposure increases the risk of a certain disease, but not the risk of other diseases, this provides evidence favoring a cause–effect relationship.
Reversibility: when the removal of a possible cause results in a reduced incidence of the disease, the likelihood that the association is causal is strengthened.
Coherence: the putative cause–effect relationship should not seriously conflict with the natural history and biology of the disease.

Source: From Hill (4), modified by Silva (3).

cancer among hard-rock underground miners in Europe (5), which was a mystery when first described but is now generally attributed to high levels of radon in the atmosphere in poorly ventilated mines. This observation preceded the discovery of radioactivity, and of radon, by more than a decade.

Credible evaluation of chance, bias, and confounding and application of the Hill criteria to establish causality require considerable experience. For further details, a textbook (3) or a treatise (6) on cancer epidemiology should be consulted.

2.2. Bioassay Data for Carcinogenicity in Experimental Animals

Bioassay data for carcinogenicity in experimental animals (generally rats and mice) are similarly evaluated according to the criteria listed in Table 3. For sufficiency of evidence, these criteria emphasize reproducibility of outcomes among studies and malignant tumors, evaluated and confirmed histologically, as experimental findings. As all kinds of tumors do occur naturally in untreated animals, at frequencies that can range from 1% or less (e.g., tumors of the brain or intestine in rats) to 50% or more, careful quantification of tumors in treated animals and untreated controls and proper statistical evaluation of the results is essential.

In the absence of adequate data in humans, in general IARC considers that "it is biologically plausible and prudent to regard agents for which there is sufficient evidence of carcinogenicity in experimental animals as if they

Table 3 IARC Criteria for Strength of Evidence for Carcinogenicity in Experimental Animals

---

Sufficient—a causal relationship has been established between exposure to the agent and increased incidence of malignant neoplasms, or an appropriate combination of benign and malignant neoplasms, in two or more species or in two or more independent studies in one species, conducted at different times or in different laboratories or under different protocols; exceptionally, a single study in one species may suffice when malignant neoplasms occur to an unusual degree with regard to incidence, site, tumor type, or age at onset.

Limited—data suggest a carcinogenic effect, but consist of a single experiment; or questions regarding adequacy of design, conduct, or interpretation of the studies are unresolved; or the effect is limited to benign tumors or lesions of uncertain neoplastic potential only, or to certain neoplasms that may occur spontaneously in high incidences in certain strains.

Inadequate—the studies cannot be interpreted as showing either presence or absence of a carcinogenic effect because of major qualitative or quantitative limitations; or no data are available.

Evidence suggesting lack of carcinogenicity—adequate studies in at least two species are negative, within the limits of the tests used.

---

presented a carcinogenic risk to humans." However, not all tumors in experimental animals are considered equally predictive of cancer hazard to humans. Some kinds of tumors occur in such high and variable incidence in the inbred strains of mice and rats that are conventionally used in bioassays (e.g., Leydig cell tumors of the testis in male Fischer 344 rats, hepatocellular tumors in male mice of many inbred strains and their F_1 hybrids) that when an apparent increase in tumor frequency in treated animals is limited to these kinds of tumors, the evidence for carcinogenicity may be considered suggestive ("limited" in the IARC vocabulary) rather than conclusive.

It is now clearly established that tumors can be induced in certain tissues through several distinct mechanisms of carcinogenic action, and that not all these mechanisms operate in all species. Animal carcinogenicity data may not predict carcinogenic risk to humans when tumors are induced in animals by a mechanism of carcinogenicity that does not operate in humans. This subject is discussed further below, and in the Appendix, and represents another exception to the basic principle that carcinogenicity in experimental animals predicts human cancer risk.

2.3. Other Relevant Data

These are data other than tumor incidence in humans and in experimental animals, and include how a substance is metabolized in experimental animals and in humans, whether the substance and/or its metabolites are genotoxic, manifestations of toxicity other than carcinogenicity, and the mode of action by which the substance acts as a carcinogen.

2.4. Overall Evaluations of Carcinogenicity

Evidence from epidemiological and experimental studies is finally combined with other relevant data to produce an overall qualitative evaluation and classification in one of the five groups defined in Table 4. This table reflects criteria that were introduced in 1992 for use of "other relevant data" in overall evaluations of carcinogenicity (7). Carcinogenic hazard identifications formulated on the basis of bioassay data in rodents can be either strengthened or weakened by additional information on the mode of action of the carcinogen in animals.

As new data are published, agents are re-evaluated. When the strength of the total evidence for carcinogenicity of an agent changes as a result of new data, the classification of the agent may also change. All evaluations, and narrative summaries of the supporting data, are available in the Internet at http://monographs.iarc.fr.

Some representative examples of *IARC Monographs* evaluations and classifications at various levels of evidence are presented in the sections that follow. These are intended to illustrate how the IARC criteria have been applied to a variety of substances and exposures, but are necessarily

Table 4 *IARC Monographs* Overall Evaluations of Carcinogenicity to Humans

Group 1—carcinogenic to humans
  Sufficient epidemiological evidence of increased risk of cancer in exposed
    humans; exceptionally, human evidence that is less than sufficient, but is
    supported by sufficient evidence of carcinogenicity in experimental animals
    together with strong evidence in exposed humans that the agent acts through
    a relevant mechanism of carcinogenicity
Group 2A—probably carcinogenic to humans
  Limited epidemiological evidence of increased cancer risk in humans, but sufficient
    evidence of carcinogenicity in experimental animals; or inadequate evidence in
    humans but sufficient evidence in experimental animals, together with strong
    evidence that the carcinogenic mechanism also operates in humans
Group 2B—possibly carcinogenic to humans
  Inadequate evidence in humans but sufficient evidence of carcinogenicity in
    experimental animals; or inadequate evidence in humans but limited evidence in
    animals supported by other relevant data
Group 3—not classifiable as to carcinogenicity to humans
  Inadequate evidence in humans and less than sufficient evidence in animals;
    exceptionally, agents for which there is inadequate evidence in humans but
    sufficient evidence in animals may be placed in this category when there is strong
    evidence that the mechanism of carcinogenicity does not operate in humans
Group 4—probably not carcinogenic to humans
  Evidence suggesting lack of carcinogenicity in both humans and animals; or
    inadequate evidence in humans, and evidence suggesting lack of carcinogenicity
    in experimental animals, consistently and strongly supported by a broad range
    of other relevant data

abbreviated. The serious student of the process of carcinogenic hazard identification will find numerous additional examples in the *Monographs* database at the above website.

3. IARC GROUP 1—CARCINOGENIC TO HUMANS

When epidemiological evidence of increased cancer risk in exposed humans
is *sufficient*, according to the definition given in Table 1, the agent is classified in Group 1—*carcinogenic to humans*. Even without any further information about the mode of action of the agent, such carcinogenic hazard
identifications carry a very high level of certainty. In rare cases where the
evidence for increased cancer risk is less than sufficient but other relevant
data including carcinogenicity in experimental animals are compelling, an
agent may also be classified in Group 1. Some examples of IARC Group 1
carcinogens are presented in Table 5.

Table 5 Some *IARC Monographs* Evaluations from Group 1—Carcinogenic to Humans[a]

Sufficient evidence in both exposed humans and experimental animals
Vinyl chloride (8,9)
 Sufficient evidence of angiosarcoma of the liver and possibly other kinds of
  tumors at other sites in occupationally exposed chemical workers
 Sufficient evidence in experimental animals: angiosarcoma of liver
  and at other sites, also tumors of lung, mammary gland, external auditory
  canal (Zymbal's gland), and kidney in mice and rats
2-Naphthylamine (10,11)
 Sufficient evidence in humans: urinary bladder carcinomas in occupationally
  exposed chemical workers
 Sufficient evidence in experimental animals other than standard bioassay
  species: hepatocellular tumors in mice; marginal effects in rats; urinary
  bladder carcinomas in dogs, monkeys, and Syrian golden hamsters
Sufficient evidence in exposed humans; less than sufficient evidence or no
data in experimental animals
Smokeless tobacco products (12,13)
 Sufficient evidence of oral cancers in individuals who chew tobacco
Analgesic mixtures containing phenacetin (14,15)
 Sufficient evidence of urothelial carcinomas of renal pelvis and urinary
  bladder in patients who ingested large quantities of phenacetin-containing
  analgesics
 Although phenacetin alone causes urinary tract tumors in rats and mice, the
  combination of phenacetin with aspirin and caffeine (formerly a standard
  formulation for over-the-counter analgesics) was tested in animals only once,
  with negative results in mice; very few urinary tract tumors were seen in rats,
  their incidence was not statistically significant.
Less than sufficient evidence in humans, sufficient evidence in experimental animals,
and strong support from other relevant data
Ethylene oxide (16,17)
 Limited evidence of increased risk of lymphoid and hematopoietic neoplasms in
  workers using ethylene oxide as a sterilant
 Sufficient evidence that ethylene oxide induced brain tumors, peritoneal
  mesotheliomas, and other tumors in rats, and lung and Harderian gland
  tumors in mice plus lymphomas in female mice when given by inhalation
 Other relevant data include evidence that ethylene oxide is a genotoxic chemical
  that causes increased frequencies of chromosomal aberrations in lymphocytes
  and micronuclei in bone marrow cells of exposed workers, forms DNA and
  hemoglobin adducts, and is a powerful mutagen and clastogen at all
  phylogenetic levels.
2,3,7,8-Tetrachlorodibenzo-*p*-dioxin (TCDD) (18)
 Limited evidence of slight increased risk of all cancers combined (relative
  risk = 1.4) in workers most highly exposed in industrial accidents
 Sufficient evidence for carcinogenicity in both mice and rats at various sites,

---

(Continued)

Table 5 Some *IARC Monographs* Evaluations from Group 1—Carcinogenic to Humans[a] (*Continued*)

including thyroid, liver, skin, oral cavity, lung, and soft connective tissues

Other relevant data supporting the concept that TCDD acts by binding to human and rodent Ah receptors, which are transcription factors, rather than by genotoxic effects

Neutron radiation (19)

Inadequate evidence in humans

Sufficient evidence for induction of leukemia and of ovarian, mammary, lung, and liver tumors in mice, and at various sites in rats, rabbits, dogs, and Rhesus monkeys

Gross chromosomal aberrations are induced in lymphocytes of people exposed to neutrons, and the spectrum of DNA damage induced by neutrons is similar to that of X rays (for which evidence of carcinogenicity to humans is sufficient), but contains more of the more serious, less readily reparable types of damage.

[a]Examples given are illustrative only and are not a comprehensive listing. For a complete and regularly updated listing of agents evaluated by the IARC Monographs Programme, and for narrative summaries of the evidence supporting each evaluation, consult the Internet posting at http://monographs.iarc.fr.

For a significant number of agents, there is sufficient evidence of carcinogenicity in both exposed humans and experimental animals. In Table 5 vinyl chloride and 2-naphthylamine are examples of such agents. Both of these are (or were, in the case of 2-naphthylamine) industrial chemicals, and human risk was from occupational exposures, but there are many other IARC Group 1 agents that do not necessarily present primarily occupational hazards. Vinyl chloride causes one relatively rare kind of tumor, hepatic angiosarcoma, in both humans and experimental animals, as well as tumors at additional sites in rodents. This overlapping tumor spectrum is not always seen; in fact, it is relatively uncommon for tumor sites in rats and mice to be the same in response to a given carcinogen, or to overlap with cancer sites in humans where those are known. For example, 2-naphthylamine is one of the most potent human urinary bladder carcinogens known, but in mice it causes only hepatocellular tumors (*limited* evidence of carcinogenicity!), and it has only marginal carcinogenic effects in rats. In certain other species that are not commonly used in bioassays, 2-naphthylamine induces bladder tumors like those seen in humans, but if the only data for carcinogenic hazard of 2-naphthylamine that were available at the time of evaluation had been conventional bioassays in rats and mice, and this compound had not yet been used industrially, it would almost certainly not have been identified as a carcinogen. Bioassays in rats and mice are very useful for identifying possible human carcinogens, but they are not infallible. When positive, they should not be overinterpreted as necessarily predicting what kind of tumor a substance would cause in a human being.

Agents can also be placed in IARC Group 1 on the strength of sufficient evidence for cancer causation in humans only. Supporting bioassays
for carcinogenicity in experimental animals are not necessary for classification in Group 1. Agents and exposures for which there are only human data
include certain biological agents that have a host range that is restricted to
humans only, and occupational circumstances or personal or cultural habits
that cannot be tested in experimental animals. Rats, for example, obsti-
nately refuse to chew tobacco, and the carcinogenicity of "tobacco habits
other than smoking" depends solely on epidemiological studies of humans
who *do* chew tobacco (12,13).

Analgesic mixtures containing phenacetin, taken as over-the-counter
analgesics, can clearly cause urothelial tumors in humans when taken in
excessive quantities for prolonged periods. The phenacetin in the mixture
(which by itself causes urothelial tumors when fed to rats in bioassays) is
almost certainly responsible for this effect, but there is no direct evidence
for this, as phenacetin *alone* has not been taken by humans for pain relief.
Accordingly, while there is *sufficient evidence* in humans that the mixture
is carcinogenic, there is only *limited evidence* for the carcinogenicity to
humans of phenacetin itself, which is therefore classified in Group 2A (see
Table 6).

Ethylene oxide and neutron radiation are two examples of agents that
are classified as human carcinogens, but with only *limited evidence* of
increased cancer risk in exposed humans (ethylene oxide) or even *inadequate
evidence* (neutrons). In both cases, animal carcinogenicity data are convincing, and other relevant data supporting genetical damage as a mode of
action are compelling.

2,3,7,8-Tetrachlorodibenzo-*p*-dioxin (TCDD) is an example of a
compound that is carcinogenic, not by a genotoxic mechanism, but by interaction with a cellular receptor. Other examples of receptor-based carcinogens are natural and synthetic estrogens.

4. IARC GROUP 2A—PROBABLY CARCINOGENIC
TO HUMANS

Agents which are carcinogenic in experimental animals and for which there
are also certain kinds of supplementary data may be classified in Group
2A—*probably carcinogenic to humans* (Table 6). Such supplementary data
may consist of *limited evidence,* of cancer in exposed humans, as in the case
of phenacetin, or may include various kinds of experimental data, for example, on genetical and related effects of an agent in microbial and mammalian
cells and in experimental animals in vivo (as for acrylamide). Certain kinds
of exposures that are not amenable to testing in experimental animals (for
example, occupational exposures in petroleum refining) may be classified

Table 6   Some *IARC Monographs* Evaluations in Group 2A—Probably
Carcinogenic to Humans

Limited evidence in exposed humans but sufficient evidence in experimental animals
   Phenacetin (14,15)
      Limited evidence of urothelial tumors of kidney and urinary bladder in patients
         who took mixtures containing phenacetin, but no data are available on the
         possible carcinogenic effects of phenacetin alone
      Sufficient evidence for tumors of urinary tract in experimental rats and mice,
         and of the nasal cavity in rats
Limited evidence in exposed humans; no data in experimental animals
   Occupational exposures in petroleum refining (20)
      Limited evidence that working in petroleum refineries entails increased risk of
         skin cancer and leukemia
      Other relevant data include the fact that various petroleum fractions are
         carcinogenic in experimental animals and that benzene and certain mineral oils
         present in or derived from petroleum are carcinogenic to humans
Inadequate evidence or no data in humans, sufficient evidence in experimental animals,
and strong support from other relevant data
   Acrylamide (17)
      No consistent evidence of increased cancer risk at any site in workers engaged in
         acrylamide manufacture (no data on possible cancer risk from exposures to
         acrylamide in foods)
      Sufficient evidence of cancers at multiple sites in rats treated with acrylamide,
         including thyroid, mesothelium, brain, and other sites
      Other relevant data: biotransformation of acrylamide to a genotoxic epoxide
         metabolite, glycidamide, occurs both in rodent species and in humans

---

in Group 2A based only on *limited evidence* for increased cancer risks in
exposed humans when other relevant data support this evaluation.

5.   IARC GROUP 2B—POSSIBLY CARCINOGENIC
TO HUMANS

Carcinogenic hazard identifications are frequently made only on the basis of
empirical carcinogenicity data in experimental animals, when there are no
data on human exposures and nothing else is known about the mode of
action of the agent. When this is the only information available, the identification is generally qualified as having a lower level of certainty than human
data. Agents for which there is *sufficient evidence* of carcinogenicity in
experimental animals by the criteria of Table 3, but for which there are
few or no other data, are classified in Group 2B as *possibly carcinogenic
to humans* (Table 7).

   For some chemicals, such as 1,2-epoxybutane, bioassay data are too
weak to meet the criteria for sufficient evidence of carcinogenicity in

Table 7   Some Representative *IARC Monographs* Evaluations from Group 2B—
Possibly Carcinogenic to Animals

Inadequate evidence or no data in humans; sufficient evidence in experimental animals
  Acrylonitrile (21)[a]
    Inadequate evidence in humans; no consistent evidence of increased lung or
      other cancer risk in exposed workers
    Sufficient evidence (brain, mammary gland, liver, and other tumors) in rats
      exposed by inhalation, in several independent studies
  Naphthalene (22)
    No data in exposed humans
    Olfactory carcinomas in rats on inhalation; lung tumors in mice
Less than sufficient evidence in experimental animals, but support from other
relevant data
  1,2-Epoxybutane (23)
    No data on exposed humans
    Limited evidence in experimental animals: nasal adenomas (benign tumors) and
      a low incidence of lung tumors including both adenomas and carcinomas in
      rats on inhalation; no significant carcinogenic effect in mice
    Other relevant data: direct-acting alkylating agent that is mutagenic in a variety
      of test systems
Limited evidence in humans; no evidence of carcinogenicity in experimental animals
  Extremely low-frequency magnetic fields (24)
    Limited evidence in humans: consistent excess risk of childhood leukemia in
      households where magnetic fields are highest
    No support of causality from either bioassays in experimental animals or data
      on putative mechanism of carcinogenic action

[a]See also the previous classification in Group 2A, in part on the basis of limited evidence of
increased lung cancer risk in occupationally exposed workers that was not confirmed by subsequent epidemiological studies with greater statistical power (25).

animals, but other relevant data support the likelihood that the agent is
potentially carcinogenic. This is especially common when the agent or its
metabolites are genotoxic. However, in the Monographs Programme, there
must be at least some empirical evidence of carcinogenicity or an agent
would not be placed in Group 2B—and, in fact, would not be selected for
evaluation in the first place.

Exposures and agents may also be classified in Group 2B on the basis
of limited epidemiological data alone, in the absence of bioassay data in
experimental animals or when the bioassays are negative. Extremely low-
frequency magnetic fields are an example; the only evidence that these fields
may be causally related to human cancer is a consistent, statistically significant increased incidence of childhood leukemia in households where such
fields are high. It was the consistency of this finding in several independent
studies that determined the outcome of *limited*, rather than *inadequate*,

evidence for increased cancer risk in exposed humans. This is also a good example of a case where the criterion of biological plausibility was considered inapplicable by the IARC Working Group (24).

6. IARC GROUP 3—NOT CLASSIFIABLE AS TO CARCINOGENICITY TO HUMANS

An agent is placed in Group 3 when there are no epidemiological data, or published studies provide inadequate evidence for increased cancer risk in humans, and experimental animal data are less than sufficient. More than half of all the agents ever evaluated by the IARC Monographs Programme are in Group 3, most of them because of various limitations in the available data.

Agents may also be placed in Group 3 when experimental carcinogenicity data are sufficient but the mechanism of carcinogenicity in animals is considered not to predict human risk. Of most practical importance are mechanisms that operate in experimental rodent species to cause tumors in a specific tissue, but that because of physiological differences between rodent species and humans do not lead to human cancer. Tumors can arise in certain tissues in rodents—sometimes in a single sex of a single species—by such "rodent-specific" mechanisms. The most important and best characterized of these modes of action are summarized in Table 8. Considerations of how such data should be used in carcinogenic hazard identification are summarized in the Appendix; these are condensed from the

Table 8 Mechanisms/Modes of Carcinogenic Action That Occur in One or Both Sexes of One or More Species of Rodents, but Are Considered Not to Predict Carcinogenic Risk to Humans

Species	Organ site	Mechanism/mode of carcinogenic action
Rat, mouse	Thyroid follicular epithelium	Thyroid-stimulating hormone (TSH) dysregulation[a]
Rat (males only)	Renal cortical epithelium	$á_2$-Urinary globulin nephropathy[a]
Rat	Urinary bladder	Urinary calculus formation[ab]
Rat	Urinary bladder	Calcium phosphate-containing urinary precipitates[a]
Rat, mouse	Liver	Peroxisome proliferation[c]

[a]For details see Capen et al. (26).
[b]Individuals with urinary tract stones do have a small excess risk of urothelial cancers; this mode of carcinogenic action in rodents is considered not to predict human risk at levels of exposure where urinary calculi do not form.
[c]For details see IARC (27).

Table 9   Some *IARC Monographs* Evaluations of Chemicals That are Carcinogenic
to Experimental Animals by Modes of Action Listed in Table 8, and Placed by the
IARC Monographs in Group 3—Not Classifiable as to Carcinogenicity to Humans

Chemical	Target tissue and mechanism of carcinogenicity in rodents	Reference
Saccharin and its salts	Rat urinary bladder: calcium phosphate-containing urinary precipitates	28
Melamine	Rat urinary bladder: urinary calculi	29
d-Limonene	Rat kidney (males only): á$_2$-urinary globulin nephropathy	30
Ethylene thiourea	Rat and mouse thyroid follicular epithelium: TSH dysregulation	31
Di (2-ethylhexyl) phthalate (DEHP)	Rat and mouse liver parenchyma: peroxisome proliferation	32

consensus statements from IARC publications on these subjects (26,27). The
full consensus statements can be found at http://monographs.iarc.fr.

Some examples of *IARC Monographs* evaluations that have been made
on the basis of such mechanistic data are listed in Table 9.

7.   IARC GROUP 4—PROBABLY NOT CARCINOGENIC TO HUMANS

When regulatory agencies conclude that an agent or exposure is not carcinogenic, typically no action is taken to broadcast such findings. The IARC
selects agents for evaluation on the basis of two criteria: there must be evidence or suspicion of carcinogenicity, and there must be human exposure,
but occasionally on review it is found that there is evidence suggesting lack
of carcinogenicity in humans or in experimental animals. When there are
adequate data both from epidemiological studies of exposed humans and
from bioassays in experimental animals, and both the human and the animal
data are negative, an agent may be placed in Group 4—*probably not
carcinogenic to humans*. At the present time there is only one substance,
caprolactam, in Group 4.

APPENDIX

IARC Monographs guidelines on the use of mode-of-action data for extrapolation of organ-specific rodent carcinogenicity findings to humans when
the mode of carcinogenic action in rodents does not exist in humans,

under realistic conditions of human exposures to the agent. This appendix is condensed from the consensus statements for the various mechanisms/modes of carcinogenic action originally published in Capen et al. (26) and in IARC (27).

Thyroid-Stimulating Hormone-Associated Follicular-Cell Neoplasms

Agents that lead to the development of thyroid neoplasia through an adaptive physiological mechanism belong to a different category from those that lead to neoplasia through genotoxic mechanisms or through mechanisms involving pathological responses with necrosis and repair.

Agents causing thyroid follicular-cell neoplasia in rodents solely through hormonal imbalance can be identified using the following criteria:

- There is a lack of genotoxic activity (agent and/or metabolite) based on an overall evaluation of in vitro and in vivo data
- The presence of hormone imbalance has been demonstrated under the conditions of the carcinogenicity assay
- The mechanism whereby the agent leads to hormone imbalance has been defined.

When tumors are observed both in the thyroid and at other sites, they should be evaluated separately on the basis of the modes of action of the agent.

Agents that induce thyroid follicular tumors in rodents through interference with a thyroid hormone homeostasis can, with a few exceptions, also interfere with thyroid hormone homeostasis in humans if given at a sufficient dose for a sufficient period of time. These agents can be assumed not to be carcinogenic in humans at exposure levels which do not lead to alterations in thyroid hormone homeostasis.

á$_2$-Urinary Globulin Nephropathy and Renal Cell Tumors in Male Rats

In making overall evaluations of carcinogenicity to humans, it can be concluded that production of renal cell tumors in male rats by agents that fulfill all of the following criteria for an á$_{2u}$-globulin-associated response is not predictive of carcinogenic hazard to humans:

- Lack of genotoxic activity (agent and/or metabolites) based on an overall evaluation of in vitro and in vivo data
- Male rat specificity for nephropathy and renal tumorigenicity
- Induction of the characteristic sequence of histopathological changes in shorter-term studies, of which protein droplet accumulation is obligatory

- Identification of the protein accumulating in tubule cells as $\acute{a}_{2u}$-globulin
- Reversible binding of the chemical or metabolite to $\acute{a}_{2u}$-globulin
- Induction of sustained increased cell proliferation in the renal cortex
- Similarities in dose–response relationship of the tumor outcome with the histopathological end points (protein droplets, $\acute{a}_{2u}$-globulin accumulation, cell proliferation).

In situations where an agent induces tumors at other sites in the male rat or tumors in other laboratory animals, the evidence regarding these other tumor responses should be used independently of the $\acute{a}_{2u}$-globulin-associated tumorigenicity in making the overall evaluation of carcinogenicity to humans.

Urinary Bladder Calculi and Urothelial Neoplasms of the Bladder in Rats

For chemicals producing bladder neoplasms in rats and mice as a result of calculus formation in the urinary bladder, the response cannot be considered to be species specific; thus, the tumor response is relevant to an evaluation of carcinogenicity to humans. There are quantitative differences in response between species and sexes. Calculus formation is dependent on the attainment in the urine of critical concentrations of constituent chemicals which form the calculus; therefore, the biological effects are dependent on reaching threshold concentrations for calculus formation. Microcrystalluria is often associated with calculus formation, but its relevance to species-specific mechanisms cannot be assessed.

Calcium Phosphate-Containing Urinary Precipitates and Urothelial Bladder Tumors in Rats

Calcium phosphate-containing precipitates in the urine of rats, such as those produced by the administration of high doses of some sodium salts, including sodium saccharin and sodium ascorbate, can result in the production of urinary bladder tumors. This sequence can be considered to be species and dose specific and is not known to occur in humans.

In making overall evaluations of carcinogenicity to humans, it can be concluded that the production of bladder cancer in rats via a mechanism involving calcium phosphate-containing precipitates is not predictive of carcinogenic hazard to humans, provided that the following criteria are met:

- The formation of the calcium phosphate-containing precipitate occurs under the conditions of the carcinogenicity bioassay which is positive for cancer induction
- Prevention of the formation of the urinary precipitate results in prevention of the bladder proliferative effect

- The agent (and/or metabolites) shows a lack of genotoxic activity, based on an overall evaluation of in vitro and in vivo data
- The agent being evaluated does not produce tumors at any other site in experimental animals
- There is evidence from studies in humans that precipitate formation or cancer does not occur in exposed populations.

In situations where an agent induces tumors at other sites in rats or tumors in other laboratory animals, the evidence regarding these other tumor responses should be used independently of information on tumors associated with calcium phosphate-containing precipitates in making the overall evaluation of carcinogenicity to humans.

Peroxisome Proliferation and Hepatocellular Tumors in Rats and Mice

The responses to the following questions are based on the interpretation of hepatocellular tumor induction in rats and mice, since the mechanisms of carcinogenesis have been evaluated in detail only in the liver. The available information on the mechanisms of tumor response elicited by some peroxisome proliferators in rats and mice at sites other than the liver suggests that peroxisome proliferation does not play a role in the formation of tumors at those sites.

1. *What mechanisms are critical to peroxisome proliferation?*

The evidence suggests that peroxisome proliferation in mouse and rat liver is mediated by activation of peroxisome proliferator-activated receptors, which are members of the steroid hormone receptor superfamily. Receptor activation may be a direct effect of the peroxisome proliferator or may be mediated through perturbation of lipid metabolism. Such receptors have also been identified in humans.

2. *Is peroxisome proliferation an indicator of cancer risk in rats and mice?*

There is a strong concordance between peroxisome proliferation and hepatocellular carcinogenesis in rats and mice. On the basis of a more limited database, a similar concordance is seen between hepatocellular proliferation induced by peroxisome proliferators and hepatocellular tumor induction.

3. *What are the mechanisms of carcinogenesis mediated by chemically induced peroxisome proliferation?*

Two major biological responses to peroxisome proliferators are associated with increased cancer induction in rats and mice. One is peroxisome proliferation, and the other is increased hepatocellular proliferation. The proposed mechanisms of peroxisome proliferator-induced hepatocellular carcinogenesis include oxidative stress, increased hepatocellular proliferation, and preferential growth of preneoplastic lesions. These mechanisms may not be mutually exclusive.

Hepatocellular carcinogenic peroxisome proliferators are generally inactive in assays for genotoxicity. Some such agents can cause morphological cell transformation and inhibit gap-junctional intercellular communication. These cellular effects appear to be independent of the process of peroxisome proliferation. Chemicals that induce peroxisome proliferation may have additional carcinogenic effects unrelated to that phenomenon.

4. *Does peroxisome proliferation also occur in humans, and do the mechanisms of carcinogenesis mediated by peroxisome proliferation in rats and mice also operate in humans?*

Data on the effects in humans of peroxisome proliferators are derived from studies of subjects receiving hypolipidaemic drugs and from studies of cultured human hepatocytes. The limited data in vivo suggest that therapeutic doses of hypolipidaemic agents produce little if any peroxisome proliferation in human liver. Hypolipidaemic fibrates and other chemicals that induce peroxisome proliferation in rat and mouse hepatocytes when given at high concentrations do not do so in cultured human hepatocytes.

Marginal, statistically nonsignificant increases in hepatocellular peroxisome proliferation in human liver have been reported after exposure to clofibrate, but a comparable increase in peroxisome proliferation was not associated with hepatocellular carcinogenesis in rats or mice.

5. *How can data on peroxisome proliferation be used in making overall evaluations of carcinogenicity to humans?*

Chemicals that show evidence of inducing peroxisome proliferation should be evaluated on a case-by-case basis. The evaluation of agents by independent expert groups is a matter of scientific judgement.

When the database supports the conclusion that a tumor response in mice or rats is secondary only to peroxisome proliferation, consideration could be given to modifying the overall evaluation, as described in the Preamble to the *IARC Monographs*, taking into account the following evidence:

- Information is available to exclude mechanisms of carcinogenesis other than those related to peroxisome proliferation.
- Peroxisome proliferation (increases in peroxisome volume density or fatty acid â-oxidation activity) and hepatocellular proliferation have been demonstrated under the conditions of the bioassay.
- Such effects have not been found in adequately designed and conducted investigations of human groups and systems.

REFERENCES

1. IARC. Some Drinking Water Disinfectants and Contaminants, Including Arsenic. Vol. 84. IARC Monographs on the Evaluation of Carcinogenic Risks to Humans. Lyon, France: International Agency for Research on Cancer., 2003.

2. IARC. Preamble. IARC Monographs on the Evaluation of Carcinogenic Risks of Chemicals to Humans. Lyon, France: International Agency for Research on Cancer, 1987; 1:42, 17:34.

3. Silva I. Cancer Epidemiology: Principles and Methods. Lyon, France: International Agency for Research on Cancer, 1999.

4. Hill AB. The environment and disease prevention: association or causation? Proc R Soc Med 1965; 58:295–300.

5. Harting F, Hesse W. Lung cancer, the mountain sickness of the Schneeberg Mines. Vierteljahrsschr Gerichtl Med 1879; 30, 31:102–132, 296–309, 313–337.

6. Schottenfeld D, Fraumeni J Jr. Cancer Epidemiologyand Prevention. 2nd ed. New York: Oxford University Press, 1996.

7. IARC. Preamble. Vol. 54. IARC Monographs on the Evaluation of Carcinogenic Risks of Chemicals to Humans. Lyon, France: International Agency for Research on Cancer, 1992:13–32.

8. IARC. Vinyl Chloride, Polyvinyl Chloride and Vinyl Chloride-Vinyl Acetate Co-polymers. Vol. 19. IARC Monographs on the Evaluation of Carcinogenic Risks of Chemicals to Humans. Lyon, France: International Agency for Research on Cancer, 1979:377–438.

9. IARC. Vinyl Chloride. IARC Monographs on the Evaluation of Carcinogenic Risks to Humans, Supplement 7—Overall Evaluations of Carcinogenicity: An Updating of IARC Monographs. Lyon, France: International Agency for Research on Cancer, 1987:1–42, 373–376.

10. IARC. 2-Naphthylamine. Vol. 19. IARC Monographs on the Evaluation of Carcinogenic Risks of Chemicals to Man. Lyon, France: International Agency for Research on Cancer, 1974:97–111.

11. IARC. 2-Naphthylamine. IARC Monographs on the Evaluation of Carcinogenic Risks to Humans, Supplement 7–Overall Evaluations of Carcinogenicity: An Updating of IARC Monographs. Lyon, France: International Agency for Research on Cancer, 1987:1–42, 261–263.

12. IARC. Tobacco Habits Other Than Smoking. Vol. 37. IARC Monographs on the Evaluation of Carcinogenic Risks of Chemicals to Humans. Lyon, France: International Agency for Research on Cancer, 1985:37–136.

13. IARC. Tobacco Products, Smokeless. IARC Monographs on the Evaluation of Carcinogenic Risks to Humans, Supplement 7–Overall Evaluations of Carcinogenicity: An Updating of IARC Monographs. Lyon, France: International Agency for Research on Cancer, 1987:1–42, 357–359.

14. IARC. Phenacetin. Vol. 24. IARC Monographs on the Evaluation of Carcinogenic Risks of Chemicals to Humans. Lyon, France: International Agency for Research on Cancer, 1980:135–161.

15. IARC. Phenacetin and Analgesic Mixtures Containing Phenacetin. IARC Monographs on the Evaluation of Carcinogenic Risks to Humans, Supplement 7—Overall Evaluations of Carcinogenicity: An Updating of IARC Monographs. Lyon, France: International Agency for Research on Cancer, 1987: 1–42, 310–312.

16. IARC. Ethylene Oxide. Vol. 54. IARC Monographs on the Evaluation of Carcinogenic Risks of Chemicals to Humans. Lyon, France: International Agency for Research on Cancer, 1994:73–159.

17. IARC. Acrylamide. Vol. 54. IARC Monographs on the Evaluation of Carcinogenic Risks of Chemicals to Humans. Lyon, France: International Agency for Research on Cancer, 1994:338–389.

18. IARC. Polychlorinated Dibenzo-para-dioxins. Vol. 69. IARC Monographs on the Evaluation of Carcinogenic Risks to Humans. Lyon, France: International Agency for Research on Cancer, 1997:33–243.

19. IARC. Neutrons. Vol. 75. IARC Monographs on the Evaluation of Carcinogenic Risks to Humans. Lyon, France: International Agency for Research on Cancer, 2000:363–448.

20. IARC. Occupational Exposures in Petroleum Refining. Vol. 45. IARC Monographs on the Evaluation of Carcinogenic Risks of Chemicals to Humans. Lyon, France: International Agency for Research on Cancer, 1989:39–117.

21. Acrylonitrile. Vol. 71. IARC Monographs on the Evaluation of Carcinogenic Risks to Humans. Lyon, France: International Agency for Research on Cancer, 1999:43–108.

22. IARC. Naphthalene. Vol. 82. IARC Monographs on the Evaluation of Carcinogenic Risks to Humans. Lyon, France: International Agency for Research on Cancer, 2003.

23. IARC. 1,2-Epoxybutane. Vol. 71. IARC Monographs on the Evaluation of Carcinogenic Risks to Humans. Lyon, France: International Agency for Research on Cancer, 1999:629–640.

24. IARC. Extremely Low Frequency Electric and Magnetic Fields. Vol. 80. IARC Monographs on the Evaluation of Carcinogenic Risks to Humans. Lyon, France: International Agency for Research on Cancer, 2002.

25. IARC. Acrylonitrile. IARC Monographs on the Evaluation of Carcinogenic Risks to Humans, Supplement 7—Overall Evaluations of Carcinigenicity: An updating of IARC Monographs. Lyon, France: International Agency for Research on Cancer, 1987:1–42, 79–80.

26. Capen CC, Dybing E, Rice JM, Wilbourne JD. Species Differences in Thyroid, Kidney and Urinary Bladder Carcinogenesis. Vol. 147. IARC Scientific Publications. Lyon, France: International Agency for Research on Cancer, 1999.

27. IARC. Peroxisome Proliferation and Its Role in Carcinogenesis. Technical Report No. 24. Lyon, France: International Agency for Research on Cancer, 1995.

28. IARC (1999) Saccharin and Its salts. IARC Monographs on the Evaluation of Carcinogenic Risks to Humans. Vol. 73. Lyon, France: IARC Press, 1999: 517–624.

29. IARC (1999) Melamine. IARC Monographs on the Evaluation of Carcinogenic Risks to Humans. Vol. 73. Lyon, France: IARC Press, 1999:329–338.

30. IARC d-Limonene. IARC Monographs on the Evaluation of Carcinogenic Risks to Humans. Vol. 73. Lyon, France: IARC Press, 1999:307–327.

31. IARC. Ethylene thiourea. IARC Monographs on the Evaluation of Carcinogenic Risks to Humans. Vol. 79. Lyon, France: IARC Press, 2001:659–701.

32. IARC. Di(2-ethylhexyl)phthalate. IARC Monographs on the Evaluation of Carcinogenic Risks to Humans. Vol. 77. Lyon, France: IARC Press, 2000: 41–148.

Cancer Risk Assessment II: Methods for Determining Cancer Etiology: Assessing Risks in Individuals

Peter G. Shields

Cancer Genetics and Epidemiology Program, Department of Medicine and Oncology, Lombardi Comprehensive Cancer Center, Georgetown University, Washington, D.C., U.S.A.

1. INTRODUCTION

Commonly, patients with cancer wonder why they have become victims. Physicians and patients alike speculate about the causes of the patients' cancer. The internet, a wide array of agencies and organizations, and the public health community are looked to in different ways to provide answers. But, for the individual, the available data that will allow for less speculation and a better understanding of causality are frequently limited. There are few biomarkers or fingerprints of a particular carcinogenic process that have been sufficiently validated to indicate what actually happened to a person. An individualized cancer risk assessment or determination of what caused cancer in an individual necessarily relies on available epidemiological data that actually provide risk estimates for populations, and have limitations for use in understanding the risks for an individual within a population.

Patients and health care providers become frustrated at the lack of answers, and intuition is relied upon. However, there are a multitude of sources that can be considered, such as epidemiological, laboratory animal, and in vitro studies. A comprehensive review may be beyond the time, resources, or expertise of a health care provider. Review articles or documents from regulatory agencies and other organizations may be available. However, it is important to consider the focus and goals of the authors for any particular document, because frequently the analysis is not aimed at providing for a causality assessment in an individual. In fact, usually such documents are intended to provide insights to protecting the public health. As such, the authors provide assessments that will focus on safety, and utilize data that will maximize such.

2. CARCINOGENESIS

Cancers result from multiple gene–environment interactions that occur over long periods of time. The environment is now defined as the area surrounding the affected critical macromolecules, specifically DNA. So, it is more important to understand what is happening at the cellular level, and the origin of exposures might be exogenous (from outside of the body) or endogenous (produced by the body).

Carcinogenesis is a multistage process of normal growth, differentiation, and development gone awry. It is driven by spontaneous and carcinogen-induced genetic and epigenetic events. Tumor initiation involves the direct effects of carcinogenic agents upon DNA that cause mutations and altered gene expression. The attendant defects lead to selective reproductive and clonal expansion of cells. This may be augmented through growth factors that control signal transduction. Progressive phenotypic changes and genomic instability occur (aneuploidy, mutations, or gene amplification). These genetic changes enhance the probability of "initiated" cells transforming into a malignancy, the odds of which are increased during repeated rounds of cell replication. During tumor progression, angiogenesis allows for a tumor to grow beyond one or two millimeters in size. Ultimately, tumor cells can disseminate through vessels invading distant tissues and establishing metastatic colonies.

The primary genes involved in driving the cancer process are proto-oncogenes and tumor suppressor genes. Proto-oncogenes are important to the regulatory mechanisms of growth, cell cycle, and terminal differentiation. Activation of proto-oncogenes enhances the probability of neoplastic transformation, which can either be an early or late event. Carcinogens can cause mutations in proto-oncogene DNA sequences or they can act as tumor promoters enhancing the activity of oncogene protein products. Examples of a proto-oncogene are those in the *RAS* family.

Tumor suppressor genes also code for products that regulate cell growth and terminal differentiation. However, they have the opposite effect by limiting growth and stimulating terminal differentiation. If inactivated, then the cell may grow or replicate uncontrollably, with limits defined only by blood supply and space. For this to occur, both copies of the tumor suppressor genes must be affected, and thus it is a recessive event. This is exemplified by inheritance of a predisposition to retinoblastoma and/or osteosarcoma, where patients possess a homozygous loss of the Rb1 gene on chromosome 13 (1–3). In the familial form, loss of one allele is inherited and the other is lost through later mutation. Loss of suppressor and antimetastasis genes can be an early or late event involving several steps, including angiogenesis and metastasis (4).

Another way of considering genes involved in the carcinogenic process is to classify them as caretaker and gatekeeper genes (5). This recognizes their respective roles in the maintenance of genomic integrity (e.g., DNA repair) and cellular proliferation, respectively. Landscaper genes are also considered that are responsible for maintaining the general environment around the cells (i.e., effects on stromal cells and signaling between cells). Some examples of caretaker genes are those that are involved in DNA repair and carcinogen metabolism, while examples of gatekeeper genes are those involved in cell cycle control and DNA replication. Dysfunctional caretaker genes increase the probability of mutations in gatekeeper genes, which are necessary to initiate the molecular pathogenesis of cancer. It is interesting that the carcinogenic effects of caretaker and gatekeeper genes appear to be tissue-specific and lead to cancer only in those organs, even though these genes are expressed in many different organs.

Carcinogenic agents affect DNA in different ways. They can covalently bind to nucleotides and form adducts. These adducts may be promutagenic, and if present at the time of DNA synthesis, can cause mutations. N-nitrosamines, for example, present in the diet and linked to esophageal and gastric carcinoma, result in nucleotide base substitutions due to mispairing at sites where adducts are formed. Some mutations may reflect specific carcinogen exposures or endogenous mechanisms, and frequently exhibit target organ specificity. For example, p53 mutations at codon 249 frequently observed in hepatocellular carcinoma from China (6) or southern Africa (7) are consistent with the type of damage caused by aflatoxin B_1 exposure, a common dietary carcinogen linked to this tumor. In contrast, several types of p53 mutations have been observed in lung cancer (8), which is consistent with a multiple carcinogen exposure etiology from tobacco smoke. To date, however, the mutational spectra of p53 or other genes cannot be used to determine what caused a cancer in a person.

Independent of carcinogen exposure, human cells are continuously undergoing spontaneous mutations at a low rate. Oxidative damage, polymerase infidelity, chromosomal rearrangement, recombinase infidelity, and telomere reduction are other sources of error. The process of cell and DNA replication can increase the rate of mutation (9). When one considers that the human body contains 10^{14} cells and that these cells undergo 10^{16} divisions over a person's life span, it is quite possible that genomic instability plays an important role in carcinogenesis (10,11).

Balancing the ongoing exposure to carcinogens, cells have the ability to repair DNA damage, such as the removal of carcinogen DNA adducts through nucleotide excision repair or gross chromosomal damage through homologous recombination. When DNA is sufficiently damaged and cannot be repaired, then cells have the ability to trigger apoptosis (cell death), in which case it is no longer viable and cannot become a cancer cell.

In almost every step of the multistage process of carcinogenesis, person-to-person differences in cancer susceptibility can be found (12). Interindividual differences for particular traits can be acquired, or inherited. Inherited susceptibilities, manifest through evolutionary changes in nucleotide sequence, may augment human cancer pathogenesis that can vary from high penetrance with an attendant high likelihood of causing cancer to low penetrance genes with an attendant increased risk of causing cancer albeit less likely than high penetrance genes. Nevertheless, the range from low to high penetrance genes is a continuum, and studies in animal models indicate that the effects of high penetrance genes can be modified by other genes (13). High penetrance genes that cause family cancer syndromes can have substantial impact in affected families (e.g., BRCA1, hereditary nonpolyposis coli or Li–Fraumeni syndrome) (13), but they affect only a small percentage of the population. In contrast, the manifestations of cancer susceptibility genes with less penetrance contribute to common sporadic cancers, and thus affect a large segment of the population.

2.1. Methods to Assess Carcinogenesis

There are many tests that are used to increase our understanding of carcinogenesis and risk; these range from in vitro and experimental animal in vivo studies to human clinical and epidemiological studies. The usefulness of each method can be contrasted with its limitations (Table 1). Short-term assays for mutagenesis provide quick and inexpensive screens for potential carcinogens. Among the most widely used is the Ames' test (14), which assesses mutagenic potential in *Salmonella typhimurium* bacteria. The Ames' test has also been used as a biomonitor in humans, as exemplified by urine mutagenicity studies from cigarette smokers (15). While other assays exist, there are none with proven increased predictive value. Although short-term assays are useful in identifying potentially carcinogenic compounds, the same sensitivity makes the results difficult to extrapolate to humans. Positive results might be unique to the strain, and factors such as metabolism, repair, and exposure cannot be assessed.

Experimental animal studies provide a short-term ability to assess the effects of a carcinogen in mammals. However, the predictivity for human risk is poor, but few better methods to study possible cancer risk and carcinogenesis exist. As used by the National Toxicology Program and others, rodent carcinogenicity studies are performed using lifetime exposures with

Table 1 Testing for Carcinogenicity

Method	Advantages	Disadvantages
In vitro testing	Economical	Uncertain in vitro to in vivo extrapolations
	Rapid results	Frequent false positives and negatives
	Human cells can be used	Mutagenicity is not the same as carcinogenicity
		Inter-laboratory variation
Animal bioassay	More predictive of human experience than short-term tests	Expensive
		Doses are higher than those experienced by humans
	Elucidates species differences	Uncertain animal-to-human extrapolation
Human clinical studies	Direct measurement of human experience	Cancer is not an endpoint
	Biomarkers show biologically effective dose and intermediate markers of cancer risk	
	Short-term results	
Epidemiology	Direct measurement of human experience	Insensitive
	Covariables examined	Does not prove causation
	Dose–response data	Unknown confounding variables
	Biomarkers can be used	
	Interindividual variation considered	

up to maximally tolerated doses (MTD), that is, those not producing clinically evident toxic effects. To infer that a carcinogenic effect is present in laboratory animals, dose–response relationships are examined, along with overall mortality rates and consistency with other species. The limitations in these experiments include the routine use of the MTD, thus potentially increasing cell replication with resultant increased endogenous mutations; interspecies, and interstrain differences; use of rodents known to have high spontaneous rates of cancer; an inability to account for metabolic differences between high- and low-dose exposure, and difficulty in interpreting data from doses that commonly exceed those received by humans (16–18). Also, the tumors of experimental animals may not resemble human cancer, or may not be malignant.

Human investigations provide the most relevant data regarding human risk. Clinical studies might be done, where exposures are unavoidable. For example, while it is conceivable to intentionally expose a person who already smokes to a modified tobacco product intended to reduce exposure, it would not be advisable to expose a person to a new chemical that has not been considered to be safe through laboratory testing. Epidemiology measures the incidence or prevalence of disease in human populations. One limitation is that epidemiology can inform us about cancer risk from prior exposures, the latency effect of most carcinogens is so long that we cannot wait to assess a cancer risk in the future, and these study repeat effects after too many people get cancer. Also, it must be realized that epidemiologic methods, by themselves, do not demonstrate causation. The assessment of causation can be aided by Sir Austin Bradford–Hill's (19) proposed criteria, summarized in Table 2.

A formal quantitative risk assessment using mathematical models is used by regulatory agencies to estimate a potential cancer risk to a population exposed to a particular carcinogen at a specific dose. Risk assessments serve public health interests as they attempt to predict the frequency of cancer in a population before epidemiologic investigations can be performed, that is, before significant exposure and adverse outcomes occur. Among the reasons that population risk assessment informs little understanding about individual cancer risk, or causality, is that the risk assessment process makes a variety of interpretations and assumptions in the public health interest, and many of these are open to debate. Examples include subjective evaluations of the literature and extrapolations from laboratory animals to humans, and the use of safety quotients to compensate for a lack of knowledge in some areas.

2.2. Gathering Risk Factor Information

The initial approach before considering the individual's situation and possible risk factors is to assess what risk factors are known, and the scientific basis that identifies these risk factors. In the case of a potential carcinogen exposure, the scientific data are considered at any level of exposure. This

Table 2 Evaluating Cancer Etiology—Bradford–Hill Criteria

Criteria	Explanation
Strength of association	What is magnitude of risk?
Consistency	Are there repeated observations by multiple investigators in different populations?
Specificity	Is the effect specific or are there other known causes?
Temporality	Does exposure precede effect?
Biological gradient	Is there a dose–response relation?
Biological plausibility	Is the effect predictable?
Coherence	Is the effect consistent with other scientific data?
Analogy	Do other similar agents act similarly?

Source: From Ref. 19.

is done by reviewing scientific textbooks and articles identified by doing computerized literature searches.

For literature searches, public websites such as the National Library of Medicine PubMed website can be useful (http://www.ncbi.nlm.nih. gov/entrez/query.fcgi). Abstracts of publications are frequently available, some articles can be downloaded for free, or at a cost, and all can be ordered through a related service on that site called Loansome Doc. Search strategies should be broad in order to identify related articles that might not be categorized appropriately. PubMed also includes links to related articles, which are sometimes helpful.

The websites for governmental agencies and other organizations can provide information, including downloads of various monographs. For example, one can view the websites of the Agency for Toxic Substances and Disease Registry (http://www.atsdr.cdc.gov)/ and its parent website for the Centers for Disease Control (http://www.cdc.gov)/, the American Conference of Governmental Hygienists (http://www.acgih.org), the Environmental Protection Agency (http://www.epa.gov), Food and Drug Administration (http://www.fda.gov), the International Agency for Research on Cancer of the World Health Organization (http://w/niosh), National Institutes of Environmental Health Sciences (http://www.niehs.nih.gov),and the Nuclear Regulatory Commission (http://www.nrc.gov). Also, one might look to links by various nonprofit and advocacy organizations.

2.3. Assessing Causality in the Individual

The methodology for the determination of cancer causality is described below. It is important to assess different types of scientific data, relying on the best studies. Sometimes, a researcher might postulate causality (i.e., as might be done through a publication of a case report, or a case series), but this is different from concluding a causal relationship of exposure to outcome. Among the types of data that might be useful, human epidemiological data are substantially more helpful than nonhuman data. If there is sufficient reason to consider that the chemical has a potential to cause the type of cancer identified for the individual (target organ specificity is important), then an assessment is made to determine the doses reported in the literature that may be associated with an increased cancer risk, and in what settings. A mechanistic understanding of the carcinogenic process (known or hypothesized) is considered in the context of the alleged exposure and disease in the patient. Animal and in vitro studies can be helpful in these mechanistic assessments. A concurrent step for assessing causality in an individual is to confirm the diagnosis, as sometimes incorrect diagnoses are made, and so would not be appropriately related to the alleged exposure in the individual. Assuming that there is sufficient reason to believe that the chemical might increase cancer risk, then one would consider the individual's potential exposure or risk factor compared to those from the literature. For example, exposure level, route of exposure, other exposures or risk factors, or the type of population would be considered.

It is helpful to consider the Bradford–Hill guidelines (19) mentioned above and described in Table 2. While not all are criteria are required to be met, there are some criteria that if violated would exclude the likelihood of causation; while fulfilling some may not lead to a definitive conclusion of causation. Among the most important criteria is consistency in the literature, that is, doing several well-designed and well-conducted epidemiology studies leading to similar findings in different populations, using different study designs. It should be noted that no single epidemiological study is definitive. A determination of a biological gradient also is important, i.e., if there is a dose–response relationship identified in scientific studies, and if those doses occur in the human exposure scenario of interest. Another is the strength of association, which allows one to consider if the reported association in an epidemiological study is believable (i.e., not too high or too low). An evaluation of temporality considers if the exposure sufficiently preceded the cancer effect to allow for latency. Specificity considers if the cancer has other reported causes and if the effect occurs in the identified target organ. Coherence refers to an evaluation and agreement of different types of scientific data (epidemiological, laboratory animal studies, cell culture models, etc.) and they do provide similar findings that lead to a mechanistic understanding of how the chemical would cause cancer in humans. Analogy looks to see if similar chemicals are known to behave similarly and what is the available scientific data for those chemicals.

2.4. Assessing the Patient

A careful history and physical examination are critical to any medical assessment, and that is true for cancer risk assessment too. The history, detailed in Table 3, needs to be thorough. What is critical is to document all potential exposures. Parenthetically, medical records are often used in litigation over potential exposures, and so the health care provider needs to document potential exposures accurately and clearly. This is true for known cancer risk factors as well.

If a known or suspected carcinogen is identified for a patient, then an evaluation of the actual exposure can be undertaken. If there are validated biomarkers for such, then these can be relied upon. Some might reflect only recent exposure, however, and do not indicate what has possibly occurred over many years or a lifetime. There is considerable research into the development and validation of biomarkers. The validation has to include the reliability of the test itself as it reflects what it is supposed to be measuring, but also its validity as a risk factor. The latter can be more complicated, and the health care provider should use caution when considering the use of a

Table 3 Assessing a Patient's History

Category	Examples of questions
Medical	History of present illness
	History of medical disorders associated with secondary malignancies
	Recent and distant medication use
	History of radiation exposure
	History of virus exposure
Family	History of cancer in different generations, including immediate and next-to-immediate members
	Assess passive smoke exposure (parents, current occupants)
	Occupational history of current and past household members
	Hereditary disorders associated with secondary malignancies
Social	Tobacco consumption (cigarettes and smokeless products)
	Alcohol use
	Risk factors for viral exposure
	Substance abuse
	All recreations and hobbies
	Diet and nutrition, including vitamin use, health fads, home gardens and locally grown food products
	Foreign travel
Occupational	All occupations, including summer and childhood work
	Parental occupation
	Any jobs with known hazards
	Any jobs where protective equipment was used
	Any jobs with cancer clusters
	Any jobs with bad odors
	Any jobs with chemicals, fumes, gases, or dusts
Environmental	All residences and types
	Residential proximity to industry, waste sites, agriculture, or other areas with potential exposure
	Source of water—well, community, and bottled
	Cancer clusters
	Use of pesticides, herbicides, and termiticides
	House building materials and renovations

test that is still experimental. A major limitation is that recommendations based on results cannot be given in an informed manner.

Environmental monitoring might be taken, and although some of these are relatively inexpensive (i.e., radon), the cost of some monitoring and testing can be prohibitive. The use of biomarkers or environmental testing must be carefully considered, including their validity. The choice of laboratory, and its competency and experience also must be considered. Resources for environmental testing might include local industrial hygienists at the company where an exposure might be alleged, or a consulting firm. Public health departments might also be helpful.

3. SUMMARY

The assessment of cancer risk in an individual can be complex. It requires an understanding of carcinogenesis, and the resources and abilities to obtain and interpret the scientific literature. It also includes a careful history and physical of the patient. Importantly, the best available means to assess considered risk factors, such as a biomarker, should be utilized. However, caution is needed for the choice of biomarker, or environmental testing, in that it must be predictive of risk. The occurrence of cancer in a patient is frequently a life-transforming event, and the health care provider needs to give the patient accurate information.

REFERENCES

1. Hansen MF, Koufos A, Gallie BL, Phillips RA, Fodstad O, Brogger A, Gedde-Dahl T, Cavenee WK. Osteosarcoma and retinoblastoma: a shared chromosomal mechanism revealing recessive predisposition. Proc Natl Acad Sci USA 1985; 82:6216–6220.
2. Cavenee WK, Murphree AL, Shull MM, Benedict WF, Sparkes RS, Kock E, Nordenskjold M. Prediction of familial predisposition to retinoblastoma. N Engl J Med 1986; 314:1201–1207.
3. Friend SH, Bernards R, Rogelj S, Weinberg RA, Rapaport JM, Albert DM, Dryja TP. A human DNA segment with properties of the gene that predisposes to retinoblastoma and osteosarcoma. Nature 1986; 323:643–646.
4. Liotta LA, Steeg PS, Stetler-Stevenson WG. Cancer metastasis and angiogenesis: an imbalance of positive and negative regulation. Cell 1991; 64:327–336.
5. Kinzler KW, Vogelstein B. Gatekeepers and caretakers. Nature 1997; 386:761–763.
6. Pawson T, Olivier P, Rozakis-Adcock M, McGlade J, Henkemeyer M. Proteins with SH2 and SH3 domains couple receptor tyrosine kinases to intracellular signalling pathways. Philos Trans R Soc Lond B Biol Sci 1993; 340:279–285.
7. Bressac B, Kew M, Wands J, Ozturk M. Selective G to T mutations of p53 gene in hepatocellular carcinoma from southern Africa. Nature 1991; 350:429–431.
8. Hollstein M, Sidransky D, Vogelstein B, Harris CC. p53 mutations in human cancers. Science 1991; 253:49–53.
9. Preston-Martin S, Pike MC, Ross RK, Jones PA, Henderson BE. Increased cell division as a cause of human cancer. Cancer Res 1990; 50:7415–7421.
10. Harris CC. Chemical and physical carcinogenesis: advances and perspectives. Cancer Res 1991; 51:5023s–5044s.
11. Loeb LA. Endogenous carcinogenesis: molecular oncology into the twenty-first century—presidential address. Cancer Res 1989; 49:5489–5496.
12. Harris CC. Interindividual variation among humans in carcinogen metabolism, DNA adduct formation and DNA repair. Carcinogenesis 1989; 10:1563–1566.

13. Ponder B. Genetic testing for cancer risk. Science 1997; 278:1050–1054.
14. Ames BN, McCann J, Yamasaki E. Methods for detecting carcinogens and mutagens with the *Salmonella*/mammalian-microsome mutagenicity test. Mutat Res 1975; 31:347–364.
15. Yamasaki E, Ames BN. Concentration of mutagens from urine by absorption with the nonpolar resin XAD-2: cigarette smokers have mutagenic urine. Proc Natl Acad Sci USA 1977; 74:3555–3559.
16. Ames BN, Magaw R, Gold LS. Ranking possible carcinogenic hazards. Science 1987; 236:271–280.
17. Lijinsky W. In vivo testing for carcinogenicity. In: Cooper CS, Grover PL, eds. Chemical Carcinogenesis and Mutagenesis I. Berlin: Springer-Verlag, 1990: 179–209.
18. Tomatis L, Bartsch H. The contribution of experimental studies to risk assessment of carcinogenic agents in humans. Exp Pathol 1990; 40:251–266.
19. Hill AB. The environment and disease: association or causation. Proc R Soc Med 1965; 58:295–300.

9

Cancer Epidemiology

James R. Cerhan

*Health Sciences Research, Mayo Clinic College of Medicine,
Rochester, New York, U.S.A.*

1. INTRODUCTION AND OVERVIEW

1.1. The Epidemiologic Method

Last (1) defines epidemiology as "the study of the distribution and determinants of health-related states or events in specified populations, and the application of this study to control of health problems." In the context of cancer, a more simplistic definition is that epidemiology attempts to answer the question of who develops cancer and why. If cancer is not random, at least at the population level, then there must be determinants of the observed patterns of cancer. This chapter will introduce the reader to the basic methods of epidemiology used to describe patterns of cancer and to test hypotheses about the causes of cancer.

Epidemiology is often divided into descriptive and analytical branches. Descriptive epidemiology describes the occurrence of disease and other health-related characteristics in human populations. These descriptive patterns are based on aggregate characteristics of disease frequency, person (age, sex, race, occupation, etc.), place (generally geographical region), and calendar time. Analytical epidemiology, in contrast, uses specific study designs (e.g., a cohort or case–control study) to test hypotheses about exposure and disease relationships, frequently incorporating biomarkers and analyzing disease mechanisms. Of note, it is descriptive epidemiology that has provided the most compelling evidence that a large proportion of human cancer should be preventable, and it is analytical epidemiology that has helped identify specific agents or risk factors for cancer (e.g., smoking, certain occupations, and so forth) that have informed preventive actions.

Epidemiology was originally developed to study infectious disease, and during the later half of the 20th century evolved to address chronic diseases such as cancer. There are several characteristics of cancer that impact epidemiologic approaches (2). Cancer is not a single disease, but a group of diseases that share several key biological and pathological characteristics. Diagnosis, treatment, and survival from cancer vary by organ site, and thus are usually discussed by site of cancer origin, and this is also true for the epidemiology of cancer. In addition, not all cancers arising from the same organ have the same characteristics or epidemiology. For example, basal cell carcinoma of the skin rarely metastasizes and causes death. In contrast, melanoma of the skin often metastasizes and causes death. Thus, both cancer site and cancer histology (i.e., both the cell or tissue of origin and the cellular/tissue appearance at diagnosis) are important to understanding cancer.

A second important concept in cancer epidemiology is the theory of multistep carcinogenesis (3,4). Experimental animal models identify several steps. *Initiation* is the first step in tumor induction, and occurs when a cell's growth and regulatory capacity are altered through genetic or epigenetic changes, such that the potential for unregulated growth is established. *Promotion*, the second stage, occurs when a promoting agent induces proliferation and, presumably, the growth advantage of the initiated cell. The third and final stage, *progression*, is a process by which the neoplastic growth begins to invade surrounding tissues or metastasize to other tissues; the cells of the primary tumor can also change as they acquire more genetic alterations. These genetic alterations commonly occur in both tumor suppressor genes (e.g., *Rb1* or *p53*) and oncogenes (e.g., *c-myc*).

In the multistep carcinogenic model, the probability of developing cancer is the combined probability of individual rare events that lead to neoplastic growth and eventually clinically evident disease. These events can be mutagenic (chemical alteration of DNA) as well mitogenic (drive proliferation). In addition, these events must either affect or overwhelm intrinsic repair and/or elimination (apoptotic) mechanisms (5). However, it seems highly likely that the carcinogenic process is more complex than simply cells acquiring multiple genetic alterations; there are likely to be determinants at the extracellular matrix and tissue levels that also influence the carcinogenic process (6). Finally, stochastic processes (i.e., some element of randomness) must also be integrated into the conceptual framework of carcinogenesis.

Epidemiologists attempt to link *exposures* to cancer risk. Exposure is broadly defined by epidemiologists, and classically includes direct contact with an infectious (e.g., the hepatitis B virus, schistosomiasis), chemical (e.g., arsenic, radon), or physical (e.g., heat, ultraviolet radiation) agent in the environment. However, exposures can also include "exposure" to higher levels of circulating estrogens (e.g., during pregnancy or with obesity), an adverse genotype (e.g., BRCA1 carrier), greater educational level, less physical activity, and so forth. Along with exposure, we often think of *dose*, which is the amount of the agent to which the host is exposed. Dose is an important concept in cancer epidemiology because for many (but not all) exposures, the greater the dose the greater the biological effect (i.e., a *dose–response* relation). Evaluation of exposure (*exposure assessment*) is a complex task and is discussed extensively elsewhere (7).

The *induction period* is defined as "the interval from the causal action of a factor to the initiation of the disease" while the *latent period* is defined as "period from disease initiation to disease detection" (1,8). However, the terms are often combined and used synonymously as the "period required for a specific cause to produce disease" (1), in part, because it is generally not possible to know when a disease was actually initiated. The latent period for most exposure–cancer associations is unknown. The cancer experience of persons exposed to short but intensive ionizing radiation (e.g., treatment with radiotherapy or a survivor of the atomic bombing of Hiroshima and Nagasaki) shows that incidence of leukemia peaks about five years after exposure, while the incidence of solid tumors rises for 15–20 years, and then shows a variable course by tumor site (9). Based on current knowledge, the latent period for most solid tumors is thought to be several decades, while the latent period for leukemias and lymphomas is probably more variable, but not likely less than five years (9).

Observation and experimentation are fundamental components of the scientific method (10). Epidemiology engages in both. The experimental arm of epidemiology includes the randomized clinical trial (individual level) and community intervention trial (group level). In observational epidemiology, researchers collect data on persons (or groups) without any actual manipulations of the exposure. The main observational study designs used in epidemiology are ecological, cross-sectional, case-control, and cohort, and they are briefly introduced in the next section. There are many branches of science that are based on mainly observational approaches, and this approach is often (mistakenly) considered an inferior form of evidence (10). There are many reasons why epidemiology cannot be a purely experimental science. For example, randomized trials are expensive, are not absolutely guaranteed to be free of chance or bias, and are often conducted on persons not representative of the general population. Most importantly, however, is that ethical and practical concerns limit the use of experimental approaches in the study of cancer etiology.

While some authors suggest that epidemiological observation may one day be displaced by laboratory investigation, this seems unlikely for several reasons (9). First, moving the study of cancer in human beings from a free-living population into the laboratory requires a level of scientific reductionism that is not likely to ever fully or adequately replicate the complexity of cancer in the human body or in human populations. Second, many hypotheses of cancer causation have been generated by the observation of the behavioral repertoire of humans, and would not likely have been suggested by a purely laboratory-based approach. Conversely, many agents that cause cancer in in vitro and in vivo experiments in the laboratory do not appear to be important determinants of risk in individuals or populations. While epidemiology is not precise enough to rule out associations of small magnitude, it does provide reliable evidence that a large effect is extremely unlikely. Epidemiological approaches are also not likely to miss the main determinants of cancer rates and trends. Thus, epidemiology provides quantititive data relating directly to humans, in whom we want to prevent disease.

1.2. Descriptive Epidemiology

Some of the earliest descriptive cancer epidemiology came from observations of exposures (11,12). In 1713, Ramazzini noted that breast cancer was unusually common among nuns, which he attributed to their celibacy and childlessness. A later observation by Rigoni-Stern in 1842 showed that over the period 1760–1839 in Verona, Italy, the ratio of uterine to breast cancer mortality for married women was 2:1, for single women other than nuns it was 1:3, and for nuns it was 1:9. In contrast, cervical cancer was a rare cause of death for nuns. The London physician, Percivall Pott, noted in 1775 that scrotal cancer was common in men who worked as chimney sweeps as boys. He hypothesized that this was due to repeated contact of the skin with combustion products of coal, and these observations became one of the foundations of the field of chemical carcinogenesis. Interestingly, rates of scrotal cancer in German chimney sweeps did not seem to be unusually high, which was attributed to the fact that German sweeps bathed frequently in contrast to English sweeps. Skin cancer among radiographers, lung cancer among miners, and bladder cancer in aniline dye workers are some of the many additional observations that accumulated and helped develop the field of descriptive cancer epidemiology.

The task of cancer surveillance is to estimate the amount of cancer in a population, and describe basic patterns of the disease (e.g., what cancer sites are most common? what is the age distribution of patients? and so forth). One approach to answer these questions is to conduct a survey of a defined population and find out who has cancer (i.e., a prevalence survey). The number of persons living with cancer in the survey divided by the number of persons in the survey is the *cancer prevalence*, giving a "snapshot" of the cancer burden in a population at a single point in time (13).

Another way to study cancer is to count the number of persons dying of cancer during a period of time, generally as identified by death certificates

(14). The number of cancer deaths in a given year divided by the number of persons in the population is the *cancer mortality rate*. From a public health perspective, this is probably the most important statistic to assess the success of a cancer program (15). A third approach to estimating the cancer burden in a population is to continuously monitor a population and count the number of newly diagnosed cases that occur (14). The number of newly diagnosed cancer cases within a defined period of time (usually 1 year) divided by the number of persons in the population is the *cancer incidence rate*.

A key to the conduct of both descriptive and analytical epidemiological studies is the availability of systematically collected data on cancer patients in a registry. Hospital-based registries collect cancer cases seen in a hospital without an underlying knowledge of the population that generated the cases. These registries are mainly kept for hospital-related needs including planning of cancer services, patient care, and clinical research (e.g., clinical trials and outcome studies). These tumor registries are most commonly found in larger, referral hospitals and therefore cancer cases are usually not representative of all cancers seen in the community, since they tend to overrepresent rarer or more unusual cases. This problem greatly limits the usefulness of hospital-based registries in understanding cancer in the general population.

In contrast, population-based registries collect all cancers occurring in a geographically defined area, which requires case finding in multiple places, including hospitals, pathology laboratories, physician offices, radiation treatment facilities, and so forth, as well as using death certificate data (16). Data on cancer cases are then related to the underlying population to derive incidence rates (below). Population data are generally derived from census data. Population-based cancer registries are much more powerful than hospital-based registries because they are linked to a defined population. Important uses of population-based registries include description of cancer patterns in space (i.e., between geographical regions) and time (trends); evaluation of the effectiveness of cancer prevention programs as well as cancer treatments; formulation and testing of etiological hypotheses using descriptive and analytical study designs; evaluation of cancer clusters; and health planning (16). In the United States, the two major sources for cancer data are the National Center for Health Statistics, which provides mortality data on all U.S. residents, and population-based cancer registries, which provide cancer incidence data. Population-based registries include many state-supported registries (17) and the Surveillance, Epidemiology and End Results (SEER) Program coordinated by the National Cancer Institute (http://seer.cancer.gov) (18).

At the international level, the International Agency for Research on Cancer (IARC) and the International Association of Cancer Registers published *Cancer Incidence in Five Continents* that includes data on 183 populations in 50 countries on 5 continents, although data from Africa and South America are limited (19). An electronic version of the database entitled *CI5VII: Electronic Database of Cancer Incidence in Five Continents Vol. VII* is also available (20). In conjunction with the World Health Organization, IARC also makes available an electronic database of cancer incidence and mortality for 25 cancer sites for all countries, entitled *GLOBO-CAN 1: Cancer Incidence and Mortality Worldwide* (21); these data are summarized by Parkin et al. (22) and Pisani et al. (23).

It is important for health planners to know the number of cases in a defined population since these numbers determine the need for medical and other services used by cancer patients. To compare populations, we need to use rates, which require both numerators (i.e., number of cases or deaths during a specified time period) and denominators (e.g., population size during the same time period that generated the cases). Prevalence, incidence, or mortality rates (see Table 1 for definitions) are used to compare populations.

Cancer rates are often termed "crude" rates when they measure frequency of cancer without taking into account the composition of the population. A better way to compare populations is to use age-specific rates. However, presenting age-specific rates is rather cumbersome, and so an alternative approach is to use a method called age standardization. Age standardized rates are the weighted average of the age-specific rates, where a common age structure or standard population is used. The choice of the standard population is arbitrary, and the SEER Program uses the 2000 U.S. population, while IARC uses the World Standard Population for *Cancer Incidence in Five Continents.*

A third cancer statistic that is commonly used is the cumulative rate, which is the sum over each year of age of the age-specific incidence rates. This method does not require the use of a standard population, which makes it a bit more intuitive. For cancer, it has been shown that the cumulative rate approximates the cumulative risk (24), which is defined as "the risk that an individual would have of developing or dying from a given cancer during a certain age span if no other causes of death were operative." The cumulative risk is presented as a percentage for a given age span (e.g., 0–64 years), and can be estimated from the cumulative rate using a conversion formula (Table 1).

Cancer incidence and mortality rates each have strengths and weaknesses when assessing the cancer burden in a population (14). Cancer incidence data almost always need to be collected using a registry set up for this purpose, while mortality data generally come from routinely collected data. Thus, incidence data are usually associated with greater quality controls than mortality data, but with a much greater investment of resources. Both incidence and mortality data, however, rely on the accuracy of clinical and pathological diagnosis by practicing physicians, which varies by place and through time. Cancer mortality data often lack histological

Table 1 Definition of Commonly Used Rates in Cancer Epidemiology

Rate	Definition (source)
Prevalence rate	The number of cancers (new and pre-existing) of a specific site/type in a specified population during a specified time period, expressed as the number of cancers per 100,000 people. Cancer cases, regardless of whether they are cured, are typically considered prevalent until death (18)
Incidence rate	The number of new cancers of a specific site/type occurring in a specified population during a year, expressed as the number of cancers per 100,000 people (18)
Mortality rate	The number of deaths with cancer as the underlying cause of death occurring in a specified population during a year, expressed as the number of cancers per 100,000 people (18)
Age-specific rate	A rate for a defined age group (18)
Age-adjusted rate or age-standardized rate	Weighted average of the age-specific cancer incidence (or mortality) rates, where the weights are the proportions of persons in the corresponding age groups of a standard population (18)
Cumulative rate	Sum of age-specific rates, giving equal weight to all age groups (24)
Cumulative risk	The cumulative rate is the probability that an individual will develop cancer during a certain specified age period (e.g., 0–64 years), in the absence of any competing cause of death. The cumulative risk, expressed as a percentage, can be estimated as $(1 - e^{-\text{Cumulative rate}}) \times 100$ (24)
Observed survival rate	The proportion of cancer patients surviving for a specified length of time after diagnosis; obtained using standard life table procedures (18)
Relative survival rate	The likelihood that a cancer patient will not die from causes associated specifically with their cancer at some specified time after diagnosis; it is essentially the observed survival rate adjusted for expected mortality; the relative survival rate will always be greater than the observed survival rate for the same group of patients (18)

confirmation, and the site of the cancer is often misspecified, particularly if the primary site is an internal organ or the cancer was metastatic. Clearly, cancer mortality data will underestimate the cancer burden in the community, as not all cancers will kill the patient and multiple cancers in the same person will be missed. Incidence data are clearly preferred for most etiological studies of cancer because mortality data cannot distinguish between effects on disease development (incidence) and disease outcome (survival). However, mortality data are more widely available globally and for a much longer period of time (i.e., much more historical data), and are thought to be the best basis for judging progress against cancer by the Extramural Committee to Assess Measures of Progress Against Cancer (15).

Figure 1 indicates the age standardization rates for the most common cancers. Cancer risk is not equally distributed across age, and the association of age with the risk of developing a site-specific cancer can provide etiological clues. The most typical age–incidence pattern is a logarithmic increase in the incidence such that cancer is extremely rare in childhood and very common in old age. This pattern, shown in Fig. 2 for selected cancer sites, is characteristic of carcinomas of the lung, colon, rectum, urinary tract, pancreas, and stomach and multiple myeloma and chronic lymphocytic leukemia. Whether cancer rates continue to rise in the oldest age groups is not clear, as many cancer rates appear to drop off after age 75 but are also unstable. The drop-off in rates among the oldest old may be a real phenomenon or an artifact due to underascertainment (i.e., missed cases) of cancer in this age group, since many elderly persons have extensive comorbidities and may not receive extensive work-ups. This age–incidence pattern suggests that life-long, cumulative exposures are likely to play an important role in these cancers, and that the latent period is likely to be decades.

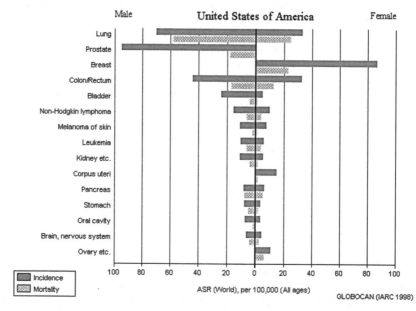

Figure 1   Age-standardized (World Standard) incidence and mortality rates for the most common cancers in the United States, 1990. *Source*: From Ref. 21.

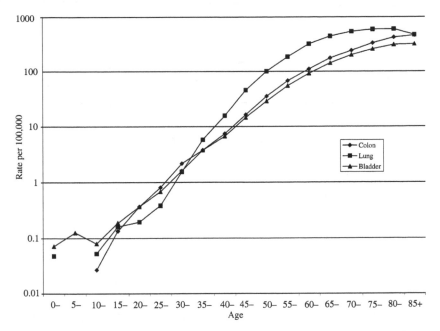

Figure 2 Age-specific incidence rates for colon, lung, and bladder cancer, males, United States (SEER Program), 1988–1992. *Source*: From Ref. 20.

While the pattern described above is the most commonly observed, there are many other age–incidence patterns. As shown in Figure 3, some cancers occur almost exclusively in childhood, such as retinoblastoma and nephroblastoma, while some cancers have two peaks in their age–incidence pattern—one in childhood and one in later life—such as Hodgkin's disease and acute lymphocytic leukemia. There are many other patterns, and these patterns suggest that there are likely to be etiological differences in quantity, timing, or quality of carcinogenic exposures as well as in the latent period for specific cancers. Evaluation of age-specific rates for breast cancer provides an interesting example. Unlike colon and many other cancers strongly related to aging, the rate of increase for breast cancer slows in women around age 50 (Fig. 4), the time of menopause when estrogen production by the ovaries ceases, suggesting (but by no means proving) a role for ovarian hormones in the etiology of breast cancer.

Cancer rarely occurs in childhood. In the United States, cancer in persons under age 15 years accounts for less than 1% of all cancers (25), while cancer in persons over age 55 accounts for 80% of cancers even though only 20% of the U.S. population is over the age of 55. One of the interesting distinctions between adult and childhood cancer is that epithelial tumors are relatively rare in children but dominate in adults (26). In contrast, tumors of

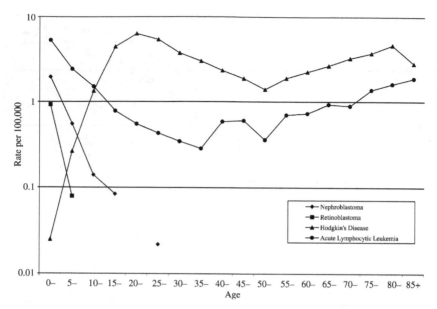

Figure 3 Age-specific incidence rates for selected cancers, females, United States (SEER Program), 1988–1992. *Source*: From Ref. 20.

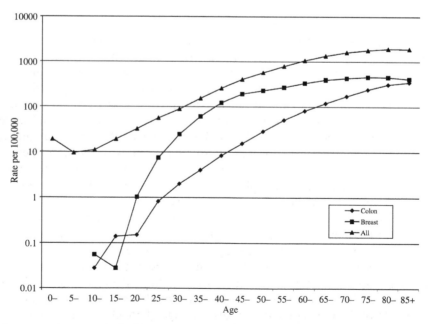

Figure 4 Age-specific incidence rates for colon, breast, and all (except skin) cancers, females, United States (SEER Program), 1988–1992. *Source*: From Ref. 20.

embryonal cells are very common in children and rare in adults. These observations also suggest broad etiologic distinctions between cancer in these age groups: childhood cancer is likely to be informed by understanding the developmental process, while cancer in adults is likely to be informed by understanding aging, repair, and senescence.

There are also notable sex differences in cancer incidence and mortality; the patterns for the top 15 cancers are shown for the United States in Figure 5. Cancer sites strongly associated with smoking (lung, bladder, kidney, oral cavity) are much more common in men, presumably due to higher smoking rates in men. Cancers thought to have a hormonal etiology—prostate in men and breast and uterine cancer in women—show a similar magnitude of incidence and mortality rates in each sex, and are in total the most common cancers seen in the United States. Colorectal cancer incidence and mortality is slightly more common in males than in females.

Time trends in mortality are generally based on death certificate data collected by governments. Thus, for long-term trends to be interpretable, there must be widespread certification of deaths for the vast majority of the population. Such data are reliably available from the late 1800s for England and Wales, and from the 1930s and 1940s for the United States and

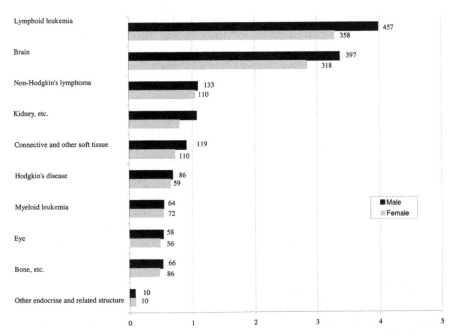

Figure 5 Age-adjusted rates (World Standard) and number of cancers for the top 10 cancer sites in children aged 0–14 years by sex, United States (SEER Program), 1988–1992. *Source*: From Ref. 20.

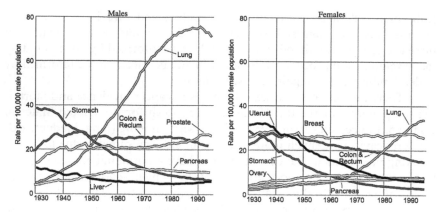

Figure 6 Age-standardized (1970 U.S. Standard) cancer mortality rates for selected sites, by sex, United States, 1930–1995. Uterus, uterine cervix and corpus combined. *Source*: From American Cancer Society, Surveillance Research, 1999 (28). Data obtained from Vital Statistics of the United States, 1990.

Scandinavian countries. Trends in cancer mortality in the United States are presented in Figure 6. Since 1930, there have been striking changes in the age-adjusted mortality rates for several cancer sites (note that crude rates are not used because the population structure of the United States has changed over this time frame). Rates for lung cancer show the most dramatic increase, from a relatively rare cause of death in 1930 to the leading cause of death after 1965. In contrast, stomach, uterine, and liver cancers have shown dramatic declines since 1930. Other cancers have shown more stable patterns in mortality over this time frame.

Long-term trends in cancer incidence rates are less available globally, since population-based cancer registration systems are a relatively new phenomenon. In the United States, Connecticut has had continuous cancer registration since 1935, and the SEER Program has conducted continuous surveillance on approximately 10% of the U.S. population since 1973. Table 2 shows the percent change in the incidence (SEER Program) and mortality (United States) rates for selected cancer sites from 1973 to 1996. Since 1973, cancer incidence for all sites (excluding nonmelanoma skin) has increased 20% and mortality has increased 3.3%. Data from the SEER Program from 1975 to 1995 suggest that for the major pediatric tumors there has been no substantial change in incidence and a dramatic decline in mortality, the latter related to treatment-related improvements in survival (27).

Some time trends are easier to explain than others, and trend data are often correlated with other data at the population level to suggest or evaluate etiological hypotheses (see ecological studies, below). For example, the trends in lung cancer incidence and mortality are thought to be almost entirely due to cigarette smoking. The reason for the decline in stomach

Table 2 Percent Change in U.S. Mortality and SEER Incidence for Selected Sites (All Races; Males and Females), 1973–1996

		Decreasing incidence			Increasing incidence	
	Site	Mortality	Incidence	Site	Mortality	Incidence
Decreasing mortality	Oral cavity and pharynx	−28.4	−11.0	Breast[a]	−7.5	25.3
	Stomach	−41.0	−34.5	Testis[a]	−70.0	41.5
	Colon and rectum	−22.6	−9.1	Urinary bladder	−24.0	7.7
	Pancreas	−3.4	−11.5	Thyroid	−21.6	42.1
	Larynx	−10.4	−16.2			
	Cervix uteri[a]	−47.3	−44.0			
	Corpus and uterus, NOS[a]	−26.7	−27.4			
	Ovary[a]	−11.2	−0.7			
	Hodgkin's disease	−64.3	−17.4			
	Leukemias	−6.2	−5.3			
Increasing mortality				All sites	3.3	20.0
				Esophagus	20.0	9.2
				Liver and intrahep	50.8	77.5
				Lung and bronchus	38.6	27.8
				Melanomas of skin	35.8	134.6
				Prostate[a]	13.0	111.9
				Kidney and renal pelvis	18.5	44.2
				Brain and other nervous	11.1	15.8
				Non-Hodgkin lymphomas	44.5	81.3
				Multiple myeloma	36.0	13.7

[a]Percent changes for sex-specific sites are only for the appropriate sex; breast data are for females only.
Source: Ref. 18. Data obtained from SEER Program—incidence National Center for Health Statistics—mortality.

cancer incidence is less clear, but is thought to be due to improvements in food preservation by the wide-scale adoption of domestic refrigeration. The rapid increase in skin melanoma is thought to be due to intermittent sun exposure occurring during recreational activities that became more prevalent starting in the 1950s. Declines in cervical cancer mortality are thought to be attributed to the introduction of effective screening using the pap smear. Evaluation of time trends can also suggest surprising trends, such as the rapid increase in the incidence of non-Hodgkin lymphoma in the United States since 1973, which is largely without explanation (28).

While time trend data provide powerful information, it must be kept in mind that changes over time may be partially or totally artifacts due to the effects of a variety of other factors (29). Changes in diagnostic practice, particularly from new medical technologies including imaging technologies, will impact incidence rates, particularly for brain and other internal tumors. There can also be changes in diagnostic criteria, and for cancer, the histopathologic classification of tumors. At the population level, changes in the availability of and/or access to medical care (e.g., the implementation of the Medicare program in the United States in the 1960s) or introduction of screening programs will also impact rates and thus time trends. Finally, declines in other diseases, particularly infectious and heart disease will impact cancer rates through effects on competing mortality.

An epidemic occurs when a disease has much higher rates than expected based on the usual (background) rates for a given population. For cancer, data on time trends presented for the United States, as well as data from elsewhere in the world (29), give no evidence that there has been an overall epidemic of cancer in the last 50 years. Total cancer rates, however, hide often dramatic changes occurring for individual cancers, and of all the changes in the 20th century, the most striking observation is the clear epidemic of lung cancer caused by cigarette smoking.

In migrant studies, the cancer rates of immigrants in a new country are compared with the cancer rates in their home country, generally using descriptive statistics (30,31). For example, in Figure 7, the incidence rates for stomach, colorectal, and breast cancer are compared for Chinese women in selected geographical locations. Rates for stomach cancer were highest in China, intermediate in Hong Kong and Singapore, and lowest in the United States; in contrast, breast cancer rates show the opposite pattern, and colorectal rates are intermediate. Migrant studies represent natural experiments in that genetic factors are essentially held constant while environmental factors, both physical (e.g., air, water, ultraviolet radiation, trace elements) and sociocultural (e.g., diet, alcohol and tobacco use, childbearing patterns, sexual habits, use of medical services), are allowed to vary. Classic studies include Japanese migration to Hawaii and the western United States, Central Europeans to the United States, Europeans to Australia, and Jews of various locations (United States, Eastern Europe, North Africa) to Israel

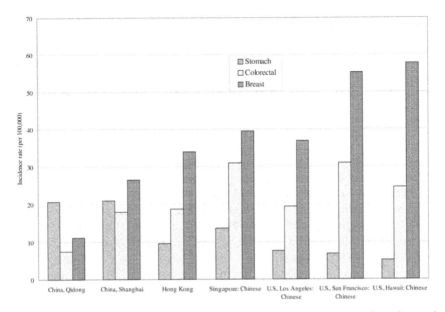

Figure 7 Age-adjusted (World Standard) incidence rates for stomach, colorectal, and breast cancer among Chinese women from selected geographical areas, 1988–1992. *Source*: From Ref. 20.

(30). Besides the relative contribution of genetics vs. environment in the etiology of cancer, migrant studies can also give insight into the timing of exposure of environmental agents in the carcinogenic process. A rapid change in cancer rates among adults migrating to a new country strongly suggests a role for agents that act in the later stages of the carcinogenic process (e.g., colon and prostate cancer rates in Japanese) or the effectiveness of the introduction of preventive strategies (e.g., cervical cancer rates in migrants to Israel) (30). In contrast, cancer rates that take several generations to approach those of the host country suggest that exposure in early life (including in utero) may be important, although the role of persistent cultural patterns must also be evaluated. It is important to be aware of the limitations of migrant studies (30,31). First, migrants are self-selected, and often vary by ethnicity, religion, socioeconomical status, and occupation from the population from which they are emigrating. These factors are risk factors for many cancers, and can confound the results. Migrants also often go from poorer, less developed areas to more industrialized areas. For valid conclusions, the data quality of the groups being compared should be comparable. Finally, if mortality rates are being compared, there is concern that migrants (particularly first-generation migrants) might return home to die.

1.3. Analytical Epidemiology

The goal of observational study designs is to make valid comparisons between individuals (or populations) with and without cancer or between those "naturally" exposed or unexposed to a factor of interest. The important strengths and limitations of the major observational study designs are summarized in Table 3.

1.3.1. Cross-Sectional Studies

In a cross-sectional study, a survey is conducted in a population during a defined time period. Both the predictor (exposure) and the outcome (in this context, having a cancer) variables are measured at the same time (note that there is no structural distinction between predictor and outcome variables; rather it is the investigator who makes the distinction). One common name for this study design is a prevalence survey. For example, the National Health and Nutrition Examination II (NHANES-II) was a cross-sectional survey of a national sample of adults who were selected to be representative of the U.S. population (32). The study provided data on the prevalence of average daily fat intake, physical activity, and many other health-related exposures. The survey also inquired about current and past disease history, and could be used to estimate the prevalence of cancer. However, as discussed earlier, the prevalence rate is of limited usefulness because it includes persons at all stages of the natural history of cancer (i.e., from recently diagnosed to long-term survivors), but underrepresents persons with rapidly fatal disease. Another major limitation of the cross-sectional study design is that it cannot easily distinguish the temporal sequence of events and whether the predictor event occured before or after the outcome. Finally, incidence rates cannot be calculated, and as discussed previously, this is one of the most useful cancer statistics.

1.3.2. Prospective and Retrospective Cohort Studies

In a cohort study, a group of people who are at risk of developing cancer are characterized as exposed or not exposed, and then they are followed through time in order to compare the rate of later cancers that develop in each group. The cohort can be a sample from the general population, workers in an industry, alumni or professional group, and so forth; a cohort is often chosen based on the ability to efficiently follow it over a long period of time. The cohort design can take place in real time (prospective) or can be historical (retrospective). The characterization of exposure can be through a questionnaire, medical records, biological testing, work records, and so forth. Methods of follow-up can include passive linkage to population-based cancer registries, mortality data, health claims databases, or active follow-up (recontact) of the cohort. The key to a valid cohort study is the nearly complete follow-up of the cohort, although as long as follow-up mechanisms do

Table 3 Comparison of Strengths and Limitations of the Major Study Designs Used in Cancer Epidemiology

Design	Strengths	Limitations
Ecological	Usually based on large populations (stable rates); capitalizes on existing and routinely collected data (mainly mortality); obtains populations markedly divergent in exposure levels; very useful to rapidly generate hypotheses for further study or to evaluate associations at the national/ international level identified in other analytical studies	Ecological fallacy; no control over subject selection; no control over measurement of exposures or evaluation/ classification of cancer; difficult to control for confounding; does not establish the sequence of events (temporality); can only be conducted once
Cross-sectional	Can potentially study multiple exposures and cancer endpoints simultaneously; control over subject selection; control over exposure measurement and evaluation/classification of cancer; can often be conducted relatively quickly; can calculate prevalence; useful to generate hypotheses; often used to initiate a cohort study	Measurement of exposure could be biased in persons with cancer; likely to miss persons with severe or rapidly fatal cancer (survivor bias); does not yield incidence; not feasible to study most cancers (due to rarity)
Cohort	Clearly establishes sequence of events; no potential for recall bias based on subsequent cancer outcome; can study several cancers simultaneously; good for studying rapidly fatal cancers (avoids survivor bias); number of cancers accumulates over time; can calculate incidence, relative risk, and excess risk	Needs large sample sizes to study site-specific cancers; not feasible for rare cancers; often can only collect a limited amount of exposure data due to feasibility and cost issues
Prospective	More control over exposure measurements and evaluation/classification of cancer; more control over subject selection	More expensive; long-term time commitment
Retrospective	Less costly and time consuming than prospective studies	Less control over selection of subjects; less control over

(Continued)

Table 3 (*Continued*)

Design	Strengths	Limitations
		measurement of exposures (what is measured; quality of measurement); often missing data on important confounders
SMR	May be the only feasible approach to study very rare exposures	Potential for bias in studying two popula- tions with data often collected in very different ways; often no data on important confounders
Case-control	Efficient for studying rarer cancers where a cohort study would not be feasible; can study multiple etiological factors simultaneously; can evaluate different latency periods for a given exposure; relatively few subjects needed; relatively short duration and inexpensive (compared to cohort studies); yields the odds ratio, generally good approximation of the relative risk	Potential for selection bias in sampling for cases and controls; limited to the study of one cancer; potential for differential recall bias in measuring exposure; does not necessarily establish sequence of events (temporality); potential for survivor bias; cannot calculate prevalence, incidence

not favor a particular exposure group, the comparison of disease experience between groups should be unbiased. The male British doctors study is one of the earliest and most famous prospective cohort studies in cancer epidemiology. The 40-year follow-up was recently published for cigarette smoking and cancer mortality (33). One of the conclusions of these data is that earlier studies appeared to underestimate the hazard of long-term smoking, and that approximately 50% of regular smokers will eventually be killed by a tobacco-related disease. There are many advantages of the cohort study design (Table 3), including the ability to clearly establish a temporal sequence, the lack of recall bias by disease status, and the ability to calculate true incidence rates and relative risks. In addition, as seen in the example of the British doctors, multiple outcomes from a single exposure can be evaluated.

A double-cohort study or standard mortality ratio (SMR), compares the rates of two separate cohorts, one highly exposed to an agent of interest and the other having low or no exposure. The most common application of this design is in occupational or environmental studies where the exposure of interest is rare in the general population. In practice, the comparison cohort is often the general population in the area where the exposed group was obtained.

There is great interest in whether radon causes lung cancer. This hypothesis was originally evaluated in underground uranium miners, but many of these men also smoked cigarettes and this was often not documented in any records, so there was a concern that any association between radon and lung cancer might be due to confounding by smoking. One approach to evaluate this possibility was to study nonsmoking uranium miners, since there would be no possibility of confounding by smoking. An example is the study of 516 nonsmoking uranium miners followed from 1950 to 1984 for lung cancer mortality (34). Lung cancer mortality rates for these men were compared to age-specific mortality rates for nonsmokers from a study of U.S. veterans. The latter group was chosen as the comparison group over the general population, since the general population rates would reflect the experience of a population with a large number of smokers, and thus would weaken the ability of the study to detect an association with lung cancer. Fourteen lung cancer deaths were observed in these 516 men through 1984, but only 1.1 deaths were expected, yielding an SMR of 13, suggesting a very strong association between radon and lung cancer mortality in nonsmokers, at least at the levels of radon exposure in these miners.

This SMR study design retains many of the advantages of the cohort study, but the use of an external comparison group, in contrast to internal comparisons in the classic cohort study, leads to the potential for bias that can occur when comparing two different populations. In the context of occupational cohort studies, where the comparison cohort is the general population, the concern is that employed persons are on average healthier and have better access to medical care than the general population. However, it should be noted that such a bias would be expected to move the SMR toward the null (i.e., make it harder to detect an association). The other major limitation of this study design is that data on confounding factors often are not available. Nevertheless, this study design is extremely useful for studying rare exposures in the population.

1.3.3. Case–Control Studies

In a case–control study, the exposure histories of cancer cases are compared with a group of individuals who are free of the cancer (controls) using the exposure odds ratio.

The advantages of the case–control study design include the ability to study multiple etiological factors, the ability to study exposures over a broad period of time (to better identify latency periods), and the efficiency in studying rare diseases. The two most common concerns in the conduct of a case–control study are selection bias and recall bias. Selection bias occurs when the case or control group is not representative of cases or controls in the underlying study base. Recall bias occurs when cases or controls *differentially* recall past exposures, leading to biased associations. A recent example of concern about differential recall bias is in the evaluation of induced abortion and breast cancer risk. There is evidence that while cases fairly accurately report induced abortions, healthy controls are likely to systematically underreport this procedure leading to a bias that suggests that there is an association (35). While case–control studies are susceptible to these types of biases, there are clear approaches to minimize their effect (36–38).

Case–control studies are also conducted from within cohort studies. This is a nested case–control study. Cases that occur during follow-up of the cohort are matched to controls who were disease free at the time the case developed their cancer. The exposure histories of cases and controls are then compared. The most useful situation for this design is when the predictor variables are expensive to evaluate and can be validly measured at a later time (e.g., DNA studies, certain serological assays). This study design is particularly useful in cancer epidemiology to evaluate the association of biomarkers with cancer risk in the context where the biomarker could potentially be affected by a cancer and thus the traditional case–control design (where cases already have a cancer when their biomarker is measured) may not be valid. The major limitation of the study design is that the time and expense of collecting and properly storing biological specimens for all cohort members must have been done at baseline, and thus there are relatively few cohorts available for such studies.

1.4. Integration of Laboratory Methodology

Epidemiologists have a long history of working closely with laboratory colleagues, dating back to the roots of infectious disease epidemiology. The explosive growth in molecular biology and other biomedical sciences has led to the rapidly evolving field called molecular epidemiology. Laboratory methods help in at least three critical areas in cancer epidemiology: exposure assessment, preclinical biological effects, and individual susceptibility (39, Fig. 8). Some of the more commonly utilized laboratory techniques in epidemiological studies of cancer etiology are listed in Table 4.

Exposure assessment is a long-standing problem in epidemiology, since questionnaire-based approaches often have great difficulty estimating average past exposure or cumulative exposure to an agent, and random measurement error is often large enough to overwhelm the ability to detect even large associations (7). Questionnaires are also subject to nonrandom error, in that cases or controls may differentially recall past exposures, and the direction of this type of bias is not always easy to predict. Biological markers of internal dose (e.g., measurement of a parent compound or metabolite in serum) or biologically effective dose (e.g., measurement of DNA or

Table 4 Common Laboratory Techniques Used in Molecular Epidemiology Studies of Cancer Etiology

Field	Biomarker to be measured in specimens	Technique
Histopathology	Grading of malignant traits in tumor tissue	Staining and blind scoring
Cytogenetics	Sister chromatid exchange	Staining and blind scoring
	Micronuclei	Staining and blind scoring
	DNA aneuploidy/hyperploidy	Flow cytometry
	Mutagen sensitivity/DNA repair capability	Bleomycin sensitivity assay, other G_2 assays
Immunology/ serology	Localization of antigenic epitopes in tissue	Immunohistochemistry
	Localization of mutated forms of gene products in cells	Immunohistochemistry
	Circulating antibodies or tumor antigens	Enzyme/radioimmunoassays
Biochemistry	Carcinogen–DNA adducts	Enzyme immunoassays, ^{32}P-postlabeling assays, fluorescent spectroscopy
	Carcinogen–protein adducts	Enzyme immunoassays, gas chromatography
	Nicotine metabolites	Enzyme immunoassays
	β-Carotene, retinol	High-performance liquid chromatography
Molecular biology	Specific DNA sequences (host or viral)	Southern blot hybridization, dot-blot hybridization, in situ hybridization, polymerase chain reaction
	Localization of specific DNA sequences in cells	In situ hybridization, polymerase chain reaction
	Specific RNA sequences or gene expression	Northern blot hybridization
	Allele losses or mutated forms of specific genes	Restriction fragment length polymorphism analysis, polymerase chain reaction, DNA sequencing
	Oncogene amplification	Southern blot amplification, dot-blot hybridization, polymerase chain reaction

Source: Franco EL. Epidemiology in the study of cancer. In: Bertino JR, ed. Encyclopedia of Cancer. Vol. 2:621–641. copyright 1996 by Academic Press.

protein adducts) of exposure to a carcinogen ("biomarkers of exposure") should allow for a much more precise and valid exposure assessment. However, much development in this field is required since issues of tissue sampling, use of surrogates for target tissues, biomarker validation, and approaches to estimating cumulative exposure are still being developed (5,40).

Preclinical biological effects (e.g., cytogenetic damage, gene mutation) and altered structure/function (e.g., premalignant alterations such as hyperproliferation or abnormal gene products) are the intermediate events between exposure and disease (39). These events can be used as specific "fingerprints" of prior exposure (e.g., mutational spectra of the *p53* tumor suppressor gene due to different environmental exposures) or as a surrogate endpoint for use in studies of chemoprevention. However, this is the least developed component of the model in Fig. 8, and the relationship of these events to preclinical and clinical cancer is still being elucidated. In addition, "fingerprints" at this point in the pathway are not necessarily specific to an exposure, since there are often multiple ways to induce the same pathological changes, and thus confounding can be introduced into the study.

Host susceptibility in this model is hypothesized to influence events at multiple points along the continuum from exposure to clinical disease (Fig. 8). Susceptibility is broadly defined, and includes effects of age and nutrition, as well as genetic effects. Genetic effects include inherited variability in the ability to activate/inactivate carcinogens (e.g., polymorphisms in cytochromes P-450 enzymes), repair DNA, and maintain genomic stability,

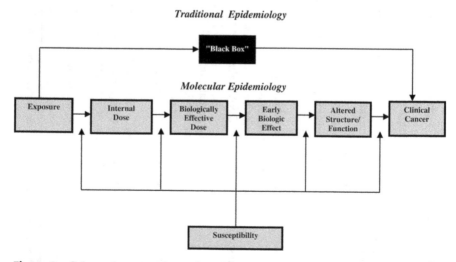

Figure 8   Schematic comparison of traditional and molecular epidemiology. *Source*: Adpated from Schulte PA, Perera FP, ed. Molecular Epidemiology: Principles and Practices. New York: Academic Press, 1993.

as well as genetic and epigenetic alterations in oncogenes and tumor suppressor genes.

The rapid inclusion of laboratory-based components to epidemiologic studies of cancer should provide better risk estimates by more accurately defining exposure, disease, and the interaction of exposure and genetic susceptibility; better accounting for individual level variability and effect modification; enhancing risk assessment; and better identifying potential points for screening and/or early intervention in the carcinogenic pathway (5,40–42). Integration of these methods into epidemiological studies also allows insight into the mechanisms of carcinogenesis, in part helping to fill in the "black box" between environmental exposure and cancer. However, many of these laboratory methods are cumbersome or expensive, and these studies require the collection of biological specimens, which often strains traditional approaches to conducting epidemiologic research. Nevertheless, the basic concepts in study design apply to studies incorporating biological data, and must be considered carefully in designing studies to prevent the introduction of bias (43,44).

1.5. Framework for Interpretation of Analytical Epidemiological Studies

1.5.1. Evaluation of Causality

Ultimately, we are interested in knowing what causes cancer. At the most basic level, a cause is something that brings about any condition or produces any effect. Unfortunately causation is in general not directly observable, and it is not possible to provide absolute proof of causation in any empirical science (8). However, the goal at hand is not absolute proof, but might be better viewed as the accumulation of sufficient evidence to convince most skeptics beyond a reasonable doubt. The two most well-known approaches to the evaluation of causation are the Henle–Koch postulates and Hill's criteria of causality (45).

The Henle–Koch postulates (1890) were developed to evaluate whether an infectious agent caused a particular disease, and they have had a major influence on how we think about causality. The postulates, listed in Table 5, while clearly useful in many situations, are limited even in infectious disease epidemiology (e.g., they do not apply to many viral, parasitic, spirochetal, and fungal diseases), and have severe limitations as useful guidelines in chronic disease (46). This is in part because they do not account for the concepts of multiple causation, biological spectrum of disease, and host response.

The most commonly used framework for evaluation of causality in cancer (and other chronic diseases) came from the Surgeon General's first report on smoking and health (47), published by Hill (45). The general approach to evaluating causality is to first rule out the likelihood of

Table 5   Criteria to Evaluate Causation

Causal criterion	Nature of inquiry
Henle-Koch's postulates (1890)	
Single cause	The parasite occurs in every case of the disease in question and under circumstances which can account for the pathological changes and clinical course of the disease
Virulence	The parasite occurs in no other disease as a fortuitous and nonpathogenic parasite
Culturability	After being fully isolated from the body and repeatedly grown in pure culture, the parasite can induce the disease anew
Hill's criteria (45)	
Strength of association	What is the relative risk?
Consistency of association	Is there an agreement among repeated observations in different places, at different times, using different methodologies, by different researchers, under different circumstances?
Temporality	Does exposure precede the outcome variable?
Biological gradient	Is there evidence of a dose–response relationship?
Plausibility	Does the causal association make biological sense?
Specificity of association	Is the outcome unique to the association?
Coherence	Is the causal association compatible with present knowledge of the disease?
Experimentation	Does controlled manipulation of the exposure change the outcome?
Analogy	Does the causal relationship conform to a previously described relationship?

noncausal explanations (i.e., bias, confounding, and chance), and then to evaluate each of the points in Table 5. Not all of the criteria are considered equally useful (8), and in literature reviews the first six criteria in Table 5 are the most commonly used (48). Further critiques of the evaluation of causality and the role of Hill's criteria can be found elsewhere (8,49).

1.5.2.   Population Attributable Risk

While there are many causes of cancer, not all causes are equally important in the primary prevention of cancer at the population level. While the magnitude of the association (i.e., size of the relative risk or odds ratio) is an important criterion in the evaluation of causality, it takes somewhat of a secondary role in evaluating the importance of an exposure at the population level. That is because the population attributable risk (PAR), which is defined as the "reduction in incidence that would be achieved if the population had been entirely unexposed, compared with its current (actual)

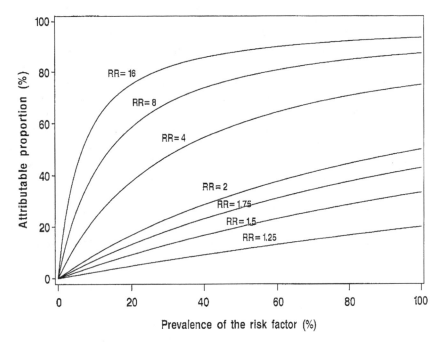

Figure 9 Relationship between relative risk and risk factor prevalence on the population attributable risk.

exposure pattern" (8), is a function of the risk ratio and the prevalence of exposure in the population. This relationship is summarized in Fig. 9. For example, a risk factor with a modest relative risk (e.g., 1.75) but a high prevalence in the population (e.g., 60%) has a PAR of 31%, while a risk factor with a high relative risk (e.g., 16) but rare (e.g., 0.1%) has a PAR of 1.5%; the former risk factor, then, explains much more of the cancer burden in the population.

A couple of caveats about using the PAR (8,50) deserve mention. First, for the PAR to be valid, the risk factor must be considered to be a causal factor of the disease, and the risk ratio is assumed to be estimated without significant bias. Second, the interpretation assumes that removal of the exposure does not affect the size of the at-risk population; however, this assumption needs to be scrutinized on a case-by-case basis as removal of an exposure may have multiple effects on the at-risk population through effects on competing mortality.

2. THE CAUSES OF CANCER

Cancer patients want to know what caused their cancer. Pragmatically, the causes of cancer in an individual can be broadly classified into environmental (cumulative exposure over a lifetime to a variety of carcinogenic and protective factors), genetic, and spontaneous (51).

1. *Spontaneous*. Often overlooked are the spontaneous causes of cancer. By spontaneous, what is meant is that a certain amount of cancer is due to "spontaneous" or "background" mutation rates (51). These mutations generally show a different pattern of DNA lesions compared to those induced by carcinogens. The exact causes of these mutations are not known, but are likely due to things such as background cosmic radiation and body temperature, and reflect the instability of DNA as a result of oxidative damage and other cellular processes. These factors would be expected to show little or no variability in terms of geographical distribution, and thus there will always be a certain background level of cancer in any population. Doll and Peto (9) have also termed this "chance," or more simply good or bad luck. At the level of the individual, spontaneous causes of cancer may play an important explanatory role. Knudson (51) has estimated that approximately 15% of cancer may be explained by spontaneous factors.

2. *Genetic*. Cancer has long been known to aggregate in families, strongly supporting a hereditary component for a certain portion of cancer. Familial cancers are generally characterized by early age at onset, bilateral tumors in paired organs, multiple primary foci within an organ, distinctive pathology, and often prominent physical findings. They may also be a part of a syndrome that includes multiple cancer sites and/or other diseases (e.g., Von Hippel–Lindau disease and renal cell carcinoma), and are caused by germline (i.e., changes in the constitutional DNA) alterations in single genes that often follow Mendelian patterns of inheritance (i.e. "major genes"). However, it must be kept in mind that cancer is a relatively common disease, and thus many persons will have a positive family history of cancer, and some cancer will cluster in families by chance alone. In addition, families often share similar environmental exposures (including residence, diet, and so forth) and this may explain some clustering of cancer within families. Thus, "familial" is not synonymous with "genetic." Geneticists and genetic epidemiologists use family studies to evaluate the relative contribution of genes vs. environment, and to identify new cancer genes.

In contrast to cancer caused by major genes, a second class of genes, often termed "susceptibility" genes (52) are also likely to be important in cancer causation. Susceptibility genes are common variants (polymorphisms) of genes generally involved in the metabolic activation and detoxification of carcinogens, but they can be involved in other pathways relevant to carcinogenesis including DNA repair. This concept is highly influenced by the field of pharmacogenetics, and examples of this approach include studies of lung cancer and debrisoquine metabolism and GST-mu deficient phenotype and bladder cancer.

An important distinction between these two types of genetic causes of cancer are that while major genes carry a high absolute and relative risk, they are uncommon in the population and thus have a low population attributable risk. In contrast, susceptibility genes are associated with a low absolute and relative risk of cancer, but because many of these variants are common in the population, they may have a high population attributable risk. Another important distinction is that the major genes are expected to be less influenced by environmental exposures relative to the susceptibility genes, which primarily influence host response to the environment. Understanding hereditary cancer is expected to give mechanistic insight into the causes of sporadic (i.e., nonhereditary) cancer. However, in the population, only about 5% of cancer is thought to be due to purely genetic (major gene) causes (51).

3. *Environmental, lifestyle, and behavioral factors.* A conclusion from the descriptive and analytical epidemiology of cancer is that cancer should be largely, although not completely, preventable and that environmental and behavioral factors should account for a large percentage of the total cases, often estimated at up to 80% of cancer (51). Doll and Peto (9,53) originally published their estimates of cancer deaths attributable to various environmental and behavioral factors in western populations in 1981, and recently updated this in 1996. As shown in Table 6, tobacco and diet are

Table 6 Estimates of the Proportion of Cancer Deaths Attributable to Environmental and Lifestyle Factors in Western Countries

Factor(s)	Best estimate of proportion (%)	Range of acceptable estimates (%)
Tobacco	33	25–40
Diet	30	20–60
Infection	9	5–15
Hormones	7	5–10
Ionizing radiation	4	2–6
Background	3.5	
Medical procedures	0.5	
Industry	<0.1	
Alcohol	3	2–4
Occupation	3	2–4
Pollution	<2	< 1–2
Atmospheric	<1	
Water	<1	
Ultraviolet light	1	0.5–1
Industrial products	<1	<1–2
Medical drugs	<1	<1–2
Food additives	<1	−2–1
Other and unknown	?	?

Source: From Ref. 9. Copyright 1996 Oxford University Press.

thought to be the most important causes of cancer, although clearly the ultimate role of diet in the etiology of cancer is still being unraveled. The next most important group of factors are infection, hormones, background ionizing radiation, occupation, and alcohol. Of relatively less importance are ultraviolet radiation, industrial products, water and air pollution, and food additives, exposures that tend to receive a disproportionate amount of media attention.

One limitation in interpreting Table 6 is that it does not take into account interactions between exposures. For example, smoking increases the risk of lung cancer, as does exposure to asbestos; however, the risk of lung cancer in smokers exposed to asbestos is much greater than expected based on each risk factor considered individually. Other well-established interactions include smoking and radon for lung cancer, smoking and alcohol for esophageal cancer, and hepatitis B infection and exposure to aflatoxin for liver cancer. Other interactions are likely.

4. *Gene–environment interaction*. While carcinogen exposure triggers the onset of cancer, a person's genetic makeup determines how they respond to the exposure. Thus, genes may increase or decrease risk from the exposure and so this is considered a gene–environment interaction. There is currently great interest in identifying interactions between genetic and environmental causes of cancer. As alluded to above, most (but by no means all) of the interest is focused on the interaction of susceptibility genes with environmental exposures. Although unknown at this time, much of the 80% of cancer thought to be due to environmental causes may be due to gene–environment interactions (39). The study of gene–environment interactions will consume much of epidemiological research over the next decade.

3. CONCLUSIONS AND FUTURE DIRECTIONS

An initial task of epidemiology is to describe the variability in cancer risk. It is clear that risk of cancer is highly variable at the population level based on observations of geographic, time trend, and migrant data, and these results strongly suggest that a large proportion of cancer is not random and there must be an explanation. Analytic epidemiology has identified many causal factors for cancer risk, and removal of the exposure has led to changes in cancer incidence. Two conclusions from these observations are that much of cancer is likely due to environmental factors and much of the cancer burden in the population should be preventable. Due to the explosion in our understanding of the molecular basis of carcino-genesis, including the quantification of genetic susceptibility and the interaction of susceptibility with environmental exposures (gene–environment interaction) these have become evolving research areas that should better define the causes and primary prevention of cancer in the population.

ACKNOWLEDGMENTS

Dr. Cerhan was supported in part by a Preventive Oncology Academic Award from the National Cancer Institute (K07 CA64220). Technical assistance was provided by Sara Butler Osborn, Robert Vierkant, and Mary Jo Janisch.

REFERENCES

1. Last JM. A Dictionary of Epidemiology. New York: Oxford University Press, 1995.
2. Harris H. General characteristics of neoplasia. In: Weatherall DJ, Ledingham JGG, Warrell DA, eds. Oxford Textbook of Medicine. 3rd ed. New York: Oxford University Press, 1996:191–196.
3. NE Day. Time as a determinant of risk in cancer epidemiology: the role of multistage models. Cancer Surv 1983; 2:577–593.
4. Armitage P. Multistage models of carcinogenesis. Environ Health Perspect 1985; 63:195–201.
5. Shields PG, Harris CC. Molecular epidemiology and the genetics of environmental cancer. J Am Med Assoc 1991; 266:681–687.
6. Bissell MJ, Weaver VM, Lelievre SA, Wang F, Petersen OW, Schmeichel KL. Tissue structure, nuclear organization, and gene expression in normal and malignant breast. Cancer Res 1999; 59:1757s–1763s; discussion 1763s–1764s.
7. Armstrong BK, White E, Saracci R. Principles of Exposure Measurement in Epidemiology. Monographs on Epidemiology and Biostatistcs. New York: Oxford University Press, 1992.
8. Rothman KJ, Greenland S. Modern Epidemiology. 2nd ed. Philadelphia, PA: Lippincott-Raven Publishers, 1998.
9. Doll R, Peto R. Epidemiology of cancer. In: Weatherall DJ, Ledingham JGG, Warrell DA, eds. Oxford Textbook of Medicine. 3rd ed. New York: Oxford University Press, 1996:197–222.
10. Herman J. Experiment and observation. Lancet 1994; 344:1209–1211.
11. Fraumeni JF, Lloyd JW, Smith EM, Wagoner JK. Cancer mortality among nuns: role of marital status in etiology of neoplastic disease in women. J Natl Cancer Inst 1969; 42:455–468.
12. Muir CS. International patterns of cancer. In: Greenwald P, Kramer BS, Weed DL, eds. Cancer Prevention and Control. New York: Marcel Dekker, Inc., 1995:37–68.
13. Chu KC, Kramer BS. Cancer patterns in the United States. In: Greenwald P, Kramer BS, Weed DL, eds. Cancer Prevention and Control. New York: Marcel Dekker, Inc., 1995:9–22.
14. Boyle P. Relative value of incidence and mortality data in cancer research. Recent Results Cancer Res 1989; 114:41–63.
15. Extramural Committee to Assess Measures of Progress Against Cancer. Measurement of progress against cancer. J Natl Cancer Inst 1990; 82:825–835.
16. Jensen OM, Parkin DM, MacLennan R, Muir CS, Skeet R. Cancer Registration: Principles and Methods. Lyon, France: IARC, 1991.

17. Howe HL, Lehnherr M, Derrick L. Cancer Incidence in North America, 1988–1992. Sacramento, CA: North American Association of Central Cancer Registries, 1996.
18. Ries LAG, Kosary CL, Hankey BF, Miller BA, Clegg LX. SEER Cancer Statistics Review, 1973–1996. Bethesda, MD: National Cancer Institute, 1999.
19. Parkin DM, Whelan SL, Feday J, Young J. Cancer Incidence in Five Continents. Lyon, France: IARC, 1997.
20. Ferlay J, Black RJ, Whelan SL, Parkin DM. CI5VII: Electronic Database of Cancer Incidence in Five Continents. International Agency for Cancer Research on Cancer, 1997.
21. Ferlay J, Parkin DM, Pisani P. GLOBOCAN 1: Cancer Incidence and Mortality Worldwide. International Association of Cancer Registries, 1998.
22. Parkin DM, Pisani P, Ferlay J. Estimates of the worldwide incidence of 25 major cancers in 1990. Int J Cancer 1999; 80:827–841.
23. Pisani P, Parkin DM, Bray F, Ferlay J. Estimates of the worldwide mortality from 25 cancers in 1990. Int J Cancer 1999; 83:18–29.
24. Day NE. Cumulative rate and cumulative risk. In: Parkin DM, Muir CS, Whelan SL, Gao YT, Ferlay J, Powell J, eds. Cancer Incidence in Five Continents. Lyon, France: IARC, 1992.
25. Landis SH, Murray T, Bolden S, Wingo PA. Cancer statistics. CA Cancer J Clin 1999; 49:8–31.
26. Miller RW, Myers MH. Age distribution of epithelial and non-epithelial cancers. Lancet 1983; 2:1250.
27. Linet MS, Ries LA, Smith MA, Tarone RE, Devesa SS. Cancer surveillance series: recent trends in childhood cancer incidence and mortality in the United States. J Natl Cancer Inst 1999; 91:1051–1058.
28. Hartge P, Devesa SS. Quantification of the impact of known risk factors on time trends in non-Hodgkin's lymphoma incidence. Cancer Res 1992; 52(suppl):5566s–5569s.
29. Muir CS, Fraumeni JF, Doll R. The interpretation of time trends. Cancer Surv 1994; 20:5–21.
30. Parkin DM, Khlat M. Studies of cancer in migrants: rationale and methodology. Eur J Cancer 1996; 32A:761–771.
31. McCredie M. What have we learned from studies of migrants? Cancer Causes Control 1998; 9:1–2.
32. National Center of Health Statistics. Plan and operation of the second national health and nutrition examination survey 1976–1980. In: Engel A, Massey J, Maurer K, eds. Hyattsville, MD: DHEW, 1981.
33. Doll R, Peto R, Wheatley K, Gray R, Sutherland I. Mortality in relation to smoking: 40 years' observations on male British doctors. Br Med J 1994; 309:901–911.
34. Roscoe RJ, Steenland K, Halperin WE, Beaumont JJ, Waxweiler RJ. Lung cancer mortality among nonsmoking uranium miners exposed to radon daughters. J Am Med Assoc 1989; 262:629–633.
35. Rookus MA, van Leeuwen FE. Induced abortion and risk for breast cancer: reporting (recall) bias in a Dutch case–control study. J Natl Cancer Inst 1996; 88:1759–1764.

36. Wacholder S, McLaughlin JK, Silverman DT, Mandel JS. Selection of controls in case–control studies. I. Principles. Am J Epidemiol 1992; 135:1019–1028.
37. Wacholder S, Silverman DT, McLaughlin JK, Mandel JS. Selection of controls in case–control studies. II. Types of controls. Am J Epidemiol 1992; 135:1029–1041.
38. Wacholder S, Silverman DT, McLaughlin JK, Mandel JS. Selection of controls in case–control studies. III. Design options. Am J Epidemiol 1992; 135:1042–1050.
39. Perera FP. Molecular epidemiology of environmental carcinogenesis. Recent Results Cancer Res 1998; 154:39–46.
40. McMichael AJ. Invited commentary—"molecular epidemiology": new pathway or new travelling companion? Am J Epidemiol 1994; 140:1–11
41. Schulte PA. A conceptual and historical framework for molecular epidemiology. In: Schulte PA, Perera FP, eds. Molecular Epidemiology: Principles and Practices. New York: Academic Press, 1993:3–44.
42. Perera FP, Weinstein IB. Molecular epidemiology and carcinogen-DNA adduct detection: new approaches to studies of human cancer causation. J Chronic Dis 1982; 35:581–600.
43. Rothman N, Stewart WF, Schulte PA. Incorporating biomarkers into cancer epidemiology: a matrix of biomarker and study design categories. Cancer Epidemiol Biomarkers Prev 1995; 4:301–311.
44. Fletcher RH. Cases and controls from different settings: ideals and practicalities. Cancer Epidemiol Biomarkers Prev 1997; 6:555–556.
45. Hill AB. The environment of disease: association or causation? Proc R Soc Med 1965; 58:295–300.
46. Fredricks DN. Sequence-based evidence of microbial disease causation: when Koch's postulates don't fit. J NIH Res 1996; 8:39–44.
47. US Department of Health, and Welfare. Smoking and Health. Washington, DC: Government Printing Office, 1964.
48. Weed DL, Gorelic LS. The practice of causal inference in cancer epidemiology. Cancer Epidemiol Biomarkers Prev 1996; 5:303–311.
49. Rothman KJ, Poole C. Causation and casual inference. In: Schottenfeld D, Fraumeni JF Jr, eds. Cancer Epidemiology and Prevention. 2nd ed. Oxford: Oxford University Press, 1996:3–10.
50. Rockhill B, Newman B, Weinberg C. Use and misuse of population attributable fractions. Am J Public Health 1998; 88:15–19.
51. Knudson AG. Genetics and etiology of human cancer. Hum Genet 1977; 8:1–66.
52. Caporaso N, Goldstein A. Cancer genes: single and susceptibility: exposing the difference. Pharmacogenetics 1995; 5:59–63.
53. Doll R, Peto R. The causes of cancer: quantitative estimates of avoidable risks of cancer in the United States today. J Natl Cancer Inst 1981; 66:1191–1308.

10

Cancer Susceptibility Genes and Common Gene Variants That Increase Cancer Risk

Ragnhild A. Lothe and Anne-Lise Børresen-Dale

Department of Genetics, Institute for Cancer Research, University Clinic of the Norwegian Radium Hospital, Oslo, Norway

Most cancers result from an interaction between genetic and environmental factors and these factors can determine an individual's cancer risk. Approximately 1% of all cancers arise in individuals with a clear hereditary cancer syndrome following Mendelian inheritance where environmental factors are thought to play a minor role (Fig. 1). Further, it is estimated that 10–15% of all cancers are due to inherited components, resulting in the so-called familial clustering of cancer. However, in most other cancers, a substantial genetic predisposition may also be present without obvious familial clustering. These genetic components include dominant mutations with a reduced penetrance, as well as more common genetic polymorphisms that influence an individual's response to environmental exposure. Most cancers however occur in the genetically low-risk population group, referred to as sporadic cases. The influence of genetic factors decreases and the impact of environmental factors increases with aging (Fig. 1). Knowledge of the spectrum of both genetic and environmental risk factors for developing cancer and how they interact, will be instrumental in future risk assessment and in prevention programs.

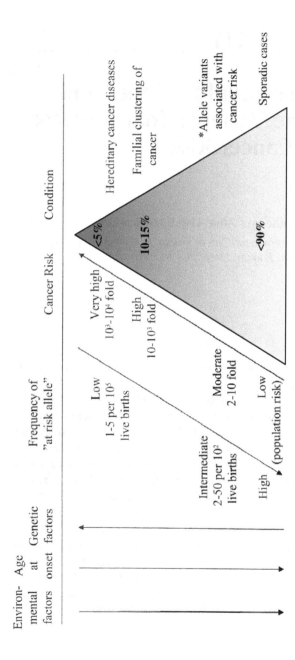

Figure 1 Environmental and genetic factors influence cancer risk. Up to 5% of all cancers are hereditary cases, 10–15% are estimated to account for familial clustering of cancer, and the rest are sporadic cases. The influence of environmental factors is low in hereditary cancer diseases and high in individuals at population risk level. The risk of cancer increases with age. The frequency of the "risk allele" is low for those genes predisposing to hereditary cancer, implying the low incidence of these diseases, whereas the cancer risk is very high, often obligatory, in the individuals carrying the mutated gene. *For allele variants associated with cancer risk, see Table 2.

1. HEREDITARY CANCER SYNDROMES

An inherited cancer syndrome is defined by Mendelian inheritance of susceptibility in a dominant, recessive, or X-linked manner. Many of the known cancer diseases follow a dominant mode of inheritance and have cancer as the main phenotype (Table 1a). Among other hereditary syndromes, both dominant and recessive, cancer can be one of several phenotypic traits (Table 1b and c). A hereditary cancer syndrome should be considered if several family members develop cancer at a young age, if both of paired organs are affected, or if affected individuals develop multiple primary cancers, including common cancers. Finally, family members with cancer who also manifest other rare conditions, particularly congenital abnormalities are suggestive of a cancer syndrome.

Many of the genes involved in these cancer syndromes have been identified (Table 1a–c) and they are referred to as "inherited cancer genes" or "susceptibility genes." Germline mutations in some of these genes approach a 100% risk of cancer during a lifetime. If a gene has incomplete penetrance, some mutation carriers will not develop the expected cancer. Environmental factors and/or other modifying genes (see below) may cause this reduced penetrance. In addition, non-carriers within a hereditary cancer family may develop sporadic cancer of the same type as the mutation carriers. These are termed phenocopies. Thus, accumulation of rare cancers in a family is more likely to be caused by an inherited predisposition than is the case for accumulation of common cancers.

2. IDENTIFICATION OF INHERITED CANCER GENES

The first step in identifying high penetrance genes is usually to do linkage analyses. These analyses are done within cancer families, to identify the chromosomal location of the predisposing gene. These studies may be difficult due to incomplete variable penetrance and different possible phenotypes. Nevertheless, by use of strict selection criteria for the families submitted to such analyses, the target genes for diseases such as hereditary breast cancer, hereditary nonpolyposis colorectal cancer, multiple endocrine neoplasia, have been localized. The chromosomal map position of the potential gene is the initial step of the positional cloning strategy, followed by cloning of the gene, identification of possible germline mutations, and finally description of the protein function. The *BRCA1* and the *BRCA2* breast cancer genes were identified through this method, for example. The cellular locations of the proteins encoded by hereditary cancer genes are shown in Fig. 2 and the protein functions are listed in Table 1.

Cytogenetical studies have also been useful in pinpointing the chromosomal location of cancer genes. Studies of constitutional (normal) cells from patients with retinoblastoma and Wilms' tumor revealed deletions of 13q14

Table 1 Cancer Diseases Caused by Germline Mutations in Known Genes

(a) Dominant hereditary cancer diseases/syndromes*

Disease	Associated tumors	Gene name	Year (Ref.)	Chromosome location	Protein function
Breast and ovarian cancers	Breast and ovarian cancers	*BRCA1*	1994 (1)	17q21	Repair of double strand breaks
Breast cancer 2	Breast cancer (male), pancreas and ovarian cancers	*BRCA2*	1995 (2)	13q12	Interacts with RAD51
Familial adenomatous polyposis (FAP)	Colorectal cancer, duodenal, gastric, and desmoid tumors	*APC*	1991 (3,4)	5q21	Complexes with β-catenin; microtubule binding
Familial melanoma	Malignant melanoma, pancreatic cancer, and dysplastic nevi	*CDKN2A*	1994 (5,6)	9p21	Inhibitor of cyclin dependent kinases
		CDK4	1996 (7)	12q13	Cyclin dependent kinase
Hereditary nonpolyposis colorectal cancer (HNPCC)	Colorectal cancer, endometrial, ovarian, gastric, and other cancers	*MSH2*	1993 (8,9)	2p16	Components of the mismatch repair system
		MLH1	1994 (10,11)	3p21	
		PMS1&2	1994 (12)	2q32	
		MSH6	1995 (13)	7p22	
Hereditary papillary renal cancer (HPRC)	Papillary renal cancer	*MET*	1997 (14)	7q31	Transmembrane receptor for hepatocyte growth factor (HGF)

Syndrome	Cancer types	Gene	Year (ref)	Location	Function
Li-Fraumeni syndrome (LFS)	Sarcoma, breast and brain cancers, leukemia	TP53	1984 (15)	17p13.1	Transcriptional regulation; responses to DNA damage
Multiple endocrine neoplasia type 1 (MEN1)	Pancreatic islet cell, parathyroid and pituitary tumors carcinoid	CHK2 / MEN1	1999 (16) / 1997 (17)	22q / 11q13	Cell cycle G2 control / Unknown
Multiple endocrine neoplasia types 2A and 2B (MEN2); familial medullary thyroid cancer	Medullary thyroid cancer. pheochromocytoma; Medullary thyroid cancer	RET	1993 (18)	10q11.2	Transmembrane receptor tyrosine kinase for glial-derived neutrophic factor (GDNF)
Retinoblastoma	Retinoblastoma, osteosarcoma	RB1	1986 (19)	13q14.2	Cell cycle and transcriptional regulation
Wilms' tumor 1	Wilms, tumor	WT1	1990 (20,21)	11p13	Transcriptional regulation
(b) Dominant hereditary syndromes with cancer as a phenotypic trait					
Cowden syndrome	Hamartoma, breast cancer, follicular thyroid cancer, glioblastoma	PTEN	1997 (22)	10q23	Tyrosine phosphatase activity; homology to tensin
Gorlin/nevoid basal cell carcinoma syndrome	Basal cell skin cancer, medulloblastoma, ovarian fibroma	PTCH	1996 (23)	9q22.3	Transmembrane receptor

(Continued)

Table 1 Cancer Diseases Caused by Germline Mutations in Known Genes (*Continued*)

Disease	Associated tumors	Gene name	Year (Ref.)	Chromosome location	Protein function
Multiple exostoses	Exostoses, chondrosarcoma	*EXT1* *EXT2*	1995 (24) 1996 (25)	8q24.1 11p12	Unknown Unknown
Neurofibromatosis type 1	Neurofibroma, malignant peripheral nerve sheath tumour, glioma	*NF1*	1990 (26–28)	17q11	GTP-ase activating protein for p21-ras
Neurofibromatosis type 2	Acoustic neuromas, meningioma, glioma, ependymoma	*NF2*	1993 (29,30)	22q12.2	Links cytoskeleton and plasma membrane
Peutz–Jegher syndrome	Intestinal hamartoma, breast cancer, gastrointestinal cancer, thyroid cancer, testicular cancer	*LKB1* = *STK*	1997 (31)	19p13.3	Serine–threonine kinase
Tuberous scleroses	Hamartoma, angio-myolipoma and fibroma	*TSC1* *TSC2*	1997 (32) 1993 (33)	9q34 16p13.3	Unknown GTP-ase activating protein for *rap1* and 5
Von Hippel–Lindau (VHL)	Renal cancer, hemangioblastoma, pheo-chromocytoma	*VHL*	1993 (34)	3p25	Transcriptional elongation

(c) Recessive hereditary syndromes with cancer as a phenotypic trait

Syndrome	Cancer	Gene	Year	Chromosome location	Function
Ataxia telangiectasia	Lymphoma, breast cancer, leukemia	ATM	1995 (35)	11q22	Induction of TP53; DNA repair
Blooms syndrome	Solid tumors	BLM	1996 (36,37)	15q26.1	DNA and RNA helicase
Fanconis anemia	Acute myelogenous leukemia	FAA	1996 (38)	16q24.3	Unknown
		FAC	1996 (39)	9q22.3	Unknown
		FAG	1998 (40)		Unknown
Xeroderma pigmentosum	Skin cancer	XPA	1989 (41)	9q22.3	Zn fmger-DNA damage recognition
		XPB(ERCC3)	1990 (42)	2q21	DNA helicase
		XPC	1992 (43)	3p25	SsDNA binding protein
		XPD(ERCC2)	1992 (44)	19q13	DNA helicase
		XPEI(DDBI)	1995 (45)	11q13–q21	Damage specific
		XPE2(DDB2)	1995 (45)	11p1–pl2	DNA binding proteins
		XPF(ERCC4)	1996 (46)	16pl3	Endonuclease
		XPG(ERCC5)	1993 (47)	13q33	Endonuclease

*Year: the year when the gene in question was isolated. Chromosome location: the map position of the gene. RG: repair gene, TSG: tumor suppressor gene, OG: oncogene, MMRG: mismatch repair gene, NER: nucleotide exision repair.

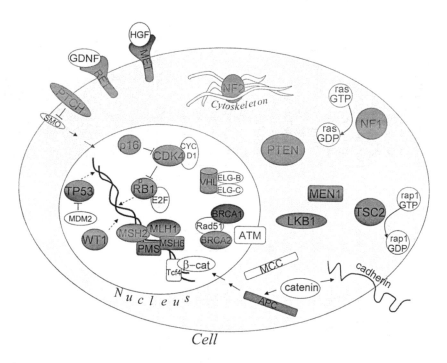

Figure 2 Cellular localization of proteins encoded by inherited cancer genes. Proteins encoded by hereditary cancer genes are shown in red and include APC, adenomatous polyposis coli; ATM, ataxia telangiectasia protein—mutated; BRCA 1 and 2, proteins encoded by breast cancer (and ovarian cancer) susceptibility genes; CDK4: cyclin dependent kinase 4; LKB1=STK11: serine threonine kinase 11; MEN: multiple endocrine neoplasia 1; MET: transmembrane receptor encoded by a susceptibility gene for hereditary papillary renal cancer; MLH1: mut L homolog 1; MSH2 and 6: mut S homologs 2 and 6; NF1 and 2: neurofibromatosis types 1 and 2; p16: cyclin dependent kinase inhibitor = CDKN2A; PMS1 and 2: mut L homologs that, if inactivated in yeast, cause a high frequency of postmeiotic segregation; PTCH: patched; PTEN: phosphatase and tensin homolog deleted on chromosome 10; RB1: retinoblastoma 1; RET: transmembrane receptor tyrosine kinase encoded by the susceptibility gene for multiple endocrine neoplasia; TSC2: tuberous sclerosis protein 2; TP53: tumor protein 53; VHL: von Hippel Lindau protein; WT1: Wilms'tumor protein 1. Other abbreviations: *β-cat: β*-catenin; CYC D1; cyclin D1; E2F: transcription factor that binds to the adenovirus E2 promoter; ELG-B and C: elongin B and C; GDNF: glial-derived neutrophic factor, HGF: hepatocyte growth factor; MCC: mutated in colorectal cancer; MDM2: mouse double minutes protein 2; SMO: smoothened; Tcf4: T-cell factor 4.

and 11p13, respectively (48,49). These two chromosome bands were later shown to harbor the predisposing genes *RB1* at 13q14.2 and *WT1* at 11p13 (19–21). Similar studies of individuals with von Recklinghausen neurofibromatosis identified two cases with balanced translocations, both involving 17q11, and these samples were then used in the cloning process of the *NF1* gene (50,51). The map position of the *APC* gene predisposing to familial adenomatous polyposis (FAP) was found at 5q21 due to an interstitial deletion in the germline of a mentally retarded patient with FAP (52). The chromosomal locations for susceptibility genes for 17 hereditary cancer diseases and 15 other syndromes with cancer as a phenotypic trait are listed in Table 1.

Individuals who are predisposed to cancer through an inherited or acquired mutation in the germline usually develop cancer at an early age, but are rarely born with cancer. For a cancer to develop in these individuals additional somatic changes are needed to initiate and establish a tumor. One hallmark of an inherited cancer gene is that they are often more frequently altered in somatic cells than in the germline. In accordance with the two-hit theory for inactivation of a tumor suppressor gene (53), deletion of the remaining allele is often found in the tumor from patients with an inherited mutated gene copy. In a sporadic case of the same type both events have to occur in the same cell line. The deletions are often identified by use of polymorphic markers within or flanking the gene in question. By comparing the heterozygous constitutional genotype with the tumor genotype, a possible loss of one allele will be detected. Cavenee et al. initially described this type of study applied on retinoblastomas in 1983 (54). Loss of hetorozygosity (LOH) studies have aided in identifying the location of several hereditary cancer genes exemplified by multiple endocrine neoplasia type 1, neurofibromatosis 2, and basal cell carcinoma syndrome (17,55,56).

3. FUNCTION OF INHERITED CANCER GENES*

Genes predisposing to hereditary cancer diseases can be subdivided into three major groups: the oncogenes that are activated through a mutated protooncogene creating a gain-of-function mutant, as opposed to an inactivated tumor suppressor gene resulting in a loss-of-function mutant. The third category is defect repair genes that indirectly cause alterations in other genes due to lack of repair. Such changes may give selective growth advantage if they affect oncogenes and tumor suppressor genes. (For a complete review, see Ref. 57.)

The proteins encoded by the inherited cancer genes are involved in a wide range of cellular processes (Fig. 2, Table 1). In the dominant inherited diseases, inactivating germline mutations are found in the tumor suppressor genes and activating mutations are found in the oncogenes. In accordance with the two-hit theory of Knudson, many of the cases with a germline mutation in a tumor suppressor gene exhibit a somatic alteration in the

---

* For review, see Ref. 57.

remaining gene copy in the tumor. Although a mutated protooncogene acts dominantly at the cellular level, additional somatic changes are necessary for development of tumors. Among the known susceptibility genes for cancer, three are classified as oncogenes, *CDK4, MET,* and *RET* (Table 1). Germline mutations in alternative components of the mismatch repair (MMR) system predispose to hereditary nonpolyposis colorectal cancer (HNPCC). Often the second allele is inactivated either by DNA sequence change or hypermethylation, and thus these genes resemble the tumor suppressor model of homozygous gene inactivation at the cellular level. Even though the tumor suppressor gene acts recessively at the cellular level, the disease follows a dominant mode of inheritance. This is due to the high probability of mutating the second allele in one cell resulting in a selective growth advantage.

The recessive cancer syndromes are similar in that they typically have defects in genes encoding proteins involved in DNA maintenance and DNA-damage repair. In these recessive conditions, homozygous gene mutation carriers have an increased cancer risk except for heterozygous *ATM* mutation carriers that have increased risk of breast cancer.

Hereditary cancer genes are often altered in sporadic tumors although the mutation frequency as well as the mutation spectrum might differ. The *APC* germline mutations cause the familial adenomatous polyposis disease with an incidence of approximately 1% among the population. However, the *APC* gene is found altered in 70% of sporadic colorectal adenomas and carcinomas. The APC protein functions in the Wingless (WNT) signaling pathway as part of the cytoplasmic protein complex that regulates the level of the β-catenin. Interestingly, where *APC* is normal in colorectal carcinomas, it tends to exhibit β-catenin mutations. Mutated *APC* or β-catenin will deregulate cell growth via T-cell factor (TCF 4) transcriptional activation. This example shows mutual exclusive mutations in different components resulting in dysfunction of the same pathway, and illustrates the intersection between important pathways in colorectal carcinogenesis. Further, TCF4 containing a poly(A) 9 tract (58) is a downstream target for MMR dysfunction. Short nucleotide repeat sequences are prone to replication errors, and defect in the (MMR) system will thus indirectly cause such changes to accumulate. Germline mutations in components of the MMR system are responsible for the HNPCC syndrome that accounts for 2–4% of the colorectal cancer cases.

The disruption of essential pathways through alternative components has been described as a somatic alteration pattern in several tumor types. Although to a lesser extent in the germline, some examples are known. In addition to the above-mentioned MMR system, defects in CDKN2A or *CDK4* cause familial melanoma, and CDKN2A is an inhibitor of *CDK4* in the cell cycle. Other examples are the proteins encoded by *BRCA1* and *BRCA2* both of which work in complex with *RAD51* (and other proteins) to repair damaged DNA (59). Mutations in *BRCA1* or *BRCA2* will lead to accumulation of DNA damage and checkpoint activation, including activation of *TP53*. However, if *TP53* is damaged, cell cycle checkpoints cannot be activated and the cells will proliferate uncontrolled. Still we do not fully understand why *BRCA1* and *BRCA2* germline mutations specifically predispose to breast and ovarian cancer. The Li–Fraumeni syndrome commonly is due to an inherited, altered *TP53* gene. p53 Mutations have not been found in all families clinically characterized as Li–Fraumeni-like. Germline mutations in the *CKH2* gene, encoding another cell cycle checkpoint protein, were responsible for predisposition in a subgroup of these families (16).

4. CANCER RISK IN CARRIERS

Carriers of germline mutations in genes described in Table 1a are known to be at high risk of developing cancer. However, there is a substantial interindividual variation in the age of onset and the risk of developing a cancer. For example, when population screening for carriers of germline mutations in *BRCA1* or *BRCA2* have been performed, mutation carriers without family history have been identified, and the penetrance estimates have varied between 28% and 80% (60). Carriers of the same mutation may show a great phenotypic variability, also within the same family. These observations imply that germline mutations in these genes are necessary to explain the Mendelian pattern of cancer in some families, but are not sufficient to completely describe the variability seen between individuals. Risk modulating factors like modifier genes or environmental exposures are therefore likely to contribute. Examples of allelic variation in genes where such modifying effects have been observed are different VNTR alleles within the *HRAS1* oncogene (61) and CAG repeats in the androgen receptor gene (62). A protective effect of cigarette smoking on mutation carriers has also been observed, and it has been speculated that cigarette smoke lowers the estrogen level (63). The Min (multiple intestinal neoplasia) mouse model provides a clear-cut example of a modifying locus. In mice, Min mutation causes premature truncation of the *APC* protein, as for *APC* mutations in familial adenomatous polyposis in humans. Mice heterozygous for Min develop multiple polyps in the intestine, but with a significant variation in the number of tumors due to the Mom (modifier of Min) locus that encodes a phospholipase A2 (64). The human homolog, *PLA2A,* does not seem to modify colorectal cancer risk (65). The *PLA2A* and several other potential target genes map to 1p36, which is frequently deleted in colorectal adenomas and carcinomas (66,67). However, the target gene in this region with potential impact on colorectal tumor development remains to be identified.

It is likely that in the future we will be able to identify a number of allelic variants that can modify the risk in mutation carriers. The ability to apply risk prediction or cancer prevention strategies in carriers with germline mutations will depend on our knowledge of risk-modulating factors and mutation carrier status.

5. FAMILIAL CLUSTERING OF CANCER

Almost all types of cancer have been reported in familial clusters, but the sites most commonly involved are the breast, ovary, endometrium, colon, lymphoid and hematopoetic tissue, and brain. The strength of familial clustering varies; it maybe caused by dominant inherited predisposition as seen in the *HNPCC* or *BRCA1* families, by common environmental factors, or by a combined influence of environmental and genetic factors. It is often difficult to distinguish between a dominant hereditary cancer syndrome with reduced penetrance and familial clustering caused by several genetic susceptibility alleles segregating in the family acting in combination with environmental factors. Breast cancer, for example, fits best a dominant gene model in which the predisposition leads to cancer at a young age. But, familial clustering of cancer cases occurring at an older age also can be seen. In these families, a dominant model is not obvious and polygenic inheritance is more likely.

Cancer is a complex disease and can be caused by a combination of multiple gene variants, each with a weak to moderate effect, interacting with each other and with the environment. Identification of the gene and gene variants involved in familial clustering of cancer is challenging. Analyses of siblings and twins, association studies using case–control or cohort analyses, are methods that have been applied. Candidate genes, in which there is biological evidence to suggest association to a specific phenotype, are screened for variations. Identified alterations are then compared to control individuals from the same population cohort.

6. COMMON GENE VARIANTS PREDISPOSING TO INCREASED CANCER RISK*

So far, familial clustering has been the main indicator of inherited cancer risk. However, a substantial predisposition may also be present without obvious familial clustering. Some genes with relatively common disease-associated variant allele frequencies may confer a small to moderate individual cancer risk. Since these variants are carried by a large number of individuals, the population attributable risk is high. Genes with allele variants reported to be associated with increased cancer risk (low to moderate) are listed in Table 2. (For review see Ref. 68.)

In analogy with strain differences in susceptibility to experimental carcinogenesis in mice, genetic variation in the metabolic activation or

---

* For review, see Ref. 68.

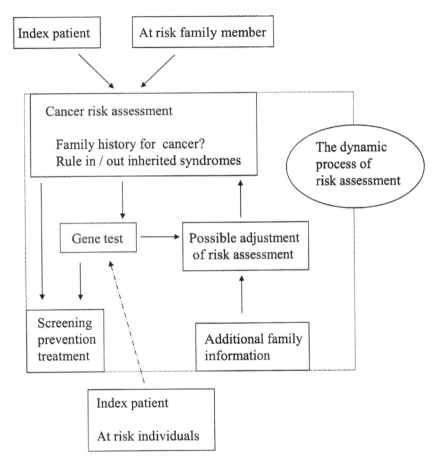

Figure 3 Cancer risk assessment in individuals with high risk. A simplified flow chart. The health institution is contacted by the index person or by potentially at-risk family members. A medical genetic evaluation of the family is performed and gene test(s) may be offered if available. The results of such testing as well as family information over time may adjust the risk assessment, implying the dynamic nature of this process. Screening, prevention, and treatment procedures should be recommended according to the existing guidelines at the time. A potential scenario is indicated by the broken arrow. If the cancer patients and family members immediately are offered relevant and complete gene tests, the results may in conjunction with family history make the diagnosis firmer as well as influence the clinical management of the patient.

detoxification of carcinogenic chemicals can be important determinants of population risk. The current candidates include the genes of the cytochrome P450 (CYP) system, which has a central role in the oxidative metabolism of many classes of exogenous and endogenous compounds, including steroid

Table 2   Genes with Genetical Polymorphisms Associated with Increased Cancer Risk

Genes involved*	Type of cancer	Mechanism	References
AR	Prostate	Hormone metabolism	69
CYP1A1	Breast, lung	Hormone/carcinogen metabolism (in smokers)	70–74
CYP1B1	Breast	Hormone metabolism	75
CYP2D6	Lung, cervical, vulva	Tobacco-specific carcinogen	76–78
CYP2E1	Breast, lung	Hormone/carcinogen metabolism	76,79
CYP17	Breast, prostate	Estrogen metabolism	72,80–82
CYP19	Breast	Estrogen metabolism	83,84
COMT	Breast	Catechol estrogen metabolism	72,85
EPHX	Colorectal	Oxidative defense	86
GST	Lung, bladder, breast, colorectal	Decreased detoxification	74,87–89
HRAS1	Lung, breast, testis	Unknown	90,91
HLA	Cervical	HPV immune response?	92
MTHFR	Colorectal, ALL	Folate inadequacy	93,94
NAT1	Colorectal	Decreased detoxification	95
NAT2	Bladder, breast	Decreased detoxification	74,96–98
TNFA	Lymphoma, breast	Increased cytokine level	99
VDR	Breast	Steroid metabolism	100

*AR, androgen receptor; CYP, cytochrome P450; CYP17, 17alpha-hydroxylase; CYP19, aromatase; COMT, catechol-O-methyltransferase; EPHX, epoxide hydroxylase; GSTs, glutation-S-transferases theta, mu, and pi; HRAS, Hras oncogene; HLA, human leucocyte antigen; MTHFR, methylen-tetra-hydro-folate-reductase; NAT, N-acetyltransferase; TNFA, tumor necrosis factor alpha; VDR, vitamin D receptor.

hormones. During the oxidative process, electrophilic and carcinogenic inter-mediates can be created. Many of these genes are highly polymorphic. One of the first genes studied was *CYP1A1,* whose product metabolizes polycyclic aromatic hydrocarbons such as benzo-a-pyrene. About 10% of the Caucasian population have a highly inducible form of *CYP1A1.* A number of studies involving different ethnic populations have been performed, and although not conclusive, certain alleles seem to be associated with increased lung cancer risk in smokers. Other *CYP* genes have been analyzed in different case control studies, and common genetic variants have been associated with increased cancer risk. In breast cancer, genes involved in the metabolism of steroid hor-mones like *CYP17, CYP19, CYP3A4,* and catechol-*O*-methyltransferase *(COMT)* have been associated with increased risk. It has also been speculated whether any of these gene variants may modify breast cancer risk in gene car-riers of *BRCA1* and *BRCA2* mutations by modulating the bioavailable steroid hormone levels. Polymorphisms in androgen and estrogen receptors are also interesting candidates in this respect.

Detoxifying enzymes, such as epoxide hydrolase, glutation-*S*-trans-ferases *(GSTs)* and *N*-acetyl-transferases *(NATs)* are highly polymorphic, and a number of studies have investigated their role in cancer risk of a vari-ety of different cancers (Table 2). The *GSTM1* deletion allele has been asso-ciated with increased risk of bladder cancer, lung cancer, and possibly breast and colorectal cancers. The null genotype had little risk of bladder cancer in the absence of exposure to tobacco smoke, while the opposite was the case for lung cancer, demonstrating the importance of gene–environment interac-tions. Individuals with the *NAT2* slow acetylator genotype have a higher risk of bladder cancer if they are exposed to carcinogens metabolized by this enzyme. Among postmenopausal women, smoking increased breast cancer risk only in those with the *NAT2* slow acetylator genotype.

Much of this research suggests that genetic variation in both metabolic activity and detoxifying enzymes plays a role in modulating cancer risk of exogenous and endogenous compounds. It is, however, difficult to estimate the exact risk of these genetic variants since, in addition to the gene–envi-ronment interaction, there also seem to be gene–gene interactions that can result in a greater-than-additive effect on risk. Many of the studies have so far suffered from small or poorly designed sample sets, and additional research using carefully defined, large samples with known exposures is needed to elucidate the role of these genes in cancer etiology.

Several other candidate genes with cancer associated alleles have been suggested. These include genes encoding proteins involved in cell cycle regu-lation and development, DNA repair and repair capacity, immune response, and angiogenesis and other correlates of metastasis. An example of a poly-morphism in a tumor suppressor gene associated with increased risk of colon cancer is the population-specific I1307K polymorphism in the *APC* gene in Ashkenazi Jews. A T-to-A transversion creates an eight-base mononucleotide tract and indirectly causes cancer predisposition in these individuals. The mutation results in an amino acid exchange that does not alter the protein, but the mononucleotide repeat sequence is hypermutable, which may lead to truncation of the APC protein. This polymorphism is characteristic to Ashkenazims (101,102).

Several approaches to identify common alleles in cancer-associated genes are emerging. Direct gene analysis of large cohorts of patients and controls is feasible with new technologies. The type of variation that most likely is responsible for a disease association is single-nucleotide polymorphism (SNP) in the coding region of the gene. A huge international effort is taken to identify SNPs in cancer related genes, and since linkage disequilibrium normally does not extend over large distances, analyses of SNPs in candidate genes seem very promising. Results from such analyses will hopefully provide a much clearer pictured of what role the genetic background contributes to by either raising or lowering the cancer risk (103).

7. HOW TO IDENTIFY CANCER PATIENTS WHO ARE GENETICALLY PREDISPOSED

7.1. High Risk

The identification of cancer predisposing genes over the past few years have led to important changes in the clinical practice for cancer risk assessments. Although evaluation of risk assessment based exclusively on the family history is still most important, gene tests for a number of cancer genes are offered and used in this process (Fig. 3). There are many challenges at the individual level, within the family, and in the society, as well as in the gene tests themselves. "Gene testing" often includes a variety of modalities like linkage analyses, analysis of one or more founder mutations, analysis of a known private family mutation, screening for unknown mutation, and/or indirect tests as immunohistochemical analyses of relevant proteins or microsatellite instability test in the patient's tumor. It often is necessary to use several techniques in order to perform the "optimal gene test," based on a stepwise analysis process requiring skilled laboratory personnel. The evaluation of the consequences of the genetic test results is best obtained by close communication between molecular biologists responsible for the laboratory work and the health professionals responsible for the genetic counseling service.

7.2. Low Risk

Low to moderate risk may be assessed for relatives to cancer patients. Moderate risk assessment can also be performed for patients without family history of cancer but with bilateral disease or multiple cancers. However, the influence the common gene variants may have on an individual's cancer risk cannot currently be determined. The microarray technology ensures the analyses of thousands of genes, providing a tool to obtain the genetic portrait of a tumor as well the individual constitutional variation. The interpretation of the computer assisted analysis is a challenge in itself, but as better software continuously is developed, our focus now also turn to the low to moderate cancer risk associated DNA now sequence alterations.

REFERENCES

1. Miki Y, Swensen J, Shattuck-Eidens D, Futreal PA, Harshman K, Tavtigian S, Liu Q, Cochran C, Bennett LM, Ding W. A strong candidate for the breast and ovarian cancer susceptibility gene BRCA1. Science 1994; 266:66–71.
2. Wooster R, Bignell G, Lancaster J, Swift S, Seal S, Mangion J, Collins N, Gregory S, Gumbs C, Micklem G. Identification of the breast cancer susceptibility gene BRCA2. Nature 1995; 378:789–792.
3. Groden J, Thliveris A, Samowitz W, Carlson M, Gelbert L, Albertsen H, Joslyn G, Stevens J, Spirio L, Robertson M. Identification and characterization of the familial adenomatous polyposis coli gene. Cell 1991; 66:589–600.
4. Kinzler KW, Nilbert MC, Su LK, Vogelstein B, Bryan TM, Levy DB, Smith KJ, Preisinger AC, Hedge P, McKechnie D. Identification of FAP locus genes from chromosome 5q21. Science 1991; 253:661–665.
5. Hussussian CJ, Struewing JP, Goldstein AM, Higgins PA, Ally DS, Sheahan MD, Clark WHJ, Tucker MA, Dracopoli NC. Germline p16 mutations in familial melanoma. Nat Genet 1994; 8:15–21.
6. Kamb A, Shattuck-Eidens D, Eeles R, Liu Q, Gruis NA, Ding W, Hussey C, Tran T, Miki Y, Weaver-Feldhaus J. Analysis of the p16 gene (CDKN2) as a candidate for the chromosome 9p melanoma susceptibility locus. Nat Genet 1994; 8:23–26.
7. Zuo L, Weger J, Yang Q, Goldstein AM, Tucker MA, Walker GJ, Hayward N, Dracopoli NC. Germline mutations in the p16INK4a binding domain of CDK4 in familial melanoma. Nat Genet 1996; 12:97–99.
8. Fishel R, Lescoe MK, Rao MR, Copeland NG, Jenkins NA, Garber J, Kane M, Kolodner R. The human mutator gene homolog MSH2 and its association with hereditary nonpolyposis colon cancer. Cell 1993; 75:1027–1038.
9. Leach FS, Nicolaides NC, Papadopoulos N, Liu B, Jen J, Parsons R, Peltomaki P, Sistonen P, Aaltonen LA, Nystrom-Lahti M. Mutations of a mutS homolog in hereditary nonpolyposis colorectal cancer. Cell 1993; 75: 1215–1225.
10. Bronner CE, Baker SM, Morrison PT, Warren G, Smith LG, Lescoe MK, Kane M, Earabino C, Lipford J, Lindblom A. Mutation in the DNA mismatch repair gene homologue hMLH1 is associated with hereditary nonpolyposis colon cancer. Nature 1994; 368:258–261.
11. Papadopoulos N, Nicolaides NC, Wei YF, Ruben SM, Carter KC, Rosen CA, Haseltine WA, Fleischmann RD, Fraser CM, Adams MD. Mutation of a mutL homolog in hereditary colon cancer. Science 1994; 263:1625–1629.
12. Nicolaides NC, Papadopoulos N, Liu B, Wei YF, Carter KC, Ruben SM, Rosen CA, Haseltine WA, Fleischmann RD, Fraser CM. Mutations of two

PMS homologues in hereditary nonpolyposis colon cancer. Nature 1994; 371:75–80.

13. Palombo F, Gallinari P, Iaccarino I, Lettieri T, Hughes M, D'Arrigo A, Truong O, Hsuan JJ, Jiricny J. GTBP, a 160-kilodalton protein essential for mismatch-binding activity in human cells. Science 1995; 268:1912–1914.

14. Schmidt L, Duh FM, Chen F, Kishida T, Glenn G, Choyke P, Scherer SW, Zhuang Z, Lubensky I, Dean M, Allikmets R, Chidambaram A, Bergerheim UR, Feltis JT, Casadevall C, Zamarron A, Bernues M, Richard S, Lips CJ, Walther MM, Tsui LC, Geil L, Orcutt ML, Stackhouse T, Zbar B. Germline and somatic mutations in the tyrosine kinase domain of the MET proto-oncogene in papillary renal carcinomas. Nat Genet 1997; 16:68–73.

15. Matlashewski G, Lamb P, Pim D, Peacock J, Crawford L, Benchimol S. Isolation and characterization of a human p53 cDNA clone: expression of the human p53 gene. EMBO 1984; 3:3257–3262.

16. Bell DW, Varley JM, Szydlo TE, Kang DH, Wahrer DC, Shannon KE, Lubratovich M, Verselis SJ, Isselbacher KJ, Fraumeni JF, Birch JM, Li FP, Garber JE, Haber DA. Heterozygous germ line hCHK2 mutations in Li-Fraumeni syndrome. Science 1999; 286:2528–2531.

17. Chandrasekharappa SC, Guru SC, Manickam P, Olufemi SE, Collins FS, Emmert-Buck MR, Debelenko LV, Zhuang Z, Lubensky IA, Liotta LA, Crabtree JS, Wang Y, Roe BA, Weisemann J, Boguski MS, Agarwal SK, Kester MB, Kim YS, Heppner C, Dong Q, Spiegel AM, Burns AL, Marx SJ. Positional cloning of the gene for multiple endocrine neoplasia-type 1. Science 1997; 276:404–407.

18. Mulligan LM, Kwok JB, Healey CS, Elsdon MJ, Eng C, Gardner E, Love DR, Mole SE, Moore JK, Papi L. Germ-line mutations of the RET proto-oncogene in multiple endocrine neoplasia type 2A. Nature 1993; 363:458–460.

19. Friend SH, Bernards R, Rogelj S, Weinberg RA, Rapaport JM, Albert DM, Dryja TP. A human DNA segment with properties of the gene that predisposes to retinoblastoma and osteosarcoma. Nature 1986; 323:643–646.

20. Call KM, Glaser T, Ito CY, Buckler AJ, Pelletier J, Haber DA, Rose EA, Kral A, Yeger H, Lewis WH. Isolation and characterization of a zinc finger polypeptide gene at the human chromosome 11 Wilms' tumor locus. Cell 1990; 60:509–520.

21. Gessler M, Poustka A, Cavenee W, Neve RL, Orkin SH, Bruns GA. Homozygous deletion in Wilms tumours of a zinc-finger gene identified by chromosome jumping. Nature 1990; 343:774–778.

22. Li J, Yen C, Liaw D, Podsypanina K, Bose S, Wang SI, Puc J, Miliaresis C, Rodgers L, McCombie R, Bigner SH, Giovanella BC, Ittmann M, Tycko B, Hibshoosh H, Wigler MH, Parsons R. PTEN, a putative protein tyrosine phosphatase gene mutated in human brain, breast, and prostate. Science 1997; 275:1943–1947.

23. Johnson RL, Rothman AL, Xie J, Goodrich LV, Bare JW, Bonifas JM, Quinn AG, Myers RM, Cox DR, Epstein EHJ, Scott MP. Human homolog of patched, a candidate gene for the basal cell nevus syndrome. Science 1996; 272:1668–1671.

24. Ahn J, Ludecke HJ, Lindow S, Horton WA, Lee B, Wagner MJ, Horsthemke B, Wells DE. Cloning of the putative tumour suppressor gene for hereditary multiple exostoses (EXT1). Nat Genet 1995; 11:137–143.
25. Stickens D, Clines G, Burbee D, Ramos P, Thomas S, Hogue D, Hecht JT, Lovett M, Evans GA. The EXT2 multiple exostoses gene defines a family of putative tumour suppressor genes. Nat Genet 1996; 14:25–32.
26. Cawthon RM, Weiss R, Xu GF, Viskochil D, Culver M, Stevens J, Robertson M, Dunn D, Gesteland R, O'Connell P. A major segment of the neurofibromatosis type 1 gene: cDNA sequence, genomic structure, and point. Cell 1990; 62:193–201.
27. Viskochil D, Buchberg AM, Xu G, Cawthon RM, Stevens J, Wolff RK, Culver M, Carey JC, Copeland NG, Jenkins NA. Deletions and a translocation interrupt a cloned gene at the neurofibromatosis type 1 locus. Cell 1990; 62:187–192.
28. Wallace MR, Marchuk DA, Andersen LB, Letcher R, Odeh HM, Saulino AM, Fountain JW, Brereton A, Nicholson J, Mitchell AL. Type 1 neurofibromatosis gene: identification of a large transcript disrupted in three NF1 patients. Science 1990; 249:181–186.
29. Trofatter JA, MacCollin MM, Rutter JL, Murrell JR, Duyao MP, Parry DM, Eldridge R, Kley N, Menon AG, Pulaski K. A novel moesin-, ezrin-, radixin-like gene is a candidate for the neurofibromatosis 2 tumor suppressor. Cell 1993; 72:791–800.
30. Rouleau GA, Merel P, Lutchman M, Sanson M, Zucman J, Marineau C, Hoang-Xuan K, Demczuk S, Desmaze C, Plougastel B. Alteration in a new gene encoding a putative membrane-organizing protein causes neurofibromatosis type 2. Nature 1993; 363:515–521.
31. Hemminki A, Markie D, Tomlinson I, Avizienyte E, Roth S, Loukola A, Bignell G, Warren W, Aminoff M, Hoglund P, Jarvinen H, Kristo P, Pelin K, Ridanpaa M, Salovaara R, Toro T, Bodmer W, Olschwang S, Olsen AS, Stratton MR, de la Chapelle A, Aaltonen LA. A serine/threonine kinase gene defective in Peutz-Jeghers syndrome. Nature 1998; 391:184–187.
32. van Slegtenhorst M, de Hoogt R, Hermans C, Nellist M, Janssen B, Verhoef S, Lindhout D, van den Ouweland A, Halley D, Young J, Burley M, Jeremiah S, Woodward K, Nahmias J, Fox M, Ekong R, Osborne J, Wolfe J, Povey S, Snell RG, Cheadle JP, Jones AC, Tachataki M, Ravine D, Kwiatkowski DJ. Identification of the tuberous sclerosis gene TSC1 on chromosome 9q34. Science 1997; 277:805–808.
33. European Chromosome 16 Tuberous Sclerosis Consortium. Identification and characterization of the tuberous sclerosis gene on chromosome 16. Cell 1993; 75:1305–1315.
34. Latif F, Tory K, Gnarra J, Yao M, Duh FM, Orcutt ML, Stackhouse T, Kuzmin I, Modi W, Geil L. Identification of the von Hippel-Lindau disease tumor suppressor gene. Science 1993; 260:1317–1320.
35. Savitsky K, Bar-Shira A, Gilad S, Rotman G, Ziv Y, Vanagaite L, Tagle DA, Smith S, Uziel T, Sfez S. A single ataxia telangiectasia gene with a product similar to PI-3 kinase. Science 1995; 268:1749–1753.

36. Straughen J, Ciocci S, Ye TZ, Lennon DN, Proytcheva M, Alhadeff B, Goodfellow P, German J, Ellis NA, Groden J. Physical mapping of the bloom syndrome region by the identification of YAC and P1 clones from human chromosome 15 band q26.1. Genomics 1996; 35:118–128.

37. Ellis NA, German J. Molecular genetics of Bloom's syndrome. Hum Mol Genet 1996; 5:1457–1463.

38. Lo TFJ, Rooimans MA, Bosnoyan-Collins L, Alon N, Wijker M, Parker L, Lightfoot J, Carreau M, Callen DF, Savoia A, Cheng NC, van Berkel CG, Strunk MH, Gille JJ, Pals G, Kruyt FA, Pronk JC, Arwert F, Buchwald M, Joenje H. Expression cloning of a cDNA for the major Fanconi anaemia gene, FAA. Nat Genet 1996; 14:320–323.

39. Strathdee CA, Gavish H, Shannon WR, Buchwald M. Cloning of cDNAs for Fanconi's anaemia by functional complementation. Nature 1992; 356: 763–767.

40. de Winter JP, Waisfisz Q, Rooimans MA, van Berkel CG, Bosnoyan-Collins L, Alon N, Carreau M, Bender O, Demuth I, Schindler D, Pronk JC, Arwert F, Hoehn H, Digweed M, Buchwald M, Joenje H. The Fanconi anaemia group G gene FANCG is identical with XRCC9. Nat Genet 1998; 20:281–283.

41. Tanaka K, Satokata I, Ogita Z, Uchida T, Okada Y. Molecular cloning of a mouse DNA repair gene that complements the defect of group-A xeroderma pigmentosum. Proc Natl Acad Sci USA 1989; 86:5512–5516.

42. Weeda G, van Ham RC, Vermeulen W, Bootsma D, van der Eb AJ, Hoeijmakers JH. A presumed DNA helicase encoded by ERCC-3 is involved in the human repair disorders xeroderma pigmentosum and Cockayne's syndrome. Cell 1990; 62:777–791.

43. Legerski R, Peterson C. Expression cloning of a human DNA repair gene involved in xeroderma pigmentosum group C. Nature 1992; 359:70–73.

44. Flejter WL, McDaniel LD, Johns D, Friedberg EC, Schultz RA. Correction of xeroderma pigmentosum complementation group D mutant cell phenotypes by chromosome and gene transfer: involvement of the human ERCC2 DNA repair gene. Proc Natl Acad Sci USA 1992; 89:261–265.

45. Dualan R, Brody T, Keeney S, Nichols AF, Admon A, Linn S. Chromosomal localization and cDNA cloning of the genes (DDB1 and DDB2) for the p127 and p48 subunits of a human damage-specific DNA binding protein. Genomics 1995; 29:62–69.

46. Sijbers AM, de Laat WL, Ariza RR, Biggerstaff M, Wei YF, Moggs JG, Carter KC, Shell BK, Evans E, de Jong MC, Rademakers S, de Rooij J, Jaspers NG, Hoeijmakers JH, Wood RD. Xeroderma pigmentosum group F caused by a defect in a structure-specific DNA repair endonuclease. Cell 1996; 86:811–822.

47. Scherly D, Nouspikel T, Corlet J, Ucla C, Bairoch A, Clarkson SG. Complementation of the DNA repair defect in xeroderma pigmentosum group G cells by a human cDNA related to yeast RAD2. Nature 1993; 363:182–185.

48. Yunis JJ, Ramsay N. Retinoblastoma and subband deletion of chromosome 13. Am J Dis Child 1978; 132:161–163.

49. Francke U, Holmes LB, Atkins L, Riccardi VM. Aniridia-Wilms' tumor association: evidence for specific deletion of 1 1p13. Cytogenet Cell Genet 1979; 24:185–192.

50. Schmidt M, Michels V, Dewald G. Cases of neurofibromatosis with rearrangements of the chromosome 17 involving band 17q11.2. Am J Med Genet 1987; 28:771–777.

51. Ledbetter DH, Rich DC, O'Connell P, Leppert M, Carey JC. Precise localization of NF1 to 17q11.2 by balanced translocation. Am J Hum Genet 1989; 44:20–24.

52. Herrera L, Kakati S, Gibas L, Pietrzak E, Sandberg AA. Gardner syndrome in a man with an interstitial deletion of 5q. Am J Med Genet 1986; 25: 473–476.

53. Knudson AGJ. Mutation and cancer: statistical study of retinoblastoma. Proc Natl Acad Sci USA 1971; 68:820–823.

54. Cavenee WK, Dryja TP, Phillips RA, Benedict WF, Godbout R, Gallie BL, Murphree AL, Strong LC, White RL. Expression of recessive alleles by chromosomal mechanisms in retinoblastoma. Nature 1983; 305:779–784.

55. Seizinger BR, Martuza RL, Gusella JF. Loss of genes on chromosome 22 in tumorigenesis of human acoustic neuroma. Nature 1986; 322:644–647.

56. Hahn H, Wicking C, Zaphiropoulous PG, Gailani MR, Shanley S, Chidambaram A, Vorechovsky I, Holmberg E, Unden AB, Gillies S, Negus K, Smyth I, Pressman C, Leffell DJ, Gerrard B, Goldstein AM, Dean M, Toftgard R, Chenevix-Trench G, Wainwright B, Bale AE. Mutations of the human homolog of Drosophila patched in the nevoid basal cell carcinoma syndrome. Cell 1996; 85:841–851.

57. Fearon ER. Human cancer syndromes: clues to the origin and nature of cancer. Science 1997; 278:1043–1050.

58. Duval A, Gayet J, Zhou XP, Iacopetta B, Thomas G, Hamelin R. Frequent frameshift mutations of the TCF-4 gene in colorectal cancers with microsatellite instability. Cancer Res 1999; 59:4213–4215.

59. Welcsh PL, Owens KN, King I. Insights into the functions of BRCA1 and BRCA2. Trends Genet 2000; 16:69–74.

60. Rebbeck TR. Inherited genetic predisposition in breast cancer: a population-based perspective. Cancer 1999; 86:1673–1681.

61. Phelan CM, Rebbeck TR, Weber BL, Devilee P, Ruttledge MH, Lynch HT, Lenoir GM, Stratton MR, Easton DF, Ponder BA, Cannon-Albright L, Larsson C, Goldgar DE, Narod SA. Ovarian cancer risk in BRCA1 carriers is modified by the HRAS1 variable number of tandem repeat (VNTR) locus. Nat Genet 1996; 12:309–311.

62. Rebbeck TR, Kantoff PW, Krithivas K, Neuhausen SL, Blackwood MA, Godwin AK, Daly MB, Norod SA, Garber JE, Lynch HT, Weber BL, Brown M. Modification of BRCA1-associated breast cancer risk by the polymorphic androgen-receptor CAG repeat. Am J Hum Genet 1999; 64:1371–1377.

63. Brunet JS, Ghadirian P, Rebbeck TR, Lerman C, Garber JE, Tonin PN, Abrahamson J, Foulkes WD, Daly M, Wagner-Costalas J, Godwin A, Olopade OI, Moslehi R, Liede A, Futreal PA, Weber BL, Lenoir GM, Lynch

HT, Narod SA. Effect of smoking on breast cancer in carriers of mutant BRCA1 or BRCA2 genes. J Natl Cancer Inst 1998; 90:761–766.

64. Moser AR, Dove WF, Roth KA, Gordon JI. The Min (multiple intestinal neoplasia) mutation: its effect on gut epithelial cell differentiation and interaction with a modifier system. J Cell Biol 1992; 116:1517–1526.

65. Riggins GJ, Markowitz S, Wilson JK, Vogelstein B, Kinzler KW. Absence of secretory phospholipase A2 gene alterations in human colorectal cancer. Cancer Res 1995; 55:5184–5186.

66. Lothe RA, Andersen SN, Hofstad B, Meling GI, Peltomaki P, Heim S, Brogger A, Vatn M, Rognum TO, Borresen AL. Deletion of lp loci and microsatellite instability in colorectal polyps. Genes Chromosomes Cancer 1995; 14:182–188.

67. Praml C, Finke LH, Herfarth C, Schlag P, Schwab M, Amler L. Deletion mapping defines different regions in Ip34.2-pter that may harbor genetic information related to human colorectal cancer. Oncogene 1995; 11:1357–1362.

68. Perera FP. Environment and cancer: who are susceptible? Science 1997; 278:1068–1073.

69. Stanford JL, Just JJ, Gibbs M, Wicklund KG, Neal CL, Blumenstein BA, Ostrander EA. Polymorphic repeats in the androgen receptor gene: molecular markers of prostate cancer risk. Cancer Res 1997; 57:1194–1198.

70. Nakachi K, Imai K, Hayashi S, Watanabe J, Kawajiri K. Genetic susceptibility to squamous cell carcinoma of the lung in relation to cigarette smoking dose. Cancer Res 1991; 51:5177–5180.

71. Xu X, Kelsey KT, Wiencke JK, Wain JC, Christiani DC. Cytochrome P450 CYP1AI Mspl polymorphism and lung cancer susceptibility. Cancer Epidemiol Biomarkers Prev 1996; 5:687–692.

72. Huang CS, Chern HD, Chang KJ, Cheng CW, Hsu SM, Shen CY. Breast cancer risk associated with genotype polymorphism of the estrogen-metabolizing genes CYP17, CYP1A1, and COMT: a multigenic study on cancer susceptibility. Cancer Res 1999; 59:4870–4875.

73. Ishibe N, Hankinson SE, Colditz GA, Spiegelman D, Willett WC, Speizer FE, Kelsey KT, Hunter DJ. Cigarette smoking, cytochrome P450 1A1 polymorphisms, and breast cancer risk in the Nurses' Health Study. Cancer Res 1998; 58:667–671.

74. Coughlin SS, Piper M. Genetic polymorphisms and risk of breast cancer. Cancer Epidemiol Biomarkers Prev 1999; 8:1023–1032.

75. Bailey LR, Roodi N, Dupont WD, Parl FF. Association of cytochrome P450 1B1 (CYP1B1) polymorphism with steroid receptor status in breast cancer. Cancer Res 1998; 58:5038–5041.

76. el-Zein R, Zwischenberger JB, Wood TG, Abdel-Rahman SZ, Brekelbaum C, Au WW. Combined genetic polymorphism and risk for development of lung cancer. Mutat Res 1997; 381:189–200.

77. Warwick AP, Redman CW, Jones PW, Fryer AA, Gilford J, Alldersea J, Strange RC. Progression of cervical intraepithelial neoplasia to cervical cancer: interactions of cytochrome P450 CYP2D6 EM and glutathione s-transferase GSTMl null genotypes and cigarette smoking. Br J Cancer 1994; 70:704–708.

78. Chen C, Cook LS, Li XY, Hallagan S, Madeleine MM, Daling JR, Weiss NS. CYP2D6 genotype and the incidence of anal and vulvar cancer. Cancer Epidemiol Biomarkers Prev 1999; 8:317–321.

79. Shields PG, Ambrosone CB, Graham S, Bowman ED, Harrington AM, Gillenwater KA, Marshall JR, Vena JE, Laughlin R, Nemoto T, Freudenheim JL. A cytochrome P4502E1 genetic polymorphism and tobacco smoking in breast cancer. Mol Carcinog 1996; 17:144–150.

80. Kristensen VN, Haraldsen EK, Anderson KB, Lonning PE, Erikstein B, Karesen R, Gabrielsen OS, Borresen-Dale AL. CYP17 and breast cancer risk: the polymorphism in the 5' flanking area of the gene does not influence binding to Sp-1. Cancer Res 1999; 59:2825–2828.

81. Feigelson HS, Shames LS, Pike MC, Coetzee GA, Stanczyk FZ, Henderson BE. Cytochrome P450c17alpha gene (CYP17) polymorphism is associated with serum estrogen and progesterone concentrations. Cancer Res 1998; 58:585–587.

82. Wadelius M, Andersson AO, Johansson JE, Wadelius C, Rane E. Prostate cancer associated with CYP17 genotype. Pharmacogenetics 1999; 9:635–639.

83. Kristensen VN, Andersen TI, Lindblom A, Erikstein B, Magnus P, Borresen-Dale AL. A rare CYP 19 (aromatase) variant may increase the risk of breast cancer. Pharmacogenetics 1998; 8:43–48.

84. Kristensen VN, Harada N, Yoshimura N, Haraldsen E, Lónning PE, Erikstein B, Kåresen R, Kristensen T, Børresen-Dale A-L. Genetic variants of CYP 19 (Aromatase) and breast cancer risk. Oncogene 2000; 19:1329–1333.

85. Thompson PA, Shields PG, Freudenheim JL, Stone A, Vena JE, Marshall JR, Graham S, Laughlin R, Nemoto T, Kadlubar FF, Ambrosone CB. Genetic polymorphisms in catechol-O-methyltransferase, menopausal status, and breast cancer risk. Cancer Res 1998; 58:2107–2110.

86. Harrison DJ, Hubbard AL, MacMillan J, Wyllie AH, Smith CA. Microsomal epoxide hydrolase gene polymorphism and susceptibility to colon cancer. Br J Cancer 1999; 79:168–171.

87. Rebbeck TR. Molecular epidemiology of the human glutathione S-transferase genotypes GSTM1 and GSTT1 in cancer susceptibility. Cancer Epidemiol Biomarkers Prev 1997; 6:733–743.

88. Helzlsouer KJ, Selmin O, Huang HY, Strickland PT, Hoffman S, Alberg AJ, Watson M, Comstock GW, Bell D. Association between glutathione S-transferase M1, P1, and T1 genetic polymorphisms and development of breast cancer. J Natl Cancer Inst 1998; 90:512–518.

89. Gertig DM, Stampfer M, Haiman C, Hennekens CH, Kelsey K, Hunter DJ. Glutathione S-transferase GSTM1 and GSTT1 polymorphisms and colorectal cancer risk: a prospective study. Cancer Epidemiol Biomarkers Prev 1998; 7:1001–1005.

90. Krontiris TG, Devlin B, Karp DD, Robert NJ, Risch N. An association between the risk of cancer and mutations in the HRAS1 minisatellite locus. N Engl J Med 1993; 329:517–523.

91. Ding S, Larson GP, Foldenauer K, Zhang G, Krontiris TG. Distinct mutation patterns of breast cancer-associated alleles of the HRAS1 minisatellite locus. Hum Mol Genet 1999; 8:515–521.

92. Helland A, Borresen AL, Kristensen G, Ronningen KS. DQA1 and DQB1 genes in patients with squamous cell carcinoma of the cervix: relationship to human papillomavirus infection and prognosis. Cancer Epidemiol Biomarkers Prev 1994; 3:479–486.

93. Ma J, Stampfer MJ, Giovannucci E, Artigas C, Hunter DJ, Fuchs C, Willett WC, Selhub J, Hennekens CH, Rozen R. Methylenetetrahydrofolate reductase polymorphism, dietary interactions, and risk of colorectal cancer. Cancer Res 1997; 57:1098–1102.

94. Skibola CF, Smith MT, Kane E, Roman E, Rollinson S, Cartwright RA, Morgan G. Polymorphisms in the methylenetetrahydrofolate reductase gene are associated with susceptibility to acute leukemia in adults. Proc Natl Acad Sci USA 1999; 96:12810–12815.

95. Bell DA, Stephens EA, Castranio T, Umbach DM, Watson M, Deakin M, Elder J, Hendrickse C, Duncan H, Strange RC. Polyadenylation polymorphism in the acetyltransferase 1 gene (NAT1) increases risk of colorectal cancer. Cancer Res 1995; 55:3537–3542.

96. Ambrosone CB, Freudenheim JL, Graham S, Marshall JR, Vena JE, Brasure JR, Michalek AM, Laughlin R, Nemoto T, Gillenwater KA, Shields PG. Cigarette smoking, N-acetyltransferase 2 genetic polymorphisms, and breast cancer risk. J Am Med Assoc 1996; 276:1494–1501.

97. Vineis P, Bartsch H, Caporaso N, Harrington AM, Kadlubar FF, Landi MT, Malaveille C, Shields PG, Skipper P, Talaska G. Genetically based N-acetyltransferase metabolic polymorphism and low-level environmental exposure to carcinogens. Nature 1994; 369:154–156.

98. Hunter DJ, Hankinson SE, Hough H, Gertig DM, Garcia-Closas M, Spiegelman D, Manson JE, Colditz GA, Willett WC, Speizer FE, Kelsey K. A prospective study of NAT2 acetylation genotype, cigarette smoking, and risk of breast cancer. Carcinogenesis 1997; 18:2127–2132.

99. Chouchane L, Ahmed SB, Baccouche S, Remadi S. Polymorphism in the tumor necrosis factor-alpha promotor region and in the heat shock protein 70 genes associated with malignant tumors. Cancer 1997; 80:1489–1496.

100. Lundin AC, Soderkvist P, Eriksson B, Bergman-Jungestrom M, Wingren S. Association of breast cancer progression with a vitamin D receptor gene polymorphism. South-East Sweden Breast Cancer Group. Cancer Res 1999; 59:2332–2334.

101. Laken SJ, Petersen GM, Gruber SB, Oddoux C, Ostrer H, Giardiello FM, Hamilton SR, Hampel H, Markowitz A, Klimstra D, Jhanwar S, Winawer S, Offit K, Luce MC, Kinzler KW, Vogelstein B. Familial colorectal cancer in Ashkenazim due to a hypermutable tract in APC. Nat Genet 1997; 17:79–83.

102. Lothe RA, Hektoen M, Johnsen H, Meling GI, Andersen TI, Rognum TO, Lindblom A, Borresen-Dale AL. The APC gene I1307K variant is rare in Norwegian patients with familial and sporadic colorectal or breast cancer. Cancer Res 1998; 58:2923–2924.

103. Kwok P-Y, Gu Z. Single nucleotid polymorphism libraries: why and how are we building them? Mol Med Today 1999; 5(12):538–543.

11

Chemical Causes of Cancer

Gary M. Williams and Alan M. Jeffrey

*Department of Pathology, New York Medical College, Valhalla,
New York, U.S.A.*

1. CHEMICAL CARCINOGENESIS

The development of neoplasms mediated by chemicals in both experimental animals and humans is a complex, multistep process (1–3), as illustrated in (Fig. 1), involving a series of genetic and epigenetic alterations (4–7). Chemicals operate in a variety of ways to either facilitate or inhibit the process of oncogenesis (8–10). As far as is currently known, the process is generally the same in humans and in animals, although many strains of rodents have much higher incidences of neoplasms (11) than occur in humans, in the absence of specific genetic susceptibility. Rodents are often much more susceptible to chemical induction of neoplasms (12) and exhibit certain responses (see section 3.2 Epigenetic Organic Carcinogens) to chemicals not observed in humans (11,13,14).

Ultimately, the outcome of exposure to a chemical carcinogen is a function of the internal or effective dose and duration of exposure to the chemical and cancer-modifying agents and intrinsic susceptibility of the exposed animal or human. The understanding of some of the differences in response between animals and humans is discussed.

1.1. Neoplastic Transformation

The first sequence of events in oncogenesis or carcinogenesis, termed initiation by Berenblum (2), consists of the transformation or conversion of a normal cell into an initiated or transformed neoplastic cell. Transformation

Sequences of Oncogenesis

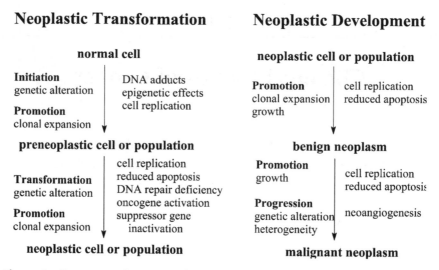

Neoplastic Transformation

normal cell

Initiation genetic alteration **Promotion** clonal expansion	DNA adducts epigenetic effects cell replication

preneoplastic cell or population

Transformation genetic alteration **Promotion** clonal expansion	cell replication reduced apoptosis DNA repair deficiency oncogene activation suppressor gene inactivation

neoplastic cell or population

Neoplastic Development

neoplastic cell or population

Promotion clonal expansion growth	cell replication reduced apoptosis

benign neoplasm

Promotion growth **Progression** genetic alteration heterogeneity	cell replication reduced apoptosis neoangiogenesis

malignant neoplasm

Figure 1 Sequences of oncogenesis. Outlines the events in neoplastic transformation and development.

is almost certainly the consequence of changes in gene expression in these cells which are either inherited, spontaneous or induced by chemicals or radiation. Mutations, and likely permanent epigenetic changes, require DNA replication, and hence the critical target cells for carcinogens are principally the renewing stem cells in tissues.

Spontaneous mutations can arise from DNA hydrolysis, errors in DNA synthesis, (6) or errors of repair process acting on intact DNA (15). Induced mutations result from chemical modification of DNA that escapes DNA damage repair and, during DNA replication, gives rise to DNA or chromosomal alterations (see Section 4.4 Mutations). Epigenetic changes in DNA expression can also be produced by one or more alterations. One is alteration of the normal pattern of cytosine methylation carried out by DNA methyltransferases, which are encoded by the cytosine DNA-methyltransferase (*DNMT*) gene family (16). Another is alteration in histone acetylation, which is mediated by histone acetyltransferase (HAT), and reduced by histone deacetylase (HDAC) (17).

Both foreign chemicals (xenobiotics) and endogenous chemicals (endobiotics) may interact with DNA either directly or indirectly to produce transformation. Endogenous agents, such as hormones, reactive oxygen species, nitric oxide, and lipid peroxidation products, as discussed later, may contribute to some sporadic or "spontaneous" cancers.

In the evolution of a neoplastic cell, focal preneoplastic populations usually precede the appearance of neoplasms and are considered to be the progenitors of the neoplastic cells that constitute tumors (1,2,18–20). Preneoplastic cells, which are not necessarily committed to progress to neoplasms, presumably lack all the requisite genetic changes that characterize neoplastic cells. In contrast, fully transformed cells are neoplastic and will form neoplasms under permissive conditions (Fig. 1). Preneoplastic lesions in both rodents and humans often express phenotypic abnormalities found in neoplastic cells; these include changes in enzyme activities and functional properties (21), alterations in expression of regulatory molecules such as erbB-2 (22), β-catenin (23,24), and fibronectin (25) and increases in inducible cyclooxygenase-2 (COX-2) (26) and nitric oxide synthase (26,27). These alterations probably are a consequence of gene mutations and, indeed, certain preneoplastic lesions are demonstrated to carry gene mutations found in the tumors that develop in association with the precursor lesions (28–30), including aberrant methylation (31). Also, preneoplastic lesions have been reported to have reduced DNA repair capacity (32). Hypermethylation of the promoter region of the DNA repair genes human Mut L homolog (*hMLH1*) and O^6-alkylguanine-DNA alkyltransferase (*AGAT*), associated with gene silencing (33), is present in a variety of neoplasms (34). Whether this could occur earlier in preneoplastic cells, thereby enhancing their susceptibility to DNA-reactive carcinogens, remains to be investigated.

Thus, preneoplastic populations represent pathological hyperplasia of altered cells resulting from dysregulation of growth control. Even at the stage of preneoplasia, impairment of growth control may result from diminished gap junctional intercellular communication (35–37), discussed further below. Promoting agents enhance the development of preneoplastic lesions, for some agents through inhibition of cell–cell communication. Increased cell proliferation and impaired DNA repair capability may be involved in rendering preneoplastic cells more susceptible to transformation with continued exposure to DNA-reactive carcinogens.

Mutations that underlie transformation are primarily those in the growth control genes, the proto-oncogenes and tumor suppressor genes, or genes that regulate expression of oncogenes and tumor suppressor genes (38,39), some of which are listed in Table 1. In addition to the mutations in growth control genes, there are numerous interactions between their gene products. Proto-oncogenes function as positive regulators of cell proliferation. They become activated oncogenes (Table 1a) by point mutation, partial deletion, amplification, or translocation. Tumor suppressor genes (Table 1b) are negative regulators of proliferation. They are inactivated mainly by deletions and point mutations. Deletions are often manifested as loss of heterozygosity (LOH). Other epigenetic mechanisms of gene silencing are under or over methylation of DNA (40) and alterations in histone

Table 1   Mutations in Growth Control Genes in Some Human Cancers

Gene	Mutation	Tumor site (type)
(a) Oncogenes		
Growth factor		
PDGF (platelet derived growth factor)	Distal deletion	Brain (meningioma)
FGF-4 (fibrobast growth factor-4; *HST-1*)	Amplification	Head and neck (squamous cell)
EGF (Epidermal growth factor)		
Growth factor receptor		
EGFRl (epidermal growth factor receptor 1; *HER-1*; human epidermal growth factor receptor-1; *ERB B-1* avian erythroblastosis)	Overexpression	Breast, lung, head and neck, esophagus, pancreas (ductal)
ERB B-2 (*HER-2/neu*; *EGFR2*)	Amplification Point mutation Transactivation	Breast, lung, prostate, esophagus, gall bladder, stomach, colon, thyroid, pancreas (ductal)
FGFR-1 (fibroblast growth factor receptor-1		Astrocytoma
FGFR-3 (fibroblast growth factor receptor-3		Multiple myeloma
HGFR (Hepatocyte growth factor receptor; *MET*, N-methyl-N'-nitro-N-nitrosoguanidine-treated)	Rearrangement Point mutation	Breast, thyroid, colon, pancreas, ovary, stomach, brain, prostate, endometrium, kidney, bone, liver
MET (mediate chemically induced transformation)	Point mutation Overexpression	Thyroid, colon, pancreas, ovary, stomach, kidney, head and neck
RET (Rearranged during transfection)	Rearrangement	Thyroid, multiple endocrine neoplasia type 2
SCFR (Stem cell growth factor receptor; *KIT*, kitten)	Deletion, insertion	Blood (myeloid leukemia), gastrointestinal tract (stromal tumors), lung (small cell), testes (seminoma), colon
Signal transduction element		
HRAS (Harvey Rasheed rat sarcoma virus)	Guanine point in codons	Bladder, lung, thyroid, head and neck

(*Continued*)

Table 1 Mutations in Growth Control Genes in Some Human Cancers (*Continued*)

Gene	Mutation	Tumor site (type)
	12, 13, 59, 61	
KRAS (Kirsten sarcoma virus)		Colon, esophagus, lung, pancreas, thyroid
NRAS (neuroblastoma)		Leukemia, breast, thyroid
BRAF (rapid *f*ibrosarcoma) B	Point mutation	Melanocyte (melanoma) colon, ovary, thyroid
CRAF (*RAF1*) (*r*apid *f*ibrosarcoma) C	Point mutation, LOH	Lung, breast, stomach, brain
SRC (Rous sarcoma virus)	Deletion, Q531 stop	Breast, colon
ABL (*A*belson *l*eukemia virus)	Translocation 9→22 (Philadelphia Chr)	Blood (chronic myelogenous leukemia)
Fos (*F*BJ murine *os*teosarcoma virus)		Brain (meningioma)
Jun (avian sarcoma virus 17: *ju-n*ana in Japanese means 17)		
PI3K (*p*hosphatidyl*i*nositol 3′-*k*inase)	Amplification	Cervix, ovary, colon, bladder
RhoA (*RAS* homolog gene family, member *A*)		Lung (nonsmallcell)
STAT3 (*s*ignal *t*ransducer and *a*ctivator of *t*ranscription)		Leukocytes (leukemia), leukocytes (lymphoma), leukocytes (multiple myeloma), head and neck, breast
Transcriptional activation factor		
CTNNB1 (β-*catenin*)	Missense, deletion, exon 3 mutation	Liver, colon, uterus (endometrium), skin, kidney, esophagus, ovary, melanoma, stomach
MYB (*my*eo*b*last)	Partial deletion	Colon, breast, blood (leukemia)
MYC (avian *my*elocytomatosis)	Translocation, amplification	Lymphoma, lung, neuroblastoma, brain (meningioma), breast
MYCN (avian *my*elocytomatosis, *n*euroblastoma derived)	Amplification	Neuroblastoma
Rel (reticuloendothe*l*iosis virus)	Chr 2p14–15 Rearrangement, amplification	Lymphoma, lung
CCND1 (*cyclin D1*)	Amplification	Breast, colon, lung, head and neck, bladder

(*Continued*)

Table 1 Mutations in Growth Control Genes in Some Human Cancers (*Continued*)

Gene	Mutation	Tumor site (type)
Antiapoptotic factor		
BCL-2 (*B*-cell *l*ymphoma)	Translocation Chr.18→14	Lymphoma, leukemia, colon, prostate
BCL-X$_L$		Prostate
HDM2 (*h*uman *d*ouble *m*inute 2; *MDM2*, *m*ouse *DM2*)	Amplification Overexpression	Soft-tissue sarcoma, osteosarcoma, esophagus, breast, bladder
Other		
NF1,2 (*n*euro*f*ibromatosis type 1,2)	Aberrant splicing	Peripheral nervous system, brain
(b) Tumor Suppressor Genes		
DNA repair		
MSH2 (*M*ut *s* *h*omolog)		Colon (hereditary nonpolyposis and sporadic), ovary
MLH1 (*M*ut *L* *h*omolog)		Colorectal, ovary
BRCA 1 (*b*reast *ca*ncer)	Deletion, promoter methylation LOH	Breast/ovary (familial), breast (sporadic)
BRCA 2 (*b*reast *ca*ncer)	Deletion LOH	Breast/ovary (familial), breast (sporadic)
Cell cycle arrest/apoptosis		
TP53 (53 kD protein)	Point mutations LOH	Colon, lung, skin, bladder, pancreas, thyroid, esophagus, adrenal cortex
ATM (*a*taxia *t*elangiectasia *m*utated)	Missense mutations In frame deletions	Lymphocyte (lymphoma, leukemia)
BAK (*B*cl-2 homologous *a*ntagonist/*k*iller)	Missense mutations	Stomach, colon, rectum
DAPK1 (*d*eath *a*ssociated *p*rotein *k*inase 1)	Promoter methylation	Lymphocyte (lymphoma), lung, colon, breast (ductal)
ING (*in*hibitor of growth)	Downregulation Chr 13q33–34 LOH	Mouth, esophagus
TGFBR (*t*ransforming growth *f*actor receptor-β) 1,2	Mutation, downregulation	Stomach, colon, breast, thyroid, prostate, pancreatic (ductal)
TNFRSF6 (*t*umor necrosis *f*actor receptor *s*uperfamily, *m*ember 6; APO1; APT1; CD95; FAS)	Splice variation, point mutation	Head and neck, lymphocyte (lymphoma)

(*Continued*)

Table 1 Mutations in Growth Control Genes in Some Human Cancers (*Continued*)

Gene	Mutation	Tumor site (type)
Cell cycle inhibitors		
INK4a/ARF (*a*lternative *r*eading *f*rame)	p16 deletion mutation, Chr. 9p21 LOH, promoter methylation	Esophagus, skin (familial melanoma), colorectum, lung, breast
RB1 (*r*etino*b*lastoma)	LOH, promoter methylation, microdeletion	Eye (rentinoblastoma), bladder, kidney, prostate, pancreatic (ductal), breast, lung (small cell)
Cell cycle control		
CDKN1A (p21$^{\text{WAF1/CIPI}}$) (*c*yclin *d*ependent *k*inase inhibitor)		
CDKN2A (p16$^{\text{ink4}}$/MTS1) (*c*yclin *d*ependent *k*inase inhibitor)	Chr. 9p21 LOH Promoter methylation	Breast, colon, lung, ovary, skin (melanoma)
CDC4	Mutation, LOH	Uterus (endometrium), breast, ovary
PHB (*prohib*itin)		Breast
PTEN (MMAC/TEP1) (phosphatase and tensin homolog)	Chr. 10q 23.3 deletions Promoter methylation	Endometrium, brain (glioma), breast, prostate, kidney, lung, skin (melanoma), thyroid, bladder
Cell signaling		
RASSF1A (*RAS* *as*sociation domain *f*amily protein *1*A)	Promoter hypermethylation LOH	Breast, lung (small cell) kidney, prostate, adrenal medulla (medulloblastoma), nervous system (neuroblastoma), striated muscle (rhabdomyosarcoma), retina (retinoblastoma), melanocyte (melanoma)
SHP-1 (*S*rc *h*omology region 2 (SH2) domain-containing *p*hosphatase)	Promoter methylation	Leukocyte (leukemia/lymphoma)
Cell differentiation		
RAR-β (*r*etinoic *a*cid receptor)	Promoter methylation	Breast, lung, mouth, colon

(*Continued*)

Table 1   Mutations in Growth Control Genes in Some Human Cancers (*Continued*)

Gene	Mutation	Tumor site (type)
DMBT 1 (*d*eleted in *m*alignant *b*rain *t*umors *Cell adhesion*	Chr 10q 25.3-q 26.1	Brain, lung, esophagus, stomach, colon-rectum
CDH1 (E-*cadh*erin-1)	LOH Promoter methylation	Breast (lobular) Stomach, breast, lung, head, and neck
Proapoptotic factor		
BAX (*B*cl-2 *a*ssociated protein *X*) *Other*	Frameshift	Colon, uterus (endometrium)
APC (*a*denomatous *p*olyposis *c*oli)	Frameshift, nonsense, promoter methylation	Colorectal, esophagus, pancreas
CNX (*c*onne*x*in)		Stomach, liver, breast, prostate
DCC (*d*eleted in *c*olon *c*ancer)	Deletion	Colon
DBC2 (*d*eleted in *b*reast *c*ancer 2)	Deletion, mutation	Breast
DLC (*d*eleted in *l*iver *c*ancer)	Chr 8 p21.3–22 LOH	Liver, colorectum, lung
DPC4 (*d*eleted in *p*ancreatic *c*ancer locus *4*)	Biallelic inactivation	Pancreas
FHIT (*f*ragile *h*istidine *t*riad)	*FRA3B* deletions	Lung, kidney, breast, cervix, esophagus, stomach, liver, estes germ cell
MCC (*m*utated in *c*olon *c*ancer)		Colon
MEN1 (*m*ultiple *e*ndocrine *n*eoplasia type *1*)		Parathyroid, pancreas, anterior pituitary
TSC-1,2 (*t*uberous *s*clerosis *c*omplex)		Kidney

TSLC1 (*t*umor *s*uppressor in *l*ung *c*ancer 1, *BL2*, *IGSF4*)	Chr 11 11q
	  23.2 LOH
	Promoter
	  methylation
		Lung (nonsmall cell), liver, pancreas

VHL (*V*on *H*ippel Lindau)	Chr. 3p LOH Promoter methylation	Kidney (clear cell), hemangioblastoma, pheochromocytoma, lung
WT (*W*ilms *t*umor)	Chr. 11p13 LOH	Kidney (Wilms)

(*Continued*)

Table 1 Mutations in Growth Control Genes in Some Human Cancers (*Continued*)

Gene	Mutation	Tumor site (type)
WWOX (WW= two tryptophans in sequence motif; domain-containing oxidoreductase; *FORII*)	Chr 16q (*FRA16D*) deletion, Chromosomal fragility	Breast, prostate, ovary, esophagus, lung

Chr, chromosome; LOH, loss of heterozygosity; FRA, chromosomal fragile site.

acetylation (17). Methylation of CpG islands not normally methylated has been implicated in the inactivation of tumor suppressor genes (41,42). Some of these genetic changes may occur in the genesis of the neoplastic cell, as discussed above, while others emerge during further neoplastic development (38). Various lines of evidence implicate at least four to seven critical mutations in growth control genes in the evolution of human cancer cells (43,44), whereas fewer may be sufficient in rodent cells. Nevertheless, it is important to recognize that over time both normal and neoplastic cells accumulate very large numbers of mutations, in the range of 10^4–10^6, as a consequence of spontaneous mutations during cell replication (45,46), although the majority of these are noninformative. Also, gene expression profiling of tumors reveals changes in expression of a large number of genes.

Tumor promoters, which are discussed later, facilitate the growth of both preneoplastic cells and neoplastic cells through a variety of mechanisms (Table 2). Promoters include both endogenous agents, such as hormones, and exogenous agents (Table 3), all of which show specificity in the species and organs affected. Their main action in transformation is to facilitate clonal expansion of responsive preneoplastic cells.

Eventually, the preneoplastic cells with the requisite genetic alterations for selective growth emerge as preneoplastic populations in which transformation to neoplastic cells occurs.

1.2. Neoplastic Development

In the second sequence of oncogenesis (Fig. 1), the neoplastic cell or population proliferates disproportionately to the surrounding tissue thereby achieving clonal expansion to eventually form a neoplasm (2,47). The clonal expansion can result from either enhancement of proliferation or reduction in programmed cell death referred to as apoptosis.

Neoplasms may be well differentiated, i.e., they express morphological and functional features of their progenitor tissue, and are benign in their biologic behavior. Qualitative changes in the biologic behavior of a neoplasm toward the malignant phenotype are known as progression (1) and is due to accumulation of changes in gene expression. As originally

Table 2   Mechanisms of Interactions in Chemical Carcinogenesis

---

Cocarcinogenesis
  Increased carcinogen delivery to target cells
  Sensitization of target cells to effects of carcinogen, e.g., enhanced cell
    proliferation
Promotion
  Inhibition of cell–cell communication
  Inhibition of immune effector cells
  Induction of tumor necrosis factor-α
  Induction of cyclooxygenase-2
  Inhibition of apoptosis in preneoplastic or neoplastic cells
Syncarcinogenesis
  Summation of genotoxic effects of two carcinogens
Photochemical skin carcinogenesis
  Increased distribution of carcinogen to skin
  Photoactivation of carcinogen
  Photochemical generation of reactive oxygen species
  Sensitization of target cells
Anticarcinogenesis
  Inhibition of carcinogen formation
  Blocking of interaction of carcinogen with target cells
  Suppression of expression of transformation

---

proposed by Loeb (48), progression may be the consequence of a mutator phenotype which introduces mutations in replicating neoplastic cells (6), adding to those occurring spontaneously and induced by carcinogen exposure. The basis for the mutator phenotype includes reduced fidelity of DNA replication and diminished DNA repair processes (33,49). The high incidence of mutations in neoplastic cells can be readily identified in short tandem repeats in DNA (microsatellites) (50,51), a phenomenon known as microsatellite instability (MSI). One basis for the mutator phenotype is mutations in mismatch repair genes whose gene products edit errors in newly replicated DNA. Mutation or transcriptional silencing of either of two of these, the *MHL1* or *MSH2* genes, leads to high levels of MSI (52,53). Transcriptional silencing can be a consequence of promoter region hypermethylation, which has been estimated to occur in about 400 genes in cancer cells (54). Another type of mutation frequently present in neoplasms is hemizygous chromosomal deletions, detected as LOH. Chromosomal fragile site loci (FRA) (55) may have a role in chromosomal instability in regions associated with tumor suppressor genes (56–58). The two most frequently expressed of the 80 fragile sites are FRA 16D and FRA 3B (56). Ultimately, most, if not all, neoplasms develop chromosome aberrations (59).

An essential alteration in neoplastic cells is dysregulation of growth control (60–62). This stems either from overexpression of the gene products

Table 3   Classification of Chemicals with Carcinogenic Activity

A. DNA-reactive
1. Activation-independent alkylating agents
   N-nitrosomethylurea, N-methyl-N'-nitro-N-nitrosoguanidine
   Epoxides: ethylene oxide, styrene oxide
   Azoxymethane, methylazoxymethanol
2. Activation-dependent
   Metabolic
       Aliphatic halides: vinyl chloride
       Aromatic amines: monocyclic-o-toludine; polycyclic-4-aminobiphenyl,
           benzidine
       Nitroaromatic compounds: 1-nitropyrene, 3-nitrofluoranthene
       Heterocyclic amines: 2-amino-3-methylimidazo[4,5-b]pyridine (PhIP)
       Aminoazo dyes: dimethylaminoazobenzene
       Polycyclic aromatic hydrocarbons: benzo[a]pyrene; substituted
           polycyclic aromatic hydrocarbons: 3-methlycholanthrene
       N-nitroso compounds: dialkyl-dimethylnitrosamine,
           diethylnitrosamine; cyclic-N-nitrosonornicotine (NNK),
           nitrosomorpholine
       Triazines, hydrazines
       Benzene
       Mycotoxins: aflatoxin B_1, aflatoxin G_1
       Plant products: pyrrolizidine alkaloids, aristolochic acid, cycasin
           Pharmaceuticals: cyclophosphamide, phenacetin, tamoxifen
   Photochemical
       Psoralens
B. Epigenetic
1. Promoter
   Liver enzyme-inducer type hepatocarcinogens: chlordane, DDT,
       pentachlorophenol, phenobarbital, polybrominated biphenyls,
       polychlorinated biphenyls
   Bladder: sodium saccharin
   Forestomach: butylated hydroxyanisole
2. Endocrine-modifier
   Hormones: estrogens-17β-estradiol; catechol estrogens-4-hydroxy-estradiol,
       2-hydroxyestradiol
   Estrogen agonists: 17α-ethinyl estradiol, diethylstillbestrol (DES)
   Prolactin inducers: chloro-s-triazines-atrazine
   Antiandrogens: finasteride, vinclozolin
   Antithyroid enhancers of thyroid tumors: thyroperoxidase inhibitors-
       amitrole, sulfamethazine; thyroid hormone conjugation enhancers-
       phenobarbital, spironolactone
   Gastrin-elevating inducers of gastric neuroendocrine tumors:
       lansoprazole, omeprazole

(Continued)

Table 3 Classification of Chemicals with Carcinogenic Activity (*Continued*)

3. Immunosuppressor
   Cyclosporin
   Purine analogs
4. Cytotoxin
   Mouse forestomach toxicants: propionic acid, diallyl phthalate, ethyl
      acrylate
   Rat nasal toxicants: chloracetanilide herbicides-alcohol
   Rat renal toxicants: potassium bromate, nitrilotriacetic acid
   Male rat α_{2u}-globulin nephropathy inducers: *d*-limonene, *p*-dichloro-
      benzene
5. Peroxisome proliferator-activated receptor α (PPAR α) agonists
   Hypolipidemic fibrates: ciprofibrate, clofibrate, gemfibrozil
   Phthalates: di(2-ethylhexyl)phthalate (DEHP), di(isononyl)phthalate
   Herbicides: lactofen
C. *Inorganics*
   Fibers: Asbestos, silica
   Arsenic, beryllium, cadmium, chromium (IV), nickel
D. *Unclassified*
   Acrylamide, acrylonitrile, dioxane

of activated oncogenes, which regulate cell survival and proliferation, or
from functional loss of the gene products of tumor suppressor genes which
inhibit cell proliferation (the full names of these genes are given in Table 1a
and b). A dynamic review of this dysfunction is available through the
Cancer Genome Anatomy Project (63). Thus, the progressive growth of
neoplasms is due to an imbalance of a higher percentage of dysregulated
neoplastic cells traversing the cell cycle (i.e., a high growth fraction), exceeding the percentage leaving the cell cycle to the resting state (G_0), differentiation, or apoptosis. Cell cycle progression is controlled by the reversible
phosphorylation and ubiquitin-mediated proteosomal degradation of key
regulatory proteins (61,64). Phosphorylation is carried out by a family of
cyclin-dependent kinases (cdks) which are regulated positively by certain
cyclins, such as cyclin D, and negatively by cdk inhibitors such as p16. In
addition, the gene products of growth control genes regulate cdks. Cyclin
E, which is involved in the initiation of DNA replication, is dysregulated
in many types of tumors (65), apparently as a consequence of mutation in
the gene *CDC4* that codes for a protein involved in targeting phosphorylated cyclin E for ubiquitination and proteasome degradation (66).

   The progressive growth of a neoplasm is a function of acquired
abnormalities either in growth control or in the response to host permissive
factors or promoters. The normal growth control genes that are mutated
in neoplasms, are proto-oncogenes (or dominant oncogenes) and tumor
suppressor genes (or recessive oncogenes).

Approximately 150 mutated oncogenes have been identified (67). The proto-oncogenes which are activated by mutation include genes whose oncoproteins function as growth factors (e.g., PDGF), growth factor recfeptors (e.g., EGFR1), signal transduction elements (e.g., H-RAS), transcriptional activation factors (e.g., β-catenin), and antiapoptotic factors (e.g., BCL-2). Most are activated in a variety of cancers, but a few have been found to be mutated only in some specific cancers, as shown in Table 1a. Additionally, oncogene expression can be upregulated by signaling cascades.

The most frequently activated oncogenes in tumors are those of the *RAS* superfamily of genes, which consists of at least six families, including *RAS, Rho*, and *Arf,* of over 90 genes. Activation of *K-RAS, H-RAS*, or *N-RAS* proto-oncogenes occurs in about 15% of many different types of human cancer (68,69). Oncogenic forms of RAS p21 protein, a guanine nucleotide binding protein, with guanosine triphosphatase activity, drive cell proliferation through several downstream effectors. In one pathway, RAS activates the *m*itogen-*a*ctivated *p*rotein *k*inase (MAPK) signaling cascade (70). MAPKs are serine/threonine kinases which phosphorylate transcriptional factors (71), including nuclear factor-κB (NF-κB), a member of the Rel/NF-κB transcription factor family (72), which is a central regulator of stress response (73,74).

The protein kinase activity altered with *RAS* mutation is one of many such alterations that are produced by oncogene mutations (75). Another family of oncogenes encodes growth factor receptors (Table 1a). These receptors, for example members of the epidermal growth factor receptor (EGFR) family, are transmembrane receptor protein-tyrosine kinases (RPTK), which regulate tyrosine phosphorylation and mediate intracellular signal-transduction pathways, including the MAPK cascade (76). RPTK activity is negatively controlled by cytoplasmic or transmembrane protein tyrosine phosphatases (PTP) (77) and inhibition of PTP produces ligand-independent RPTK activation. Another growth factor receptor, peroxisome proliferation activated receptor (PPAR)-γ, which is a member of the membrane hormone receptor superfamily, is widely expressed in many tumors (78).

Cellular responses to growth factors or cytokines are also mediated by proteins known as signal transducers and activators of transcription (STAT) (79). STATs are activated through tyrosine phosphorylation, which can be produced by nonreceptor tyrosine kinases such as scr and abl oncoproteins. STATs are constitutively activated in various types of tumors (80) (Table 1a), which can result in overexpression of cyclin D1 (81).

CTNNB1 encodes β-catenin, a multifunctional protein which operates in cell adhesion by binding to E-cadherin and, in cell proliferation, through the Wnt signaling pathway (82). β-Catenin is degraded by ubiquination following phosphorylation by glycogen synthase kinase (GSK)3β as part of a multiprotein complex including the APC and axin proteins. Mutations in *CTNNB1*, *APC*, or *AXIN* genes lead to stabilized β-catenin which complexes with members of the T-cell transcription factor (TCF)/lymphoid enhancer factor (LEF) family of DNA binding proteins and acts as a transcription factor for target genes, possibly including *MYC* (83), whose gene product is involved in proliferation, apoptosis, and cell differentiation (84) and also is an inducer of telomerase (see below).

Myb has been identified as an activator of transcription of the cyclooxygenase-2 (*COX*-2) gene (85), also referred to as prostaglandin endoperoxide synthase, an inducible enzyme which is implicated in carcinogen metabolism (86) and cancer progression through induction of neoangiogenesis (see below).

Thus, activated oncogenes are involved in cancer development in a variety of ways. In some cancers sustained overexpression of the encoded oncoprotein is required to maintain the neoplastic phenotype.

The other type of gene involved in neoplastic transformation is the tumor suppressor gene of which over 170 are known (67). These encode proteins that restrain cell proliferation either by inhibiting cell cycle progression (e.g., p53), exerting cell cycle control (e.g., pRB), mediating cell differentiation (e.g., RAR-β) or serving as receptors for growth inhibition factors (e.g., transforming growth factor-β receptor, TGFBR). Also, a few tumor suppressor genes are involved in response to genetic damage. Some tumor suppressor genes have multiple functions. Examples are given in Table 1b. The function of tumor suppressor genes is lost by inactivation of both alleles. This occurs through point mutation or deletion, partial or complete (class I) or downregulation (class II) resulting from promoter methylation. Most tumor suppressor genes have been found to be mutated in a variety of tumors, but some are mutated only in specific tumors.

Abnormalities of *TP53* are the most frequent tumor suppressor gene alterations in human cancers (87) (Table 1b); the gene is mutated in 10–70% of common cancers (88), with a high fraction of missense mutations, which result in full-length mutant proteins. *TP53* codes for a gene product, p53, that is a 53 kD transcription factor which controls cell cycle arrest and apoptosis (89). The p53 protein transactivates other genes by interacting with the p53 responsive element (RE) present in their promoter regions (90). Among these genes, p53 regulates the expression of *BAX*, and *APAF-1* (apoptosis activating factor), which direct apoptosis, and *CDKN1A*, which encodes p21$^{\text{WAF1/CIP1}}$, an inhibitor of cyclin E- and A-dependent kinases, and *GADD45*, thereby producing cell cycle arrest. Alterations of *TP53*-type function may be even more frequent than evidenced by *TP53* mutations since *TP53* is one of a gene family including *TP63* and *TP73*, which have some similar functions (91). *TP53* function is regulated by several proteins whose genes may be altered in neoplastic cells. The product of the oncogene *HDM2* (*MDM2* in mice named for double minute centromeric extrachromosomal nuclear bodies), *HDM2* protein, is involved in the degradation of p53 protein through a protesome mechanism (92), and hence *HDM2* overexpression abrogates p53 function. Mutations in *TP53* and *HDM2* do not commonly occur in the same tumor (93). Conversely, several proteins enhance p53 activity. The tumor suppressor gene product of *INK* can attenuate the interaction between p53 and MDM2 (94) and the product of the oncogene *ARF* inactivates *HDM2*. Two isoforms of the *ING* tumor suppressor gene bind to p53 and enhance its activity (95).

The second most frequently inactivated tumor suppressor locus is *INK4a/ARF* (96). One of the gene products, p14^{ARF}, activates *TP53* in response to activated oncogenes by neutralizing the effects of *HDM2*, thereby preventing transformation. The other product p16^{INK4a} is an inhibitor of cyclin D-dependent kinase, maintaining Rb protein in the unphosphorylated state, thereby inhibiting cell cycle progression (97).

Also, a key alteration in many types of neoplasm is loss of function of the *RB1* tumor suppressor gene (Table 1). Its protein product, pRB, in its hypophosphorylated form binds several transcription factors, especially E2 factors (E2F), required for cell cycle progression from G_1 to S phase in which DNA is replicated.(98). When pRB is phosphorylated by the cyclin/CDK complexes in late G_1, its function is blocked, allowing E2F to activate expression of genes whose products facilitate cell cycle transition (99). Loss of function of *RB1* occurs through mutation of the gene, by mutations in the *INK4a/ARF* gene, amplification of cyclin D1/CDK4 activity or by hypermethylation in its promoter region (100). Subsequent to identification of silencing of Rb by promoter methylation, at least eight other tumor suppressor genes have been shown to be silenced by this alteration (Table 1b), which maybe a consequence of the overall increase in DNA methyltransferase activity found in tumors (101). Other members of the *RB* gene family, which include *p107* and *Rb2/p130*, encode proteins with similar functions as pRB (102) and may play a role in neoplasia.

The receptor for growth inhibition factors, transforming growth factor receptor β (TGFBR), contains a protein kinase with serine/threonine specificity (RSK), which phosphorylates Smads [merger of *Sma*II gene in *C. elegans* and *Mad* (mothers against decapentaplegic) gene in *Drosophila*], which are signal mediation proteins which act as transcriptional regulators.

In individual cancers, various oncogenes and tumor suppressor genes are abnormal. Some of those identified in human cancers are given in Table 1. No oncogene is activated in all types of cancer and likewise, no tumor suppressor gene is deleted in all types. Among the genes mutated in cancers, *K-RAS* and *TP53* are the only two consistently mutated in a high proportion of cancers of different types. Cancers can exhibit a variety of genetic alterations, depending upon the extent of progression. For example, the sequential development of gene changes in colon cancer has been described by Fearon and Vogelstein (103). Recently, Hahn et al. (44) have provided evidence that changes in at least four distinct signaling pathways may be required for transformation of human cells. Certainly, the more mutations in the regulatory pathways that a tumor incurs, the more aggressive its behavior can become. Interestingly, pediatric tumors exhibit relatively few mutations (104), but high frequencies of promoter methylation, especially in *RASSF1A* (105) (Table 1b).

Tumor cells can also acquire resistance to apoptosis or programmed cell death, which results from a variety of factors. For one, loss of matrix attachment leads to death of epithelial cells, a phenomenon termed anoikis (106). Also, a rapid process of apoptosis (2–8 hr) is evoked by various factors including extracellular factors such as tumor necrosis factor (TNF) family members, including TNF-α, Fas ligand (Fas L; also known as TNFSF6, *tumor necrosis factor super family, member 6*; APT1 APO1 or CD95) and *TNF-related apoptosis-inducing ligand* (TRAIL) (107), whereas a slower intrinsic process (8–48 hr) is mediated by intracellular factors such as proapoptotic products of the *BCL-2* gene family (108). This slower form of apoptosis is initiated by mitochondrial release of proapoptotic factors and cytochrome C, which can result from translocation of BAX to mitochondria (109). Apoptosis is effected by caspases, which comprise three families of *cysteine aspartate proteases* (hence caspase) residing in the cytosol as inactive zymogens (110). Specific caspases are involved in either the initiation or execution phases of cell death. Members of one family, caspases 8 and 10, associate through a death effector domain with the cell membrane death receptors of TNF-α, Fas L or TRAIL. Another family of caspases, 1, 2, 4, 5, and 9, have a caspase recruiting domain. The downstream effector caspases are 3, 6, and 7, which are activated by members of the other two families. Deregulation of the death receptor pathway to apoptosis is frequent in many types of pediatric tumors due to methylation and gene silencing of *CASP8* (111). Apoptosis can be inhibited by prevention of increased mitochondrial permeability transition and/or stabilization of the barrier function of the outer mitochondrial membrane (112) or through interaction with Apaf (*apoptosis activation factor*)-1 to inhibit activation of caspases (113). Antiapoptotic members of the *BCL-2* gene family include *BCL-2*, *BCL-X_L*, and *MCL-1* which encode proteins that prevent release of proapoptotic factors, thereby conferring resistance to apoptosis. Because elevated expression of *BCL-2* and *BCL-X_L* results in enhanced cell survival, they are considered to be proto-oncogenes (Table 1a), although in some circumstances *BCL-2* inhibits tumorigenesis (114). Inactivating mutations in the proapoptotic *BAX* and *BAK* genes are found in some cancers (115), and hence these are considered to be tumor suppressor genes (Table 1b). Another proapoptotic protein is *death-associated protein* (DAP) which is localized to the cytoskeleton and mediates interferon-γ-induced cell death (116). The gene for DAP kinase (*DAPK1*) is considered to be a tumor suppressor gene (Table 1b). Activation of RPTKs, including EGFR, ILGF-1R and Met, can alleviate anoikis (117). Overexpression of *COX-2* can also inhibit apoptosis (118). Thus, tumor cells can acquire resistance to apoptosis through alteration of a number of signaling pathways, several of which are regulated by p53 (90).

The *transforming growth factor* (*TGF*) gene family proteins are involved in various cell functions including growth, differentiation, apoptosis, and migration (119). TGF-β1 is growth inhibitory to certain cancers, but they can lose their responsiveness through mutations of the receptor (TβR). The alterations, however, are complex; in some tumors TGF-β1 is overexpressed and TGF-β1 and RAS can counteract one another collaborate (120).

Enhanced cell proliferation is facilitated by reduced intercellular gap junction communication (35–37). The gap junction is a membrane channel between adjacent cells that is composed of junctional hemichannels, connexons, in the cell membranes of communicating cells. Connexons are made up of subunit proteins, connexins, of about 15 different types, which are expressed differently in connexons formed in various tissues. The gap junctions allow transport of hydrophylic molecules of low molecular weight (up to 1 kD). A decrease or loss of connexin expression and gap junction formation occurs often in tumors, particularly connexin 43 (121). Thus, the connexin gene family (*CNX*) may be considered tumor suppresor genes (122). Also, expression of oncogene-coded kinases that produce connexin phosphorylation downregulates gap-junctional communication.

In addition to alterations that drive cell proliferation, neoplastic cells acquire a variety of phenotypic alterations that support growth. Important among these is an increased glycolysis for generation of ATP, known as the Warburg effect, which facilitates growth in a hypoxic micro environment. An inducible isozyme of 6-phosphofructo-2 kinase has been implicated in this phenomenon (123). Also, upregulation of glutamine synthetase (124), which catalyzes synthesis of glutamine, and downregulation of 10-formyltetrahydrofolate dehydrogenase (125), which regulates purine biosynthesis through controlling the levels of 10-formyltetrahydrofolate, contribute to tumor cell growth. Additionally, some tumors have diminished biotransformation activities, although not all Phase I and II enzymes are equally affected (126–130) and some enzymes may be increased (126). The basis for most such differences is not known, but it is established that glutathione *S*-transferase P1 gene, *GSTP1*, can be silenced by promoter methylation (131).

For tumor cells to continue to proliferate, an important element is the maintenance of the length of their telomeres, the terminal portion of the chromosome consisting of TTAGGG repeats. Due to the inability of DNA polymerase to replicate the extreme ends of the lagging strand of DNA, telomeres are shortened by approximately 50–200 bp with each cell division in normal cells, eventually leading to senescence. Telomere length is maintained by a ribonucleoprotein complex, telomerase, consisting of the enzyme *t*elomerase *r*everse *t*ranscriptase (TERT) and a 451 nucleotide RNA template for the hexanucleotide repeats that are added to the ends of replicating chromosomes. Telomerase is active in cells of many tumors due to increased expression of TERT (132). The oncoprotein myc binds to the *TERT* promoter and induces telomerase activity (133,134).

In addition to these intrinsic alterations in neoplastic cells, the development of a tumor can be facilitated by host factors. Among these, hormones, such as estrogen and *i*nsulin-like growth *f*actor-1 (IGF-1), are implicated in the development of several types of cancer, including colon, breast, prostate, and lung (135–137). Also, enhanced expression of hormone receptors, such as estrogen receptor (ER) or *i*nsulin-like growth *f*actor-*b*inding *p*rotein (IGFBP) 2 (138), increases tumor response to trophic hormones, although IGFBPs are both positive and negative regulators of insulin-like growth factor signaling (139). Cytokines, such as interlukin-6 (IL-6), have been implicated in the pathogenesis of several types of tumors through activation of STATs (140,141).

As the neoplastic population expands, establishment of a new blood supply is necessary to sustain the increased number of cells (142). Tumor vascularization is stimulated by a number of factors including vascular endothelial growth factor (VEGF) (142,143), and prostaglandin E_2 (PGE_2) produced from arachidonic acid by COX-2, which is elevated in tumor cells including those of the colon, lung, stomach, pancreas, and breast (144,145), as well as in their neovasculature (146). *COX-2* is upregulated by Myb and TNF-α. Angiogenic factors may be elaborated by the tumor cells or by other cells, such as mast cells stimulated by stem cell factor produced by tumor cells (147). The angiogenesis inhibitor endostatin, which is a cleavage product of collagen XVIII, has produced antitumor effects (148).

Neoplasms also must evade the host immune system and overcome other host factors that restrain growth. Some tumors express factors inhibitory to immune effector cells such as TGF-β, interleukin-10, and Fas-L (149). Also, tumor cells can develop defects in proteosome function that results in impairment of presentation of antigenic peptides and lack of recognition by cytotoxic T lymphocytes.

The malignant phenotype in neoplasms is defined by the ability to invade adjacent tissue and to metastasize to remote sites. Invasiveness requires altered expression of specific cellular properties leading to decreased cell adhesion or degradation of the adjacent extracellular matrix (ECM) (19,150). Cell adhesion molecules include the tight junctions, the connexins, which couple cells by formation of gap junctions (35), cadherins, which are cell surface glycoproteins that bridge the extracellular space (151) and integrins, which are signaling receptors which connect the ECM to the actin fiber cytoskeleton, thereby regulating the cytoskeleton (152). E-cadherin is the major epithelial cell–cell adhesion molecule which is connected to the cytoskeleton by association with the cytoplasmic proteins, catenins. E-cadherin is downregulated in a variety of carcinomas and its gene

CDH1 displays LOH in some carcinomas (153). A variety of alterations of the ECM occur in tumors. Fibronectin is reported to be decreased, even in preneoplastic lesions (25). Recently, DMBT1 (deleted in malignant brain tumor-1), a mucin-like molecule, which is the product of the putative tumor supressor gene *DMBT1* (Table 1b) was found to be reduced in digestive tract cancers (154). Proteases that degrade the extracellular matrix include the zinc-dependent matrix metaloproteases (MMP), of which gelatinase A (MMP-2) is the most abundant and plasmin/urokinase urokinase plasminogen activator (uPA) (150), an activator of MMP9 which is involved in basement membrane transgression. MMP activities are inhibited by homologous tissue inhibitors of MMP (TIMPs) (155). In some tumors, MMP activities are directed by overexpression of members of the protein kinase C family, which consists of 11 serine–threonine kinases, or the mitogen-activated protein (MAP) kinases. Also, NF-κB, which is increased in malignancies, is a transcriptional activator of MMP9 and uPA (156).

Each type of malignancy has a specific pattern of metastasis which is determined both by lymphatic and blood drainage from the tumor, and also by factors produced by disseminated cells allowing them to establish metastases (157,158). Genes regulating metastasis of tumor cells have been categorized as either metastasis-promoting (*CDH2, CXCRy, MTA1*) or metastasis-suppressing (*CD9, CD44, Nm 23, KiSS1, Kal1/CD82, CDH1, MAP2K4, MKK4, TIMP*, and *BRMS1*) (159). Several of these (*CD9, CD44*, and *CD82*) code for transmembrane proteins. One possible mechanism for metastasis inhibition is the maintenance of gap junction intracellular communication (160).

In addition to the alterations in genes critical to neoplastic development and progression, neoplasms acquire a variety of alterations in other genes, a phenomenon referred to as aberrant gene expression. Such genes include those for hormones that would not normally be produced by the cell type of origin of the neoplasm, such as secretion of vasopressin by small cell lung carcinomas and those for proteins such as bone morphogenetic protein (BMP) which can produce osseous differentiation in nonoesteogenic tumors.

In summary, neoplastic development, in which the neoplastic cell arising from transformation evolves into a malignant neoplasm, comprises the phenomena of clonal expansion of the neoplastic population, which is facilitated by promotion, and the progression of genetic abnormalities in the evolving neoplasm.

2. INTERACTIVE CARCINOGENESIS

Interaction between a carcinogen and other chemicals, including a second carcinogen, can enhance or reduce carcinogenesis through different mechanisms listed in Table 2. As described above, replicating cells are susceptible to neoplastic transformation by carcinogens and, because of that, factors that increase cell replication can enhance the response of a tissue to a carcinogen, while those that suppress replication can diminish susceptibility.

Chemicals that are not themselves carcinogenic, but that enhance carcinogenicity are referred to as cocarcinogens (8,9). These generally operate in concert with carcinogens either by increasing the exposure of target cells to the carcinogen or by enhancing the effect of the carcinogen on the target cell, such as by increasing cell proliferation. An example of human cocarcinogenesis is the enhancement of tobacco-induced oral cancer by heavy alcohol consumption (161).

Agents that operate after carcinogen exposure to facilitate manifestation of carcinogenicity are referred to as promoters (8). As described above, these operate in the sequence of neoplastic development, often by increasing cell proliferation whereby a selective growth advantage is achieved by neoplastic cells. A wide variety of experimental agents with promoting activity is known (Table 3). Various possible mechanisms of tumor promotion are listed in Table 2. One that characterizes a wide spectrum of promoters is inhibition of cell–cell communication (36,122,162), which results in liberation of tumor cells from the growth regulatory signals of surrounding normal cells, as discussed above. Promoters also modulate gene expression, including in critical genes such as *COX-2* (163).

Under the influence of promoting agents, which include endogenous substances such as hormones and growth factors, as well as xenobiotics, the growth of initiated or transformed neoplastic cells is facilitated to form a neoplastic population with progressive growth capability (2). The promoting action of chemicals is generally characterized by increased cell proliferation in both the affected tissue and the preneoplastic or neoplastic cells present in it. In response to promoters, preneoplastic populations, in some tissues, exhibit reduced apoptosis (164).

Unlike cocarcinogens, promoters are often weakly carcinogenic in the target tissue (Table 3), probably through promotion of cryptogenically transformed cells. A likely example of human tumor promotion is increased risk of breast cancer with hormone replacement therapy (165).

Both cocarcinogenisis and promotion are highly species and tissue specific.

Syncarcinogenesis refers to the additive or synergistic effect of two carcinogens applied simultaneously or sequentially (8). Syncarcinogenesis is well recognized for DNA-reactive carcinogens with the same target organ (166), but apparently occurs infrequently among pairs of carcinogens (167). Typically, syncarcinogenesis results from summation of the genetic effects produced by each carcinogen in the target tissue (168), which could possibly be a consequence of the accumulation of different DNA adducts,

Table 4 Classification of Chemicals and Mixtures Judged to Be Carcinogenic to Humans by the International Agency Research Cancer[a]

DNA-Reactive	
Aflatoxins	Myleran [1,4-butanediol dimethanesulfonate]
4-Aminobiphenyl	MOPP (nitrogen mustard, vincristine, procarbazine, and prednisone)
2-Aminonaphthalene	Phenacetin-containing analgesic mixtures
5-Azacytidine	Soot
Benzidine	Sulfur mustard
Betel quid with tobacco	Tamoxifen
Bis(chloromethyl)ether	Tobacco smoke and products
Chlorambucil	Thiotepa
Chlornaphazine [*N,N*-bis(2-chloroethyl)-2-naphthylamine] [triethylenethiophosphoramide]	Ethylene oxide
Chromium compounds, hexavalent	Treosulphan
Coal-tars	Vinyl chloride
Cyclophosphamide	
Melphalan	
Methyl CCNU [1-(2-chloroethyl)-3-(4-methylcyclohexyl)-1-nitrosourea]	
Epigenetic	
Azathioprine	Postmenopausal estrogen therapy
2,3,7,8-Tetrachlorodibenzo-*p*-dioxin (TCDD)[b]	Cyclosporin A
Oral contraceptives, combined and sequential	
Unclassified	
Alcoholic beverages	Diethylstilbestrol
Arsenic and arsenic compounds	Mineral oils
Asbestos	Nickel compounds
Benzene	Shale-oils
Cadmium compounds	Silica
Chromium compounds	Wood dust

[a]WWW.IARC.fr
[b]Based on relevent mechanism

saturation of DNA repair, or the interference of one type of adduct with the repair of another. A possible example in human carcinogenesis is cigarette smoking in which there is exposure to several carcinogens, formed during tobacco consumption.

A type of interaction of potential importance in skin carcinogenesis is photochemical carcinogenicity, which results from the combined action of a chemical carcinogen and ultraviolet radiation. The interaction can be of various types. An example of one type is the photoactivation of psoralens to DNA binding species (169) that induce skin cancer (170). In humans, skin cancer has occurred with 8-methoxypsoralen-UVA (PUVA) treatment of skin conditions (171). Another type of interaction is the photodegradation of chemicals, such as the fluoroquinolone antibiotics, resulting in formation of reactive oxygen species, which may be implicated in the mouse skin photochemical carcinogenicity of some of these chemicals (172). UVA is the predominant UV radiation reaching the earth's surface and could contribute to human skin through such a mechanism, involving either endogenous photosensitizers, such as riboflavin, or exogenous ones.

Mechanisms of anticarcinogenesis are of several types (10,173,174). Examples of experimental inhibition of the formation of an ultimate carcinogen include inhibition by vitamin C of *N*-nitrosation of amines to form carcinogens (175) and inhibition of formation of sulfate esters of aromatic amines by acetaminophen (176). Other anticarcinogens that increase detoxification of carcinogens include oltipraz (177), the phenolic antioxidants, butylated hydroxyanisole and butylated hydroxytoluene (178) and the isothiocyantes, sulforaphane (179). Agents that block the effects of carcinogens, possibly by free radical scavenging, include phenolic antioxidants (178). Among agents that suppress tumor development, the most generally effective experimentally is caloric restriction (180). Other suppressing agents include antiestrogens, such as tamoxifen (181) and nonsteroidal anti-inflammatory drugs (182). Several of these agents are now in clinical development, as discussed below in Section 6, *Cancer Prophylaxis*.

These types of interactive carcinogenesis contribute to the multifactorial nature of cancer in humans, as discussed below.

3. TYPES OF CHEMICAL CARCINOGENS

A wide variety of chemicals, both natural and synthetic, have carcinogenic activity in rodents (183–185). The diversity of carcinogens reflects the fact that the multistep process of oncogenesis can be influenced by chemicals in various ways, mainly involving either DNA reactivity of the chemical, leading to genetic alteration, or epigenetic modulation of cell growth or function, as discussed above. Accordingly, carcinogens have been broadly characterized as either DNA-reactive or epigenetic (9,186). Examples of the types of chemicals that can be assigned to these two categories and those for which data are insufficient for classification are given in Table 3. These are described further below.

3.1. DNA-Reactive Organic Carcinogens

DNA-reactive carcinogens are defined by their ability to bind covalently to DNA (186). This reactivity is a consequence of their molecular structure which gives rise to an electrophilic reactant, either directly or after bioactivation, capable of reacting covalently with cellular nucleophiles, particularly DNA (187). These aspects are discussed further in Section 4.2, *Types of Interactions with DNA*. As a consequence of their DNA-reactivity, carcinogens of this type produce mutations in the target tissue and this is the most rigorous basis for their categorization. They also are generally positive in genotoxicity assays, although activity in certain tests such as those for chromosomal effects are not necessarily indicative of DNA reactivity. DNA-reactive carcinogens operate primarily in the first steps of oncogenesis by binding to the DNA of target cells to effect initiation and neoplastic transformation. DNA-reactive agents can also enhance tumor development by producing cytotoxicity leading to compensatory cell proliferation, thereby causing further progression in neoplastic cells through additional DNA modification in these highly susceptible proliferating cells.

In experimental systems, most DNA-reactive carcinogens produce neoplasms, usually malignant, in several species, in several organs, and often in high incidence with short latencies. They can be carcinogenic with no other observable toxic effect and with a single exposure. A number of DNA-reactive carcinogens are active transplacentally in rodents (188). Several DNA-reactive carcinogens have been active in nonhuman primates (189), including transplacentally (190).

Owing to their mechanism of action, DNA-reactive carcinogens are presumptive human carcinogens with sufficient exposure (191) and, indeed, most human carcinogens are DNA reactive (Table 4).

The category of DNA-reactive carcinogens comprises mainly the classic organic carcinogens that operate as alkylating agents, e.g., epoxides, aliphatic nitrosamines, or arylating agents, e.g., polycyclic aromatic hydrocarbons (PAH) and aromatic amines (Table 3). DNA-reactive carcinogens with intrinsic reactivity occur mainly as products of the chemical and pharmaceutical industries or as products of pyrolysis in which very reactive chemicals are formed.

3.2. Epigenetic Organic Carcinogens

Epigenetic carcinogens have structures that do not give rise to reactive electrophiles and thus they lack the ability to bind covalently to DNA and are generally negative in genotoxicity assays, particularly in those that directly measure DNA damage.

Some epigenetic carcinogens may be indirectly genotoxic and produce neoplastic transformation by generating reactive chemical compounds intracellularly, such as reactive oxygen species (192,193) or other reactive compounds such as nitric oxide (194,195) α,β-unsaturated aldehydes (enals) (196,197), and dialdehydes from lipid peroxidation (198). Also, epigenetic agents may enhance spontaneous transformation rates by increasing cell proliferation. Many operate in the sequence of neoplastic development as promoters by facilitating tumor development from cryptogenically transformed cells.

Epigenetic carcinogens often are active in only one species and have limited sites of activity, for example tissues that are hormonally responsive. To be effective, they usually require prolonged exposure at levels sufficient to produce the cellular effect that underlies their carcinogenic activity. While only a few have been tested in primates, none has been active (189).

A few epigenetic carcinogens have been tumorigenic in humans (Table 4) under conditions in which they produce the cellular effect that underlies their carcinogenicity in rodents, i.e., hormonal perturbation and immunosuppression. Thus, epigenetic carcinogens in animal models do not necessarily represent human cancer hazards except under specific exposure conditions (191).

Epigenetic carcinogens are extremely diverse in their structures, with varied modes of action (Table 3). Some require bioactivation, for example the chloracetanilide herbicides are bioactivated to cytotoxic products, but many elicit their critical cellular effect in their parent form and are metabolically detoxified.

3.3. Inorganics

Inorganic carcinogens include fibers, such as asbestos, and metals and their salts, including arsenic, chromium, and nickel (Table 3). The mode of action of these is not well defined. For the metals, it has been suggested that inhibition of DNA repair processes (199,200), in the case of arsenic leading to cocarcinogenesis (201), or disruption of normal oxidation/reduction balance affecting signaling molecules (202), are involved in their carcinogenicity. Such mechanisms would require substantial exposure to effect carcinogenicity and these proposed mechanisms have not been demonstrated with exposures comparable to implicated environmental exposures.

4. CARCINOGEN BIOTRANSFORMATION AND CELLULAR EFFECTS

4.1. Bioactivation and Reactivity

Many DNA-reactive carcinogens require bioactivation to form reactive electrophiles, the ultimate carcinogen, and hence are activation-dependent (Table 3). In target cells, bioconversion generally takes place in the cytoplasmic smooth endoplasmic reticulum catalyzed by the cytochrome P450 (CYP) oxidases. Initial oxidation reactions, referred to as Phase I bioconversion, function to convert xenobiotics to more water soluble forms which are either excretable directly or may be conjugated in Phase II reactions to excretable products (Fig. 2). Epoxide hydrolase, another Phase I microsomal enzyme, adds functional groups (hydroxyl) to substrates (cyclic ethers) which are often chemically quite reactive but otherwise unsuited for conjugation reactions, apart from reaction with glutathione. Subsequent to oxidation or at already available suitable molecular sites, bioconversion is further carried out by Phase II conjugation reactions, catalyzed principally by cytosolic enzymes glutathione *S*-transferases (GST), glucuronyl transferases (GT), sulfotransferases (ST), and *N*-acetyltransferases (NAT). Other conjugates are potentially formed which are often species specific. The Phase I and II enzyme systems exhibit polymorphisms, as discussed below.

The main role of the biotransformation systems is in excretion of endogenous substrates such as steroid hormones. In the biotransformation of xenobiotics, most products are less toxic than the parent compound and are readily excreted, mainly in urine or bile. However, oxidation of DNA-reactive carcinogens occurs at molecular sites that lead to formation of an electrophile, an ultimate carcinogenic species. Thus, although both Phase I and Phase II reactions generally lead to detoxification, some chemicals such as PAHs (Phase I) or dibromoethane, tamoxifen and many carcinogenic aromatic amines are activated by Phase I and Phase II bioconversion leading to reactive species. Hence, most Phase I and II enzymes can either activate or detoxify depending upon the substrate.

Besides tissue biotransformation capabilities, the gastrointestinal tract contains organisms capable of a wide variety of chemical biotransformations (203,204). A classical example is the activation by bacteria of cycasin,

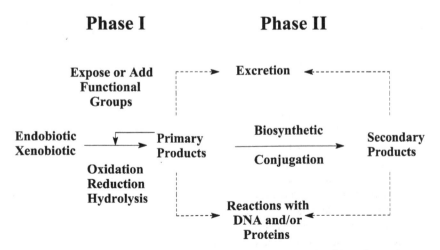

Figure 2   Relationship between drug metabolism and DNA adduct formation.

the β-glycoside of methylazoxymethanol, which occurs in the cycad nut. Cycasin is only carcinogenic when hydrolyzed to the aglycone by bacterial gut flora. More recent studies have shown that bacterial gut flora are involved in the specific activation of several nitroarenes and more generally by causing enterohepatic circulation of conjugates excreted in the bile. In addition to their role in the overall biotransformation of potential carcinogens, bacteria also produce mutagens such as the fecapentaenes, which may act as promoters (205).

The CYPs, which are involved in Phase I biotransformation, are a super family currently subdivided into 76 different families in animals with genes coding for more than 1000 enzymes with broad versatility in oxidative, peroxidative, and reductive activities for both endogenous and exogenous substrates (206) and are inducible by a variety of xenobiotics (207). The CYPs that are most important in carcinogen bioactivation are 1A1 (PAH), 1A2 (arylamines), 1B1 (arylamines, PAH), 2A6 (aflatoxin, nitrosamines), and 2E1 (benzene, nitrosamines, vinyl chloride). CYPs involved in hormone metabolism include 1A2, 4, 5, and 17. Another Phase I enzyme, epoxide hydrolase catalyzes the inactivation of chemically reactive epoxides to dihydrodiols, but dihydrodiol products are intermediates in the activation of many carcinogenic PAH to bay region diol epoxides.

The Phase II GSTs are a supergene family with several classes including five cytosolic classes, GSTA, GSTK, GSTM, GSTP, and GSTT and one microsomal class, MGST (208,209). Each GST enzyme has substrate specificity for conjugation with glutathione, although considerable overlaps exist.

NATs are the products of two active genes *NAT1* and *NAT2* (210). They acetylate xenobiotics at accessible nitrogen and oxygen sites. In the case of aromatic amines, acetylation results in either detoxification or activation (211); certain aromatic amines are acetylated by NAT2 in the liver to less reactive forms (211), while alternatively they can be *N*-hydroxylated by CYP1A2 and reach the bladder where they undergo *O*-acetylation by NAT1 resulting in the formation of highly reactive metabolites (212).

Likewise, GTs are a family of enzymes (213). An important GT substrate which undergoes glucuronidation and urinary excretion is the metabolite 4-(methynitrosoamino)-1-(3-pyridyl)-1-butanal (NNAL) of the tobacco specific nitrosamine 4-(methylnitrosamino)-1-(3-pyridyl)-1-butanone (NNN) (214). GTs, but not NATs, are inducible by xenobiotics. Genes for these, and other enzymes, exhibit polymorphisms (215,216), often due to single nucleotide polymorphisms (SNPs). The polymorphic enzymes exhibit different catalytic activities which influence the disposition of carcinogens.

The liver has the greatest capacity for biotransformation, reflecting its situation as the first pass organ for absorbed chemicals from the gastrointestinal tract. Other organs, notably the intestinal tract, lung, and kidney express in lesser levels the Phase I and Phase II enzymes. The content and composition of biotransformation enzymes within an organ is a major determinant of susceptibility to chemical carcinogens (217). However, the variability of phenotypic expression of biotransformation enzymes in tissues is high (218), possibly due in part to hormonal or xenobiotic influences on activity levels (219).

Biotransformation processes are generally qualitatively similar between animal species and humans (206), although quantitative differences, sometimes major, exist. For example, the selective estrogen receptor modulator, tamoxifen, is readily bioactivated in rat liver by hydroxylation and sulfate conjugation leading to DNA reactivity (220,221) and is a potent hepatocarcinogen (222), whereas in mice and humans these reactions appear to take place only to a limited extent (220). Consequently, significant carcinogenicity has been observed in humans only in the endometrium (223) and it is unresolved whether this involves DNA reactivity, since the evidence for adduct formation is contradictory (224–226). Also, species may differ in the organ expression of Phase I and II enzymes; for example, CYP1A1 which is involved in biotransformation of PAH is highly expressed in rodent liver, whereas in humans the lung is the principal organ of expression, which appears to be a determinant for the risk of lung cancer from cigarette smoking.

Humans and some animals exhibit variations in genes encoding biotransformation enzymes that influence toxicity and carcinogenicity (227–231). Most of these allelic variations are due to single nucleotide polymorphisms (SNPs) which affect the catalytic activity of the encoded protein. Among the Phase I reactions, *CYP1A1* SNP has been linked to lung cancer risk in cigarette smokers (232). In a population exposed to PAH environmentally and through cigarette smoking, PAH adducts in lung tissue were greater in individuals with a combined *CYP1A1* polymorphism and *GST M1* (null) phenotype (233). *CYP1B1* polymorphisms, which are numerous (234), include an SNP which is a susceptibility factor for head and neck cancers in cigarette smokers (235). Among male Japanese cigarette smokers, the normal genotype of *CYP2A6* gene was associated with greater risk for lung cancer than a polymorphism which results in a lack of CYP2A6 activity (236). A polymorphism in *CYP2E1*, which catalyzes the activation of many nitrosamines (237), has been associated with increased risk of rectal cancer (238).

Polymorphisms in the CYPs involved in steroid metabolism have been linked to cancer risk in hormone-dependent tissues. *CYP1B1* polymorphisms result in differences in estrogen hydroxylation which may relate to individual susceptibility to breast cancer (239). Also a polymorphism in *CYP17* (A2/A2 genotype), which encodes the enzyme responsible for testosterone biosynthesis, has been associated with elevated risk of prostate cancer in white men with a family history of cancer (240).

A polymorphism in *EPHX1* that encodes microsomal epoxide hydrolase has been associated with increased risk of oral, pharynx, and larynx cancers (241), although this has not been confirmed (242). A mutant allele *ALDH2*2*, prevalent in East Asians, which results in a loss of aldehyde dehydrogenase activity and accumulation of acetaldehyde in alcoholic patients, has been associated with increases in esophageal and oropharyngo-laryngeal squamous cell carcinomas (243).

The most widely expressed polymorphism is in the Phase II NAT con-jugating enzymes, rendering individuals either rapid or slow acetylators (244). There are over 25 alleles for the *NAT2* gene, of which *NAT2*4* is asso-ciated with the rapid acetylator phenotype (245). Slow acetylation is due to lack of expression of the *NAT2* gene or an SNP (246). With reduced or absent NAT2 activity, acetylation is carried out by NAT1, resulting in slow acetylation. Slow acetylation activity has been associated with elevated risk for bladder cancer in workers exposed to aromatic amines in some studies but the results are inconsistent (247,248). Also, slow acetylation status increases the risk of bladder cancer risk in cigarette smokers (249). Slow acetylation status has been associated with risk of sporadic colorectal cancer (250), risk of breast cancer in postmenopausal women who are cigarette smokers (251). Likewise, GSTs display polymorphisms (209); about half of Caucasians are homozygous for deletion of GSTM1 and lack any func-tional enzyme. A positive association has been identified between the null phenotype of GSTM1 and cancers of the lung (252), bladder (229,253), and breast (254). The null phenotype is also associated with a high rate of *TP53* transversion mutations in lung and bladder cancer.

The association of these various polymorphisms in biotransformation enzymes with cancer risks clearly implicates an important role for their sub-strates in cancer etiology.

4.2. Types of Interactions with DNA

Intrinsically reactive or bioactivated carcinogens that form electrophiles (Fig. 3) react with all cellular nucleophiles and, since protein is the most abundant nucleophile and has very reactive sites, most adducts are formed on proteins. In addition, adducts are also formed at nucleophilic sites on DNA, most often guanine residues (Fig. 3), although the other bases and the phosphotriester backbone (255) are normally also modified. Modification of the guanine N7 position results in a protonated imidazole ring which is unstable and can easily result in depurination or opening of the imidazole ring to give relatively stable adducts as happens, for example with aflatoxin B_1 (256). This unifying concept of DNA adduct formation for initiating carcino-gens was proposed by James and Elizabeth Miller (187). In another type of interaction planar chemicals can intercalate between bases without DNA binding (257).

DNA is also continuously modified by endogenous processes (258), including methylation of cytosine at position 5 by DNMT (16). The base–sugar bonds in DNA are susceptible to hydrolysis resulting in loss of bases at a rate of about 10^4 per cell per day creating apurinic/apyrimidinic sites

Electrophiles

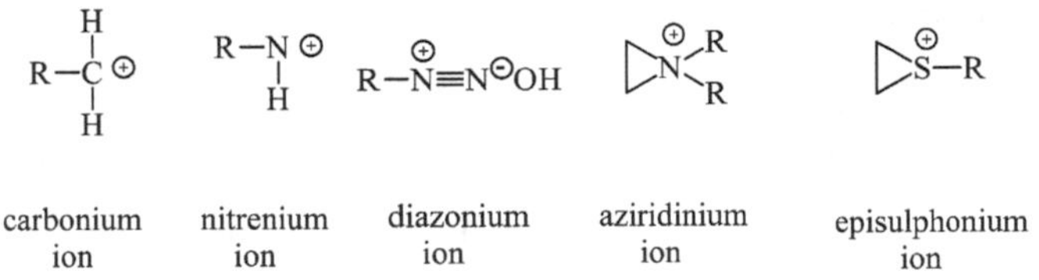
carbonium ion
nitrenium ion
diazonium ion
aziridinium ion
episulphonium ion

Nucleophilic sites

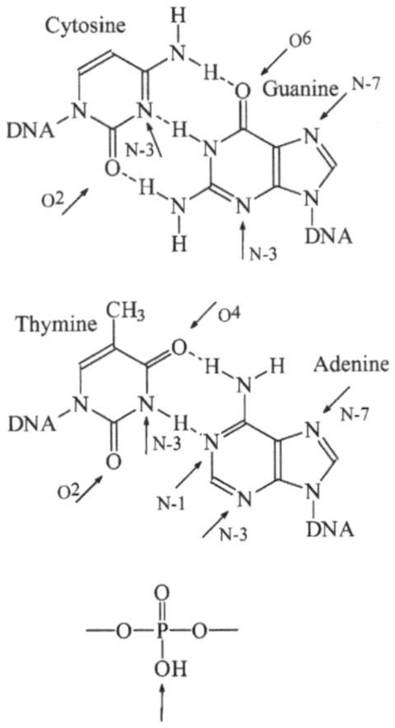
Cytosine
Guanine
O6
N-7
N-3
O2
DNA
Thymine
Adenine
O4
N-1

Base	Site	% total alkylation	
		DMN	DEN
Adenine	N-1	0.8	~0.1
	N-3	9	4
	N-7	1.5	0.6
Guanine	N-3	0.6	1.5
	O^6	6	8
	N-7	69	12
Cytosine	O^2	~0.1	2
	N-3	0.5	~0.3
Thymine	O^2	~0.1	7
	N-3	0.3	0.4
	O^4	~0.1	2.5
Phosphate	Triester	12	58

Figure 3 Structure of electrophiles and the nucleophilic sites in DNA with which they react. Electrophiles are the generalized structures of common electrophilic species which react with DNA. These electrophiles react with nucleophilic sites in DNA. Guanine residues are the most common target and the most frequently modified sites are indicated with arrows. Sometimes more than one site may be involved or the initial DNA adduct may undergo rearrangements (Fig. 6). *Source*: Data from Ref. 471.

(Fig. 4) (259). Deamination of 5-methylcytosine to thymine (Fig. 4) is a frequent reaction while deamination of cytosine to uracil is less frequent. Nitric oxide can deaminate 5-methylcytosine to produce thymine (260), which represents a greater challenge for DNA repair pathways (261). Keto/enol tautomerism may be responsible for some G→A point mutations (262). Oxygen metabolism generates reactive oxygen species such as hydroxyl radicals and singlet oxygen that produce in oxidation of dGTP and bases in DNA (263). The oxidation of deoxyguanine residues in DNA to 7,8-dihydro-8-oxodeoxyguanine (8-oxodG) (Fig. 5) has been reported to occur in

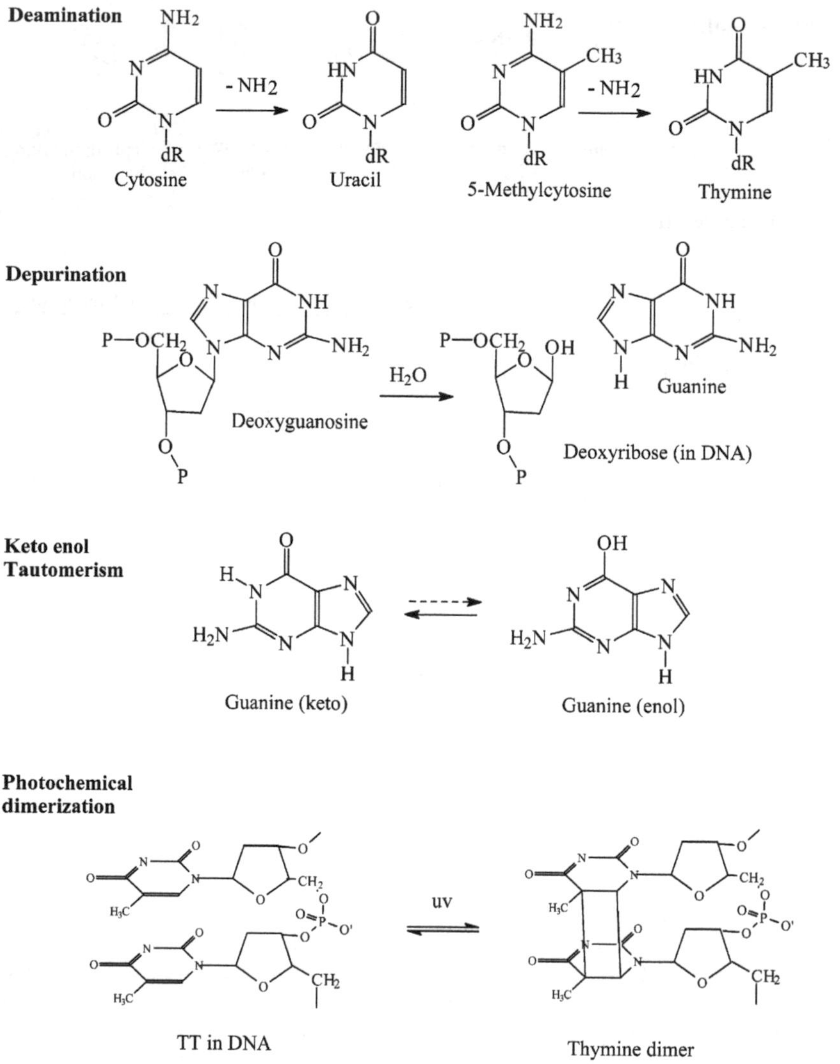

Figure 4 DNA deductions and rearrangements. Deamination and depurination are significant events. The role of keto/enol tautomerism in guanine and thymine residues is less clear. Photochemical damage to DNA can result from effects such as rearrangements of thymine residues to form dimers, photochemical oxidations in the presence of endogenous (riboflavin) or exogenous (fluoroquinolones) to form a variety of modification including 8-oxo-2′-deoxyguanosine (Fig. 5).

up to 1 in 10^3 residues (264), although there is considerable uncertainty about precise levels due to artifacts in DNA preparation. A variety of other oxidized bases have also been found (198). Peroxidation of unsaturated fatty acids leads to formation of α,β-unsaturated aldehydes which produce cyclic

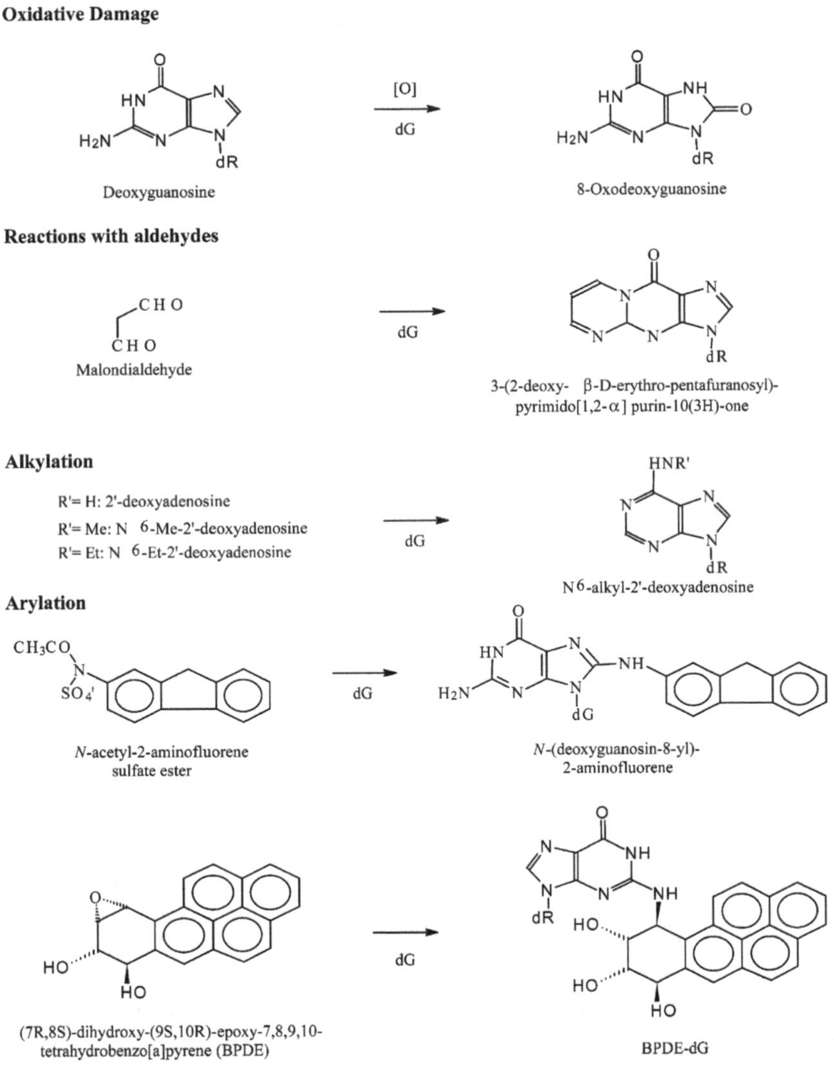

Oxidative Damage

Deoxyguanosine   [O] dG   8-Oxodeoxyguanosine

Reactions with aldehydes

Malondialdehyde   dG

3-(2-deoxy- β-D-erythro-pentafuranosyl)-
pyrimido[1,2-α] purin-10(3H)-one

Alkylation

R'= H: 2'-deoxyadenosine
R'= Me: N 6-Me-2'-deoxyadenosine
R'= Et: N 6-Et-2'-deoxyadenosine

dG

N^6-alkyl-2'-deoxyadenosine

Arylation

N-acetyl-2-aminofluorene
sulfate ester   dG

N-(deoxyguanosin-8-yl)-
2-aminofluorene

(7R,8S)-dihydroxy-(9S,10R)-epoxy-7,8,9,10-
tetrahydrobenzo[a]pyrene (BPDE)   dG   BPDE-dG

Figure 5 Examples of structure of DNA adducts. DNA adducts found in vivo range from the addition of small molecules such as oxygen (top) to bulky adducts such as those derived from the reaction with (7R,8S)-dihydroxy-(9R,10R)-epoxy-7,8,9,10-tetrahydrobenzo[a]pyrene (bottom).

adducts with a propano ring moiety in DNA (Fig. 5) (196,265). These are all premutagenic lesions as detailed below. Additionally, cytosine is methylated by DNMT using *S*-adenosylmethionine as the methyl donor (16). Methylene tetrahydrofolate reductase (MTHFR) plays a central role in converting folate to methyl donors and polymorphisms in *MTHFR* reduce DNA methylation (266). Chemicals, such as 5-azacytidine, can modify methylation patterns (266,267).

Using the sensitive ^{32}P-postlabeling assay for DNA adducts, nonpolar adducts of two types, referred to as I-compounds for indigenous compounds, have been found in tissues of rodents not exposed to exogenous carcinogens (268–270). In these animals, Type I I-compounds are affected by age, gender, diet, hormone, and chemicals. Type II compounds are oxidative adducts.

Two main types of interactions of chemical carcinogens with DNA have been recognized: noncovalent and covalent (271). Several types of noncovalent interaction occur. For example, bleomycin forms a complex with DNA and, together with chelated iron and oxygen, causes base loss. Planar molecules like actinomycin D intercalate between the base pairs of DNA, without covalent DNA binding (257). Covalent interactions of carcinogens with DNA may result from the intrinsic reactivity of a particular chemical with DNA. This occurs with antineoplastic alkylating agents which are designed for this property, or with reactive industrial chemicals. Such carcinogens have been designated as ultimate carcinogens or activation-independent DNA-reactive carcinogens (Table 3). Other compounds, of both natural and synthetic origins, which lack this intrinsic reactivity, need metabolic activation by one or more Phase I enzymes, as discussed above, to form DNA-reactive products. Such carcinogens are known as precarcinogens or activation-dependent DNA-reactive carcinogens (Table 3).

4.2.1. Chemistry and Conformation of DNA Adducts

Once the ultimate reactive carcinogens are formed, there are numerous factors that can influence their reactivity with DNA, including the reaction mechanism (S_N1 or S_N2), the hardness of the nucleophilic center in the nucleoside or nucleotide (oxygen generally being hard and poorly reactive in contrast to nitrogen which is intermediate and sulfur, which is soft and reactive) and the presence of adjacent groups which can influence the reactivity of a compound either electronically or sterically. Most alkylating reagents modify the purine (guanine and adenine) ring nitrogens, especially at the N-7 position, and both purine and pyrimidine (thymine and cystosine) oxygens. Alkylation can also occur on the phosphate backbone of DNA (255), but the biological significance of this is uncertain. Their repair has been better studied in *E. coli* than mammalian systems. Arylhydroxylamines, formed by reduction of nitroarenes or oxidation of arylamines, react at the C-8 and N-7 position of purines, possibly by rearrangement of transient N-7 adducts (Fig. 6). PAH diol epoxides react mainly with the exocyclic amino groups (Fig. 5). DNA is chiral and therefore any reactive carcinogen containing one or more chiral centers may show preferential isomeric reactivity.

The biotransformation enzymes described above, while often having broad substrate specificity, can show remarkable specificity in the chirality

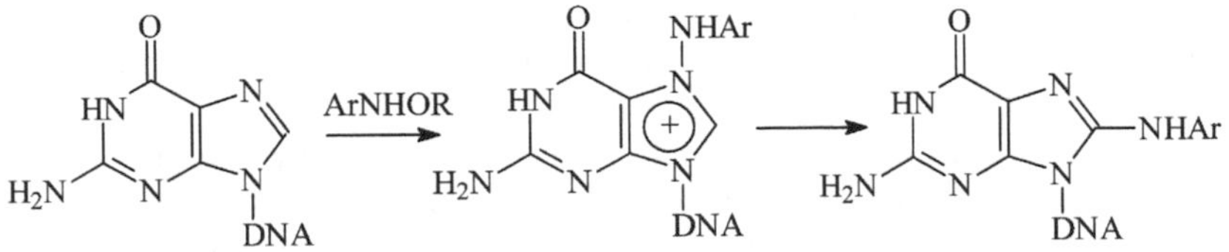

Figure 6 Formation of C-8 arylamine-DNA adduct via rearrangement of a transient N-7 adduct.

of products formed; for example, in biotransformation of B[a]P, the dihydrodiols are always trans, whereas one of the four possible isomers of B[a]P diolepoxide (BPDE), the *R,S*-dihydrodiol *S,R*-epoxide, is formed predominately and also reacts with DNA preferentially (272). No proteins have been described which specifically assist in the binding of the ultimate carcinogens to DNA, although the structure of chromatin is important (273) and numerous enzyme systems are involved in repair of such damage (see below). Consequently, shortly after exposure to DNA-reactive carcinogens, patterns of DNA adducts formed in vivo and in vitro are generally similar.

The reactivity of PAH diol epoxides with DNA, compared to hydrolysis by water to tetraols, varies considerably. For example, binding of BPDE in contrast to the sterically hindered fjord diol epoxide of benzo[c]-phenanthrene, ranges from about 10% to 75% of the diol epoxide added, respectively. The binding pattern of adducts also changes from only minor quantities of adenine adducts formed from BPDE compared to large amounts for benzo[c]phenanthrene. Not surprisingly, for a given PAH, the various isomeric diol epoxides differ markedly in their DNA binding and ratios of guanine and adenine adducts. Examples of the various types of interaction with DNA are illustrated in Fig. 5.

In addition to the chemical structure of DNA adducts, their conformation is important in determining their potential to escape repair and induce mutations during replication. Studies of two examples, DNA adducts formed from the reaction of BPDE or *N*-acetoxy-2-acetylaminofluorene (274), show quite different conformations. The former causes little disruption of the DNA helix as the pyrene moiety lies in the minor groove of the DNA helix, while the latter displaces the normal base to become intercalated into and opens the DNA helix. Some PAH diolepoxide adducts that bind to adenine residues also intercalate into DNA (275,276). Alkylation at the N-7 guanines is initially in the major groove while N3 adenine adducts are in the minor groove. Cross-linking agents such as cisplatin cause major disruptions of the DNA helix by binding in the minor groove, displacing the opposite cytosines, causing bending and considerable unwinding of the helix (277).

There are few studies of the binding of carcinogens to specific genes. Among these, B[a]P has been shown to bind preferentially to mutational hotspots in *TP53* (278).

Measurement of DNA adducts is an important tool in biomonitoring or molecular epidemiology of exposure to DNA-reactive carcinogens (279–283) to provide information on the summation of the effects of exposure, absorption, bioactivation of the genotoxin to the final DNA adduct, and rate of repair (279). Tobacco smokers have been the primary source of DNA since their exposure to known carcinogens is much higher than any other population. Industrial exposures and the effects of food contaminants, such as aflatoxin B_1, have also been monitored. These measurements have been used primarily to monitor cohort exposure, but, as improvement takes place in the ability to measure adduct levels more accurately and understand their significance, information on individual risk should be possible. Since DNA adduct levels are extremely low, highly sensitive techniques are needed. These include primarily immunological approaches such as the ELISA assay (280), or radiochemical techniques, particularly ^{32}P-postlabeling (284). Other techniques such as fluorescence or electrochemical analysis may be used depending upon the type of adduct being detected. The level of adduct formation resulting from exogenous exposures is of the order of one adduct per 10^7–10^9 normal DNA bases (285). Protein adduct detection is a valuable surrogate for DNA adduct formation since many carcinogens form adducts with both hemoglobin and serum albumin, which are readily accessible (286).

The presence of DNA adducts in both animal and human tissues has been applied to risk assessment of specific chemicals. Quantification of adducts in animals exposed to a specific, often single, dose of the ^{14}C-labeled chemical carcinogen, has been used to establish a chemical binding index (CBI) for the ratio of adducts formed per mole of DNA per kg body weight for the particular compound administered (287,288). In a few exceptional circumstances, it may be possible to extend these studies to humans (289). These values range over many orders of magnitude, but if above unity, i.e., significant levels of DNA adduct formation, the compounds are generally known to be DNA-reactive carcinogens.

Determination of adduct profiles after short-term administration may be misleading since many chemical carcinogens produce multiple DNA adducts which may show marked differences in repair rates. For example, N-7 and O^6-alkyl guanine lesions are better repaired than O^4-alkyl thymine (290) and C-8 adducts of N^2-acetylaminofluorene (AAF) are better repaired than N-7 adducts (291,292). Hence, with continued administration of carcinogen, the pattern of adducts can change as more slowly repaired ones accumulate.

It is important to keep in mind that formation of DNA adducts may not be sufficient to induce tumors. One line of evidence for this is the fact that DNA adducts are often formed in nontarget tissues for carcinogens.

4.2.2. Isolation and Structure Determination of DNA Adducts

Major challenges still exist in the structural elucidation of many adducts of DNA-reactive carcinogens formed in vivo. Their presence is often known, but, since the levels of modification of DNA are typically less than one adduct in 10^6 normal nucleotides and often three or four orders of magnitude less, the quantities of these adducts that can be isolated are, consequently, extremely small. In general, clues as to possible structures of an adduct have been inferred from the structure of the chemical producing the adduct, its metabolism, and the possible structure of the ultimate carcinogenic metabolite. The latter can then be prepared synthetically or biosynthetically, at least in a transient state, and reacted directly with DNA or homopolymers in vitro. Digestion of the DNA to the modified nucleotides will often provide sufficient material for comparison with adducts formed in vivo and subsequent structural elucidation. Only a few adducts have been prepared by direct chemical synthesis. Structure identification is normally by nuclear magnetic resonance (NMR) and mass spectrometry (MS) analysis. However, if isolated at the deoxyribonucleotide level, adducts with chiral centers will frequently separate as diastereomeric pairs with often approximately mirror image circular dichroism spectra. Such pairing of spectra simplifies the identification of multiple adducts, and can provide information on their absolute steriochemistry. Formation of some DNA adducts results in unstable products; for example aflatoxin forms several DNA adducts including those at N-7 position of guanine residues (256). This charged product is released from DNA either by depurination to yield 2,3-dihydro-2-(*N*-7-guanyl)-3-hydroxyaflatoxin B_1 which can be found in the urine of exposed animals or, by opening of the imidazole ring of the guanine, forms chemically stable adducts. Anthramycin reacts with DNA to produce adducts which are unstable during DNA digestion but whose structure can be determined in oligonucleotides (293).

As an approach to the identification of unknown DNA adducts, we, in collaboration with Dr. Esmans's group at the University of Antwerp, have used nanoliter HPLC coupled to ms/ms following the loss of the deoxyribose moiety to identify "unknown" DNA adducts. Digests of DNA isolated from the liver of rats treated with AAF and having adduct levels of about 3 in 10^7 were initially separated on OASIS HLB columns. Both acetylated and deacetylated adducts were detected as the specific adducts present when scanning for the constant neutral loss (CNL) of 116 M/e (unpublished results). Once identified by the CNL spectra, much stronger spectra could be obtained by scanning for these specific ions and, in conjunction with high resolution mass analysis, provides valuable initial clues as to adduct structure when reference materials are not available.

The most structural information regarding the conformation of DNA adducts comes from NMR data involving nuclear Overhauser effect spectroscopy (NOESY) and correlation spectroscopy (COSY) analysis, which have provided very detailed three-dimensional information regarding the solution conformation of the DNA adducts. Such analyses complement and provide proof for molecular modeling studies (294). It is, however, often difficult to prepare sufficient material for this type of analysis and the sequences of oligonucleotides into which the adduct can be incorporated may also be limited if the reactive ultimate carcinogen is used to modify the oligonucleotides.

4.3. DNA Damage Responses and Repair

Prokaryotic and eukaryotic cells possess a variety of enzymes capable of repairing DNA alterations in order to maintain its integrity (295,296). In resting mammalian cells, these operate with high efficiency and fidelity thereby restoring damaged DNA to its original molecular state. However, in cycling cells, complete repair may not be achieved in DNA that is being replicated and consequently, misincorporation can occur opposite unrepaired sites. Also, DNA damage and evoked repair processes may lead to apoptosis.

In addition to the proteins directly involved in DNA repair, the repair process is assisted by other DNA damage-responsive proteins including some encoded by tumor suppressor genes (297) (Table 1b). Of particular importance is p53, which, with DNA damage, is phosphorylated by DNA-dependent protein kinases (DNA-PK) leading to decreased interaction with dm2 protein, which targets p53 for proteolytic degradation (298,299). The resulting stabilization of p53 leads to increased activation of target genes including *CDKN1A*, *GADD45* (growth arrest and DNA damage 45) and *HDM2*. P21$^{WAF1/CIP1}$ inhibits activation of cyclin E/cdk 2 complexes thereby preventing phosphorylation of pRB and blocking progression from G_1 to S phase (300). Gadd45 protein interacts with the replication factor, proliferating cell nuclear antigen (PCNA) to arrest DNA synthesis (301). Dm2 protein maintains p53 under negative control, which is subject to an autoregulatory feedback loop (298). Thus, with increased functional p53, cell cycle progression is arrested, allowing a greater opportunity for DNA repair. Likewise, ATM, a pleiotropic kinase, is activated by double-strand DNA breaks and activates several factors that arrest cell cycling (302). The enzyme poly (ADP-ribosyl) polymerase (PARP), which catalyzes post-translational modification of proteins, also is activated by DNA strand breaks and appears to be involved in DNA repair by interacting with effectors of repair (303). PARP occupies DNA break sites to prevent recombination between homologous ends of DNA (304). The double-stranded RNA-activated protein kinase (RPK), which is a component of the cellular reaction to stress (21), has been shown to function in regulation of DNA damage response, possibly by modulation of DNA repair processes (305).

The DNA repair capacity of eukaryotic cells is maintained by six main eukaryotic repair processes are as follows: (a) nucleotide excision repair (NER) in which a region of DNA including the damaged nucleotide is removed; (b) base excision repair (BER) in which the damaged base and a few adjacent bases are removed by DNA glycosylases such as the alkylpurine-DNA-*N*-glycosylase (APNG); (c) alkylguanine-DNA alkyl transferase (AGAT) repair in which alkylation products on the O^6 position of guanine are removed by a repair protein without excision of the base; (d) mismatch repair (MMR) in which an incorrect base misincorporated during DNA replication is edited by an exonuclease; (e) postreplication repair in which gaps in newly replicated DNA created by polymerase bypass are closed; and (f) nonhomologous end-joining (NHEJ) of double-strand breaks or homologous recombination repair (HRR) of double-strand breaks. These processes are mediated by numerous proteins.

The first step in repair is lesion recognition. In NER, the xeroderma pigmentosum group C (XPC) protein complex 3 is the initiator (306). For some types of lesions, p53 is involved (307). Lesion recognition is followed by removal of the damaged DNA, which in NER involves about 20 proteins, including the excision repair cross-complementation (ERCC) group proteins (308). In NER, in which lesion-containing segments of approximately 30 nucleotides in length are removed, there are two subpathways, global genome repair (GNER) which occurs over the entire genome and transcription-coupled repair (TCNER) which is directed preferentially to the template strand of actively transcribed DNA and thereby serves to prevent interruption of RNA transcription. Following removal of bases or nucleotides, polymerases (most likely pol-δ and ε in the case of NER and β in the case of BER, although polymerases can participate) positioned by the replication factor PCNA gap fill the eliminated bases or nucleotides and finally, ligases rejoin the strands, restoring the DNA to its original structure, if no mutations have been introduced.

Nucleotide exision repair is elicited by a variety of DNA lesions, notably bulky adducts from arylating agents (309) and photoproducts (310). BER and AGAT processes are elicited by smaller alkylating agents (311), with NER serving as backup. Oxidative DNA damage is repaired by a BER glycosylase encoded by the *OGG1* (8-*oxo*guanine glycosylase 1) gene (312) and possibly NER (313). BER also repairs strand breaks through the protein XRCC1 (x-ray repair cross-complementing group 1) (314). If repair processes are complete before the cell replicates, its DNA, the DNA damage will not have a biological consequence, unless it is sufficient to affect gene transcription or cell viability (i.e., trigger apoptosis). When unrepaired DNA serves as the template for synthesis of new DNA, mutations can occur, as detailed below.

Some adducts are repaired better than others, as noted above. For example, N-7 and O^6-alkylation of guanine are better repaired than O^4-alkyl thymine, which is therefore more persistent (290). The basis for the efficient repair of O^6-alkylation is that it is a substrate for the AGAT repair process. The dealkylation by AGAT is stoichiometric and the repair molecule is inactivated by transferring the alkyl group to one of its cysteine residues (315). AGAT is also inactivated by reaction with nitric oxide (316).

The types and amounts of DNA damage can also initiate toxicity or apoptosis. DNA alkylation can elicit MMR leading to apoptosis (317) through the reduction of the antiapoptotic protein Bcl-2 (318) or inhibition of transcription by the MLH1 MMR protein (319). Also, if DNA damage is so extensive that repair fails, damaged cells are eliminated by apoptosis (320), involving both p53-dependent and -independent pathways. Among the latter, poly(ADP-ribose) polymerase activity depletes cellular energy pools leading to cell death (321).

The factors that regulate the many DNA repair genes are poorly understood. Some, such as AGAT, may be regulated by methylation of promoter regions (322). Transcripts of repair genes such as those for MMR are at the highest level during maximal DNA synthesis (323), which would, of course, serve to make available high levels of repair enzymes to protect the integrity of DNA in a critical state. Some DNA repair genes can be upregulated (324). The MAPK signaling pathway plays a role in upregulation of some genes through phosphorylation of transcription factors including members of the activator protein (AP) and specificity protein (SP) families, which have regulatory elements within the enhancer region of promoter sequences of many DNA repair genes (325)

DNA repair capacity varies between tissues and species, with human cells being generally the most proficient and about sixfold greater than rodent cells (326,327). As a specific example, adducts of 2-aminofluorene and AAF introduced into phage are largely repaired within 4 hr when the phage are transfected into human cells (328). In contrast, in the rat liver, some AAF adducts persist for weeks after exposure (292).

Despite the general proficiency of DNA repair in humans, variations in repair capacity exist among individuals, for example in AGAT (329). One basis for such variation is genetic polymorphisms in the DNA repair genes, several of which have been identified. These include an SNP in the polymerase β gene which has been identified in bladder cancer cells (330). Allelic variations in the *XRCC1* gene (331), whose gene product is involved in BER, have been associated with reduced DNA repair capacity (332), and higher risks of skin (333) and bladder (334) cancers. An SNP in the *XRCC3* gene, which codes for homologous double-stranded repair, is associated with increased melanoma risk (335). An SNP in *OGG-1*, resulting in reduced repair of oxidative DNA damage, is associated with a two-fold increase in risk of lung cancer (336). Lastly, an SNP in the promoter region of the

DNMT gene is associated with increased risk of lung cancer, possibly related to reduced DNA repair (337).

A variety of DNA repair deficient conditions arise from germ line mutations, including the hereditary nonpolyposis colorectal cancer (HNPCC) condition in which one of five mismatch repair genes *MLH1*, *PMS1*, *PMS2*, *MSH2*, and *MSH6* is mutated (338,339), xeroderma pigmentosum in which *XP* genes are mutated and NER is impaired (340) and ataxia telangiectasia in which the *ATM* gene is mutated resulting in deficient double-strand break recognition (341) and familial breast/ovarian cancer in which mutations are present, the *BRACA1* and *BRAC2* tumor suppressor genes whose encoded proteins are involved in postreplicational homologous recombination DNA repair (342).

As noted above, neoplastic cells display abnormalities in repair systems, including mismatch repair (33), AGAT (33), BRCA1 function in double-strand break repair (343), and DNA polymerase β (49). Recently, the *HR6B* (human homolog of yeast *Rad6*) DNA repair gene, which encodes ubiquitin-conjugating enzymes (E2), has been reported to be overexpressed in breast cancers, leading to genetic instability (344).

4.4. Mutations

At the molecular level, a mutation is a permanent change in the linear structure of DNA. Carcinogens can mutate critical genes either by producing DNA alteration such as point mutations, frameshifts, deletions and translocations or structural or numerical (aneuploidy) chromosomal alterations. DNA alterations occur only when damaged DNA is used as the template for DNA synthesis or when DNA polymerases introduce errors not corrected by mismatch repair. In either case, the proliferative status of the cell is critical.

As an example of point mutations, the non-Watson–Crick base pairing due to O^6-alkylation of guanine residues, a highly promutagenic lesion, is shown in Fig. 7. This mispairing with T (345) leads to the G→A transitions of one purine for another, which is found in genes mutated by many alkylating agents. The oxidation product 8-oxodG leads to G→T transversions in which a pyrimidine replaces the purine. Unrepaired apurinic sites lead to A→T and G→T base substitutions, while deamination of C to U can yield C→T mutations. A major form of DNA modification in mammalian cells is methylation of the C5 of cytosines in CpG dinucleotides (346). 5MeC can undergo spontaneous deamination to thymine resulting in 5MeC→T mutations (Fig. 4). A high frequency of mutations in the *TP53* gene in tumors occurs at presumably methylated CpG sites (88).

Point mutations are generally missense mutations that result in amino acid substitutions in the encoded proteins. Owing to the redundancy of the gene code, they may be silent or change to stop signals.

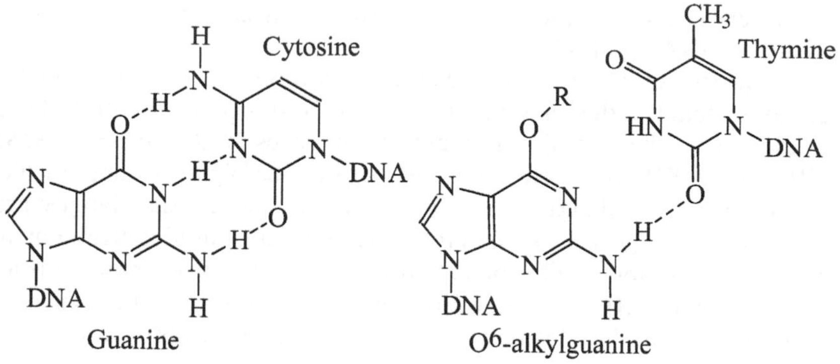

Figure 7 DNA base pairing. Normal Watson–Crick G:C base paring (*left*). Mispairing of thymine with an O^6-allylguanine base in DNA resulting from misincorporation during DNA synthesis (*right*). *Source*: From Ref. 472.

Individual adducts have different mutagenic potential. For example, the acetylated C-8 guanine adduct of AAF, dG-AAF, leads primarily to misincorporation of dTMP whereas the deacetylated adduct, dG-AF, mispairs with dAMP, dTMP, and dCMP approximately equally (347).

The critical mutations for cancer occur in growth control genes, proto-oncogenes, tumor suppressor genes, or genes regulating tumor suppressor genes, leading to dysregulation of these genes. The mutated growth control genes identified in the most common human cancers are given in Table 1, together with the type of mutation.

In oncogenes, specific point mutations lead to activation. For example, in the *RAS* gene family, activating mutations occur at codons 12, 13, and 61 (348) and rarely in codons 22 (349) and 59 (350).

In tumor suppressor genes or their regulatory genes, mutations are usually deletions (LOH) or point mutations leading to functional loss of the gene product. As noted, promoter methylation also leads to silencing.

Signature mutations for specific carcinogens are uncommon. In liver cancers that arise in geographic regions where mycotoxin contamination of foods is prevalent, mutations in *TP53* are mainly G→T transversion in the third base of codon 249 (87). Also, in nonsmall cell lung cancer, frequent *TP53* mutations occur in codons 157, 158, 245, 248, and 273 at methylated CpG sites which preferentially bind PAHs (351). Interestingly, the pattern of mutations in *TP53* in human bladder cancer were mostly G→A transitions in codons 175, 248, and 273 (352). In contrast, the proximate form of a rodent bladder carcinogen, 4-aminobiphenyl, produced predominantly mostly G→T transversion at five preferential adduction sites, raising the question as to the involvement of aromatic amines in human carcinogenesis (353). Measurement of mutated alleles in nontumorous tissue, like measurement of adducts, can suggest linkage of exposure to a carcinogen with cancer known to arise at the site (354).

Although some specific carcinogen-associated mutations have been identified, the cells of neoplasms harbor 10^4–10^6 mutations from various sources, as noted above, and thus many remain to be characterized.

4.5. Spectrum of Chemicals with Carcinogenic Activity

A number of chemicals were found to cause cancer in humans before they were tested for carcinogenicity in animals, for example, bis(chloromethyl) ether, 2-naphthylamine, and vinyl chloride. The demonstration of the carcinogenic activity of chemicals in animals (2) began with the report in 1916 by Yamagiwa and Ichikawa of induction of skin cancer in rabbits by coal tar. Subsequent salient advances included induction of liver cancer in rats by *o*-aminoazotoluene described by Yoshida in 1934 and the induction of urinary bladder tumors in dogs by 2-naphthylamine reported by Hueper and coworkers in 1938. Hundreds of chemicals have now been identified to produce increases in neoplasia in rodent tests (9,183,184). A brief listing of some examples, including both naturally occurring, i.e., mycotoxins, as well as synthetic chemicals, notably industrial chemicals and pharmaceuticals, is provided in Table 4 .

Relatively few of the many rodent carcinogens for which there is human exposure have been implicated in human cancer (Table 4). This may reflect lack of robust epidemiological data, but where good data are available, explanations lie in the fact that humans are not susceptible to some of the mechanisms operating in rodents or the exposures of humans are orders of magnitude less than in animal experiments. In particular, no food additive that elicits tumors in rodents, e.g., saccharin, has been associated with cancer in humans and likewise, no rodent carcinogenic organic pesticide, e.g., DDT, or other organochlorine compound, e.g., polychlorinated biphenyls, with the possible exception of TCDD (Table 4), has been found to cause human cancer (13). As noted, most identified human carcinogens are of the DNA-reactive type.

4.5.1. Industrial Chemicals

The first association of human cancer with a chemical exposure was the classic observation by Pott in 1775 of scrotal skin cancer in chimney sweeps, which is now known to be due to DNA-reactive PAH in chimney soot. Soot and related coal-tars are recognized as human carcinogens (Table 4) and are carcinogenic in rodents, particularly when applied to mouse skin. Subsequently, several other industrial chemicals were found to cause cancer in humans, i.e., 4-aminobiphenyl, benzene, bis(chloromethyl) ether, 2-naphthylamine, and vinyl chloride. All of these are of the DNA-reactive type. 2,3,7,8-Tetrachlorodibenzo-*p*-dioxin (TCDD) has been concluded by IARC to cause cancer in humans (355), based on mechanistic considerations, although the data in humans were judged to be limited. In rodents, TCDD appears to act as an epigenetic agent (74). Similarly, polychlorinated biphenyls are rodent liver promoters (356) and have not been conclusively associated with cancer risk to humans (357–359). Several minerals with occupational exposure, including chromium and nickel salts, have also been associated with increases in cancer. Numerous other industrial chemicals are known to produce cancer in animals, for example acrylamide, acrylonitrile, phthalates, but have not been established to cause cancer even in the most highly exposed worker populations. Likewise, a number of pesticides that are carcinogenic in rodents have been suggested to be associated with increased cancer, for example 2,4-dichlorophenoxy acetic acid and soft-tissue sacromas (360,361), but the evidence is not conclusive (362,363). Studies of agricultural workers do reveal increases in rates of several cancers such as non-Hodgkins lymphoma (364,365).

4.5.2.   Natural Substances

Endogenous hormones, such as estradiol and its catechol metabolites and thyroid stimulating hormone, are carcinogenic in animal models when administered at super physiologic doses or when persistently elevated by physiologic perturbations. Considerable evidence exists that the cumulative exposure to estrogen increases risk of breast cancer (366) and the catechol metabolites of estrogens also have been implicated, possibly as indirectly genotoxic (367). A class of mutagen and potential carcinogen formed in the body is the fecapentaenes, which are conjugated ether lipids produced by intestinal bacteria (368). Their role in human cancer remains unresolved.

Several substances found in nature have been associated with cancer in humans. The most important occur as lifestyle exposures. Tobacco, in various forms of voluntary use results in exposure to tobacco-specific nitrosamines, and PAH, both of which are DNA reactive (369). Also, alcohol, which as noted above, can act as a cocarcinogen, under conditions of excessive use leads to liver injury and cancer in humans, as well as increases in cancers of the oral cavity, pharynx, larynx, and esophagus (161). In addition, the human diet contains a number of carcinogens and anticarcinogens (370).

A variety of microbial and plant products are carcinogenic. The aflatoxins are products of the mold *Aspergillus* and contaminate certain crops such as peanuts and corn (371). Aflatoxin B_1 is a potent hepatocarcinogen in rats and has been implicated as causing human liver cancer (371). Among the many plant products which are carcinogenic in animals, those that have produced toxicity in humans are the pyrrolizidine alkaloids and aristolochic acid. DNA adducts have been found in patients consuming herbs containing aristolochic acid (372).

High levels of inorganic arsenic in well water (i.e., $> 50\,\mu g/L$) in rural areas of Asia and South America have been associated with increased human cancer risks, notably skin cancer (373) and also lung, bladder, liver, and kidney (374). The mode of action of arsenic carcinogenesis is not understood, as discussed above, and no mechanistic data are available from individuals exposed to arsenic (375).

Carcinogens are also formed during processing of food. Urethane is formed during fermentation. The cooking of protein-containing food results in generation by pyrolysis of at least 14 distinct potent carcinogenic heterocyclic amines (376). Three of these, 2-amino-1-methyl-1H-6-phenyl-imidazo[4,5-b] pyridine (PhIP), 2-amino-3-methyl-3H-imidazo[4,5-f] quinoline (IQ), and 2-amino-3,4-dimethyl-3H-imidazo[4,5-f] quinoline (MeIQ) have been shown to induce mammary cancer in rodents. Colon cancer has been induced in rodents by IQ and MeIQ, as well as 2-amino-6-methyldipyrido [1,2-a:3',2;-d]imidazole (Glu-P-1). Recently, acrylamide has been found in fried starch-containing foods (377). Some of these are suspect human carcinogens, as discussed below.

4.5.3. Medicines

Iatrogenic cancer, mainly leukemia, was first observed with alkylating agents used to treat cancer. The carcinogenic chemotherapeutics include chlorambucil, cyclophosphamide, methyl-CCNU, myleran, MOPP, nitrogen mustards, and thiotepa (378), all of which are DNA reactive (Table 4). Other pharmaceuticals, which are DNA-reactive in rodents such as tamoxifen, induce cancer in treated patients (223). A few epigenetic carcinogens, mainly hormones and immunosuppressants (Table 4), have also been associated with increased cancer risk under conditions in which they produce the pharmacological effect that underlies their carcinogenicity in rodents. For example, use of combination oral contraceptives leads to increased risk of hepatocellular carcinoma, but reduced risk for endometrial and ovarian cancer (379). Postmenopausal estrogen therapy conveys small increased risks for breast and endometrial cancers (379). Medical use of arsenic (Fowler's solution) has been associated with bladder cancer (380). Otherwise, over 80 medicines known to increase tumors in rodents (381) by epigenetic mechanisms have been used extensively without indication of increased cancer risk.

4.5.4. Food Additives

Several agents used in food such as saccharin and butylated hydroxytoluene are tumorigenic in rodents under specific conditions. None of these has been linked to human cancer. Sodium nitrite, which is used in the preservation of cured meats, has been the subject of several studies, but has not been found to be carcinogenic (382).

5. CHEMICALS AND HUMAN CANCER

The environmental agents sunlight and chemicals, particularly those derived from smoking and diet, are believed to be the major causes of human cancers (383,384). Nevertheless, cancer is a multifactorial disease and individual genetic susceptibility is important (385), as well as interaction between carcinogens and enhancing or inhibitory factors.

Excess body weight appears to increase the risk of several types of cancer, notably kidney and endometrium. This may relate to hormonal abnormalities (386).

Age is also an important determinant. Certain cancers such as leukemia and bone cancer have their greatest incidence in childhood when these tissues are highly proliferative. Most other cancers peak later in life, which may reflect prolonged accumulation of DNA alterations and increased carcinogen sensitivity (387).

To date, 88 specific chemicals or mixtures have been established by the International Agency for Research on Cancer to cause cancer in humans (Table 4), some of which have been discussed above. Most of these are of the DNA-reactive type and virtually all of them, apart from cigarette smoke and mycotoxins, affect humans either through occupational or therapeutic exposures, which are substantial compared to general environmental exposures to chemicals. These industrial chemicals and pharmaceuticals, however, account for only a small fraction of human cancer (Table 5).

The few epigenetic carcinogens implicated in human cancer are mainly hormones or immunosuppressants, which are associated with increased risk of cancer only under conditions of exposure in which they produce the pharmacological effects that is the basis for their carcinogenicity in rodents. No food additive or pesticide that has produced increases in tumors in rodents through an epigenetic mechanism has been definitively identified to be a cause of human cancer (Table 4), although a number of associations have been reported for pesticides (364).

Inorganic carcinogens, mainly asbestos and arsenic, account for only a small proportion of cancers. In both cases, substantial chronic exposures were involved; for asbestos, occupational exposure is implicated (388), while for arsenic, both occupational exposure and consumption of highly contaminated well water is involved (375).

The calculated contribution of various agents to cancer incidence in the United States is given in Table 5. These numbers are based upon the numbers of new cancer cases estimated by the American Cancer Society to occur in 2005 (389) and the fraction of each type of cancer that can be attributed to implicated etiologic agents. The etiologic agents or risk factors include both carcinogens and enhancing or promoting factors.

The cancer with the highest incidence is skin cancer, including basal and squamous cell cancers, making sunlight the most effective human

Table 5   Estimated Causes of Cancer Incidence in the United States 2002

Type	Percent of total (excluding skin)[a]
Lifestyle cancers	
Diet related:	
High fat, low fiber, low vegetables and fruits, high, broiled or fried foods?—large bowel, breast, pancreas, prostate, ovary, endometrium	25–30
Low vegetables and fruits—stomach[b]	2–3
Tobacco related: lung, larynx, oral cavity, bladder, pancreas, kidney, stomach, cervix	20–25
Tobacco and alcohol related: oral cavity, esophagus, lung	2–3
Alcohol: liver, pharynx, larynx, esophagus, breast	3–4
Sunlight: melanoma of the skin	1–2
Lifestyle and occupational exposures	
Tobacco and asbestos, tobacco and mining, tobacco and uranium/radium: respiratory tract, lung	1–2
Occupational cancers	
Various carcinogens, e.g., aromatic amines—bladder and other organs	≈1
Asbestos—mesothelioma	>0.5
Bacteria-related cancers	
Helicobacter pylori—stomach	1–2
Virus-related cancers	
Hepatitis B,C—liver; human papilloma—cervix, penis, anus; Epstein–Barr—B-cell lymphoma, Hodgkins lymphoma; HIV-1, Kaposi's sarcoma, non-Hodgkins lymphoma	2–5
Genetically determined cancers	
Tumor suppressor gene mutations: *APC*, familial adenomatous polyposis, colon; *BRCA1, 2*, familial breast, ovary; *CDKN2A*, familial melanoma; *LKB1*, various in Peutz–Jeghers syndrome; *MEN1*, multiple endocrine; *RB1*, retinoblastoma; *WT1*, Wilms tumor	3–5
Other genetic predispositions: mismatch repair genes in hereditary nonpolyposis colorectal cancer, colorectal, endometrial, stomach; hemochromatosis, liver cancer; steroidogenesis (*HSD3B*), prostate; *ATM* dysfunction in processing of double-strand breaks in Ataxia telangiectasia, lymphorecticular; defects in *BLM* DNA helicase in Bloom's syndrome, various; rare	

(Continued)

Table 5 Estimated Causes of Cancer Incidence in the United States 2002 (*Continued*)

Type	Percent of total (excluding skin)[a]
HRAS-VNTR alleles, sporadic ovary	
Iatrogenic:	
Radiation—leukemia, thyroid, brain	≈ 1
Medicines—leukemia, endometrium	≈ 1
Unknown	
Leukemia, lymphoma, brain	3–25[c]

[a]1,284,900 total cases exculding basal cell and squamous cell cancers of the skin which account for about 1,000,000 cases
[b]*Helicobactor pylori* has an interactive role
[c]This large variation is a function of the broad range calculated for the main diet and tobacco associated cancers
Source: Ref. 389

carcinogen. After this, the most frequent cancer incidence in women is breast and in men, prostate. Both of these are believed to be attributable in part to diet.

The main causative agents of human cancer are lifestyle factors, including damaging sunlight exposure, unhealthy diets, tobacco smoking, and excess alcohol consumption (384,390,391). In the United States, body weight and obesity contribute significantly to cancer mortality (392). Many types of human cancer result from specific carcinogens as the initiating agents and contributing enhancing or inhibiting elements. Table 6 gives the agents proven or suspected to influence the occurrence of the major cancers worldwide. In addition, a significant fraction of cancer is genetically determined and genetic predisposition influences susceptibility to exposures, as discussed below.

Specific carcinogens have been implicated in the etiology of several cancers. For lung cancer due to tobacco smoking, there is strong evidence for the involvement of DNA-reactive carcinogens, particularly polycyclic aromatic hydrocarbons, such as benzo[a]pyrene, and possibly tobacco-specific nitrosamines (369). For breast, large intestine and prostate cancers attributable to diet, certain of the carcinogenic heterocyclic amines formed during cooking of food have been implicated as carcinogens for the mammary gland and large intestine and possibly the prostate (376). Specifically, PhIP, IQ, and MeIQ, discussed above, are suspected human mammary carcinogens (393). The risk calculated for ingestion of heterocyclic amines, however, is small (394) and accordingly other factors appear to be involved in these diet-related cancers. For bladder cancer associated with cigarette smoking, the DNA-reactive carcinogens 4-aminobiphenyl and

Table 6 Agents Proven or Implicated to Influence Human Cancers Worldwide

Cancer	Carcinogen[a,b]	Enhancing or promoting factors	Protective factors
Lung	Tobacco smoke, including second hand (polycyclic aromatic hydrocarbons ?nitrosamines) Occupational exposures, PAHs	?High fat diet,[c] asbestos	Fruits and vegetables (vitamin A, cryptoxanthin), soy foods
Large intestine	?Heterocyclic amines	High fat diet,[b] alcohol low folate or methionine intake	Calcium, vitamin D, soy foods, tea, adequate fiber; estrogen replacement therapy, cyclo-oxygenase 2 inhibitors
Breast	Meat cooked at high temperatures (?heterocyclic amines)	High fat diet,[b] high alcohol intake, combination oral contraceptives, postmenopausal estrogen	Pregnancy, breast feeding, vitamin A, olive oil consumption (?hydroxytyrosol), ?soy foods (?iso-flavones), ?calcium, ?vitamin D ?Eicosapentaenoic acid;-antiestrogens,? cyclo-oxygenase-2 inhibitors
Prostate	?Heterocyclic amines	High fat diet IGF-1[b]	Soy foods (?iso-flavones), cooked tomato (lycopene), ?selenium ?eicosapentaenoic acid
Pancreas	Tobacco smoke ?heterocyclic amines	High fat,[b] meat diet	Soy foods, tea, vegetables, fruits

(Continued)

Table 6 Agents Proven or Implicated to Influence Human Cancers Worldwide (*Continued*)

Cancer	Carcinogen[a,b]	Enhancing or promoting factors	Protective factors
Stomach	?Reactive chloro or nitroso compounds ?tobacco smoke	High intake of salted and preserved foods, *Helicobacter pylori*	Fruits and vegetables (vitamin C) soy foods, tea
Esophagus	Tobacco smoke, ?nitrosamines	Alcohol (?acetaldehyde)	Vegetables, tea, ?soy foods
Cervix	Human papilloma virus? tobacco smoke	Estrogen	
Liver	Aflatoxins	Hepatitis B, C, alcohol, combination oral contraceptives	Antioxidants
Biliary tract		Primary sclerosing cholangitis, hepatolithiasis, liver fluke infestation	
Thyroid	Radiation	?Low or high iodine intake	
Endometrium		?Tamoxifen	Obesity, (?17-?-estradiol) Post-menopausal estrogen, tamoxifen
Kidney	Combination oral contraceptives ?Tobacco smoke	Obesity (?IGF-1), ?high animal protein	
Urinary bladder	Tobacco smoke (aromatic amines[a]), aromatic amines, arsenic	Schistosomiasis	Vegetables, especially cruciferous (?isothiocynate sulforaphane), fruits

Ovary	Hormones	Nulliparity	Fruits, ?vegetables, vitamin A,?β-carotene; combination oral contraceptives
Testes		Gonadal abnormalities	
Brain	Radiation		
Leukemia	Radiation, chemotherapy, benzene		?Vegetables
T-cell adult	T-cell lymphotrophic virus 1		
Lymphoma			
Non-Hodgkins	HIV-1	Psoriasis	
Hodgkins	Epstein–Barr virus	Psoriasis	
Skin	Sunlight, PUVA therapy	Arsenic	Sun screens, vitamin A
Oral cavity	Tobacco smoke, chewing tobacco, betel quid	Alcohol (?acetaldehyde)	Fruits and vegetables, vitamin A
Pharynx, larynx	Tobacco smoke	Alcohol (?acetaldehyde)	Vegetables, vitamin A

[a]Presumed agent.
[b]?=implicated.
[c]Monounsaturated oils, olive, peanut, or canola oils do not promote, n-3-polyunsaturated oils are protective.
Source: Updated from Ref. 391.

2-naphthylamine have been implicated (395). The likely role of aromatic amines is supported by the observation of increased risk in slow acetylators (249), as discussed above. In the stomach, foods high in salt, nitrates, and nitrites, under certain conditions, may contribute to the formation of *N*-nitroso carcinogens, although the evidence for current cancer causation by these is not conclusive (396). Aflatoxins are fungal products that cause liver cancer in both experimental animals and in humans consuming contaminated foods (371).

In addition to specific carcinogens, enhancing agents (promoters), largely derived from diet, are involved in human cancers (384,397). The role of diet in the etiology of breast (398,399), colon (400), and prostate (401) cancers has been detailed. Diets associated with these cancers are characterized by being high in calories, high in fat, and low in starch and fiber, although the relationship of these dietary components to cancer risk remains unresolved (402–404). In animal models, high energy and fat intake have enhancing effects on breast and colon cancer (405). Accordingly, it has been postulated that the incidence of these cancers in humans may be influenced by the promoting stimulus of high fat diets, but this remains unproven. Nevertheless, in each tissue, specific effectors appear to be involved in human carcinogenesis, some related to diet. In postmenopausal breast cancer, estrogen is clearly involved, probably through stimulation of ductal epithelial cell proliferation (366) mediated by estrogen receptor α (406). In the large intestine, high levels of excreted bile acids have been implicated in colon cancer as part of a complex set of interacting factors (407), including elevated blood levels of insulin-like growth factor-1 (IGF-1) (136), which is regulated by growth hormone and nutritional status. For prostate cancer also, the blood level of IGF-1 is a risk factor (408). In individuals with a genetic susceptibility to insulin resistance, excessive weight gain and/or a diet high in fat can trigger hyperinsulinemia which may contribute to breast and colon cancer risk (409). The specificity of the effects of fats is exemplified by the fact that they differ in their modulating effects on experimental cancer, with n-6 fatty acids enhancing cancer development and long chain n-3 fatty acids inhibiting (410,411). The mechanism of the anticancer effect of n-3 fatty acids may involve inhibition of translation initiation (412).

Microbial agents play a definite role in several human cancers, both as carcinogenic and enhancing agents (413). It is estimated that about 80% of liver cancer worldwide is attributable to infection with hepatitis B virus (HBV) and/or hepatitis C virus (HCV) (413). Hepatitis B plays a major role in liver cancer in sub-Saharan Africa, and parts of Asia, while rising rates in Japan (414), the United States (415), and parts of Europe (416) are attributed to increases in HCV infection. Stomach cancer often arises on a background of chronic gastritis and frequently involves *Helicobacter pylori* (417,418). The human papilloma virus (HPV) (types 16 and 18) is involved in cervical cancer by producing oncoproteins that inactivate tumor suppressor genes (419). The E6 protein promotes degradation of p53 through the ubiquitin–proteosome pathway (420), while the HPV 16 E7 oncoprotein binds to Rb (421). In persons infected with human immunodeficiency virus (HIV) type 1, the incidences of Kaposi's sarcoma and Non-Hodgkin's lymphoma are greatly increased (422). Human T-lymphotropic virus-I (HTLV-1) infection is prevalent in southwest Japan, the Caribbean, parts of South American and Central and West Africa and is associated with adult T-cell leukemia/lymphoma (423). Other cancer-associated microbial agents include *Schistosoma hematobium*, whose chronic bladder infestation leads to increased risk of bladder cancer, and the flukes, *Clonorchis sinensis* and *Opisthorchis viverrini*, whose infestation of the biliary tract leads to increased occurrence of cholangiocarcinoma (424).

The carcinogenicity of these microbial agents, as well as that of some other forms of chronic tissue injury, may relate to oxidative damage. With chronic inflammation, high levels of nitric oxide are produced by the inducible nitric oxide synthetase (iNOS) which is highly expressed in activated macrophages (425). Nitric oxide may be an endogenous carcinogen (194) and it also inhibits the ogg1 protein repair enzyme involved in excision of 8-oxoguanine (426).

A factor contributing to an increasing fraction of human cancers is family cancer syndromes, which number about 35, resulting from both autosomal dominant and autosomal recessive patterns of inheritance (427,428). Polymorphisms in tumor suppressor genes, such as *TP53*, appear to elevate risks of some cancers (429). Germ line mutations in tumor suppressor genes, such as *BRCA1* and *BRCA2* in familial breast cancer and *APC* in colon cancer arising in the condition adenomatous polyposis coli, clearly predispose to cancer (Table 5). Also, germ line mutations in DNA repair genes, discussed above, increase cancer risks; examples include the hereditary non-polyposis colorectal cancer mutation which leads to increased colorectal, endometrial, stomach, and other cancers (339,430), the xeroderma pigmentosum mutation which increases risk of sunlight-induced skin cancer 2000-fold (431) and the ataxia telangiectasia mutation which conveys extreme predisposition to lymphoreticular malignancies (432) and is associated with an increased risk of breast cancer (433). In addition, it is likely that numerous tumor susceptibility alleles or quantitative trait loci exist (434). Finally, inheritance of predisposing factors can elevate cancer risk as in male germ cell tumors for which cryptorchidism, spermatogenic or testicular dysgenesis, Klinefelter's syndrome, and a positive family history can elevate risk several fold (435).

For the cancers for which a specific initiating carcinogen has not been identified, a potential explanation gaining in support is that the accumulation of oxidative DNA damage leads to cancer (192,263). Oxidation of DNA is established to be mutagenic (436) and is clearly carcinogenic, as demonstrated by the example of ionizing radiation. A variety of rodent carcinogens give rise to oxidative DNA damage (193,437), suggesting that similar effects could occur in humans. Levels of 8-oxodG in human tissues range from one adduct per 10^7 nucleotides to one adduct per 10^3 nucleotides (264). Although the exact levels of this promutagenic lesion may be uncertain, the existence of repair enzymes to remove it clearly indicates that DNA oxidation is an important biological problem. Further support for a role of oxidative damage in human cancer comes from the fact that diets high in fruits and vegetables protect against a variety of cancers (438), as listed in Table 6, and have been shown to reduce endogenous oxidation of DNA (439). Moreover, a novel "signature mutation" for oxidative DNA damage, discontinuous loss of heterozygosity, has been identified as an effect of H_2O_2 (440) and this mutation purportedly resembles a mutation pattern found in human cancers such as those of the head and neck, lung, prostate, breast, and colorectum (see Ref. 440 for references).

As noted, in addition to enhancing agents, a variety of inhibitors have been identified (Table 6). Among these, high consumption of fruits and vegetables, especially cruciferous vegetables, is associated with reduced risks for several cancers (438,441). Soy foods (442) and tea (443) consumption also appear to be protective. However, consumption of a high fiber diet has not been shown to reduce occurrence of colorectal adenomas (444,445).

6. CANCER PROPHYLAXIS

The most effective approach to prevention of cancer is designated as primordial prevention in which exposure to causative agents such as such as cigarette smoking, high risk diets, excessive alcohol consumption, and damaging sunlight exposure is abrogated. Since cancer is a disease which has a prolonged development time, and evidence exists for influences on some cancers of exogenous agents acting very early in life, primordial prevention really must begin in childhood through appropriate education and behavior modification (222). Next in the hierarchy of prophylaxis is primary prevention of cancer which is achieved with reduction or elimination of existing exposures to causative agents before the inception of cancer. Again, managerial preventive medicine is an important modality here. Secondary prevention involves the application of factors to reduce the effects of carcinogenic exposures. For example, prophylaxis for several types of cancer is furthered by consumption of a diet rich in protective components, as detailed in Table 6. Important among these are fruits and vegetables consumed at three or more servings per day (446–448), which reduce risks of colon, pancreas, bladder, lung, oral cavity, larynx, esophagus, and stomach cancer (449). The protective agents involved appear to be vitamin A and carotenoids, particularly cryptoxanthin. Also, high intake of fish, which contain n-3 fatty acids, particularly eicosapentaenoic acid and docosahexaenoic acid is associated with reduced risks of breast, prostate, and colorectal cancers (450).

These foods together with food sources of monounsaturated fats (olive oil) characterize Mediterranean-type diets, which convey reduced risks of several cancers (451). A diet devised to provide these components is the Fiber First Diet which implements adequate fiber content derived from vegetables, fruits, whole grain breads, and wheat bran cereals and reduces fat intake (391). Consumption of soy-containing foods is associated with reduced risk of prostate cancer (452) possibly due to *iso*-flavones. Several vitamins appear to reduce cancer risks (Table 6) and hence it is important that diets provide recommended intakes (453), or otherwise regular use of a multivitamin is indicated.

One component of secondary prevention is the use of anticancer or chemopreventive agents whose mechanisms were discussed earlier. A wide variety of experimental cancer preventive agents, both naturally occurring and synthetic, is known (177,391,454,455). Several of these have shown promise in humans (456), mostly as inhibitors of the growth of neoplastic cells. Among agents of this type, retinoids have been evaluated for suppression of oral cancer but high relapse rates and serious side effects occur (457). The selective estrogen receptor modulator tamoxifen reduces breast cancer risk (223,458). Also, breast (459) and colon (460) cancer risks are reduced by regular use of nonsteriodal anti-inflammatory drugs. Of particular interest is specific COX-2 inhibitors such as celecoxib, whose anticancer activity may result from a variety of effects (461), including reduction of enzyme-derived prostaglandins, particularly PGE_2. Another strategy, the enhancement of carcinogen detoxification, is being pursued with agents such as oltipraz (177).

With potent pharmaceuticals, however, there are complexities to be recognized. For example, tamoxifen, although reducing breast cancer risk, also increases endometrial cancer risk (223). Thus, efforts in chemoprevention are being directed toward synthesis of analogs with greater specificity for specific molecular targets. An example is the rexinoids which bind selectively to retinoid X receptors (RXR) but not retinoic acid receptors (RAR) (462). Similarly, vitamin D analogs that do not produce hypercalcemia are under investigation (463).

The utility for cancer prevention of supplemental intake of specific components of foods that are associated with reduced cancer risks also merits further investigation. Although substantial observational epidemiologic data exist for a preventive role of diets high in carotenoids, intervention studies with β carotene at 20–50 mg daily either showed an increase in lung cancer or no reduction (464). In contrast, selenium supplementation was found to reduce the risk of prostate cancer (465,466), and lung cancer in individuals with low selenium levels (467).

For cancers related to infections, primordial protection can be achieved by good public health measures. Also, primary prevention can be afforded by therapy for parasites (424) and bacteria (418) and vaccines for viruses such as HBV (468) and HPV (469).

The opportunities and challenges to chemoprevention were formulated by the Chemoprevention Working Group several years ago (470). While further progress is to be expected, it remains that prevention offers the best prospect for reduction of cancer attributable to chemical and microbial agents.

7. CONCLUDING REMARKS

It is clear from the above review that many of the agents involved in human cancer have been identified and critical factors that influence their effects have been elucidated. Various appropriate intervention strategies are available and others are being developed. Accordingly, it can be anticipated that control or reductions in many cancers can be achieved in the near future.

REFERENCES

1. Foulds L. Neoplastic Development. New York: Academic Press, 1969.
2. Berenblum I. Carcinogenesis as a Biological Problem. Amsterdam: North–Holland Publishing Co., 1974.
3. Clayson DB. Chemical Carcinogenesis. Boston: Little, Brown and Co, 1962.
4. Knudson AG Jr, Hethcote HW, Brown BW. Mutation and childhood cancer: a probabilistic model for the incidence of retinoblastoma. Proc Natl Acad Sci USA 1975; 72:5116–5120.
5. Feinberg AP. Cancer epigenetics takes center stage. Proc Natl Acad Sci USA 2001; 98:392–394.
6. Loeb KR, Loeb LA. Significance of multiple mutations in cancer. Carcinogenesis 2000; 21:379–385.
7. Jones PA, Baylin SB. The fundamental role of epigenetic events in cancer. Nat Rev Genet 2002; 3:415–428.
8. Williams GM. Interactive carcinogenesis in the liver. In: Bannasch P, Keppler D, Weber G, eds. Falk Symposium: Liver Cell Carcinoma. Boston,1989;51: Academic Press, 197–216.
9. Williams GM, Weisburger JH. Chemical carcinogenesis. In: Klaassen CD, Amdur MO, Doull J, eds. toxicology. New York, NY: McGraw–Hill, 1991; 127–200.
10. Wattenberg GM. Chemoprevention of Cancer. Cancer Res 1985; 45:1–8.
11. Williams GM, Iatropoulos MJ. Principles of testing for carcinogenic activity. Hayes W, ed. Principles and Methods of Toxicology. New York: Taylor & Francis, 2001; 959–1000.
12. Williams GM, Reiss B, Weisburger JH. A comparison of the animal and human carcinogenicity of several environmental, occupational and therapeutic chemicals. In: Flamm G, Lorentzen R, eds. Mechanisms and Toxicology of Chemical Carcinogens and Mutagens. Princeton, NJ: Princeton Scientific Publishers 1985; 9:207–248.

13. Williams GM. Chemicals with carcinogenic activity in the rodent liver; mechanistic evaluation of human risk. Cancer Lett 1997; 117:175–188.
14. International Agency for Research on Cancer Species Differences in Thyroid, Kidney and Urinary Bladder Carcinogenesis. Lyon, France: IARC Scientific Publications, 1999; 147.
15. Muniappan BP, Thilly WG. The DNA polymerase β replication error spectrum in the adenomatous polyposis coli gene contains human colon tumor mutational hotspots. Cancer Res 2002; 62:3271–3275.
16. Bestor TH. The DNA methyltransferases of mammals. Hum Mol Genet 2000; 9:2395–2402.
17. Cress WD, Seto E. Histone deacetylases, transcriptional control, and cancer. J Cell Physiol 2000; 184:1–16.
18. Pitot HC. Multistage carcinogenesis. In: Bertino JR, ed. Encyclopedia of Cancer. San Diego : Academic Press, 1997;2:1108–1119.
19. Birchmeier C, Meyer D, Riethmacher D. Factors controlling growth, motility, and morphogenesis of normal and malignant epithelial cells. Int Rev Cytol 1995; 160:221–266.
20. Williams BR. PKR; a sentinel kinase for cellular stress. Oncogene 1999; 18:6112–6120.
21. Williams GM. Chemically induced preneoplastic lesions in rodents as indicators of carcinogenic activity. IARC Sci Publ 1999; 146:185–202.
22. Gusterson BA, Machin LG, Gullick WJ, Gibbs NM, Powles TJ, Price P, McKinna A, Harrison S. Immunohistochemical distribution of c–erbB-2 in infiltrating and in situ breast cancer. Int J Cancer 1988; 42:842–845.
23. Hao XP, Pretlow TG, Rao JS, Pretlow TP. β-catenin expression is altered in human colonic aberrant crypt foci. Cancer Res 2001; 61:8085–8088.
24. Sellin JH, Umar S, Xiao J, Morris AP. Increased β-catenin expression and nuclear translocation accompany cellular hyperproliferation in vivo. Cancer Res 2001; 61:2899–2906.
25. Maruyama H, Tanaka T, Gebhardt R, Berghem L, Williams GM. Decreased fibronectin in rat liver altered foci and adenomas induced by N^2-fluorenylacetamide. Lab Invest 1988; 58:630–635.
26. Wilson KT, Fu S, Ramanujam KS, Meltzer SJ. Increased expression of inducible nitric oxide synthase and cyclooxygenase-2 in Barrett's esophagus and associated adenocarcinomas. Cancer Res 1998; 58:2929–2934.
27. Hao XP, Pretlow TG, Rao JS, Pretlow TP. Inducible nitric oxide synthase (iNOS) is expressed similarly in multiple aberrant crypt foci and colorectal tumors from the same patients. Cancer Res 2001; 61:419–422.
28. Smith AJ, Stern HS, Penner M, Hay K, Mitri A, Bapat BV, Gallinger S. Somatic APC and K–ras codon 12 mutations in aberrant crypt foci from human colons. Cancer Res 1994; 54:5527–5530.
29. Xu XC, Ro JY, Lee JS, Shin DM, Hong WK, Lotan R. Differential expression of nuclear retinoid receptors in normal, premalignant, and malignant head and neck tissues. Cancer Res 1994; 54:3580–3587.
30. Sakurazawa N, Tanaka N, Onda M, Esumi H. Instability of X chromosome methylation in aberrant crypt foci of the human colon. Cancer Res 2000; 60:3165–3169.

31. Belinsky SA, Nikula KJ, Palmisano WA, Michels R, Saccomanno G, Gabrielson E, Baylin SB, Herman JG. Aberrant methylation of p16(INK4a) is an early event in lung cancer and a potential biomarker for early diagnosis. Proc Natl Acad Sci USA 1998; 95:11891–11896.

32. Mori H, Sugie S, Ohbayashi F, Shima H, Yoshimi N, Takahashi M, Williams GM. Reduced DNA repair response of cells from carcinogen–induced rat liver altered foci exposed to chemical carcinogens in culture. Carcinogenesis 1985; 6:1087–1090.

33. Esteller M, Catasus L, Matias-Guiu X, Mutter GL, Prat J, Baylin SB, Herman JG. *hMLH1* promoter hypermethylation is an early event in human endometrialtumorigenesis. Amer J pathol 1999; 155:1767–1772.

34. Herman JG, Umar A, Polyak K, Graff JR, Ahuja N, Issa JP, Markowitz S, Willson JK, Hamilton SR, Kinzler KW, Kane MF, Kolodner RD, Vogelstein B, Kunkel TA, Baylin SB. Incidence and functional consequences of *hMLH1*promoter hypermethylation in colorectal carcinoma. Proc Natl Acad Sci USA 1998; 95:6870–6875.

35. Loewenstein WR, Rose B. The cell–cell channel in the control of growth. Semin Cell Biol 1992; 3:59–79.

36. Trosko JE, Madhukar BV, Chang CC. Endogenous and exogenous modulation of gap junctional intercellular communication: toxicological and pharmacological implications. Life Sci 1993; 53:1–19.

37. Yamasaki H, Mesnil M, Omori Y, Mironov N, Krutovskikh V. Intercellular communication and carcinogenesis. Mutat Res 1995; 333:181–188.

38. Vogelstein B, Kinzler KW. The multistep nature of cancer. Trends Genet 1993; 9:138–141.

39. Murakami Y, Sekiya T. Accumulation of genetic alterations and their significance in each primary human cancer and cell line. Mutat Res 1998; 400: 421–437.

40. Jones PA, Laird PW. Cancer epigenetics comes of age. Nat Genet 1999; 21:163–167.

41. Jones PA. DNA methylation errors and cancer. Cancer Res 1996; 56: 2463–2467.

42. Rountree MR, Bachman KE, Herman JG, Baylin SB. DNA methylation, chromatin inheritance, and cancer. Oncogene 2001; 20:3156–3165.

43. Renan MJ. How many mutations are required for tumorigenesis? Implications from human cancer data. Mol Carcinog 1993; 7:139–146.

44. Hahn WC, Counter CM, Lundberg AS, Beijersbergen RL, Brooks MW, Weinberg RA. Creation of human tumour cells with defined genetic elements. Nature 1999; 400:464–468.

45. Boland CR, Ricciardiello L. How many mutations does it take to make a tumor? Proc Natl Acad Sci USA 1999; 96:14675–14677.

46. Tomlinson I, Sasieni P, Bodmer W. How many mutations in a cancer? Amer J Pathol 2002; 160:755–758.

47. Nowell PC. The clonal evolution of tumor cell populations. Science 1976; 194:23–28.

48. Loeb LA. Mutator phenotype may be required for multistage carcinogenesis. Cancer Res 1991; 51:3075–3079.

49. Washington SL, Yoon MS, Chagovetz AM, Li SX, Clairmont CA, Preston BD, Eckert KA, Sweasy JB. A genetic system to identify DNA polymerase β mutator mutants. Proc Natl Acad Sci USA 1997; 94:1321–1326.

50. Ionov Y, Peinado MA, Malkhosyan S, Shibata D, Perucho M. Ubiquitous somatic mutations in simple repeated sequences reveal a new mechanism for colonic carcinogenesis. Nature 1993; 363:558–561.

51. Wooster R, Cleton-Jansen AM, Collins N, Mangion J, Cornelis RS, Cooper CS, Gusterson BA, Ponder BA, von Deimling A, Wiestler OD, Cornelisse CJ, Denilee P, Stratton MR. Instability of short tandem repeats (microsatellites) in human cancers. Nat Genet 1994; 6:152–156.

52. Perucho M. Cancer of the microsatellite mutator phenotype. Biol Chem 1996; 377:675–684.

53. Dietmaier W, Wallinger S, Bocker T, Kullmann F, Fishel R, Ruschoff J. Diagnostic microsatellite instability: definition and correlation with mismatch repair protein expression. Cancer Res 1997; 57:4749–4756.

54. Costello JF, Fruhwald MC, Smiraglia DJ, Rush LJ, Robertson GP, Gao X, Wright FA, Feramisco JD, Peltomaki P, Lang JC, Schuller DE, Yu L, Bloomfield CD, Caligiuri MA, Yates A, Nishikawa R, Su HH, Petrelli NJ, Zhang X, O'Dorisio MS, Held WA, Cavenee WK, Plass C. Aberrant CpG-island methylation has non-random and tumour-type-specific patterns. Nat Genet 2000; 24:132–138.

55. Yunis JJ, Soreng AL. Constitutive fragile sites and cancer. Science 1984; 226:1199–1204.

56. Smith DI, Huang H, Wang L. Common fragile sites and cancer (Review). Int J Oncol 1998; 12:187–196.

57. Zimonjic DB, Druck T, Ohta M, Kastury K, Croce CM, Popescu NC, Huebner K. Positions of chromosome 3p14.2 fragile sites (FRA3B) within the *FHIT* gene. Cancer Res 1997; 57:1166–1170.

58. Mangelsdorf M, Ried K, Woollatt E, Dayan S, Eyre H, Finnis M, Hobson L, Nancarrow J, Venter D, Baker E, Richards RI. Chromosomal fragile site FRA16D and DNA instability in cancer. Cancer Res 2000; 60:1683–1689.

59. Mitelman data base, http://cgap.nci.nih.gov/Chromosomes/Mitelman

60. Weinstein IB, Begemann M, Zhou P, Han EK, Sgambato A, Doki Y, Arber N, Ciaparrone M, Yamamoto H. Disorders in cell circuitry associated with multistage carcinogenesis: exploitable targets for cancer prevention and therapy. Clin Cancer Res 1997; 3:2696–2702.

61. Sherr CJ. Cancer cell cycles. Science 1996; 274:1672–1677.

62. Weinstein IB. Disorders in cell circuitry during multistage carcinogenesis: the role of homeostasis. Carcinogenesis 2000; 21:857–864.

63. National Cancer Institute, The Cancer Genome Anatomy Project. http://cgap.nci.nih.gov/Pathways/BioCarta/

64. Tyers M, Jorgeson P. Proteolysis and the cell cycle: with this RING I do thee destroy. Curr Opin Genet Dev 2000; 10:54–64.

65. Donnellan R, Chetty R. Cyclin E in human cancers. *FASEB J* 1999; 13:773–780.

66. Spruck CH, Strohmaier H, Sangfelt O, Muller HM, Hubalek M, Muller-Holzner E, Marth C, Widschwendter M, Reed SI. hCDC4 gene mutations in endometrial cancer. Cancer Res 2002; 62:4535–4539.
67. DNA-Tumor Suppressor and Oncogene Database. http://embryology.med. unow.edu.au/DNA/DNA10.htm.
68. Bos JL. RAS oncogenes in human cancer: a review. Cancer Res 1989; 49: 4682–4689.
69. Cooper GM. Oncogenes. Boston, MA: Jones & Bartlett, 1995.
70. Kolch W. Meaningful relationships: the regulation of the Ras/Raf/ MEK/ERK pathway by protein interactions. Biochem J 2000; 351(Pt 2): 289–305.
71. Chang L, Karin M. Mammalian MAP kinase signalling cascades. Nature 2001; 410:37–40.
72. Luque I, Gélinas C. Rel/NF-κB and IκB factors in oncogenesis. Semin Cancer Biol 1997; 8:103–111.
73. Mercurio F, Manning AM. Multiple signals converging on NF-κB. Curr Opin Cell Biol 1999; 11:226–232.
74. Ramakrishna G, Perella C, Birely L, Diwan BA, Fornwald LW, Anderson LM. Decrease in K-ras p21 and increase in Raf1 and activated Erk 1 and 2 in murine lung tumors initiated by *N*–nitrosodimethylamine and promoted by 2,3,7,8-tetrachlorodibenzo-*p*-dioxin. Toxicol Appl Pharmacol 2002; 179:21–34.
75. Blume-Jensen P, Hunter T. Oncogenic kinase signalling. Nature 2001; 411:355–365.
76. Hackel PO, Zwick E, Prenzel N, Ullrich A. Epidermal growth factor receptors: critical mediators of multiple receptor pathways. Curr Opin Cell Biol 1999; 11:184–189.
77. Bixby JL. Ligands and signaling through receptor-type tyrosine phosphatases. IUBMB Life 2001; 51:157–163.
78. Ikezoe T, Miller CW, Kawano S, Heaney A, Williamson EA, Hisatake J, Green E, Hofmann W, Taguchi H, Koeffler HP. Mutational analysis of the peroxisome proliferator–activated receptor gamma gene in human malignancies. Cancer Res 2001; 61:5307–5310.
79. Bromberg J, Darnell JE Jr. The role of STATs in transcriptional control and their impact on cellular function. Oncogene 2000; 19:2468–2473.
80. Bowman T, Garcia R, Turkson J, Jove R. STATs in oncogenesis. Oncogene 2000; 19:2474–2488.
81. Masuda M, Suzui M, Yasumatu R, Nakashima T, Kuratomi Y, Azuma K, Tomita K, Komiyama S, Weinstein IB. Constitutive activation of signal transducers and activators of transcription 3 correlates with cyclin D1 overexpression and may provide a novel prognostic marker in head and neck squamous cell carcinoma. Cancer Res 2002; 62:3351–3355.
82. Cadigan KM, Nusse R. Wnt signaling: a common theme in animal development. Genes Dev 1997; 11:3286–3305.
83. Barker N, Morin PJ, Clevers H. The Yin-Yang of TCFβ-catenin signaling. Adv Cancer Res 2000; 77:1–24.
84. Dang CV. c-Myc target genes involved in cell growth, apoptosis, and metabolism. Mol Cell Biol 1999; 19:1–11.

85. Ramsay RG, Friend A, Vizantios Y, Freeman R, Sicurella C, Hammett F, Armes J, Venter D. Cyclooxygenase-2, a colorectal cancer nonsteroidal anti-inflammatory drug target, is regulated by c-MYB. Cancer Res 2000; 60:1805–1809.
86. Wiese FW, Thompson PA, Kadlubar FF. Carcinogen substrate specificity of human COX-1 and COX-2. Carcinogenesis 2001; 22:5–10.
87. Hussain SP, Harris CC. Molecular epidemiology of human cancer. Recent Results Cancer Res 1998; 154:22–36.
88. Soussi T. The p53 tumor suppressor gene: from molecular biology to clinical investigation. Ann N Y Acad Sci 2000; 910:121–137.
89. Levine AJ. p53, the cellular gatekeeper for growth and division. Cell 1997; 88:323–331.
90. el Deiry WS. Regulation of p53 downstream genes. Semin Cancer Biol 1998; 8:345–357.
91. Wu G, Nomoto S, Hoque MO, Dracheva T, Osada M, Lee C-CR, Dong SM, Guo Z, Benoit N, Cohen Y, Rechthand P, Califano J, Moon C-S, Ratovitski E, Jen J, Sidransky D, Trink B. ΔNp63 α and TAp63 α regulate transcription of genes with distinct biological functions in cancer and development. Cancer Res 2003; 63:2351–2357.
92. Fuchs SY, Adler V, Buschmann T, Wu X, Ronai Z. Mdm2 association with p53 targets its ubiquitination. Oncogene 1998; 17:2543–2547.
93. Momand J, Jung D, Wilczynski S, Niland J. The MDM2 gene amplification database. Nucleic Acids Res 1998; 26:3453–3459.
94. Leung KM, Po LS, Tsang FC, Siu WY, Lau A, Ho HT, Poon RY. The candidate tumor suppressor ING1b can stabilize p53 by disrupting the regulation of p53 by MDM2. Cancer Res 2002; 62:4890–4893.
95. Shiseki M, Nagashima M, Pedeux RM, Kitahama–Shiseki M, Miura K, Okamura S, Onogi H, Higashimoto Y, Appella E, Yokota J, Harris CC. p29ING4 and p28ING5 bind to p53 and p300, and enhance p53 activity. Cancer Res 2003; 63:2373–2378.
96. Ruas M, Peters G. The p16INK4a/CDKN2A tumor suppressor and its relatives. Biochim Biophys Acta 1998; 1378:F115–F177.
97. Sherr CJ. The INK4a/ARF network in tumour suppression. Nat Rev Mol Cell Biol 2001; 2:731–737.
98. Weinberg RA. The retinoblastoma protein and cell cycle control. Cell 1995; 81:323–330.
99. Dyson N. The regulation of E2F by pRB-family proteins. Genes Dev 1998; 12:2245–2262.
100. Greger V, Passarge E, Hopping W, Messmer E, Horsthemke B. Epigenetic changes may contribute to the formation and spontaneous regression of retinoblastoma. Hum Genet 1989; 83:155–158.
101. Baylin SB, Esteller M, Rountree MR, Bachman KE, Schuebel K, Herman JG. Aberrant patterns of DNA methylation, chromatin formation and gene expression in cancer. Hum Mol Genet 2001; 10:687–692.
102. Paggi MG, Giordano A. Who is the boss in the retinoblastoma family? The point of view of Rb2/p130, the little brother. Cancer Res 2001; 61:4651–4654.

103. Fearon ER, Vogelstein B. A genetic model for colorectal tumorigenesis. Cell 1990; 61:759–767.
104. Davidoff AM, Hill DA. Molecular genetic aspects of solid tumors in childhood. Semin Pediatr Surg 2001; 10:106–118.
105. Harada K, Toyooka S, Maitra A, Maruyama R, Toyooka KO, Timmons CF, Tomlinson GE, Mastrangelo D, Hay RJ, Minna JD, Gazdar AF. Aberrant promoter methylation and silencing of the RASSF1A gene in pediatric tumors and cell lines. Oncogene 2002; 21:4345–4349.
106. Frisch SM, Francis H. Disruption of epithelial cell–matrix interactions induces apoptosis. J Cell Biol 1994; 124:619–626.
107. Nagata S. Apoptosis by death factor. Cell 1997; 88:355–365.
108. Korsmeyer SJ. BCL-2 gene family and the regulation of programmed cell death. Cancer Res 1999; 59:1693s–1700s.
109. Reed JC, Jurgensmeier JM, Matsuyama S. Bcl-2 family proteins and mitochondria. Biochim Biophys Acta 1998; 1366:127–137.
110. Salvesen GS, Dixit VM. Caspase activation: the induced–proximity model. Proc Natl Acad Sci USA 1999; 96:10964–10967.
111. Harada K, Toyooka S, Shivapurkar N, Maitra A, Reddy JL, Matta H, Miyajima K, Timmons CF, Tomlinson GE, Mastrangelo D, Hay RJ, Chaudhary PM, Gazdar AF. Deregulation of caspase 8 and 10 expression in pediatric tumors and cell lines. Cancer Res 2002; 62:5897–5901.
112. Kluck RM, Bossy-Wetzel E, Green DR, Newmeyer DD. The release of cytochrome C from mitochondria: a primary site for Bcl–2 regulation of apoptosis. Science 1997; 275:1132–1136.
113. Hu Y, Benedict MA, Wu D, Inohara N, Nunez G. Bcl-XL interacts with Apaf-1 and inhibits Apaf-1-dependent caspase-9 activation. Proc Natl Acad Sci USA 1998; 95:4386–4391.
114. de La Coste A, Mignon A, Fabre M, Gilbert E, Porteu A, Van Dyke T, Kahn A, Perret C. Paradoxical inhibition of c-myc-induced carcinogenesis by Bcl-2 in transgenic mice. Cancer Res 1999; 59:5017–5022.
115. Kondo S, Shinomura Y, Miyazaki Y, Kiyohara T, Tsutsui S, Kitamura S, Nagasawa Y, Nakahara M, Kanayama S, Matsuzawa Y. Mutations of the bak gene in human gastric and colorectal cancers. Cancer Res 2000; 60:4328–4330.
116. Raveh T, Kimchi A. DAP kinase-a proapoptotic gene that functions as a tumor suppressor. Exp Cell Res 2001; 264:185–192.
117. Kari C, Chan TO, Rocha dQ, Rodeck U. Targeting the epidermal growth factor receptor in cancer: apoptosis takes center stage. Cancer Res 2003; 63:1–5.
118. Tsujii M, DuBois RN. Alterations in cellular adhesion and apoptosis in epithelial cells overexpressing prostaglandin endoperoxide synthase 2. Cell 1995; 83:493–501.
119. Massague J. The transforming growth factor-β family. Ann Rev Cell Biol 1990; 6:597–641.
120. Park BJ, Park JI, Byun DS, Park JH, Chi SG. Mitogenic conversion of transforming growth factor-β1 effect by oncogenic Ha–Ras–induced activation of the mitogen-activated protein kinase signaling pathway in human prostate cancer. Cancer Res 2000; 60:3031–3038.

121. Wilgenbus KK, Kirkpatrick CJ, Knuechel R, Willecke K, Traub O. Expression of Cx26, Cx32 and Cx43 gap junction proteins in normal and neoplastic human tissues. Int J Cancer 1992; 51:522–529.
122. Budunova IV, Williams GM. Cell culture assays for chemicals with tumor-promoting or tumor–inhibiting activity based on the modulation of intercellular communication. Cell Biol Toxicol 1994; 10:71–116.
123. Atsumi T, Chesney J, Metz C, Leng L, Donnelly S, Makita Z, Mitchell R, Bucala R. High expression of inducible 6-phosphofructo-2 kinase/fructose-2,6-bisphosphatase (iPFK-2; PFKFB3) in human cancers. Cancer Res 2002; 62:5881–5887.
124. Gebhardt R, Williams GM. Glutamine synthetase and hepatocarcinogenesis. Carcinogenesis 1995; 16:1673–1681.
125. Krupenko SA, Oleinik NV. 10-formyltetrahydrofolate dehydrogenase, one of the major folate enzymes, is down-regulated in tumor tissues and possesses suppressor effects on cancer cells. Cell Growth Differ 2002; 13:227–236.
126. Iscan M, Coban T, Bulbul D, Eke BC, Aygormez S, Berberoglu U. Xenobiotic metabolizing and antioxidant enzymes in normal and neoplastic human breast tissue. Eur J Drug Metab Pharmacokinet 1998; 23:497–500.
127. Janot F, Massaad L, Ribrag V, de WI, Beaune PH, Luboinski B, Parise O Jr, Gouyette A, Chabot GG. Principal xenobiotic-metabolizing enzyme systems in human head and neck squamous cell carcinoma. Carcinogenesis 1993; 14:1279–1283.
128. Albin N, Massaad L, Toussaint C, Mathieu MC, Morizet J, Parise O, Gouyette A, Chabot GG. Main drug-metabolizing enzyme systems in human breast tumors and peritumoral tissues. Cancer Res 1993; 53:3541–3546.
129. Roy D, Liehr JG. Characterization of drug metabolism enzymes in estrogen-induced kidney tumors in male Syrian hamsters. Cancer Res 1988; 48:5726–5729.
130. Massaad L, de WI, Ribrag V, Janot F, Beaune PH, Morizet J, Gouyette A, Chabot GG. Comparison of mouse and human colon tumors with regard to phase I and phase II drug-metabolizing enzyme systems. Cancer Res 1992; 52:6567–6575.
131. Lee WH, Morton RA, Epstein JI, Brooks JD, Campbell PA, Bova GS, Hsieh WS, Isaacs WB, Nelson WG. Cytidine methylation of regulatory sequences near the π-class glutathione S-transferase gene accompanies human prostatic carcinogenesis. Proc Natl Acad Sci USA 1994; 91:11733–11737.
132. Shay JW, Bacchetti S. A survey of telomerase activity in human cancer. Eur J Cancer 1997; 33:787–791.
133. Wang J, Xie LY, Allan S, Beach D, Hannon GJ. Myc activates telomerase. Genes Dev 1998; 12:1769–1774.
134. Wu KJ, Grandori C, Amacker M, Simon-Vermot N, Polack A, Lingner J, Dalla-Favera R. Direct activation of TERT transcription by c-MYC. Nat Genet 1999; 21:220–224.
135. Hankinson SE, Willett WC, Colditz GA, Hunter DJ, Michaud DS, Deroo B, Rosner B, Speizer FE, Pollak M. Circulating concentrations of insulin-like growth factor-I and risk of breast cancer. Lancet 1998; 351:1393–1396.

136. Ma J, Pollak MN, Giovannucci E, Chan JM, Tao Y, Hennekens CH, Stampfer MJ. Prospective study of colorectal cancer risk in men and plasma levels of insulin-like growth factor (IGF)-I and IGF-binding protein-3. J Natl Cancer Inst 1999; 91:620–625.

137. Wolk A, Mantzoros CS, Andersson SO, Bergstrom R, Signorello LB, Lagiou P, Adami HO, Trichopoulos D. Insulin-like growth factor 1 and prostate cancer risk: a population-based, case-control study. J Natl Cancer Inst 1998; 90:911–915.

138. Hoeflich A, Reisinger R, Lahm H, Kiess W, Blum WF, Kolb HJ, Weber MM, Wolf E. Insulin-like growth factor-binding protein 2 in tumorigenesis: protector or promoter? Cancer Res 2001; 61:8601–8610

139. Hwa V, Oh Y, Rosenfeld RG. The insulin-like growth factor-binding protein (IGFBP) superfamily. Endocr Rev 1999; 20:761–787.

140. Catlett-Falcone R, Landowski TH, Oshiro MM, Turkson J, Levitzki A, Savino R, Ciliberto G, Moscinski L, Fernandez-Luna JL, Nunez G, Dalton WS, Jove R. Constitutive activation of Stat3 signaling confers resistance to apoptosis in human U266 myeloma cells. Immunity 1999; 10:105–115.

141. Smith PC, Hobisch A, Lin DL, Culig Z, Keller ET. Interleukin-6 and prostate cancer progression. Cytokine Growth Factor Rev 2001; 12:33–40.

142. Hanahan D, Folkman J. Patterns and emerging mechanisms of the angiogenic switch during tumorigenesis. Cell 1996; 86:353–364.

143. Beckner ME. Factors promoting tumor angiogenesis. Cancer Invest 1999; 17:594–623.

144. Molina MA, Sitja-Arnau M, Lemoine MG, Frazier ML, Sinicrope FA. Increased cyclooxygenase-2 expression in human pancreatic carcinomas and cell lines: growth inhibition by nonsteroidal anti-inflammatory drugs. Cancer Res 1999; 59:4356–4362.

145. Dannenberg AJ, Altorki NK, Boyle JO, Dang C, Howe LR, Weksler BB, Subbaramaiah K. Cyclo-oxygenase 2: a pharmacological target for the prevention of cancer. Lancet Oncol 2001; 2:544–551.

146. Chiarugi V, Magnelli L, Gallo O. Cox-2, iNOS and p53 as play-makers of tumor angiogenesis. Int J Mol Med 1998; 2:715–719.

147. Zhang W, Stoica G, Tasca SI, Kelly KA, Meininger CJ. Modulation of tumor angiogenesis by stem cell factor. Cancer Res 2000; 60:6757–6762.

148. Perletti G, Concari P, Giardini R, Marras E, Piccinini F, Folkman J, Chen L. Antitumor activity of endostatin against carcinogen-induced rat primary mammary tumors. Cancer Res 2000; 60:1793–1796.

149. Hahne M, Rimoldi D, Schroter M, Romero P, Schreier M, French LE, Schneider P, Bornand T, Fontana A, Lienard D, Cerottini J, Tschopp J. Melanoma cell expression of Fas(Apo-1/CD95) ligand: implications for tumor immune escape. Science 1996; 274:1363–1366.

150. Dano K, Romer J, Nielsen BS, Bjorn S, Pyke C, Rygaard J, Lund LR. Cancer invasion and tissue remodeling—cooperation of protease systems and cell types. APMIS 1999; 107:120–127.

151. Behrens J. Cadherins and catenins: role in signal transduction and tumor progression. Cancer Metastasis Rev 1999; 18:15–30.

152. Howe A, Aplin AE, Alahari SK, Juliano RL. Integrin signaling and cell growth control. Curr Opin Cell Biol 1998; 10:220–231.
153. Cleton-Jansen AM. E-cadherin and loss of heterozygosity at chromosome 16 in breast carcinogenesis: different genetic pathways in ductal and lobular breast cancer? Breast Cancer Res 2002; 4:5–8.
154. Mollenhauer J, Herbertz S, Helmke B, Kollender G, Krebs I, Madsen J, Holmskov U, Sorger K, Schmitt L, Wiemann S, Otto HF, Grone HJ, Poustka A. Deleted in Malignant Brain Tumors 1 is a versatile mucin-like molecule likely to play a differential role in digestive tract cancer. Cancer Res 2001; 61:8880–8886.
155. Woessner JF, Nagase H. Matrix Metalloproteinases and TIMPs. Oxford, UK: Oxford University Press, 2004.
156. Andela VB, Schwarz EM, Puzas JE, O'Keefe RJ, Rosier RN. Tumor metastasis and the reciprocal regulation of prometastatic and antimetastatic factors by nuclear factor kappaB. Cancer Res 2000; 60:6557–6562.
157. Woodhouse EC, Chuaqui RF, Liotta LA. General mechanisms of metastasis. Cancer 1997; 80:1529–1537.
158. Fidler IJ. Critical determinants of cancer metastasis: rationale for therapy. Cancer Chemother Pharmacol 1999; 43(suppl):S3–S10.
159. Welch DR, Wei LL. Genetic and epigenetic regulation of human breast cancer progression and metastasis. Endocrine-related Cancer 2002; 5:155–197.
160. Saunders MM, Seraj MJ, Li Z, Zhou Z, Winter CR, Welch DR, Donahue HJ. Breast cancer metastatic potential correlates with a breakdown in homospecific and heterospecific gap junctional intercellular communication. Cancer Res 2001; 61:1765–1767.
161. International Agency for Research on Cancer Alcohol drinking. IARC Monographs on the Evaluation of Carcinogenic Risks to Humans. Lyons: IARC, 1988; 44:35–321.
162. Krutovskikh V, Yamasaki H. Gap junctional intercellular communication as a method to detect and predict carcinogenicity. In: Kitchin KT, ed. Carcinogenicity: Testing, Predicting, and Interpreting Chemical Effects. New York, NY: M.Dekker, 1999; 267–88.
163. Herschman HR. Primary response genes induced by growth factors and tumor promoters. Annu Rev Biochem 1991; 60:281–319.
164. Schulte-Hermann R, Bursch W, Grasl-Kraupp B, Mullauer L, Ruttkay-Nedecky B. Apoptosis and multistage carcinogenesis in rat liver. Mutat Res 1995; 333:81–87.
165. Collaborative Group on Hormonal Factors in Breast Cancer. Breast cancer and hormone replacement therapy: collaborative reanalysis of data from 51 epidemiological studies of 52,705 women with breast cancer and 108,411 women without breast cancer. Collaborative Group on Hormonal Factors in Breast Cancer. Lancet, 1997; 350:1047–1059.
166. Williams GM, Katayama S, Ohmori T. Enhancement of hepatocarcinogenesis by sequential administration of chemicals: summation versus promotion effects. Carcinogenesis 1981; 2:1111–1117.
167. Gough M. Antagonism—no synergism—in pairwise tests of carcinogens in rats. Regul Toxicol Pharmacol 2002; 35:383.

168. Schmahl D. Combination effects in chemical carcinogenesis. Arch Toxicol Suppl 1980; 4:29–40.

169. Dall'Acqua F, Vedaldi D, Bordin F, Rodighiero G. New studies on the interaction between 8-methoxypsoralen and DNA in vitro. J Invest Dermatol 1979; 73:191–197.

170. Forbes PD, Davies RE, Urbach F. Phototoxicity and photocarcinogenesis: comparative effects of anthracene and 8-methoxypsoralen in the skin of mice. Food Cosmet Toxicol 1976; 14:303–306.

171. Stern RS, Laird N, Melski J, Parrish JA, Fitzpatrick TB, Bleich HL. Cutaneous squamous-cell carcinoma in patients treated with PUVA. N Engl J Med 1984; 310:1156–1161.

172. Johnson BE, Gibbs NK, Fergurson J. Quinolone antibiotics with potential to photosensitize skin tumorigenesis. J Photochem Photobiol B 1997; 37:171–173.

173. Van Duuren BL, Melchionne S. Inhibition of tumorigenesis. Prog Exp Tumor Res 1969; 12:55–94.

174. Falk HL. Anticarcinogenesis—an alternative. Prog Exp Tumor Res 1971; 14:105–137.

175. Mirvish SS, Grandjean AC, Reimers KJ, Connelly BJ, Chen SC, Morris CR, Wang X, Haorah J, Lyden ER. Effect of ascorbic acid dose taken with a meal on nitrosoproline excretion in subjects ingesting nitrate and proline. Nutr Cancer 1998; 31:106–110.

176. Yamamoto RS, Williams GM, Richardson HL, Weisburger EK, Weisburger JH. Effect of *p*-hydroxyacetanilide on liver cancer induction by *N*-hydroxy-*N*-2-fluorenylacetamide. Cancer Res 1973; 33:454–457.

177. Kensler TW, Groopman JD, Sutter TR, Curphey TJ, Roebuck BD. Development of cancer chemopreventive agents: oltipraz as a paradigm. Chem Res Toxicol 1999; 12:113–126.

178. Williams GM, Iatropoulos MJ. Anticarcinogenic effects of synthetic phenolic antioxidants. In: Baskin S, Salem H, eds. Oxidants, Antioxidants, and Free Radicals. Washington, DC: Taylor & Francis, 1997; 341–351.

179. Zhang Y, Talalay P. Mechanism of differential potencies of isothiocyanates as inducers of anticarcinogenic Phase 2 enzymes. Cancer Res 1998; 58:4632–4639.

180. Kritchevsky D. Caloric restriction and experimental carcinogenesis. Toxicol. Sci 1999; 52:13–16.

181. Lerner LJ, Jordan VC. Development of antiestrogens and their use in breast cancer: Eighth Cain Memorial Award lecture. Cancer Res 1990; 50:4177–4189.

182. Smalley WE, DuBois RN. Colorectal cancer and nonsteroidal anti-inflammatory drugs. Adv Pharmacol 1997; 39:1–20.

183. Gold LS, Zeiger E. Handbook of Carcinogenic Potency and Genotoxicity Data. Boca Raton, FL: CRC Press, 1996.

184. International Agency for Research on Cancer. Monograph Series 1971–2005, www.iacr.fr

185. National Toxicology Program. http://ntp-server.niehs.nih.gov/

186. Williams GM. DNA reactive and epigenetic carcinogens. Exper Tox Path 1992; 44:457–464.

187. Miller JA. The metabolism of xenobiotics to reactive electrophiles in chemical carcinogenesis and mutagenesis: a collaboration with Elizabeth Cavert Miller and our associates. Drug Metab Rev 1998; 30:645–674.
188. Tomatis L. Prenatal exposure to chemical carcinogens and its effect on subsequent generations. Natl Cancer Inst Monogr 1979:159–184.
189. Thorgeirsson UP, Dalgard DW, Reeves J, Adamson RH. Tumor incidence in a chemical carcinogenesis study of nonhuman primates. Regul Toxicol Pharmacol 1994; 19:130–151.
190. Rice JM, Williams GM, Palmer AE, London WT, Sly DL. Pathology of gestational choriocarcinoma induced in patas monkeys by ethylnitrosourea given during pregnancy. Placenta Suppl 1981; 3:223–230.
191. Williams GM. Definition of human cancer hazard. In: Nongenotoxic Mechanisms in Carcinogenesis. Banbury Report. New York: Cold Spring Harbor Laboratory, 1987; 25:367–380.
192. Floyd RA. The role of 8-hydroxyguanine in carcinogenesis. Carcinogenesis 1990; 11:1447–1450.
193. Kasai H. Analysis of a form of oxidative DNA damage, 8-hydroxy-2′-deoxyguanosine, as a marker of cellular oxidative stress during carcinogenesis. Mutat Res 1997; 387:147–163.
194. Ohshima H, Bartsch H. Chronic infections and inflammatory processes as cancer risk factors: possible role of nitric oxide in carcinogenesis. Mutat Res 1994; 305:253–264.
195. Tamir S, Burney S, Tannenbaum SR. DNA damage by nitric oxide. Chem Res Toxicol 1996; 9:821–827.
196. Esterbauer H, Schaur RJ, Zollner H. Chemistry and biochemistry of 4-hydroxynonenal, malonaldehyde and related aldehydes. Free Radic Biol Med 1991; 11:81–128.
197. Comporti M. Lipid peroxidation and biogenic aldehydes: from the identification of 4-hydroxynonenal to further achievements in biopathology. Free Radic Res 1998; 28:623–635.
198. Marnett LJ. Oxyradicals and DNA damage. Carcinogenesis 2000; 21:361–370.
199. Li JH, Rossman TG. Inhibition of DNA ligase activity by arsenite: a possible mechanism of its comutagenesis. Mol Toxicol 1989; 2:1–9.
200. Hartwig A, Schwerdtle T. Interactions by carcinogenic metal compounds with DNA repair processes: toxicological implications. Toxicol Lett 2000; 127:47–54.
201. Rossman TG, Uddin AN, Burns FJ, Bosland MC. Arsenite is a cocarcinogen with solar ultraviolet radiation for mouse skin: an animal model for arsenic carcinogenesis. Toxicol Appl Pharmacol 2001; 176:64–71.
202. Buzard GS, Kasprzak KS. Possible roles of nitric oxide and redox cell signaling in metal-induced toxicity and carcinogenesis: a review. J Environ Pathol Toxicol Oncol 2000; 19:179–199.
203. Rowland IR, Mallett AK, Wise A. The effect of diet on the mammalian gut flora and its metabolic activities. Crit Rev Toxicol 1985; 16:31–103.
204. Chadwick RW, George SE, Claxton LD. Role of the gastrointestinal mucosa and microflora in the bioactivation of dietary and environmental mutagens or carcinogens. Drug Metab Rev 1992; 24:425–492.

205. Zarkovic M, Qin X, Nakatsuru Y, Oda H, Nakamura T, Shamsuddin AM, Ishikawa T. Tumor promotion by fecapentaene-12 in a rat colon carcinogenesis model. Carcinogenesis 1993; 14:1261–1264.

206. Guengerich FP. Human cytochrome P450 enzymes. In: Ortiz de Montellano PR, ed. Cytochrome P450: Structure, Mechanism and Biochemistry. New York, NY: Plenum Press, 1995; 473–535.

207. Schuetz EG. Induction of cytochromes P450. Curr Drug Metab 2001; 2: 139–147.

208. Hayes JD, Pulford DJ. The glutathione *S*-transferase supergene family: regulation of GST and the contribution of the isoenzymes to cancer chemoprotection and drug resistance. Crit Rev Biochem Mol Biol 1995; 30:445–600.

209. Eaton DL, Bammler TK. Concise review of the glutathione *S*-transferases and their significance to toxicology. Toxicol Sci 1999; 49:156–164.

210. Hein DW. Molecular genetics and function of NAT1 and NAT2: role in aromatic amine metabolism and carcinogenesis. Mutat Res 2002; 506–507:65–77.

211. McQueen CA, Maslansky CJ, Williams GM. Role of the acetylation polymorphism in determining susceptibility of cultured rabbit hepatocytes to DNA damage by aromatic amines. Cancer Res 1983; 43:3120–3123.

212. Kadlubar FF, Badawi AF. Genetic susceptibility and carcinogen-DNA adduct formation in human urinary bladder carcinogenesis. Toxicol Lett 1995; 82–83: 627–632.

213. Mackenzie PI, Owens IS, Burchell B, Bock KW, Bairoch A, Belanger A, Fournel-Gigleux S, Green M, Hum DW, Iyanagi T, Lancet D, Louisot P, Magdalou J, Chowdhury JR, Ritter JK, Schachter H, Tephly TR, Tipton KF, Nebert DW. The UDP glycosyltransferase gene superfamily: recommended nomenclature update based on evolutionary divergence. Pharmacogenetics 1997; 7: 255–269.

214. Ren Q, Murphy SE, Dannenberg AJ, Park JY, Tephly TR, Lazarus P. Glucuronidation of the lung carcinogen 4-(methylnitrosamino)-1-(3-pyridyl)-1-butanol (NNAL) by rat UDP-glucuronosyltransferase 2B1. Drug Metab Dispos 1999; 27:1010–1016.

215. Upton A, Johnson N, Sandy J, Sim E. Arylamine *N*-acetyltransferases—of mice, men and microorganisms. Trends Pharmacol Sci 2001; 22:140–146.

216. Raucy JL, Allen SW. Recent advances in P450 research. Pharmacogenomics J 2001; 1:178–186.

217. Coles B, Ketterer B. The role of glutathione and glutathione transferases in chemical carcinogenesis. Crit Rev Biochem Mol Biol 1990; 25:47–70.

218. Coles BF, Anderson KE, Doerge DR, Churchwell MI, Lang NP, Kadlubar FF. Quantitative analysis of interindividual variation of glutathione *S*-transferase expression in human pancreas and the ambiguity of correlating genotype with phenotype. Cancer Res 2000; 60:573–579.

219. Waxman DJ, Chang TKH. Hormonal regulation of liver cytochrome P450 enzymes. In: Ortiz de Montellano PR, ed. Cytochrome P450: Structure, Mechanism and Biochemistry. New York, NY: Plenum Press, 1995; 391–417.

220. Phillips DH, Davis W, Venitt S, Glatt H. Tamoxifen metabolism and activation: The reason for interspecies differences. Eur J Cancer 1998; 34:s13–s14.

221. Shibutani S, Dasaradhi L, Terashima I, Banoglu E, Duffel MW. α-Hydroxy-tamoxifen is a substrate of hydroxysteroid (alcohol) sulfotransferase, resulting in tamoxifen DNA adducts. Cancer Res 1998; 58:647–653.

222. Williams CL, Bollella M, Williams GM. Cancer prevention beginning in childhood. In: DeVita VT, Hollman S, Rosenberg SA, eds. Cancer Prevention. Philadelphia, PA: J. B. Lippincott Co, 1993; 1–13.

223. International Agency for Research on Cancer. Tamoxifen. IARC Monographs on the Evaluation of Carcinogenic Risks to Humans. Lyon, France: IARC 1996; 66:253–367.

224. Carmichael PL, Ugwumadu AH, Neven P, Hewer AJ, Poon GK, Phillips DH. Lack of genotoxicity of tamoxifen in human endometrium. Cancer Res 1996; 56:1475–1479.

225. Hemminki K, Rajaniemi H, Lindahl B, Moberger B. Tamoxifen-induced DNA adducts in endometrial samples from breast cancer patients. Cancer Res 1996; 56:4374–4377.

226. Shibutani S, Suzuki N, Terashima I, Sugarman SM, Grollman AP, Pearl ML. Tamoxifen-DNA adducts detected in the endometrium of women treated with tamoxifen. Chem Res Toxicol 1999; 12:646–653.

227. Nebert DW, McKinnon RA, Puga A. Human drug-metabolizing enzyme polymorphisms: effects on risk of toxicity and cancer. DNA Cell Biol 1996; 15: 273–280.

228. Gonzalez FJ. The role of carcinogen-metabolizing enzyme polymorphisms in cancer susceptibility. Reprod Toxicol 1997; 11:397–412.

229. Hengstler JG, Arand M, Herrero ME, Oesch F. Polymorphisms of *N*-acetyltransferases, glutathione *S*-transferases, microsomal epoxide hydrolase and sulfotransferases: influence on cancer susceptibility. Recent Results Cancer Res 1998; 154:47–85.

230. Autrup H. Genetic polymorphisms in human xenobiotica metabolizing enzymes as susceptibility factors in toxic response. Mutat Res 2000; 464: 65–76.

231. Clapper ML. Genetic polymorphism and cancer risk. Curr Oncol Rep 2000; 2:251–256.

232. Raunio H, Husgafvel-Pursiainen K, Anttila S, Hietanen E, Hirvonen A, Pelkonen O. Diagnosis of polymorphisms in carcinogen-activating and inactivating enzymes and cancer susceptibility—a review. Gene 1995; 159:113–121.

233. Butkiewicz D, Cole KJ, Phillips DH, Harris CC, Chorazy M. GSTM1, GSTP1, CYP1A1 and CYP2D6 polymorphisms in lung cancer patients from an environmentally polluted region of Poland: correlation with lung DNA adduct levels. Eur J Cancer Prev 1999; 8:315–323.

234. Thier R, Bruning T, Roos PH, Bolt HM. Cytochrome P450 1B1, a new keystone in gene-environment interactions related to human head and neck cancer? Arch Toxicol 2002; 76:249–256.

235. Ko Y, Abel J, Harth V, Brode P, Antony C, Donat S, Fischer HP, Ortiz-Pallardo ME, Thier R, Sachinidis A, Vetter H, Bolt HM, Herberhold C, Bruning T. Association of CYP1B1 codon 432 mutant allele in head and neck squamous cell cancer is reflected by somatic mutations of p53 in tumor tissue. Cancer Res 2001; 61:4398–4404.

236. Ariyoshi N, Miyamoto M, Umetsu Y, Kunitoh H, Dosaka-Akita H, Sawa-mura Y, Yokota J, Nemoto N, Sato K, Kamataki,T. Genetic polymorphism of *CYP2A6* gene and tobacco-induced lung cancer risk in male smokers. Cancer Epidemiol Biomarkers Prev 2002; 11:890–894.

237. Yang CS, Yoo JS, Ishizaki H, Hong JY. Cytochrome P450IIE1: roles in nitro-samine metabolism and mechanisms of regulation. Drug Metab Rev 1990; 22:147–159.

238. Le Marchand L, Donlon T, Seifried A, Wilkens LR. Red meat intake, CYP2E1 genetic polymorphisms, and colorectal cancer risk. Cancer Epidemiol Biomarkers Prev 2002; 11:1019–1024.

239. Hanna IH, Dawling S, Roodi N, Guengerich FP, Parl FF. Cytochrome P450 1B1 CYP1B1 pharmacogenetics: association of polymorphisms with func-tional differences in estrogen hydroxylation activity. Cancer Res 2000; 60:3440–3444.

240. Stanford JL, Noonan EA, Iwasaki L, Kolb S, Chadwick RB, Feng Z, Ostran-der EA. A polymorphism in the *CYP17* gene and risk of prostate cancer. Cancer Epidemiol Biomarkers Prev 2002; 11:243–247.

241. Jourenkova-Mironova N, Mitrunen K, Bouchardy C, Dayer P, Benhamou S, Hirvonen A. High-activity microsomal epoxide hydrolase genotypes and the risk of oral, pharynx, and larynx cancers. Cancer Res 2000; 60:534–536.

242. Wenghoefer M, Pesch B, Harth V, Broede P, Fronhoffs S, Landt O, Bruning T, Abel J, Bolt HM, Herberhold C, Vetter H, Ko YD. Association between head and neck cancer and microsomal epoxide hydrolase genotypes. Arch Toxicol 2003; 77:37–41.

243. Yokoyama A, Kato H, Yokoyama T, Tsujinaka T, Muto M, Omori T, Haneda T, Kumagai Y, Igaki H, Yokoyama M, Watanabe H, Fukuda H, Yoshimizu H. Genetic polymorphisms of alcohol and aldehyde dehydro-genases and glutathione *S*-transferase M1 and drinking, smoking, and diet in Japanese men with esophageal squamous cell carcinoma. Carcinogenesis 2002; 23:1851–1859.

244. Weber WW. The molecular basis of hereditary acetylation polymorphisms. Drug Metab Dispos 1986; 14:377–381.

245. Hein DW, Doll MA, Fretland AJ, Leff MA, Webb SJ, Xiao GH, Devana-boyina US, Nangju NA, Feng Y. Molecular genetics and epidemiology of the NAT1 and NAT2 acetylation polymorphisms. Cancer Epidemiol Biomar-kers Prev 2000; 9:29–42.

246. Zhu Y, Doll MA, Hein DW. Functional genomics of $C^{190}T$ single nucleotide polymorphism in human *N*-acetyltransferase 2. Biol Chem 2002; 383:983–987.

247. Green J, Banks E, Berrington A, Darby S, Deo H, Newton,R. *N*-acetyltrans-ferase 2 and bladder cancer: an overview and consideration of the evidence for gene-environment interaction. Br J Cancer 2000; 83:412–417.

248. Johns LE, Houlston RS. *N*-acetyl transferase-2 and bladder cancer risk: a meta-analysis. Environ Mol Mutagen 2000; 36:221–227.

249. Risch A, Wallace DM, Bathers S, Sim E. Slow *N*-acetylation genotype is a sus-ceptibility factor in occupational and smoking related bladder cancer. Hum Mol Genet 1995; 4:231–236.

250. Roberts-Thomson IC, Ryan P, Khoo KK, Hart WJ, McMichael AJ, Butler RN. Diet, acetylator phenotype, and risk of colorectal neoplasia. Lancet 1996; 347:1372–1374.

251. Ambrosone CB, Freudenheim JL, Graham S, Marshall JR, Vena JE, Brasure JR, Michalek AM, Laughlin R, Nemoto T, Gillenwater KA, Shields PG. Cigarette smoking, N-acetyltransferase 2 genetic polymorphisms, and breast cancer risk. JAMA 1996; 276:1494–1501.

252. McWilliams JE, Sanderson BJ, Harris EL, Richert-Boe KE, Henner WD. Glutathione *S*-transferase M1 GSTM1 deficiency and lung cancer risk. Cancer Epidemiol Biomarkers Prev 1995; 4:589–594.

253. Salagovic J, Kalina I, Stubna J, Habalova V, Hrivnak M, Valansky L, Kohut A, Biros E. Genetic polymorphism of glutathione *S*-transferases M1 and T1 as a risk factor in lung and bladder cancers. Neoplasma 1998; 45:312–317.

254. Mitrunen K, Jourenkova N, Kataja V, Eskelinen M, Kosma VM, Benhamou S, Vainio H, Uusitupa M, Hirvonen A. Glutathione *S*-transferase M1, M3, P1, and T1 genetic polymorphisms and susceptibility to breast cancer. Cancer Epidemiol Biomarkers Prev 2001; 10:229–236.

255. Swenson DH, Farmer PB, Lawley PD. Identification of the methyl phosphotriester of thymidylyl-3′,5′-thymidine as a product from reaction of DNA with the carcinogen *N*-methyl-*N*-nitrosourea. Chem Biol Interact 1976; 15:91–100.

256. Groopman JD, Croy RG, Wogan GN. In vitro reactions of aflatoxin B_1-adducted DNA. Proc Natl Acad Sci USA 1981; 78:5445–5449.

257. Glazer AN, Mathies RA. Energy-transfer fluorescent reagents for DNA analyses. Curr Opin Biotechnol 1997; 8:94–102.

258. Lindahl T. The Croonian Lecture, 1996: endogenous damage to DNA. Philos Trans R Soc Lond B Biol Sci 1996; 351:1529–1538.

259. Nakamura J, Swenberg JA. Endogenous apurinic/apyrimidinic sites in genomic DNA of mammalian tissues. Cancer Res 1999; 59:2522–2526.

260. Wink DA, Kasprzak KS, Maragos CM, Elespuru RK, Misra M, Dunams TM, Cebula TA, Koch WH, Andrews AW, Allen JS, Keefer LK. DNA deaminating ability and genotoxicity of nitric oxide and its progenitors. Science 1991; 254:1001–1003.

261. Sibghat U, Day RS III. DNA-substrate sequence specificity of human G:T mismatch repair activity. Nucleic Acids Res 1993; 21:1281–1287.

262. Gorb L, Podolyan Y, Leszczynski J, Siebrand W, Fernandez-Ramos A, Smedarchina Z. A quantum-dynamics study of the prototropic tautomerism of guanine and its contribution to spontaneous point mutations in *Escherichia coli*. Biopolymers 2001; 61:77–83.

263. Ames BN. Endogenous oxidative DNA damage, aging, and cancer. Free Radic Res Commun 1989; 7:121–128.

264. Cadet J, Douki T, Ravanat JL. Artifacts associated with the measurement of oxidized DNA bases. Environ Health Perspect 1997; 105:1034–1039.

265. Burcham PC. Genotoxic lipid peroxidation products: their DNA damaging properties and role in formation of endogenous DNA adducts. Mutagenesis 1998; 13:287–305.

266. Friso S, Choi SW, Girelli D, Mason JB, Dolnikowski GG, Bagley PJ, Olivieri O, Jacques PF, Rosenberg IH, Corrocher R, Selhub J. A common mutation in

the 5,10-methylenetetrahydrofolate reductase gene affects genomic DNA methylation through an interaction with folate status. Proc Natl Acad Sci USA 2002; 99:5606–5611.

267. Villar-Garea A, Esteller M. DNA demethylating agents and chromatin-remodelling drugs: which, how and why? Curr Drug Metab 2003; 4:11–31.

268. Bartsch H. DNA adducts in human carcinogenesis: etiological relevance and structure–activity relationship. Mutat Res 1996; 340:67–79.

269. Randerath K, Randerath E, Zhou GD, Li D. Bulky endogenous DNA modifications I-compounds—possible structural origins and functional implications. Mutat Res 1999; 424:183–194.

270. Farmer PB, Shuker DE. What is the significance of increases in background levels of carcinogen-derived protein and DNA adducts? Some considerations for incremental risk assessment. Mutat.Res 1999; 424:275–286.

271. Colvin ME, Hatch FT, Felton JS. Chemical and biological factors affecting mutagen potency. Mutat.Res 1998; 400:479–492.

272. Roche CJ, Jeffrey AM, Mao B, Alfano A, Kim SK, Ibanez V, Geacintov NE. Dependence of conformations of benzo[a]pyrene diol epoxide-DNA adducts derived from stereoisomers of different tumorigenicities on base sequence. Chem Res Toxicol 1991; 4:311–317.

273. MacLeod MC. Interaction of bulky chemical carcinogens with DNA in chromatin. Carcinogenesis 1995; 16:2009–2014.

274. Jeffrey AM, Kinoshita T, Santella RM, Grunberger D, Katz L, Weinstein IB. The chemistry of polycyclic aromatic hydrocarbon-DNA adducts. In: Pullman P, Ts'o POP, Gelboin H, eds. Carcinogens Fundamental Mechanisms and Environmental Effects. Amsterdam Holland D.: Reidel Publishing Co, 1980; 565–579.

275. Suri AK, Mao B, Amin S, Geacintov NE, Patel DJ. Solution conformation of the (+)-trans-anti-benzo[g]chrysene-dA adduct opposite dT in a DNA duplex. J Mol Biol 1999; 292:289–307.

276. Li Z, Kim HY, Tamura PJ, Harris CM, Harris TM, Stone MP. Intercalation of the $(1S,2R,3S,4R)$-N^6-[1-1,2,3,4-tetrahydro-2,3, 4-trihydroxybenz[a]anthracenyl]-2'-deoxyadenosyl adduct in an oligodeoxynucleotide containing the human N-ras codon 61 sequence. Biochemistry 1999; 38:16045–16057.

277. Malinge JM, Giraud-Panis MJ, Leng, M. Interstrand cross-links of cisplatin induce striking distortions in DNA. J Inorg Biochem 1999; 77:23–29.

278. Denissenko MF, Pao AP, Tang MS, Pfeifer GP. Preferential formation of benzo[a]pyrene adducts at lung cancer mutational hotspots in P53. Science 1996; 274:430–432.

279. Hemminki K. DNA adducts and mutations in occupational and environmental biomonitoring. Environ Health Perspect 1997; 105(Suppl 4):823–827.

280. Santella RM. Immunological methods for detection of carcinogen–DNA damage in humans. Cancer Epidemiol. Biomarkers Prev 1999; 8:733–739.

281. Bartsch H. Studies on biomarkers in cancer etiology and prevention: a summary and challenge of 20 years of interdisciplinary research. Mutat Res 2000; 462:255–279.

282. Vineis P, Perera F. DNA adducts as markers of exposure to carcinogens and risk of cancer. Int J Cancer 2000; 88:325–328.

283. Warren AJ, Shields PG. Carcinogen-DNA adducts as biomarkers and genetic susceptibility. In: Williams GM, Aruoma OI, eds. Molecular Drug Metabolism and Toxicology. London: OICA International (UK) Ltd, 2000; 167–180.

284. Randerath K, Randerath E. ^{32}P-Postlabelling methods for DNA adduct detection: overview critical evaluation. Drug Metab Rev 1994; 26:67–85.

285. Povey AC. DNA adducts: endogenous and induced. Toxicol Pathol 2000; 28:405–414.

286. Poirier MC, Santella RM, Weston A. Carcinogen macromolecular adducts and their measurement. Carcinogenesis 2000; 21:353–359.

287. Lutz WK. In vivo chemical binding of organic chemicals to DNA as a quantative indicator in the process of chemical carcinogenesis. Mutat Res 1979; 65:289–356.

288. Lutz WK. Quantitative evaluation of DNA binding data for risk estimation and for classification of direct and indirect carcinogens. J Cancer Res Clin Oncol 1986; 112:85–91.

289. Garner RC, Lightfoot TJ, Cupid BC, Russell D, Coxhead JM, Kutschera W, Priller A, Rom W, Steier P, Alexander DJ, Leveson SH, Dingley KH, Mauthe RJ, Turteltaub KW. Comparative biotransformation studies of MeIQx and PhIP in animal models and humans. Cancer Lett 1999; 143:161–165.

290. Swenberg JA, Dyroff MC, Bedell MA, Popp JA, Huh N, Kirstein U, Rajewsky MF. O^4-ethyldeoxythymidine, but not O^6-ethyldeoxyguanosine, accumulates in hepatocyte DNA of rats exposed continuously to diethylnitrosamine. Proc Natl Acad Sci USA 1984; 81:1692–1695.

291. Howard PC, Casciano DA, Beland FA, Shaddock JG Jr. The binding of N-hydroxy-2-acetylaminofluorene to DNA and repair of the adducts in primary rat hepatocyte cultures. Carcinogenesis 1981; 2:97–102.

292. Culp SJ, Poirier MC, Beland FA. Biphasic removal of DNA adducts in a repetitive DNA sequence after dietary administration of 2-acetylaminofluorene. Environ Health Perspect 1993; 99:273–275.

293. Graves DE, Pattaroni C, Krishnan BS, Ostrander JM, Hurley LH, Krugh TR. The reaction of anthramycin with DNA. Proton and carbon nuclear magnetic resonance studies on the structure of the anthramycin–DNA adduct. J Biol Chem 1984; 259:8202–8209.

294. Mao B, Gu Z, Gorin A, Chen J, Hingerty BE, Amin S, Broyde S, Geacintov NE, Patel DJ. Solution structure of the (+)-cis-anti-benzo[a]pyrene-dA [BP]dA adduct opposite dT in a DNA duplex. Biochemistry 1999; 38:10831–10842.

295. Lindahl T, Wood RD. Quality control by DNA repair. Science 1999; 286:1897–1905.

296. Petit C, Sancar A. Nucleotide excision repair: from E. coli to man. Biochimie 1999; 81:15–25.

297. Weinert T. DNA damage and checkpoint pathways: molecular anatomy and interactions with repair. Cell 1998; 94:555–558.

298. Freedman DA, Levine AJ. Regulation of the p53 protein by the MDM2 oncoprotein—thirty-eighth G.H.A. Clowes Memorial Award Lecture. Cancer Res 1999; 59:1–7.

299. Ashcroft M, Taya Y, Vousden KH. Stress signals utilize multiple pathways to stabilize p53. Mol Cell Biol 2000; 20:3224–3233.

300. Harper JW, Adami GR, Wei N, Keyomarsi K, Elledge SJ. The p21 Cdk-interacting protein Cip1 is a potent inhibitor of G1 cyclin-dependent kinases. Cell 1993; 75:805–816.

301. Cox LS, Lane DP. Tumour suppressors, kinases and clamps: how p53 regulates the cell cycle in response to DNA damage. Bioessays 1995; 17:501–508.

302. Abraham RT. Cell cycle checkpoint signaling through the ATM and ATR kinases. Genes Dev 2001; 15:2177–2196.

303. D'Amours D, Desnoyers S, D'Silva I, Poirier GG. Poly (ADP-ribosyl)ation reactions in the regulation of nuclear functions. Biochem J 1999; 342(Pt 2):249–268.

304. Lindahl T, Satoh MS, Poirier GG, Klungland A. Post-translational modification of poly ADP-ribose polymerase induced by DNA strand breaks. Trends Biochem Sci 1995; 20:405–411.

305. Bergeron J, Benlimame N, Zeng-Rong N, Xiao D, Scrivens PJ, Koromilas AE, Alaoui-Jamali MA. Identification of the interferon-inducible double-stranded RNA-dependent protein kinase as a regulator of cellular response to bulky adducts. Cancer Res 2000; 60:6800–6804.

306. Sugasawa K, Ng JM, Masutani C, Iwai S, van der Spek PJ, Eker AP, Hanaoka F, Bootsma D, Hoeijmakers JH. Xeroderma pigmentosum group C protein complex is the initiator of global genome nucleotide excision repair. Mol Cell 1998; 2:223–232.

307. Lloyd DR, Hanawalt PC. p53-dependent global genomic repair of benzo[a]-pyrene-7,8-diol-9,10-epoxide adducts in human cells. Cancer Res 2000; 60:517–521.

308. de Laat WL, Jaspers NG, Hoeijmakers JH. Molecular mechanism of nucleotide excision repair. Genes Dev 1999; 13:768–785.

309. Hanawalt PC. Genomic instability: environmental invasion and the enemies within. Mutat Res 1998; 400:117–125.

310. Moriwaki S, Kraemer KH. Xeroderma pigmentosum—bridging a gap between clinic and laboratory. Photodermatol Photoimmunol Photomed 2001; 17:47–54.

311. Singer B, Hang B. What structural features determine repair enzyme specificity and mechanism in chemically modified DNA? Chem Res Toxicol 1997; 10:713–732.

312. Boiteux S, Radicella JP. The human OGG1 gene: structure, functions, and its implication in the process of carcinogenesis. Arch Biochem Biophys 2000; 377:1–8.

313. Satoh MS, Lindahl T. Enzymatic repair of oxidative DNA damage. Cancer Res 1994; 54:1899s–1901s.

314. Nilsen H, Krokan HE. Base excision repair in a network of defence and tolerance. Carcinogenesis 2001; 22:987–998.

315. Pegg AE. Repair of O^6-alkylguanine by alkyltransferases. Mutat Res 2000; 462:83–100.

316. Liu L, Xu-Welliver M, Kanugula S, Pegg AE. Inactivation and degradation of O^6-alkylguanine-DNA alkyltransferase after reaction with nitric oxide. Cancer Res 2002; 62:3037–3043.

317. Hickman MJ, Samson LD. Role of DNA mismatch repair and p53 in signaling induction of apoptosis by alkylating agents. Proc Natl Acad Sci USA 1999; 96:10764–10769.

318. Ochs K, Kaina B. Apoptosis induced by DNA damage O^6-methylguanine is Bcl-2 and caspase-9/3 regulated and Fas/caspase-8 independent. Cancer Res 2000; 60:5815–5824.

319. Yanamadala S, Ljungman M. Potential role of MLH1 in the induction of p53 and apoptosis by blocking transcription on damaged DNA templates. Mol Cancer Res 2003; 1:747–754.

320. Kastan MB, Onyekwere O, Sidransky D, Vogelstein B, Craig RW. Participation of p53 protein in the cellular response to DNA damage. Cancer Res 1991; 51:6304–6311.

321. Ha HC, Snyder SH. Poly (ADP-ribose) polymerase is a mediator of necrotic cell death by ATP depletion. Proc Natl Acad Sci USA 1999; 96:13978–13982.

322. Esteller M. Epigenetic lesions causing genetic lesions in human cancer: promoter hypermethylation of DNA repair genes. Eur J Cancer 2000; 36:2294–2300.

323. van der Meijden CM, Lapointe DS, Luong MX, Peric-Hupkes D, Cho B, Stein JL, van Wijnen AJ, Stein GS. Gene profiling of cell cycle progression through S-phase reveals sequential expression of genes required for DNA replication and nucleosome assembly. Cancer Res 2002; 62:3233–3243.

324. Yacoub A, Park JS, Qiao L, Dent P, Hagan MP. MAPK dependence of DNA damage repair: ionizing radiation and the induction of expression of the DNA repair genes XRCC1 and ERCC1 in DU145 human prostate carcinoma cells in a MEK1/2 dependent fashion. Int J Radiat Biol 2001; 77:1067–1078.

325. Zhong X, Thornton K, Reed E. Computer based analyses of the 5'-flanking regions of selected genes involved in the nucleotide excision repair complex. Int J Oncol 2000; 17:375–380.

326. Hart RW, Setlow RB. Correlation between deoxyribonucleic acid excision-repair and life-span in a number of mammalian species. Proc Natl Acad Sci USA 1974; 71:2169–2173.

327. Cortopassi GA, Wang E. There is substantial agreement among interspecies estimates of DNA repair activity. Mech Ageing Dev 1996; 91:211–218.

328. Mah MC, Boldt J, Culp SJ, Maher VM, McCormick JJ. Replication of acetyl-aminofluorene-adducted plasmids in human cells: spectrum of base substitutions and evidence of excision repair. Proc Natl Acad Sci USA 1991; 88: 10193–10197.

329. Myrnes B, Giercksky KE, Krokan H. Interindividual variation in the activity of O^6-methyl guanine-DNA methyltransferase and uracil-DNA glycosylase in human organs. Carcinogenesis 1983; 4:1565–1568.

330. Eydmann ME, Knowles MA. Mutation analysis of 8p genes POLB and PPP2CB in bladder cancer. Cancer Genet Cytogenet 1997; 93:167–171.

331. Shen MR, Jones IM, Mohrenweiser H. Nonconservative amino acid substitution variants exist at polymorphic frequency in DNA repair genes in healthy humans. Cancer Res 1998; 58:604–608.

332. Lunn RM, Langlois RG, Hsieh LL, Thompson CL, Bell DA. XRCC1 polymorphisms: effects on aflatoxin B_1-DNA adducts and glycophorin A variant frequency. Cancer Res 1999; 59:2557–2561.

333. Nelson HH, Kelsey KT, Mott LA, Karagas MR. The XRCC1 Arg399Gln polymorphism, sunburn, and non-melanoma skin cancer: evidence of gene–environment interaction. Cancer Res 2002; 62:152–155.

334. Stern MC, Umbach DM, van Gils CH, Lunn RM, Taylor JA. DNA repair gene XRCC1 polymorphisms, smoking, and bladder cancer risk. Cancer Epidemiol Biomarkers Prev 2001; 10:125–131.

335. Winsey SL, Haldar NA, Marsh HP, Bunce M, Marshall SE, Harris AL, Wojnarowska F, Welsh KI. A variant within the DNA repair gene XRCC3 is associated with the development of melanoma skin cancer. Cancer Res 2000; 60:5612–5616.

336. Le Marchand L, Donlon T, Lum-Jones A, Seifried A, Wilkens LR. Association of the hOGG1 Ser326Cys polymorphism with lung cancer risk. Cancer Epidemiol Biomarkers Prev 2002; 11:409–412.

337. Shen H, Wang L, Spitz MR, Hong WK, Mao L, Wei Q. A novel polymorphism in human cytosine DNA-methyltransferase-3B promoter is associated with an increased risk of lung cancer. Cancer Res 2002; 62:4992–4995.

338. Fishel R, Lescoe MK, Rao MR, Copeland NG, Jenkins NA, Garber J, Kane M, Kolodner R. The human mutator gene homolog MSH2 and its association with hereditary nonpolyposis colon cancer. Cell 1993; 75:1027–1038.

339. Peltomaki P, Vasen HF. Mutations predisposing to hereditary nonpolyposis colorectal cancer: database and results of a collaborative study. The International Collaborative Group on Hereditary Nonpolyposis Colorectal Cancer. Gastroenterology 1997; 113:1146–1158.

340. Bootsma D, Kraemer KH, Cleaver JE, Hoeijmakers JHJ. Nucleotide excision repair syndromes: xeroderma pigmentosum, Cockayne syndrome, and trichothiodystrophy. In: Vogelstein B, Kinzler KW, eds. The Genetic Basis of Human Cancer. New York: McGraw-Hill Book Co, 1998; 245–274.

341. Bishop AJ, Barlow C, Wynshaw-Boris AJ, Schiestl RH. Atm deficiency causes an increased frequency of intrachromosomal homologous recombination in mice. Cancer Res 2000; 60:395–399.

342. Chen JJ, Silver D, Cantor S, Livingston DM, Scully R. *BRCA1, BRCA2*, and *Rad51* operate in a common DNA damage response pathway. Cancer Res 1999; 59:1752s–1756s.

343. Dobrovic A, Simpfendorfer D. Methylation of the BRCA1 gene in sporadic breast cancer. Cancer Res 1997; 57:3347–3350.

344. Shekhar MP, Lyakhovich A, Visscher DW, Heng H, Kondrat N. *Rad6* overexpression induces multinucleation, centrosome amplification, abnormal mitosis, aneuploidy, and transformation. Cancer Res 2002; 62:2115–2124.

345. Tan HB, Swann PF, Chance EM. Kinetic analysis of the coding properties of O^6-methylguanine in DNA: the crucial role of the conformation of the phosphodiester bond. Biochemistry 1994; 33:5335–5346.

346. Ordway JM, Curran T. Methylation matters: modeling a manageable genome. Cell Growth Differ 2002; 13:149–162.

347. Suzuki N, Ohashi E, Hayashi K, Ohmori H, Grollman AP, Shibutani S. Translesional synthesis past acetylaminofluorene-derived DNA adducts catalyzed by human DNA polymerase κ and Escherichia coli DNA polymerase IV. Biochemistry 2001; 40:15176–15183.

348. Minamoto T, Mai M, Ronai Z. K-ras mutation: early detection in molecular diagnosis and risk assessment of colorectal, pancreas, and lung cancers—a review. Cancer Detect Prev 2000; 24:1–12.

349. Miyakura Y, Sugano K, Fukayama N, Konishi F, Nagai H. Concurrent mutations of K-ras oncogene at codons 12 and 22 in colon cancer. Jpn J Clin Oncol 2002; 32:219–221.

350. Munirajan AK, Mohanprasad BK, Shanmugam G, Tsuchida N. Detection of a rare point mutation at codon 59 and relatively high incidence of H-ras mutation in Indian oral cancer. Int J Oncol 1998; 13:971–974.

351. Smith LE, Denissenko MF, Bennett WP, Li H, Amin S, Tang M, Pfeifer GP. Targeting of lung cancer mutational hotspots by polycyclic aromatic hydrocarbons. J Natl Cancer Inst 2000; 92:803–811.

352. Hainaut P, Hollstein M. p53 human cancer: the first ten thousand mutations. Adv Cancer Res 2000; 77:81–137.

353. Besaratinia A, Bates SE, Pfeifer GP. Mutational signature of the proximate bladder carcinogen *N*-hydroxy-4-acetylaminobiphenyl: inconsistency with the p53 mutational spectrum in bladder cancer. Cancer Res 2002; 62:4331–4338.

354. Hussain SP, Harris CC. p53 mutation spectrum and load: the generation of hypotheses linking the exposure of endogenous or exogenous carcinogens to human cancer. Mutat Res 1999; 428:23–32.

355. International Agency for Research on Cancer 2,3,7,8-Tetrachlorodibenzo-*p*-dioxin. IARC Monographs on the Evaluation of Carcinogenic Risks to Humans. Lyon, France: IARC, 1997; 69:33–343.

356. Silberhorn EM, Glauert HP, Robertson LW. Carcinogenicity of polyhalogenated biphenyls: PCBs and PBBs. Crit Rev Toxicol 1990; 20:440–496.

357. International Agency for Research on Cancer Polychlorinated biphenyls. IARC Monographs on the Evaluation of Carcinogenic Risks to Humans Overall Evaluation of Carcinogenicity: An Updating of IARC monographs Volumes 1 to 42. Lyon, France: IARC, 1987; suppl 7:322–326.

358. Bosetti C, Negri E, Fattore E, La Vecchia C. Occupational exposure to polychlorinated biphenyls and cancer risk. Eur J Cancer Prev 2003; 12:251–255.

359. Laden F, Ishibe N, Hankinson SE, Wolff MS, Gertig DM, Hunter DJ, Kelsey KT. Polychlorinated biphenyls, cytochrome P450 1A1, and breast cancer risk in the Nurses' Health Study. Cancer Epidemiol Biomarkers Prev 2002; 11:1560–1565.

360. Eriksson M, Hardell L, Berg NO, Moller T, Axelson O. Soft-tissue sarcomas and exposure to chemical substances: a case-referent study. Br J Ind Med 1981; 38:27–33.

361. Hardell L, Eriksson M. Soft-tissue sarcomas, phenoxy herbicides, and chlorinated phenols. Lancet 1981; 2:250.

362. Smith JG, Christophers AJ. Phenoxy herbicides and chlorophenols: a case control study on soft tissue sarcoma and malignant lymphoma. Br J Cancer 1992; 65:442–448.

363. Hardell L. Phenoxy herbicides, chlorophenols, soft-tissue sarcoma STS and malignant lymphoma. Br J Cancer 1993; 67:1154–1156.

364. Zahm SH, Ward MH, Blair A. Pesticides and cancer. Occup Med 1997; 12:269–289.
365. Zheng T, Blair A, Zhang Y, Weisenburger DD, Zahm SH. Occupation and risk of non-Hodgkin's lymphoma and chronic lymphocytic leukemia. J Occup Environ Med 2002; 44:469–474.
366. Henderson BE, Feigelson HS. Hormonal carcinogenesis. Carcinogenesis 2000; 21:427–433.
367. Yager JD, Liehr JG. Molecular mechanisms of estrogen carcinogenesis. Annu Rev Pharmacol Toxicol 1996; 36:203–232.
368. Kingston DG, Van Tassell RL, Wilkins TD. The fecapentaenes, potent mutagens from human feces. Chem ResToxicol 1990; 3:391–400.
369. Hecht SS. Tobacco and cancer: approaches using carcinogen biomarkers and chemoprevention. Ann N Y Acad Sci 1997; 833:91–111.
370. Commitee on Comparative Toxicity of Naturally Occurring Carcinogens, Carcinogens and Anticarcinogens in the Human Diet: A Comparison of Naturally Occurring and Synthetic Substances. www.nap.edu/books/ 0309053919/html/index.html
371. International Agency for Research on Cancer Some naturally occurring substances: food items and constituents, heterocyclic aromatic amines and mycotoxins, Aflatoxins. IARC Monographs on the Evaluation of Carcinogenic Risks to Humans. IARC, 1993; 56:245–395.
372. Stiborova M, Frei E, Breuer A, Bieler CA, Schmeiser HH. Aristolactam I a metabolite of aristolochic acid I upon activation forms an adduct found in DNA of patients with Chinese herbs nephropathy. Exp Toxicol Pathol 1999; 51:421–427.
373. International Agency for Research on Cancer arsenic and arsenic Compounds. IARC Monographs on the Evaluation of Carcinogenic Risks to Humans. Vol. 1–42. Lyons: IARC, 1987; suppl 7:100–106.
374. Chen CJ, Chen CW, Wu MM, Kuo TL. Cancer potential in liver, lung, bladder and kidney due to ingested inorganic arsenic in drinking water. Br J Cancer 1992; 66:888–892.
375. International Agency for Research on Cancer, Some Drinking-water Disinfectants and Contaminants, including Arsenic. http://www-cie.iarc.fr/ht-htdocs/announcements/vol84.htm
376. Sugimura T. Overview of carcinogenic heterocyclic amines. Mutat Res 1997; 376:211–219.
377. Weiss G. CANCER RISKS: acrylamide in food: uncharted territory. Science 2002; 297:27.
378. Levine EG, Bloomfield CD. Leukemias and myelodysplastic syndromes secondary to drug, radiation, and environmental exposure. Semin Oncol 1992; 19:47–84.
379. International Agency for Research on Cancer Post-menopausal estrogen therapy. IARC Monographs on the Evaluation of Carcinogenic Risks to Humans. Lyon, France: IARC, 1999; 72:399–530.
380. Cuzick J, Sasieni P, Evans S. Ingested arsenic, keratoses, and bladder cancer. Am J Epidemiol 1992; 136:417–421.

381. Davies ST, Monro A. Marketed human pharmaceuticals reported to be tumorigenic in rodents. J Am Coll Toxicol 1995; 14:90–107.
382. WHO, Guidelines for drinking-water quality. http://www.who.int/ water_sanitation_health/GDWQ/Chemicals/nitratenitritesum.htm
383. Ames BN, Gold LS, Willett WC. The causes and prevention of cancer. Proc Natl Acad Sci USA 1995; 92:5258–5265.
384. Weisburger JH, Williams GM. Causes of cancer. Murphy GP, Lawrence W, Lenhard RE, eds. American Cancer Society Textbook of Clinical Oncology. Atlanta: American Cancer Society Inc, 1995:10–39.
385. Lynch HT, Fusaro RM, Lynch JF. Cancer genetics in the new era of molecular biology. Ann N Y Acad Sci 1997; 833:1–28.
386. Gascón F, Valle M, Martos R, Zafra M, Morales R, Castaño MA. Childhood obesity and hormonal abnormalities associated with cancer risk. Eur J Cancer Prev 2004; 13:193–197.
387. Richie JP, Williams GM. Aging and cancer. In: Ingram DK, Baker GT III, Shock NW, eds. The Potential for Nutritional Modulation of the aging process. Trumbull, CT: Food & Nutrition Press, Inc, 1991:51–66.
388. Selikoff IJ, Seidman H. Asbestos-associated deaths among insulation workers in the United States and Canada, 1967–1987. Ann N Y Acad Sci 1991; 643: 1–14.
389. American Cancer Society. http://www.cancer.org/downloads/ STT/CAFF 2005f4pwsecured.pdf
390. Doll R, Peto R. The causes of cancer: quantitative estimates of avoidable risks of cancer in the United States today. J Natl Cancer Inst 1981; 66:1191–1308.
391. Williams GM, Williams CL, Weisburger JH. Diet and cancer prevention: the fiber first diet. Toxicol Sci 1999; 52(suppl):72–86.
392. Calle EE, Rodriguez C, Walker-Thurmond K, Thun MJ. Overweight, obesity, and mortality from cancer in a prospectively studied cohort of US adults. N Engl J Med 2003; 348:1625–1638.
393. Snyderwine EG. Some perspectives on the nutritional aspects of breast cancer research. Food-derived heterocyclic amines as etiologic agents in human mammary cancer. Cancer 1994; 74:1070–1077.
394. Layton DW, Bogen KT, Knize MG, Hatch FT, Johnson VM, Felton JS. Cancer risk of heterocyclic amines in cooked foods: an analysis and implications for research. Carcinogenesis 1995; 16:39–52.
395. Vineis P, Terracini B. Biochemical epidemiology of bladder cancer. Epidemiology 1990; 1:448–452.
396. Eichholzer M, Gutzwiller F. Dietary nitrates, nitrites, and N-nitroso compounds and cancer risk: a review of the epidemiologic evidence. Nutr Rev 1998; 56:95–105.
397. Hill MJ. Nutrition and human cancer. Ann NY Acad Sci 1997; 833:68–78.
398. Howe GR, Hirohata T, Hislop TG, Iscovich JM, Yuan JM, Katsouyanni K, Lubin F, Marubini E, Modan B, Rohan T, Toniolo P, Shunzhang Y. Dietary factors and risk of breast cancer: combined analysis of 12 case–control studies. J Natl Cancer Inst 1990; 82:561–569.

399. Velie E, Kulldorff M, Schairer C, Block G, Albanes D, Schatzkin A. Dietary fat, fat subtypes, and breast cancer in postmenopausal women: a prospective cohort study. J Natl Cancer Inst 2000; 92:833–839.
400. Potter JD, Slattery ML, Bostick RM, Gapstur SM. Colon cancer: a review of the epidemiology. Epidemiol Rev 1993; 15:499–545.
401. Kolonel LN. Nutrition and prostate cancer. Cancer Causes Control 1996; 7:83–44.
402. Willett WC. Dietary fat and breast cancer. Toxicol Sci 1999; 52:127–146.
403. Cassidy A, Bingham SA, Cummings JH. Starch intake and colorectal cancer risk: an international comparison. Br J Cancer 1994; 69:937–942.
404. Byrne C, Rockett H, Holmes MD. Dietary fat, fat subtypes, and breast cancer risk: lack of an association among postmenopausal women with no history of benign breast disease. Cancer Epidemiol Biomarkers Prev 2002; 11:261–265.
405. Welsch CW. Interrelationship between dietary lipids and calories and experimental mammary gland tumorigenesis. Cancer 1994; 74:1055–1062.
406. Russo J, Lareef H, Tahin Q, Russo IH. Pathways of carcinogenesis and prevention in the human breast. Eur J Cancer 2002; 38(suppl 6):S31–S32.
407. Haines A, Hill MJ, Thompson MH, Owen RW, Williams RE, Meade TW, Wilkes H, Griffin M. A prospective study of faecal bile acids and colorectal cancer. Eur J Cancer Prev 2000; 9:317–323.
408. Chan JM, Stampfer MJ, Giovannucci E, Gann PH, Ma J, Wilkinson P, Hennekens CH, Pollak M. Plasma insulin-like growth factor-I and prostate cancer risk: a prospective study. Science 1998; 279:563–566.
409. Stoll BA. Association between breast and colorectal cancers. Br J Surg 1998; 85:1468–1472.
410. Ip C. Review of the effects of trans fatty acids, oleic acid, n-3 polyunsaturated fatty acids, and conjugated linoleic acid on mammary carcinogenesis in animals. Amer J Clin Nutrition 1997; 66:1523S–1529S.
411. Das UN. Essential fatty acids and their metabolites and cancer. Nutrition 1999; 15:239–240.
412. Palakurthi SS, Fluckiger R, Aktas H, Changolkar AK, Shahsafaei A, Harneit S, Kilic E, Halperin JA. Inhibition of translation initiation mediates the anticancer effect of the n-3 polyunsaturated fatty acid eicosapentaenoic acid. Cancer Res 2000; 60:2919–2925.
413. Pisani P, Parkin DM, Munoz N, Ferlay J. Cancer and infection: estimates of the attributable fraction in 1990. Cancer Epidemiol. Biomarkers Prev 1997; 6:387–400.
414. Okuda K. New trends in hepatocellular carcinoma. Int J Clin Lab Res 1993; 23:173–178.
415. El Serag HB, Mason AC. Rising incidence of hepatocellular carcinoma in the United States. N Engl J Med 1999; 340:745–750.
416. La Vecchia C, Lucchini F, Franceschi S, Negri E, Levi F. Trends in mortality from primary liver cancer in Europe. Eur J Cancer 2000; 36:909–915.
417. Correa P. Helicobacter pylori and gastric cancer: state of the art. Cancer Epidemiol Biomarkers Prev 1996; 5:477–481.
418. Sepulveda AR, Coelho LG. Helicobacter pylori and gastric malignancies. Helicobacter 2002; 7(suppl 1):37–42.

419. Kubbutat MHG, Vousden KH. Role of E6 and E7 oncoproteins in HPV-induced anogenital malignancies. Semin Virol 2002; 7:295–304.

420. Scheffner M, Werness BA, Huibregtse JM, Levine AJ, Howley PM. The E6 oncoprotein encoded by human papillomavirus types 16 and 18 promotes the degradation of p53. Cell 1990; 63:1129–1136.

421. Dyson N, Howley PM, Munger K, Harlow E. The human papilloma virus-16 E7 oncoprotein is able to bind to the retinoblastoma gene product. Science 1989; 243:934–937.

422. International Agency for Research on Cancer Human immunodeficiency viruses. IARC Monographs on the Evaluation of Carcinogenic Risks to Humans. Lyon, France: IARC 1996; 67:31–259.

423. International Agency for Research on Cancer T-lymphotropic Viruses. IARC Monographs on the Evaluation of Carcinogenic Risks to Humans. Lyon, France: IARC, 1996; 66:261–390.

424. Abdel-Rahim AY. Parasitic infections and hepatic neoplasia. Dig Dis 2001; 19:288–291.

425. Tozer GM, Everett SA. Nitric oxide in tumour biology and cancer therapy. Part 1: physiological aspects. Clin Oncol R Coll Radiol 1997; 9:282–293.

426. Jaiswal M, LaRusso NF, Nishioka N, Nakabeppu Y, Gores GJ. Human Ogg1, a protein involved in the repair of 8-oxoguanine, is inhibited by nitric oxide. Cancer Res 2001; 61:6388–6393.

427. Knudson AG. Hereditary predisposition to cancer. Ann N Y Acad Sci 1997; 833:58–67.

428. Lindor NM, Greene MH. The concise handbook of family cancer syndromes. Mayo Familial Cancer Program. J Natl Cancer Inst 1998; 90:1039–1071.

429. Kawaguchi H, Ohno S, Araki K, Miyazaki M, Saeki H, Watanabe M, Tanaka S, Sugimachi K. p53 polymorphism in human papillomavirus-associated esophageal cancer. Cancer Res 2000; 60:2753–2755.

430. Dunlop MG, Farrington SM, Carothers AD, Wyllie AH, Sharp L, Burn J, Liu B, Kinzler KW, Vogelstein B. Cancer risk associated with germline DNA mismatch repair gene mutations. Hum Mol Genet 1997; 6:105–110.

431. Kraemer KH, Lee MM, Andrews AD, Lambert WC. The role of sunlight and DNA repair in melanoma and nonmelanoma skin cancer. The xeroderma pigmentosum paradigm. Arch Dermatol 1994; 130:1018–1021.

432. Morrell D, Cromartie E, Swift M. Mortality and cancer incidence in 263 patients with ataxia-telangiectasia. J Natl Cancer Inst 1986; 77:89–92.

433. Swift M, Morrell D, Massey RB, Chase CL. Incidence of cancer in 161 families affected by ataxiatelangiectasia. N Engl J Med 1991; 325:1831–1836.

434. Balmain A. Cancer as a complex genetic trait: tumor susceptibility in humans and mouse models. Cell 2002; 108:145–152.

435. Chaganti RS, Houldsworth J. Genetics and biology of adult human male germ cell tumors. Cancer Res 2000; 60:1475–1482.

436. Lindahl T. Instability and decay of the primary structure of DNA. Nature 1993; 362:709–715.

437. Williams GM, Jeffrey AM. Oxidative DNA damage: Endogenous and chemically induced. Reg Toxicol Pharmacol 2000; 32:283–292.

438. Steinmetz KA, Potter JD. Vegetables, fruit, and cancer. II. Mechanisms. Cancer Causes Control 1991; 2:427–442.
439. Simic MG, Bergtold DS. Dietary modulation of DNA damage in human. Mutat Res 1991; 250:17–24.
440. Turker MS, Gage BM, Rose JA, Elroy D, Ponomareva ON, Stambrook PJ, Tischfield JA. A novel signature mutation for oxidative damage resembles a mutational pattern found commonly in human cancers. Cancer Res 1999; 59:1837–1839.
441. Michaud DS, Spiegelman D, Clinton SK, Rimm EB, Willett WC, Giovannucci EL. Fruit and vegetable intake and incidence of bladder cancer in a male prospective cohort. J Natl Cancer Inst 1999; 91:605–613.
442. Adlercreutz H. Phyto-oestrogens and cancer. Lancet Oncol 2002; 3:364–373.
443. Weisburger JH, Chung FL. Mechanisms of chronic disease causation by nutritional factors and tobacco products and their prevention by tea polyphenols. Food Chem Toxicol 2002; 40:1145–1154.
444. Jacobs ET, Giuliano AR, Roe DJ, Guillen-Rodriguez JM, Hess LM, Alberts DS, Martinez ME. Intake of supplemental and total fiber and risk of colorectal adenoma recurrence in the wheat bran fiber trial. Cancer Epidemiol Biomarkers Prev 2002; 11:906–914.
445. Asano T, McLeod RS. Dietary fibre for the prevention of colorectal adenomas and carcinomas. Cochrane Database Syst Rev CD003430. 2002.
446. Potter JD, Steinmetz K. Vegetables, fruit and phytoestrogens as preventive agents. IARC Sci Publ 1996; 139:61–90.
447. La Vecchia C, Tavani A. Fruit and vegetables, and human cancer. Eur J Cancer Prev 1998; 7:3–8.
448. Giovannucci E. Tomatoes, tomato-based products, lycopene, and cancer: review of the epidemiologic literature. J Natl Cancer Inst 1999; 91:317–331.
449. World Cancer Research Fund International. Food, Nutrition and the Prevention of Cancer: a Global Perspective. World Cancer Research Fund International, 2002.
450. de Deckere EA. Possible beneficial effect of fish and fish n-3 polyunsaturated fatty acids in breast and colorectal cancer. Eur J Cancer Prev 1999; 8:213–221.
451. Trichopoulou A, Katsouyanni K, Stuver S, Tzala L, Gnardellis C, Rimm E, Trichopoulos D. Consumption of olive oil and specific food groups in relation to breast cancer risk in Greece. J Natl Cancer Inst 1995; 87:110–116.
452. Strom SS, Yamamura Y, Duphorne CM, Spitz MR, Babaian RJ, Pillow PC, Hursting SD. Phytoestrogen intake and prostate cancer: a case control study using a new database. Nutr Cancer 1999; 33:20–25.
453. Institute of Medicine, Dietary Reference Intakes for Vitamin A, Vitamin K, Arsenic, Boron, Chromium, Copper, Iodine, Iron, Manganese, Molybdenum, Nickel, Silicon, Vanadium, and Zinc. http://www.nap.edu/books/0309072794/html/
454. Kelloff GJ. Perspectives on cancer chemoprevention research and drug development. Adv Cancer Res 2000; 78:199–334.
455. Sporn MB, an Suh N. Chemoprevention of cancer. Carcinogenesis 2000; 21:525–530.

456. Greenwald P, Kelloff G, Burch-Whitman C, Kramer BS. Chemoprevention. CA Cancer J Clin 1995; 45:31–49.

457. Scheer M, Kuebler AC, Zoller JE. Chemoprevention of oral squamous cell carcinomas. Onkologie 2004; 27:187–193.

458. Fisher B, Costantino JP, Wickerham DL, Redmond CK, Kavanah M, Cronin WM, Vogel V, Robidoux A, Dimitrov N, Atkins J, Daly M, Wieand S, Tan-Chiu E, Ford L, and Wolmark N. Tamoxifen for prevention of breast cancer: report of the National Surgical Adjuvant Breast and Bowel Project P-1 Study. J Natl Cancer Inst 1998; 90:1371–1388.

459. Harris RE, Chlebowski RT, Jackson RD, Frid DJ, Ascenseo JL, Anderson G, Loar A, Rodabough RJ, White E, McTiernan A. Breast cancer and nonsteroidal anti-inflammatory drugs: prospective results from the Women's Health Initiative. Cancer Res 2003; 63:6096–6101.

460. Janne PA, Mayer RJ. Chemoprevention of colorectal cancer. N Engl J Med 2000; 342:1960–1968.

461. Masferrer JL, Leahy KM, Koki AT, Zweifel BS, Settle SL, Woerner BM, Edwards DA, Flickinger AG, Moore RJ, Seibert K. Antiangiogenic and antitumor activities of cyclooxygenase-2 inhibitors. Cancer Res 2000; 60: 1306–1311.

462. Mukherjee R, Davies PJ, Crombie DL, Bischoff ED, Cesario RM, Jow L, Hamann LG, Boehm MF, Mondon CE, Nadzan AM, Paterniti JR Jr, Heyman RA. Sensitization of diabetic and obese mice to insulin by retinoid X receptor agonists. Nature 1997; 386:407–410.

463. Mehta RG, Mehta RR. Vitamin D and cancer. J Nutr Biochem 2002; 13: 252–264.

464. Albanes D. β-carotene and lung cancer: a case study. Amer J Clin. Nutr 1999; 69:1345S–1350S.

465. Clark LC, Dalkin B, Krongrad A, Combs GF Jr, Turnbull BW, Slate EH, Witherington R, Herlong JH, Janosko E, Carpenter D, Borosso C, Falk S, Rounder J. Decreased incidence of prostate cancer with selenium supplementation: results of a double-blind cancer prevention trial. Br J Urol 1998; 81: 730–734.

466. Duffield-Lillico AJ, Dalkin BL, Reid ME, Turnbull BW, Slate EH, Jacobs ET, Marshall JR, Clark LC. Selenium supplementation, baseline plasma selenium status and incidence of prostate cancer: an analysis of the complete treatment period of the Nutritional Prevention of Cancer Trial. BJU Int 2003; 91: 608–612.

467. Reid ME, Duffield-Lillico AJ, Garland L, Turnbull BW, Clark LC, Marshall JR. Selenium supplementation and lung cancer incidence: an update of the nutritional prevention of cancer trial. Cancer Epidemiol Biomarkers Prev 2002; 11:1285–1291.

468. Montesano R. Hepatitis B immunization and hepatocellular carcinoma: The Gambia Hepatitis Intervention Study. J Med Virol 2002; 67:444–446.

469. Furumoto H, Irahara M. Human papilloma virus HPV and cervical cancer. J Med Invest 2002; 49:124–133.

470. Chemoprevention Working Group Prevention of cancer in the next millennium: report of the Chemoprevention Working Group to the American Association for Cancer Research. Cancer Res 1999; 59:4743–4758.
471. Singer B. In vivo formation and persistence of modified nucleosides resulting from alkylating agents. Environ Health Perspect 1985; 62:41–48.
472. Kalnik MW, Li BF, Swann PF, Patel DJ. O^6-ethylguanine carcinogenic lesions in DNA: an NMR study of O^6-EtG.T pairing in dodecanucleotide duplexes. Biochemistry 1989; 28:6170–6181.

12

Viral Causes of Cancer

Michie Hisada and Charles S. Rabkin

Viral Epidemiology Branch, Division of Cancer Epidemiology and Genetics, National Cancer Institute, Bethesda, Maryland, U.S.A.

1. INTRODUCTION

A viral etiology of cancer was first recognized in 1911 when a cell-free filtrate from a chicken sarcoma, later identified and named as Rous sarcoma virus, was demonstrated to induce a tumor in another chicken to which the filtrate was transmitted. A number of mammalian oncoviruses were identified subsequent to this observation. A cause of a disease may be an agent, event, condition, or characteristic that plays a vital role in the occurrence of the disease. Cause must be distinguished from pathogenesis, in that the implication of the former is not limited to what happens but also includes the mechanisms by which it happens. Cause must also be distinguished from mere association, as causation implies the temporal relationship where the causal event precedes the disease consequences by direct or indirect mechanism. A formal model of disease causation by an infectious agent was enunciated in 1840 by Jakob Henle and further developed by his successor Robert Koch. In this formulation, there are three basic conditions by which the association between the agent and the disease can be considered no longer accidental but causal.

1. The agent occurs in every case of the disease in question and under circumstances that can account for the pathological changes and clinical course of the disease.
2. The agent occurs in no other disease as a fortuitous and non-pathogenic parasite.

3. The agent can induce the disease anew, after being fully isolated from the body and repeatedly grown in pure culture.

While correctly identifying many human pathogens, the Henle–Koch criteria, if strictly applied, would exclude other presumed pathogens, particularly many viruses. To overcome some of these limitations, the classical Henle–Koch postulates were modified and expanded to nine criteria proposed by Sir Austin Bradford Hill (1):

1. Exposures strongly associated with disease are more likely to be a true cause (strength of association).
2. Relationships can be demonstrated in multiple studies in different populations and/or different study designs. Strength of association may differ, but direction should be the same (consistency).
3. One exposure is associated with one disease (specificity).
4. Exposure precedes disease (temporality).
5. Changes in exposure relate to changes in risk (dose–response relationship).
6. The proposed causal mechanism—direct or indirect—is biologically plausible (plausibility).
7. The cause–effect interpretation does not seriously conflict with the generally known facts of the natural history and biology of the disease (coherence).
8. Experimental removal or blockage of the cause prevents the disease (experimental evidence).
9. Similarity to other disease–agent associations provides support for causation by another agent (analogy).

The concepts of sufficient and component causes—where a sufficient cause is a set of minimal conditions that inevitably produce disease whereas each of the contributing conditions to a sufficient cause is considered a component cause—provided further foundation for causal associations in epidemiological studies (2). In contrast, a condition invariably associated with all cases of a particular disease became known as a necessary cause.

Viral-associated cancers in humans became a major focus of cancer research when Epstein–Barr virus (EBV)—the first human oncovirus—was found in 1964 (3). Followed by this discovery, a series of human oncogenic viruses were found through the 1980s and 1990s, including hepatitis viruses (HBV and HCV), human retroviruses (HTLV-I and HIV), human herpesviruses, and human papillomaviruses. Evans and Mueller (4) noted common characteristics for the epidemiology of virus-associated cancers:

1. The long induction period between initial infection and the onset of cancer.

2. Most candidate viruses are ubiquitous but cancer incidence is rare.
3. The initial infection is often subclinical and the time of infection is rarely known.
4. Most viral-related cancers require cofactors.
5. The causes of cancer may vary by age and by geographic area.
6. Different viral strains may have different oncogenic potentials.
7. The host factors, especially age of infection, genetic characteristics, and immune status, play a critical role in susceptibility to cancer.
8. A virus may play a role at different points in a complex, multistage process of pathogenesis by altering the host's immune system or by causing a variety of events at the molecular level.
9. Many human cancers cannot be reproduced in experimental animals with the putative virus.
10. A virus-induced cancer could have the same histologic features with cancers caused by a toxin, chemical, altered gene, or other causal factors.

To establish associations between a putative viral cause and a human cancer, the following guidelines were proposed:

1. The geographic distribution of virus infection is similar to that of the associated tumor when adjusted for the age of infection and the presence of cofactors.
2. Viral markers (antibody titers or antigenemia) are higher in cases than in matched controls in the same geographic setting, as shown in case–control studies.
3. The viral marker precedes the tumor and a significantly higher incidence of the tumor follows in persons with the marker than in those without it.
4. Prevention of the viral infection (e.g., by vaccination) or control of the host's response to the virus (such as by delaying the time of infection) decreases the tumor incidence.
5. The virus transforms human cells in vitro.
6. The viral genome is present in tumor cells but not in normal cells.
7. The virus induces the tumor in a susceptible experimental animal, while neutralization of the virus prior to injection prevents tumor development.

As evident in these guidelines, mere detection of a virus in a tumor is not strong evidence for a causal association. In seroepidemiological studies, the following provide additional support in relating a virus to a cancer (5):

1. Specific antibody is present more frequently in cancer patients than in healthy controls in the same geographic area.
2. Antibody levels (i.e., geometric mean titer or prevalence of elevated titers) are higher in cancer patients than in seropositive controls.
3. Antibody profiles by epitope or immunoglobulin subclass suggest persistence or reactivation of the putative agent.
4. Antibody is specific for the virus being considered and other viral antibodies are not elevated.
5. Sera obtained prior to cancer show antibody to be absent (if the cancer is due to primary infection) or elevated (if cancer is a consequence of reactivation).
6. Variation in the virus–cancer association is explainable by differences in distribution of co-factors.

This chapter outlines the well-established associations of viruses with cancers in humans. We primarily focus on the epidemiology and mechanisms of these associations as well as on biomarkers of cancer risk in humans.

2. EPSTEIN–BARR VIRUS

Since its discovery in the 1960s, EBV and its oncogenesis have been extensively studied. The unique feature of this virus is its association with multiple types of cancer of different cellular origins. EBV infection is not associated with apparent immune suppression, but in some instances EBV-associated malignancies appear to develop in the presence of subclinical immune suppression (6).

2.1. Molecular Biology

EBV is a member of the herpes family of viruses. It has a linear, double-stranded DNA genome consisting of about 100 genes, surrounded by a viral capsid and a lipid envelope. The virus infects B-lymphocytes and can replicate via both lytic and latent pathways. EBV-infected cells express a variety of EBV-encoded products, including EBV-encoded RNA (EBERs), nuclear antigens (EBNA), and latent membrane proteins (LMP). Correspondingly, infected individuals produce antibodies to composites of these viral products, including viral capsid antigen (VCA), early antigen (EA), and EBNA.

2.2. Epidemiology of EBV Infection

EBV is primarily transmitted by the oral route. Infection leads to a life-long carrier state, characterized by latent infection of a subset of B-lymphocytes and persistent shedding of infectious virus in saliva. Infection is nearly ubiquitous by adulthood in all populations worldwide, with age-specific seroprevalence of younger individuals varying by socioeconomic status, family size, and hygiene. In developing countries, 70%–95% of children are infected with EBV by the age of 5 years, whereas in industrialized countries infection is normally delayed until young adulthood. Primary infection in early childhood is usually asymptomatic, whereas infection later in life often results in a self-limiting lymphoproliferative syndrome, recognized clinically as infectious mononucleosis.

2.3. EBV-Associated Malignancies in Humans

Since the normal reservoir of latent infection is the B lymphocyte, EBV-infected lymphocytes in tumor tissue may be either incidental or an effect of the tumor rather than evidence for an etiological role of this virus in cancer development. Thus, the causality of association with a given tumor should be judged with consideration to other factors, such as the proportion of EBV-positive cases in a given tumor type, the proportion of tumor cells that carry the virus in any given case, the monoclonality of EBV in the tumor (indicating that the malignant clone expanded from a single EBV-infected cell), and evidence of active infection such as the expression of EBV proteins. Based on these and other criteria, four major tumor types have well-established associations with EBV: Burkitt's lymphoma (BL), other non-Hodgkin's lymphomas (NHL), Hodgkin's lymphomas (HL), and nasopharyngeal carcinoma (NPC).

EBV infection of B-lymphocytes in vitro efficiently induces transformation into immortalized cell lines. In EBV-transformed B-cells, 13 viral genes are expressed: six nuclear antigens, three LMPs, two small nontranslated RNAs, and two other transcripts. The viral proteins regulate maintenance of episomal viral DNA and viral gene expression, drive cellular proliferation, and block apoptosis.

2.3.1. Burkitt's Lymphoma

Patients with BL have high titers of antibodies to EBV VCA and EA, preceding the appearance of tumor by months to years (7). Viral DNA is present in tumor cells and is monoclonal. Viral protein expression is almost entirely restricted to a nuclear antigen, EBNA-1. Notably, the frequency of association between EBV and BL varies geographically. In most developed countries, 20% or fewer tumors contain EBV, while in equatorial Africa about 95% are positive. A characteristic chromosomal translocation between the *c-myc* protooncogene and an immunoglobulin gene is invariably present in BL, although the molecular features of these translocations vary geographically in parallel with differences in EBV prevalence in tumors. In equatorial Africa, infection with *Plasmodium falciparum*, a malaria parasite, is an important cofactor for the incidence of BL, which accounts for 30–70% of childhood cancers (8). Incidence outside of this region, with the exception of AIDS-related cases, is much less than 1 per 100,000 children per year (9).

2.3.2. Other Non-Hodgkin's Lymphomas

EBV is particularly important in tumors occurring in immunosuppressed individuals, who are at elevated risk for these malignancies. In patients with congenital immunodeficiency or receiving immunosuppressive therapy, NHLs are nearly always EBV-positive. In HIV-positive subjects, EBV is uniformly found in NHL of the central nervous system and also in a fraction of systemic NHL. In the absence of immunosuppression, EBV is strongly associated with some uncommon types of NHL, particularly sinonasal angiocentric T-cell lymphoma and other peripheral T-cell tumors.

2.3.3. Hodgkin's Lymphoma

Monoclonal EBV genome and latent viral protein expression may be found in the putative tumor cells (Reed–Sternberg cells) of one-third of HL cases. In particular, HL occurring in association with immunodeficiency, such as in HIV infection, is usually EBV-positive. HL patients also have altered antibody profiles to EBV prior to the disease onset (10).

2.3.4. Nasopharyngeal Carcinoma

Incidence rates are two to three times higher in males than females, and reach 25–40 per 100,000 in the highest incidence areas of southern China, but are <1 per 100,000 in most parts of the world (9). EBV DNA and viral products are regularly found in malignant cells but not in normal nasopharyngeal epithelium. Patients with this tumor have elevated levels of IgA antibodies to EBV VCA and EA. Consumption of Chinese-style salted fish appears to be an important cofactor in high-risk populations (11).

3. HUMAN T-LYMPHOTROPIC VIRUS TYPE I

In the early 1980s, HTLV-I was isolated by cell culture from a patient with T-cell lymphoma in the United States (12) and a patient with adult T-cell leukemia (ATL) in Japan (13). A number of other diseases in addition to ATL were subsequently associated with this infection, including HTLV-I-associated myelopathy/tropical spastic paraparesis (HAM/TSP), HTLV-I associated uveitis (HU), and infective dermatitis (ID) in children (6). The infection causes subclinical immune suppression, which is evidenced by an increased frequency and severity of opportunistic infections in HTLV-I-positive individuals (14,15).

3.1. Molecular Biology

HTLV-I is an enveloped, type C retrovirus with an RNA dimer of two identical subunits (16). The viral genome contains three structural genes (*gag, pol,* and *env*) and two regulatory genes (*tax* and *rex*) flanked by two long terminal repeats (LTRs). The *gag* gene encodes core proteins p19 and p24, *pol* encodes RNA-dependent DNA polymerase (reverse transcriptase), and *env* encodes the small transmembrane (gp21) and large external envelope (gp46) glycoproteins. The *tax* and *rex* regulatory genes transactivate viral replication and control expression of viral proteins. The virus uses reverse transcriptase to synthesize DNA copies of its genome within the host cell that integrate into the host's genome as aprovirus.

3.2. Epidemiology and Biomarkers of HTLV-I Infection

HTLV-I infection can be detected by the presence of antibodies to core, envelope, and Tax proteins in serum, as measured by an enzyme-linked immunosorbent assay (ELISA) or a particle agglutination assay (PAA). A recombinant western blot (WB) assay is used as a confirmatory test, in which reactivity to *gag* (p19 or p24) and *env* (gp21 or gp46) gene products is considered indicative of true positivity.

HTLV-I infection affects several million people worldwide (6). Endemic areas include southern Japan, the Caribbean, parts of West Africa, the Middle East, South America, and the Pacific Melanesian islands. Seroprevalence varies from <1% among populations in the United States and Europe to ~5% in the Caribbean islands (17,18) and ~30% in rural Kyushu, Japan (19,20). Seroprevalence increases with age and is twice as high in females than in males (6). The virus is usually acquired early in life by way of breast feeding (21). Early age of infection is considered to be a risk factor for ATL (22). Among adults, the virus may be transmitted via sexual contact (23) or transfusion of cellular components of blood products (24). Thus, effective prevention strategies against HTLV-I infection include screening of blood products to eliminate contaminated units, curtailment of breastfeeding by HTLV-I-positive mothers, and use of barrier contraceptives by HTLV-I-discordant sexual partners.

A high proviral load and high levels of antibody to the whole virus (anti-HTLV-I) and the Tax regulatory protein (anti-Tax) are the primary markers of increased infectivity (23,25). These biomarkers are also markers of HTLV-I pathogenesis, since both ATL and HAM/TSP patients generally have a high proviral load (26) and high anti-HTLV-I titer. A population-based prospective study of asymptomatic HTLV-I carriers found that carriers who later developed ATL had a higher anti-HTLV-I titer as compared to those who did not develop the disease, but the ATL patients lacked anti-Tax antibody prior to diagnosis (27). The lack of *tax* mRNA expression and anti-Tax antibody (28) are particularly useful markers for distinguishing those at risk of ATL from those at risk of HAM/TSP, as the latter tend to express a high level of *tax* mRNA (29,30). In addition, the level of soluble interleukin 2 receptor (sIL-2R), presence of circulating "flower cell"-like abnormal lymphocytes, and mono- or oligoclonal expansion of HTLV-I infected cells (31–33), may be used as intermediate markers of ATL risk.

Determinants of cytotoxic T-lymphocyte (CTL) response, such as the human leukocyte antigens (HLA), have also been hypothesized to play a role in HTLV-I disease pathogenesis (34). *DRB1**1501 and *DQB1**0602 appear to be associated with risk of ATL both in Japanese and Caribbean populations (35). However, the possible influence of linkage disequilibrium in these associations greatly complicates their proper interpretation.

3.3. HTLV-I Associated Malignancies in Humans

The oncogenicity of HTLV-I is not related to host cell protooncogenes. Instead, Tax regulatory protein, which promotes transcription of viral mRNA and of host cellular genes that modulate cell growth (36,37), is thought to play an important role (38–40). Multiple pathways appear to be involved in HTLV-I oncogenesis. Tax indirectly binds to the enhancer-binding transcription factors, resulting in the activation of these factors. Tax also binds to IkB protein resulting in repression of the cyclin-dependent kinase inhibitor, tumor suppressor, and apoptosis-associated proteins (41). Furthermore, Tax protein inactivates the p53 tumor suppressor protein by post-translational phosphorylation (42,43) and inhibits DNA repair mechanisms (44,45), which may explain, at least in part, the propensity for transformation of HTLV-I-infected T-cells.

Because Tax protein is a known target for CTL activity (46,47), ATL cells that do not express *tax* are likely to escape CTL-mediated cell killing. Genetic events that alter immunogenicity of the tax protein, such as mutations in the *tax* gene or changes in viral transcription and translation, may play an additional role (48,49). However, the lack of *tax* mRNA and Tax protein expression in ATL cells (47,50) suggests that HTLV-I-induced oncogenesis becomes independent of *tax* gene activity after a critical period of cellular transformation.

3.3.1. Adult T-Cell Leukemia/Lymphoma

ATL is a rapidly progressive malignancy of activated CD4-, CD25-positive T-lymphocytes (51). The integrated HTLV-I proviral genome is frequently defective in ATL cells, which may help them escape from immune surveillance (52). The disease is characterized by the presence of circulating "flower cells," which are leukemic cells with cleaved, convoluted nuclei. The tumor cells express CD2, CD3, and CD5 as well as the activation markers IL-2R (CD25 Tac antigen) and HLA-DR, but may lack CD7. Based on the total leukocyte count, level of flower cells, presence of clonal provirus integration, presence of immune suppression, and other biochemical data, the disease may be classified into different clinical subtypes (53). The incidence of ATL among HTLV-I carriers is estimated to be 2–4 per 100,000 person-years, with a lifetime risk of ~5% (54,55). Risk seems to be higher in men as compared to women in Japan, but no such difference is evident in the Caribbean. The average age of disease onset is much later in Japan than in the Caribbean (60 vs. 40 years), perhaps due in part to differences in life expectancy, as well as host and environmental factors.

The broad clinical spectrum of ATL sometimes overlaps with that of mycosis fungoides (MF) (56), a T-cell NHL with a propensity for skin involvement, or with the MF variant, Sezary syndrome (SS) (57). The tumor cells of MF and SS can be distinguished from ATL cells by their lack of expression of activation markers. The majority of MF patients do not have antibody to HTLV-I (58). A possible role of HTLV-I in the development of MF has been speculated because portions of its genome were found in skin lesions and peripheral lymphocytes of MF patients (59,60). However, these observations could not be confirmed by other investigators (61,62), and the association of HTLV-I with MF remains inconclusive.

4. HUMAN IMMUNODEFICIENCY VIRUSES

HIV type 1 (HIV-1) was discovered in 1983 (63) and definitively associated with acquired immunodeficiency syndrome (AIDS) in 1984 (64). A related but distinct virus, HIV type 2 (HIV-2), was later discovered in AIDS patients from West Africa (65). HIV-2 infected persons can have the same immunological and clinical spectrum of disease as HIV-1, although there is some evidence that HIV-2 may be less pathogenic than HIV-1 (6).

4.1. Molecular Biology

Human immunodeficiency virus is also a type C retrovirus, with a single-stranded RNA genome (6). HIV targets CD4+ T-lymphocytes and macrophages and replicates via a DNA intermediate integrated into the host genome. HIV-2 is likely identical to the primate infection, simian immunodeficiency virus (SIV). The genome contains three structural genes (*gag*, *pol*, and *env*), two regulatory genes (*tat* and *rev*), and four accessory genes (*nef*, *vif*, *vpr*, and *vpu/vpx*).

4.2. Epidemiology and Biomarkers of Infection

The virus is transmitted sexually, parenterally through contaminated blood products and injection equipment, as well as vertically from mother-to-child in utero or via breast milk. Risk of transmission is associated with viral load in the infected person. Prevalence of infection varies by age, sex, geographical area, risk behavior, and calendar year. In the United States and Europe, homosexual men, the earliest affected group, still account for the largest number of HIV- carriers, followed by injection drug users, as well as their sexual partners and children. In Africa, heterosexual contact is the predominant mode of transmission, with extensive incidence of mother-to-child transmission. In Asia, all modes of transmission are frequent.

The first biomarker for HIV infection was antibody to the virus detected by ELISA and Western blot. Western blot, which simultaneously assesses antibodies to multiple antigenic determinants, is a better tool to handle cross reactivity and detect HIV infection with higher specificity. Early studies of HIV seropositivity in the 1980s in several populations documented elevated prevalence of HIV antibodies in groups at higher risk of AIDS, including homosexual men, injection drug users, and transfusion recipients (66). These studies provided insight into the exposure–biomarker relationship and demonstrated that within groups at higher risk of HIV, HIV seropositivity was quantitatively associated with AIDS risk behaviors or exposures (67). Later, careful epidemiological studies revealed an association of HIV antibody with AIDS and AIDS-related complex (64,68).

Today, an improved laboratory assay for detecting HIV antibody is a useful, valid biomarker of widespread application in risk assessment to identify high-risk groups and in screening and early intervention (69). HIV testing also has stimulated enormous attention to the issues of confidentiality, insurability, employability, informed consent, and individual rights, as well as behavioral modification regarding sexual practice.

4.3. HIV-Associated Malignancies in Humans

The strongest associations of HIV infection with cancers are observed in Kaposi's sarcoma (KS), NHL, and, to a lesser extent, HL. NHL and KS are also seen in other immunosuppressed groups, such as transplant recipients. Smooth muscle tumors (leiomyosarcoma and leiomyomas) in children and conjunctival squamous cell carcinoma in equatorial Africa also appear to be associated with HIV, despite prevailing lack of association in other populations. With rare exceptions, HIV is not present in the tumor cells, suggesting an indirect induction of tumor via immune alterations. In contrast, the angiogenic and spindle cell stimulatory effects of the HIV-1 *tat* gene product *in vitro* may indicate direct induction of KS, explaining the uniquely elevated risk of this condition in HIV infection.

4.3.1. Kaposi's Sarcoma

HIV-infected individuals are at greatly increased risk of KS, an otherwise rare tumor associated with the cofactor human herpesvirus type 8 (HHV-8). Homosexual/bisexual men with HIV are at 5–10-fold greater risk than other HIV-infected groups (70), which may reflect differences in HHV-8 prevalence. Highly active antiretroviral therapy appears to strongly diminish the risk of KS. The nature of KS is uncertain, but a recent study has indicated that it is a disseminated monoclonal neoplasm.

4.3.2. Non-Hodgkin's Lymphoma

NHL incidence is greatly increased in HIV infection and the risk increases with duration of infection. Unlike KS, NHL incidence has increased similarly (up to 100-fold) in all HIV transmission groups. In AIDS-related tumors, EBV coinfection is uniformly found in the primary lymphoma of the brain as well as in a fraction of systemic lymphomas; HHV-8 coinfection is found in a rare subtype, primary effusion lymphoma (PEL).

4.3.3. Hodgkin's Lymphoma

The association of HIV with HL is weaker than that with KS or NHL (RR 5–10). HIV-associated HL is more likely to have mixed cellularity or lymphocyte-depleted histology and in most instances the tumors contain EBV, as discussed above.

4.3.4. Anogenital Dysplasia

Although invasive cervical cancer in an HIV-infected person is one of the AIDS-defining malignancies, there is little evidence that cervical cancer is specifically associated with HIV apart from shared risk factors with human papillomavirus (HPV). Nevertheless, dysplasia and in situ carcinoma of the cervix do appear to be increased with HIV infection and associated immune alteration. Similarly, the incidence of HPV-associated anal dysplasia appears accelerated in HIV infection. Anal cancer incidence, however, does not appear to be substantially increased.

4.3.5. Other Neoplasms

Smooth muscle tumors are the second most common neoplasm in HIV-infected children (71), yet no increase has been demonstrable in HIV-infected adults. These tumors uniformly contain EBV. Conjunctival squamous cell carcinoma, an HPV-associated tumor, has been noted to be increased with HIV in equatorial Africa, but is extremely rare in other locales. Testicular germ-cell tumors may be increased in HIV, although this association is not firmly established. Most other tumors, including those most common in the general population, do not appear increased in HIV infection.

5. HUMAN HERPESVIRUS TYPE 8

A condition invariably associated with all cases of a particular disease is considered to be a necessary cause. This concept is particularly relevant to the question of causation of a few malignancies by HHV-8, or

KS-associated herpesvirus, where the virus is found in 100% of the tumors. The HHV-8 genome is detectable in virtually all cases of KS, PEL and a subset of Castleman's disease (9).

5.1. Molecular Biology

HHV-8 is a herpesvirus with a 165-kb genome, which encodes a number of homologs of cell growth regulatory proteins. One of these proteins, cyclin D, may play a role in virally induced cellular transformation. In vivo, HHV-8 infects B-cells, macrophages, and dendritic cells, with lytic replication occurring in subpopulations of infected cells. Specific patterns of latent gene expression characterize KS and PEL.

5.2. Epidemiology and Biomarkers of HHV-8 Infection

The prevalence of HHV-8 in populations without KS is controversial. Current serologic assays for HHV-8 antibody have uncertain sensitivity and specificity for detecting asymptomatic infection, and frequently disagree in individual samples. Thus, the HHV-8 antibody prevalence determined by these tests for a low risk population may either over- or underestimate the true prevalence of infection. Geographic variation in HHV-8 seroprevalence reflects variation in incidence of endemic KS. In contrast, geographical variation in AIDS-related cases is minimal. Male homosexual contact likely accounts for the high seroprevalence among gay men, whereas heterosexual contact does not appear to spread the infection. Other modes of transmission remain uncertain.

5.3. HHV8-Associated Malignancies in Humans

The universal presence of the HHV-8 genome in tumor tissue of both KS and PEL suggests direct oncogenic effects of HHV-8. The viral homolog of D-type cyclins, which can disrupt cell cycle control, is expressed in both these tumor types, as are other proteins of less-defined function. Lytic replication occurs in a subset of HHV-8-infected KS spindle cells, upregulating expression of several viral growth factors and a growth factor regulatory protein that may stimulate expansion of latently infected cells nearby. PEL similarly expresses virally encoded growth factors and their regulatory proteins and receptors. The large number of HHV-8 genes corresponding to human genes regulating cell growth may reflect a viral strategy for replication that as a corollary mediates HHV-8 oncogenesis.

5.3.1. Kaposi's Sarcoma

KS was most common in eastern European and Mediterranean populations and in central and eastern Africa in endemic forms before the onset of the AIDS epidemic. It is also known to occur in excess in persons with iatrogenic immune suppression. Today, KS is the most common tumor in persons with AIDS. In immunocompromised hosts, HHV-8 seropositivity and the presence of viremia are predictors for subsequent development of KS (72). The pathological features of the tumor are similar in both endemic and AIDS-associated cases, with proliferating "spindle cells" thought to be the primary abnormality, including thin-walled neovascular formations, extravasated red blood cells, and inflammatory lymphocytes.

5.3.2. Primary Effusion Lymphoma

This lymphoma is a rare, distinct subtype of NHL morphologically resembling immunoblastic and anaplastic large-cell lymphomas. A B-cell origin is suspected based on clonal immunoglobulin gene rearrangement. Although first recognized in association with AIDS, cases have also been reported in HIV-negative individuals. Like KS, these tumors always contain HHV-8.

6. HUMAN PAPILLOMAVIRUS

The malignant papillomatous tumors induced in cottontail rabbits by the Shope papillomavirus serve as a valuable model for papillomavirus-associated carcinogenesis (73). The presence of papillomaviruses in humans, or HPV, has been recognized in association with warts of various sites (74,75). Over 70 HPV types have been identified, each sharing less than 90% homology in the nucleotide sequence of specific regions of the genome (E6, E7, and L1 open reading frames) (76). Each type appears to be associated with specific clinical lesions, but not all types are associated with cancer. HPV types strongly associated with cancer are often referred as "high-risk" types (type 16, 18, 31, and 33 among others), while others are classified as "low-risk" types. The genomic DNA of high-risk HPVs can immortalize primary human genital keratinocytes, the normal host cells for the HPVs (77–79). Because of the virus' tropism for squamous epithelial cells, most cancers associated with HPV are of epithelial origin.

6.1. Molecular Biology

HPVs are small, nonenveloped DNA viruses that have a circular double-stranded genome of approximately 8000 bp. Only one DNA strand is transcribed. The HPV genome consists of three distinct sections, the early, late, and long control regions (LCRs). The early region (E) encodes viral proteins involved in viral DNA replication, transcriptional regulation, and cellular transformation. Within this region, the E2 gene encodes a viral regulatory factor that represses the promoter for transcription of the E6 and E7 genes (80,81). The late region (L) encodes the two viral capsid proteins. The LCR, with no apparent open reading frame, contains *cis* elements of the viral genome required for viral DNA replication and gene expression. The HPV genome is generally maintained as an episome in benign precancerous lesions, but integration into the host DNA frequently accompanies carcinogenic progression of these lesions. Viral integration occurs at multiple sites throughout the host genome, although it is unclear whether integration near protooncogenes such as *c-myc* is relevant for oncogenesis.

6.2. Epidemiology and Biomarkers of HPV Infection

HPV infection is common worldwide although seroprevalence varies, ranging from <5% in Europe to nearly 50% in Africa in asymptomatic women with normal Pap smears (82). While less data are available on men, HPV seroprevalence appears to be similar in both sexes. Seroprevalence is higher among younger than older individuals, indicating that the infection may resolve over time.

Although HPV infection in particular tissues (e.g., cervical scrapings) can be detected by the presence of DNA sequences with polymerase chain reaction (PCR) assays, such methods are less suitable than serological assays for large population studies. However, different HPV types generally cannot be distinguished by available serologic assays because of cross reactivity between types, which presents a major challenge for epidemiological studies. A new ELISA assay utilizing HPV-16 virus-like particles (VLPs) is a promising specific approach for detecting HPV-16 infection serologically.

6.3. HPV-Associated Malignancies in Humans

HPVs are found in over 90% of all invasive cervical cancers, the leading cause of cancer death in women in developing countries. Other anogenital cancers (e.g., anal, vulvar, and penile) are also strongly associated with HPV infection. These cancers share similar anatomic features, pathology, and associations with sexual behavior. In addition, HPV is found in some rare types of skin cancer, including cases associated with immune suppression.

In cervical cancer, integration of the HPV genome precedes the clonal outgrowth of the tumor, indicating that the virus plays an essential role in the malignant progression to cancer. Disruption of the E1 or E2 regulatory genes of HPV-16 results in an increased immortalization capacity of the viral genome (81). Not surprisingly, expression of E1 and E2 is frequently absent in HPV-transformed cells, whereas the E6 and E7 genes are selectively retained and highly expressed.

The E6 and E7 protein products act together to immortalize primary human cells (82–84). E6 of high-risk HPV types complexes with the tumor suppressor protein p53 (85), and reduces the steady state levels of p53 (86,87). On the other hand, E7 protein of high-risk HPV interacts with the tumor suppressor protein pRB and related proteins, leading to their destabilization and modulation of the E2F family of transcription factors. Thus, by disrupting a regulatory network, E7 causes overexpression of E2F, which results in cell cycle progression and induced morphological changes. E7 also interacts with the AP-1 family of transcription factors and the cyclin-dependent kinase inhibitors (CKIs) to further disrupt the cell cycle.

7. HEPATITIS B VIRUS AND HEPATITIS C VIRUS

Hepatitis B virus (HBV) was one of the first DNA viruses found to be associated with human cancer. HBV is associated with acute and chronic hepatitis, liver cirrhosis and hepatocellular carcinoma (HCC). Chronic sequelae of HBV infection are highest in carriers who had been infected during childhood (88), while symptoms of acute infection are more likely to manifest in persons who are infected later in life.

The pathogenesis of HCV is distinct from that of HBV in that the former is associated with a variety of systemic autoimmune diseases, such as mixed cryoglobulinemia, in addition to liver disease. While HCV infection alone does not appear to suppress the host's immune response, there is some evidence that HCV infection may compound preexisting cellular immune suppression among persons with HTLV-I infection (89), and may accelerate the progression of liver diseases.

7.1. Molecular Biology

HBV is a partially double-stranded DNA virus and replicates through an RNA intermediate by the use of a reverse transcriptase (90). The HBV genome is circular, 3200 kb in length, and consists of four partially overlapping reading frames. The virus predominantly infects hepatocytes and establishes persistent infection. The virus can integrate into the host DNA, which is an important step in viral oncogenesis, although it is uncertain whether integration occurs in acute infection.

HCV, on the other hand, is a positive-sense, single-stranded RNA virus, without reverse transcriptase. Unlike HBV, the virus does not integrate into the host genome (91). The large single open reading frame encodes a polypeptide precursor of roughly 3000 amino acids. Viral isolates from different geographical regions significantly differ. Multiple subtypes and quasispecies may exist in an individual at the same time.

7.2. Epidemiology and Biomarkers of HBV and HCV Infections

HBV infection can be detected by the presence of surface antigen (HBsAg), envelope antigen (HBeAg) and antibody (HBeAb), and core antibody (HBcAb). High titer ($>2^{12}$) of HBcAb is often reflective of perinatally acquired infection and usually chronic carriage of HBV. Antibody to surface antigen (HBsAb), on the other hand, may result from immunization against HBV, and thus is not a suitable marker of natural infection. The prevalence of HBV varies geographically. The highest rates (>8%) are seen in China, Southeast Asia, and sub-Saharan Africa, while the lowest rates (<2%) are found in western Europe, North and South America, and Australia. Intermediate prevalences (2–8%) are found in eastern and southern Europe, the Middle East, Japan, and south Asia. Perinatal infection will result in chronic carriage of HBV in more than 90% of infected children, while acquisition later in life will result in chronic carriage in only about 10% of infected persons.

HCV infection can be detected by third-generation antibody assays as well as by more sensitive branched DNA- or PCR-based methods. Approximately 0.5–2% of the general population is seropositive for HCV worldwide. In addition, pockets of high prevalence have been reported in Japan, where up to 10–20% of the population is infected (92,93). The major route of transmission appears to be parenteral exposure to contaminated blood and needles (94), although sexual transmission also may play a role (92). It is thought that about 85% of those infected with HCV will develop a persistent infection, although most remain asymptomatic (95).

7.3. HBV- and HCV-Associated Malignancies in Humans

Random integration of HBV could function as a tumor initiator, promoter, and/or progressor in a given patient (96). HBV is thought to cause cancer indirectly through chronic inflammation. The virus may also affect growth-controlling genes at distant sites by transactivation, as is the case with HTLV-I. The protein product of a truncated sequence of the pre-S2/S region of HBV transactivates the *c-myc* promoter in vitro (97). HBV X-protein, on the other hand, increases transcription of *c-fos* and *c-myc* (98) and activates the transcription factor AP-1 through which many oncogenes function (99). HBV X also binds to p53 and blocks p53-mediated apoptosis (100). Mutations of p53 have been found in over 60% of HCC cases, but such mutations are likely a late event that primarily affects cancer progression (101).

The mechanisms by which HCV causes HCC are less understood. This nonintegrating virus is less likely than HBV to serve as an initiator, but rather, indirectly through cirrhosis and inflammation, may function as a promoter in the development of HCC (102). Coinfection with both HCV and HBV may have a synergistic effect on hepatic carcinogenesis (103). In cases of HCV-associated HCC, p53 has been found to be overexpressed only in the less-differentiated area of the tumor, indicating that p53 contributes to dedifferentiation during tumor progression (104). Many HCC cases also have mutations of the *RB* tumor suppressor gene.

7.3.1. Hepatocellular Carcinoma

The association of HBV with HCC was first recognized (105) through detection of HBsAg in sera from HCC patients, and confirmed by many others around the world (96,106,107). HCC cells have multiple integrated copies of the HBV genome, but no common integration site has been identified (108). Early age of infection is an important risk factor for the development of HCC among chronic HBV carriers (109–111). It is estimated that 60% of liver cancer worldwide may be attributable to chronic HBV infection, with the proportion much higher in developing countries than in industrialized nations (112).

It is not known whether cancer risk is age-dependent in the case of HCV-associated HCC. Overall, about one-fourth of liver cancer cases worldwide are estimated to be attributable to HCV (112). Over 70% of HBV-negative HCC cases have anti-HCV antibodies. Seventy to 95% of HCV-seropositive HCC patients also have a detectable level of serum HCV RNA by PCR (113). HCV RNA also is detectable in up to two-thirds of HCV-antibody negative HCC patients (114), indicating that a high proportion of HCC cases in endemic areas may be attributable to HCV. Interestingly, the incidence of HCC in Japan has doubled in the past 25 years, mostly due to HCV-associated cases (115). In endemic areas such as Japan, Greece, and Singapore, the estimated mortality from HCC is approximately 15–25 per 100,000 per year in men, but only 5–7 per 100,000 per year in women (116). The incidence of HCC is much higher in Japanese men (greater than 22 per 100,000) than in Caucasian men in the United States (less than 0.6 per 100,000), although the general population prevalence of HCV is similar (~1%) in the two countries. The reasons for this difference are uncertain, but environmental exposures, such as alcohol and smoking behavior and genetic factors, may each play a role.

8. CONCLUSIONS

Approximately 10–15% of newly diagnosed cancer cases worldwide are estimated to be attributable to infectious agents (112,117,118). The estimated proportion is twice as high in developing countries as compared to that in developed countries (112). These estimated proportions may be on the rise, as new infectious agents of uncertain pathogenesis continue to be identified every year. Furthermore, infectious causes have been speculated for some chronic diseases associated with malignancies, including ulcerative colitis, Crohn's disease, rheumatoid arthritis, sarcoidosis, and multiple sclerosis. These observations raise the possibility that the proportion of cancer attributable to infectious agents may become even higher as the underlying etiologies of these diseases unfold. With the aging trends of the world's population, infectious agents and viruses in particular are increasingly important causes of malignancy.

REFERENCES

1. Bradford Hill A. The environment and disease: association or causation? J R Soc Med 1965; 58:295–300
2. Rothman KJ. Modern Epidemiology. Boston: Little, Brown and Company, 1986.
3. Epstein MA, Achong BG, Barr YM. Virus particles in cultured lymphoblasts from Burkitt's lymphoma. Lancet 1964; 1:702–703.
4. Evans AS, Mueller NE. Viruses and cancer. Causal associations. Ann Epidemiol 1990; 1:71–92.
5. Evans AS. Causation and disease: the Henle–Koch postulates revisited. Yale J Biol Med 1976; 49:175–195.
6. IARC Working Group on the Evaluation of Carcinogenic Risks to Humans; Human Immunodeficiency Viruses and Human T-Cell Lymphotropic Viruses. Lyon, France, 1–18 June 1996. IARC Monogr Eval Carcinog Risks Hum 1996; 67:1–424.
7. De The G, Geser A, Day NE, Tukei PM, Williams EH, Beri DP, Smith PG, Dean AG, Bronkamm GW, Feorino P, Henle W. Epidemiological evidence for causal relationship between Epstein–Barr virus and Burkitt's lymphoma from Ugandan prospective study. Nature 1978; 274:756–761.
8. Geser A, Brubaker G, Drapen CC. Effect of a malaria suppression program on the incidence of African Burkitt's lymphoma. Am J Epidemiol 1989; 129: 740–752.
9. IARC Working Group on the Evaluation of Carcinogenic Risks to Humans. Epstein–Barr Virus and Kaposi's Sarcoma Herpesvirus/Human Herpesvirus 8. Lyon, France, 17–24 June 1997. IARC Monogr Eval Carcinog Risks Hum 1997; 70:1–492.
10. Gutensohn N, Cole P. Childhood social environment and Hodgkin's disease. N Engl J Med 1981; 304:135–140.
11. Yu MC, Huang TB, Henderson BE. Diet and nasopharyngeal carcinoma: a case–control study in Guangzhou, China. Int J Cancer 1989; 43:1077–1082.
12. Poiesz BJ, Ruscetti FW, Gazder AF, Bunn PA, Minna JD, Gallo RC. Detection and isolation of type C retrovirus particles from fresh and cultured lymphocytes of a patient with cutaneous T-cell lymphoma. Proc Natl Acad Sci USA 1980; 77:7415–7419.
13. Yoshida M, Miyoshi I, Hinuma Y. Isolation and characterization of retrovirus from cell lines of human adult T-cell leukemia and its implication in the disease. Proc Natl Acad Sci USA 1982; 79:2031–2035.
14. Nakada K, Yamaguchi K, Furugen S, Nakasone T, Nakasone K, Oshiro Y, Kohakura M, Hinuma Y, Seiki M, Yoshida M, Matutes E, Catovsky D, Ishii T, Takatsuki K. Monoclonal integration of HTLV-I proviral DNA in patients with strongyloidiasis. Int J Cancer 1987; 40:145–148.
15. Plumelle Y, Pascaline N, Nguyen D, Panelatti G, Jouannelle A, Jouault H, Imbert M. Adult T-cell leukemia-lymphoma: a clinico-pathologic study of twenty six patients from Martinique. Haematol Pathol 1993; 7:241–262.
16. Cann AJ, Chen ISY. Human T-cell leukemia virus types I and II. In: Fields BN, Knipe DM, Howley PM, eds. Fields Virology. 3d ed. Philadelphia: Lippincott-Raven, 1996.

17. Blattner WA, Saxinger C, Riedel D, Hull B, Taylor G, Cleghorn F, Gallo R, Blumberg B, Bartholomew C. A study of HTLV-I and its associated risk factors in Trinidad and Tobago. J Acquir Immune Defic Syndr 1990; 3:1102–1108.

18. Murphy EL, Figueroa JP, Gibbs WN, Holding-Cobham M, Cranston B, Malley K, Bodner AJ, Alexander SS, Blattner WA. Human T-lymphotropic virus type I (HTLV-I) seroprevalence in Jamaica. I: demographic determinants. Am J Epidemiol 1991; 133:1114–1124.

19. Mueller N, Okayama A, Stuver S, Tachibana N. Findings from the Miyazaki cohort study. J Acquir Immune Defic Syndr Hum Retrovirol 1996; 13(suppl 1):S2–S7.

20. Iwata Ito S, Saito H, Ito M, Nagatomo M, Yamasaki T, Yoshida S, Suto H, Tajima K. Mortality among inhabitants of an HTLV-I endemic area in Japan. Jpn J Cancer Res 1994; 85:231–237.

21. Hino S, Yamaguchi K, Katamine S, Sugiyama H, Amagasaki T, Kinoshita K, Yoshida Y, Doi H, Tsuji Y, Miyamoto T. Mother-to-child transmission of human T-cell lymphotropic virus type I associated with prolonged breast-feeding. Jpn J Cancer Res (Gann) 1985; 76:474–480.

22. Tajima K, Hinuma Y. Epidemiology of HTLV-I/II in Japan and the world. In: Takatsuki K, Hinuma Y, Yoshida M, eds. Gann Monograph on Cancer Research. Vol. 39. Tokyo: Japan Scientific Societies Press, 1992:129–147.

23. Stuver SO, Tachibana N, Okayama A, Shioiri S, Tsunetoshi Y, Tsuda K, Mueller NE. Heterosexual transmission of human T cell leukemia/lymphoma lymphoma virus type I among married couples in southwestern Japan: an initial report from the Miyazaki cohort study. J Infect Dis 1993; 167:57–65.

24. Manns A, Wilks RJ, Murphy EL, Haynes G, Figueroa JP, Barnett M, Hanchard B, Blattner WA. A prospective study of transmission by transfusion of HTLV-I and risk factors associated with seroconversion. Int J Cancer 1992; 51:886–891.

25. Ureta-Vidal A, Angelin-Duclos C, Tortevoye P, Murphy E, Lepere JF, Buigues RP, Jolly N, Joubert M, Carles G, Pouliquen JF, de The G, Moreau JP, Gessain A. Mother-to-child transmission of human T-cell-leukemia/lymphoma virus type I: implication of high antiviral antibody titer and high proviral load in carrier mothers. Int J Cancer 1999; 82:832–836.

26. Yamaguchi K, Seiki M, Yoshida M, Nishimura H, Kawano F, Takatsuki K. The detection of human T-cell leukemia virus proviral DNA and its application for classification and diagnosis of T-cell malignancy. Blood 1984; 63:1235–1240.

27. Hisada M, Okayama A, Shioiri S, Spiegelman DL, Stuver SO, Mueller NE. Risk factor for adultT-cell leukemia among carriers of human T-lymphotropic virus type I. Blood 1998; 92:3557–3561.

28. Yokota T, Cho MJ, Tachibana N, McLane MF, Takatsuki K, Lee TH, Mueller N, Essex M. The prevalence of antibody to p42 of HTLV-I among ATLL patients in comparison to healthy carriers in Japan. Int J Cancer 1989; 43:970–974.

29. Higashiyama Y, Katamine S, Kohno S, Mukae H, Hino S, Miyamoto T, Hara K. Expression of human T lymphotropic virus type 1 (HTLV-1) tax/rex gene

in fresh bronchoalveolar lavage cells of HTLV-1-infected individuals. Clin Exp Immunol 1994; 96:193–201.

30. Furukawa Y, Osame M, Kubota R, Tara M, Yoshida M. Human T-cell leukemia virus type-1 (HTLV-1) Tax is expressed at the same level in infected cells of HTLV-1-associated myelopathy or tropical spastic paraparesis patients as in asymptomatic carriers but at a lower level in adult T-cell leukemia. Blood 1995; 85:1865–1870.

31. Etoh K, Yamaguchi K, Tokudome S, Watanabe T, Okayama A, Stuver S, Mueller N, Takatsuki K, Matsuoka M. Rapid quantification of HTLV-I provirus load: detection of monoclonal proliferation of HTLV-I-infected cells among carriers. Int J Cancer 1999; 81:859–864.

32. Tachibana N, Okayama A, Ishihara S, Shioiri S, Murai K, Tsuda K, Goya N, Matsuo Y, Essex M, Stuver S, Mueller N. High HTLV-I proviral DNA level associated with abnormal lymphocytes in peripheral blood from asymptomatic carriers. Int J Cancer 1992; 51:593–595.

33. Hisada M, Okayama A, Tachibana N, Stuver SO, Spiegelman DL, Tsubouchi H, Mueller NE. Predictors of level of circulating abnormal lymphocytes among human T-lymphotropic virus type I carriers in Japan. Int J Cancer 1998; 77:188–192.

34. Sonoda S, Fujiyoshi T, Yashiki S. Immunogenetics of HTLV-I/II and associated diseases. J Acquir Immune Defic Syndr Hum Retrovirol 1996; 13(suppl 1):S119–S123.

35. Manns A, Hanchard B, Morgan OSC, Wilks R, Cranston B, Nam JM, Blank M, Kuwayama M, Yashiki S, Fujiyoshi T, Blatmer W, Sonoda S. Human leukocyte antigen class II alleles associated with human T-cell lymphotropic virus type I infection and adult T-cell leukemia/lymphoma in a black population. J Natl Cancer Inst 1998; 90:617–622.

36. Buckle GJ, Hafler DA, Hollsberg P. HTLV-I-induced T-cell activation. J Acquir Immune Defic Syndr Hum Retrovirol 1996; 13(suppl 1):S107–S113.

37. Yoshida M. Molecular biology of HTLV-I: recent progress. J Acquir Immune Defic Syndr Hum Retrovirol 1996; 13(suppl 1):S63–S68.

38. Rosen C, Park R, Sodroski J, Haseltine WA. Multiple sequence elements are required for regulation of human T-cell leukemia virus gene expression. Proc Natl Acad Sci USA 1987; 84:4919–4923.

39. Seiki M, Inoue, J, Hidaka M, Yoshida M. Two cis-acting elements responsible for posttranscriptional trans-regulation of gene expression of human T-cell leukemia virus type I. Proc Natl Acad Sci USA 1988; 85:7124–7128.

40. Franchini G. Molecular mechanisms of human T-cell leukemia/lymphotropic virus type I infection. Blood 1995; 86:3619–3639.

41. Yoshida M. HTLV-1 oncoprotein Tax deregulates transcription of cellular genes through multiple mechanisms. J Cancer Res Clin Oncol 1995; 121:521–528.

42. Pise-Masison CA, Radonovich M, Sakaguchi K, Appella E, Brady JN. Phosphorylation of p53: a novel pathway for p53 inactivation in human T0 cell lymphotropic virus type 1-transformed cells. J Virol 1998; 72:6348–6355.

43. Pise-Masison CA, Choi KS, Radonovich M, Dittmer J, Kim SJ, Brady JN. Inhibition of p53 transactivation function by the human T-cell leymphotropic virus type 1 tax protein. J Virol 1998; 72:1165–1170.

44. Philpott SM, Buehring GC. Defective DNA repair in cells with human T-cell leukemia/bovine leukemia viruses: role of tax gene. J Natl Cancer Inst 1999; 91:933–942.
45. Miyake H, Suzuki T, Hirai H, Yoshida M. Trans-activator tax of human T-cell leukemia virus type 1 enhances mutation frequency of the cellular genome. Virology 1999; 253:155–161.
46. Jacobson S, Shida H, McFarlin DE, Fauci AS, Koenig S. Circulating CD8+ cytotoxic T lymphocytes specific for HTLV-I pX in patients with HTLV-I associated neurological disease. Nature 1990; 348:245–248.
47. Kannagi M, Matsushita S, Harada S. Expression of the target antigen for cytotoxic T lymphocytes on adult T-cell-leukemia cells. Int J Cancer 1993; 54: 582–588.
48. Niewiesk S, Daenke S, Parker C, Taylor G, Weber J, Nightingale S, Bangham CR. Naturally occurring variants of human T-cell leukemia virus type I Tax protein impair its recognition by cytotoxic T-lymphocytes and the transactivation of Tax. J Virol 1995; 69:2649–2653.
49. Koralnik I, Gessain A, Klotman M, Lo Monico A, Berneman ZN, Franchini G. Protein isoforms encoded by the pX region of human T-cell leukemia/lymphotropic virus type I. Proc Natl Acad Sci USA 1992; 89:8813–8817.
50. Franchini G, Wong-Staal F, Gallo RC. Human T-cell leukemia virus (HTLV-I) transcripts in fresh and cultured cells of patients with adult T-cell leukemia. Proc Natl Acad Sci USA 1984; 81:6207–6211.
51. Uchiyama T, Yodoi J, Sagawa K, Takatsuki K, Uchino H. Adult T-cell leukemia: clinical and hematologic features of 16 cases. Blood 1977;50: 481–492.
52. Korber B, Okayama A, Donnelly R, Tachibana N, Essex M. Polymerase chain reaction analysis of defective human T-cell leukemia virus type I proviral genomes in leukemic cells of patients with adult T-cell leukemia. J Virol 1991; 65:5471–5476.
53. Yamaguchi K, Kiyokawa T, Nakada K, Yul LS, Asou N, Ishii T, Sanada I, Seiki M, Yoshida M, Matutes E, Catovsky D, Takatsuki, Polyclonal integration of HTLV-I proviral DNA in lymphocytes from HTLV-I seropositive individuals: an intermediate state between the healthy carrier state and smouldering ATL. Br J Haematol 1988; 68:169–174.
54. Kondo T, Kono H, Miyamoto N, Yoshida R, Toki H, Matsumoto I, Hara M, Inoue H, Inatsuki A, Funatsu T, Yamano N, Bando F, Iwao Em Miyoshi I, Hinuma Y, Hanaoka M. Age-, and sex-specific cumulative rate and risk of ATLL for HTLV-I carriers. Int J Cancer 1989; 43:1061–1064.
55. Cleghorn FR, Manns A, Falk R, Hartge P, Hanchard B, Jack N. Williams E, Jaffe E, White F, Bartholomew C. Effect of human T-ymphotropic virus type I infection on non-Hodgkin'slymphoma incidence. J Natl Cancer Inst 1995; 87:1009–1014.
56. Shimoyama M. and the Members of the Lymphoma Study Group (1984–1987). Diagnostic criteria and classification of clinical subtypes of adult T-cell leukemia-lymphoma. Br J Haematol 1991; 79:428–437.
57. Lorincz AL. Cutaneous T-cell lymphoma (mycosis fungoides). Lancet 1996; 347:871–876.

58. Posner LE, Robert-Guroff M, Kalyanaraman VS, Poiesz BJ, Ruscetti FW, Fossieck B, Bunn PA Jr, Minna JD, Gallo RC. Natural antibodies to the human T cell lymphoma virus in patients with cutaneous T cell lymphomas. J Exp Med 1981; 154:333–346.

59. Hall WW, Liu CR, Schneewind H, Takahashi H, Kaplan MH, Roupe G, Vahlne A. Deleted HTLV-I provirus in blood and cutaneous lesions of patients with mycosis fungoides. Science 1991; 253:317–320.

60. Zucker-Franklin D, Coutavas EE, Rush MG, Zouzias DC. Detection of human T-lymphotropic virus-like particles in cultures of peripheral blood lymphocytes from patients with mycosis fungoides. Proc Natl Acad Sci USA 1991; 88:7630–7634.

61. Wood G, Savekar A, Schaffer J, Crooks CF, Henghold W, Fivenson DP, Kim YH, Smoller BR. Evidence against a role for HTLV-I in the pathogenesis of American cutaneous T-cell lymphoma. J Invest Dermatol 1996; 107:301–307.

62. Li G, Vowels B, Benoit B, Rook AH, Lessin SR. Failure to detect humanT-lymphotropic virus type-I proviral DNA in cell lines and tissues from patients with cutaneous T-cell lymphoma. J Invest Dermatol 1996; 107:308–313.

63. Barre-Sinoussi F, Chermann JC, Rey F, Nugeyre MT, Chamaret S, Gruest J, Dauguet C, Axler-Blin C, Vezinet-Brun F, Rouzioux C, Rozenbaum W, Montagnier L. Isolation of a T-lymphotropic retrovirus from a patient at risk for acquired immune deficiency syndrome (AIDS). Science 1983; 220:868–871.

64. Gallo RC, Salahuddin SZ, Popovic M, Shearer GM, Kaplan M, Haynes BF, Palker TJ, Redfield R, Oleske J, Safai B. Frequent detection and isolation of cytopathic retroviruses (HTLV-III) from patients with AIDS and at risk for AIDS. Science 1984; 224:500–503.

65. Clavel F, Guetard D, Brun-Vezinet F, Chamaret S, Rey MA, Santos-Ferreira MO, Laurent AG, Dauguet C, Katlama C, Rouzioux C, Klatzmann D, Champalimaud JL, Montagnier L. Isolation of a new human retrovirus from West African patients with AIDS. Science 1986; 233:343–346.

66. Weiss SH, Goedert JJ, Sarngadharan MG, Bodner AJ, Gallo RC, Blattner WA. Screening test for HTLV-III (AIDS agent) antibodies. Specificity, sensitivity, and applications. JAMA 1985; 253:221–225.

67. Goedert JJ, Sarngadharan MG, Biggar RJ, Weiss SH, Winn DM, Grossman RJ, Greene MH, Bodner AJ, Mann DL, Strong DM. Determinants of retrovirus (HTLV-III) antibody and immunodeficiency conditions in homosexual men. Lancet 1984; 2:711–716.

68. Jaffe HW, Darrow WW, Echenberg DF, O'Malley PM, Getchell JP, Kalyanaraman VS, Byers RH, Drennan DP, Braff EH, Curran JW. The acquired immunodeficiency syndrome in a cohort of homosexual men. A six-year follow-up study. Ann Intern Med 1985; 103:210–214.

69. van Griensven GJ, de Vroome EM, Goudsmit J, Coutinho RA. Changes in sexual behaviour and the fall in incidence of HIV infection among homosexual men. Br Med J 1989; 298:218–221.

70. Beral V, Peterman TA, Berkelman RL, Jaffe HW. KS among persons with AIDS: a sexually transmitted infection? Lancet 1990; 335:123–128.

71. Granovsky MO, Mueller BU, Nicholson HS, Rosenberg PS, Rabkin CS. Cancer in human immunodeficiency virus-infected children: a case series from the

Children's Cancer Group and the National Cancer Institute. J Clin Oncol 1998; 16:1729–1735.

72. Whitby D, Howard MR, Tenant-Flowers M, Brink NS, Copas A, Boshoff C, Hatzioannou T, Suggett FE, Aldam DM, Denton AS. Detection of Kaposi sarcoma associated herpesvirus in peripheral blood of HIV-infected individuals and progression to Kaposi's sarcoma. Lancet 1995; 346:799–802.

73. Shope RE, Hurst EW. Infectious papillomatosis of rabbits; with a note on the histopathology. J Exp Med 1933; 58:607–624.

74. Ciuffo G. Innesto positivo confiltrato di verruca vulgare. G Ital Mal Venereol 1907; 48:12–17.

75. Rowson KEK, Mahy WJ. Human papova (wart) virus. Bacterio Rev 1967; 31:110–131.

76. Delius H, Hofmann B. Primer-directed sequencing of human papillomavirus types. Curr Top Microbiol Immunol 1994; 186:13–32.

77. Baker CC, Phelps WC, Lindgren V, Braun MJ, Gonda MA. Structural and transcriptional analysis of human papillomavirus type 16 sequences in cervical carcinoma cell lines. J Virol 1987; 61:962–971.

78. Schlegel R, Phelps WC, Zhang YL, Barbosa M. Quantitative keratinocyte assay detects two biological activities of human papillomavirus DNA and identifies viral types associated with cervical carcinoma. EMBO J 1988; 7: 3181–3187.

79. Woodworth CD, Bowden PE, Doninger J, Pirisi L, Barnes W, Lancaster WD, Dipaolo JA. Characterization of normal human exocervical epithelial cells immortalized in vitro by papillomavirus type 16 and 18 DNA. Cancer Res 1998; 48:4620–4628.

80. Thierry F, Yaniv M. The BPV1 E2 trans-acting protein can be either an activator or a repressor of the HPV18 regulatory region. EMBO J 1987; 6: 3391–3397.

81. Romanczuk H, Howley PM. Disruption of either the E1 or the E2 regulatory gene of human papillomavirus type 16 increases viral immortalization capacity. Proc Natl Acad Sci USA 1992; 89:3159–3163.

82. IARC Working Group on the Evaluation of Carcinogenic Risks to Humans: Human Papillomaviruses. Lyon, France, 6–13 June 1995. IARC Monogr Eval Carcinog Risks Hum 1995; 64:1–378.

83. Hawley-Nelson P, Vousden KH, Hubbert NL, Lowy DR, Schiller JT. HPV16 E6 and E7 proteins cooperate to immortalize human foreskin keratinocytes. EMBO J 1989; 8:3905–3910.

84. Muenger K, Phelps WC, Bubb V, Howley PM, Schlegel R. The E6 and E7 genes of the human papillomavirus type 16 together are necessary and sufficient for transformation of primary human keratinocytes. J Virol 1989; 63: 4417–4421.

85. Werness BA, Levine AJ, Howley PM. Association of human papillomavirus types 16 and 18 E6 proteins with p53. Science 1990; 248:76–79.

86. Hubbert NL, Sedman SA, Schiller JT. Human papillomavirus type 16 E6 increases the degradation rate of p53 in human keratinocytes. J Virol 1992; 66:6237–6241.

87. Scheffner M, Munger K, Byrne JC, Howley PM. The state of the p53 and retinoblastoma genes in human cervical carcinoma cell lines. Proc Natl Acad Sci USA 1991; 88:5523–5527.

88. Beasley RP, Hwang LY, Lin CC, Chien CS. Hepatocellular carcinoma and hepatitis B virus. A prospective study of 22 707 men in Taiwan. Lancet 1981; 2:1129–1133.

89. Hisada M, Shima T, Okayama A, Mueller N, Tsubouchi H, Stuver S. Suppression of skin reactivity to purified protein derivative by hepatitis C virus among HTLV-I carriers in Japan. J Acquir Immune Defic Syndr Hum Retrovirol 1998; 19:421–425.

90. IARC Working Group on the Evaluation of Carcinogenic Risks to Humans. Hepatitis Viruses. Lyon, France, 8–15 June 1993. IARC Monogr Eval Carcinog Risks Hum 1994; 59:1–255.

91. Tabor E. Hepatitis C virus and hepatocellular carcinoma. AIDS Res Hum Retroviruses 1992; 8:793–796.

92. Tanaka K, Stuver SO, Ikematsu H, Okayama A, Tachibana N, Hirohata T, Kashiwagi S, Tsubouchi H, Mueller NE. Heterosexual transmission of hepatitis C virus among married couples in southwestern Japan. Int J Cancer 1997; 72:50–55.

93. Nakashima K, Ikematsu H, Hayashi J, Kishihara Y, Mitsutake A, Kashiwagi S. Intrafamilial transmission of hepatitis C virus among the population of an endemic area of Japan. JAMA 1995; 274:1459–1461.

94. Alter MJ. Epidemiology of hepatitis C. Eur J Gastroenterol Hepatol 1996; 8: 319–323.

95. Alter HJ. To C or not to C: these are the questions. Blood 1995; 85:1681–1685.

96. Trichopoulos D, Tabor E, Gerety RJ, Xirouchaki E, Sparros L, Munoz N, Linsell CA. Hepatitis B and primary hepatocellular carcinoma in a European population. Lancet 1978; ii:1217–1219.

97. Kekule AS, Lauer U, Meyer M, Caselmann WH, Hofschneider PH, Koshy R. The preS2/S region of integrated hepatitis B virus DNA encodes a transcriptional transactivator. Nature 1990; 343:457–461.

98. Balsano C, Avantaggiati ML, Natoli G. Transactivation of c-*fos* and c-*myc* protooncogenes by both full-length and truncated versions of the HBV-X protein. In: Hollinger FB, Lemon SM, Margolis H, eds. Viral Hepatitis and Liver Disease. Baltimore: Williams & Wilkins, 1991:572–576.

99. Kekule AS, Lauer U, Weiss L, Hofschneider PH, Koshy R. Trans-activation by hepatitis B virus X protein is mediated via a tumor promoter pathway. Arch Virol (suppl.) 1992; 4:63–64.

100. Wang XW, Gibson MK, Vermeulen W, Yeh H, Forrester K, Sturzbecher HW, Hoeijmakers JH, Harris CC. Abrogation of p53-induced apoptosis by the hepatitis B virus X gene. Cancer Res 1995; 55:6012–6016.

101. Tabor E. Tumor suppressor genes, growth factor genes, and oncogenes in hepatitis B virus-associated hepatocellular carcinoma. J Med Virol 1994; 42: 357–365.

102. Tabor E. Viral hepatitis and liver cancer. In: Goldin RD, Thomas HC, Gerber MA, eds. Pathology of Viral Hepatitis. London: Arnold, 1998:161–177.

103. Donato F, Boffetta P, Puoti M. A meta-analysis of epidemiologic studies on the combined effect of hepatitis B and C virus infections in causing hepatocellular carcinoma. Int J Cancer 1998; 75:347–354.
104. Nakashima Y, Hsia CC, Yuwen H, Minemura M, Nakashima O, Kojiro M, Tabor E. P53 overexpression in small hepatocellular carcinomas containing two different histologic grades. Int J Oncol 1997; 12:455–459.
105. Sherlock S, Fox RA, Niazi SP, Scheuer PJ. Chronic liver disease and primary liver-cell cancer with hepatitis-associated (Australia) antigen in serum. Lancet 1970; i:1243–1247.
106. Tabor E, Gerety RJ, Vogel CL, Bayley AC, Anthony PP, Chan CH, Barker LF. Hepatitis B virus infection and primary hepatocellular carcinoma. J Natl Cancer Inst 1977; 58:1197–1200.
107. Yarrish RL, Werner BG, Blumberg BS. Association of hepatitis B virus infection with hepatocellular carcinoma in American patients. Int J Cancer 1980; 26:711–715.
108. Harrison TJ, Lin Y, Stamps, AC, Dusheiko GM, Zuckerman AJ. Hepatitis B virus-associated hepatocellular carcinoma in African patients. Cancer Detect Prev 1990; 14:457–460.
109. Higginson J. The geographical pathology of primary liver cancer. Cancer Res 1963; 23:1624–1633.
110. Heyward WL, Bender TR, Lanier AP, Francis DP, McMahon BJ, Maynard JE. Serological markers of hepatitis B virus and alpha-fetoprotein levels preceding primary hepatocellular carcinoma in Alaskan Eskimos. Lancet 1982; ii:889–891.
111. Norman JE, Beebe GW, Hoofnagle JH, Seeff LB. Mortality follow-up of the 1942 epidemic of hepatitis B in the U.S. Army. Hepatology 1993; 18:790–879.
112. Pisani P, Parkin DM, Munoz N, Ferlay J. Cancer and infection: estimates of the attributable fraction in 1990. Cancer Epidemiol Biomarkers Prev 1997; 6: 387–400.
113. Tabor E, Kobayashi K. Commentary: hepatitis C virus, a causative infectious agent of non-A, non-B hepatitis: prevalence and structure. Summary of a conference on hepatitis C virus as a cause of hepatocellular carcinoma. J Natl Cancer Inst 1992; 84:86–90.
114. Park YM, Yoon SK, Chung KW, Kim BS. Detection of HCV RNA using reverse transcription and nested polymerase chain reaction in chronic non-A, non-B liver diseases in Korea. Gastroenterol Jpn 1993; 28(suppl 5):12–16.
115. Nishioka K, Watanabe J, Furuta S, Tanaka E, Iino S, Suzuki H, Tsuji T, Yano M, Kuo G, Choo QL, Houghton M, Oda T. A high prevalence of antibody to the hepatitis C virus in patients with hepatocellular carcinoma in Japan. Cancer 1991; 67:429–433.
116. Bosch FX, Munoz N. Hepatocellular carcinoma in the world: epidemiologic questions. In: Tabor E, Di Disceglie AM, Purcell RH, eds. Etiology, Pathology, and Treatment of Hepatocellular Carcinoma in North America. The Woodlands, TX: Portfolio, 1991:35–54.
117. zur Hausen H. Viruses in human cancers. Science 1991; 254:1167–1173.
118. Parkin DM, Stjernsward J, Muir CS. Estimates of the worldwide frequency of twelve major cancers. Bull World Health Organ 1984; 62:163–182.

13

Uncertainty in the Estimation of Radiation-Related Cancer Risk

Charles E. Land

Radiation Epidemiology Branch, Division of Cancer Epidemiology and Genetics, National Cancer Institute, Bethesda, Maryland, U.S.A.

1. OVERVIEW

Ionizing radiation is an established and well-quantified cancer risk factor, based on a large body of experimental and epidemiological studies. The application of quantitative estimates of radiation-related risk must take into account a number of differences between the exposures and populations on which the estimates are based and those exposures and populations of immediate interest. This problem is discussed in the context of quantitative uncertainty analysis, a method that is increasingly being applied to areas related to radiation risk protection, and relies on the recent work of several expert committees involved in issues of radiation protection. Particular issues discussed are uncertainties and biases associated with dose reconstruction error in studied populations, transfer of estimates between populations with different baseline cancer rates, low-dose extrapolation of risk estimates, and projection to different qualities of radiation. Depending on the application, taking account of these and other uncertainties can substantially change estimates of risk and their associated uncertainties.

2. INTRODUCTION

A history of exposure to ionizing radiation is an established human cancer risk factor in the sense that, for cancer sites making up the majority of the human cancer burden, there is solid scientific evidence of increased risk associated with high levels of exposure. Some level of exposure to ionizing radiation is unavoidable, e.g., from natural background, and there are undeniable benefits associated with many medical and industrial uses of radiation. The human evidence on risk is based on epidemiological studies of populations exposed for medical and occupational reasons and, especially, on follow-up studies of a large cohort of atomic bomb survivors from Hiroshima and Nagasaki, Japan. There is also a substantial body of research in experimental radiobiology. The experimental evidence is particularly informative about variation in effect as a function of the amount and quality of radiation energy deposited in tissue and its distribution in time and space, and as a function of time following exposure, for different animal models. Although radiation-related cancer risk is among the most comprehensively documented risks associated with a common environmental carcinogen, estimates are subject to considerable uncertainty, which must be taken into account in any activity where radiation-related risk is a consideration. Some of this uncertainty is observational in nature and can be quantified on the basis of statistical data analyses. However, the analyses are usually conditional upon assumptions that are themselves uncertain. Quantitative uncertainty analysis involves an assessment of all the uncertainties involved in risk estimation, many of which may require subjective input based on expert judgment, and the cumulative effect of all these uncertainties on estimated risk and its policy implications. A more detailed discussion of this methodology as applied to radiation-related risk can be found in reports of the National Council on Radiation Protection and Measurement (NCRP) (1,2) the Environmental Protection Agency (3), the Colorado State Health Department (4), and the National Cancer Institute (NCI) and Centers for disease Control and Prevention (CDC) (5). The present paper illustrates some, but not all, of the uncertain factors that need to be taken into account when applying our knowledge of ionizing radiation effects to radiation protection and informed consent.

3. IONIZING RADIATION

The term "radiation" covers the electromagnetic spectrum, which includes static fields like the earth's magnetic field, fields generated by 50- or 60-cycle alternating currents, radio waves, microwaves, infrared, visible, and ultraviolet (UV) light, and ionizing radiation, which has the highest frequencies and energies. It is well established that exposure to the more energetic wavelengths, like UV light and ionizing radiation, is associated with increased risk of cancer at certain sites. Ionizing radiation is sufficiently energetic to remove electrons from atoms, creating ions that are highly reactive with other molecules, and thus may weaken or disrupt chemical bonds. If that disruption occurs in the genetical material of a somatic cell, and is not properly repaired, a possible outcome is a mutation that may contribute to the process of carcinogenesis. A more usual outcome is cell death, which is why ionizing radiation is used successfully to treat some kinds of cancer.

Radiation dose, corresponding to the amount of energy absorbed per unit volume of tissue, is expressed in units of gray (Gy). However, some types of radiation, such as neutrons and alpha particles, produce patterns of ionizing events that are more dense, and therefore more likely to cause lasting damage, than more sparsely ionizing forms of radiation such as x rays and gamma rays. The concept of "dose equivalent," expressed in sieverts (Sv), was introduced to facilitate comparison of exposures involving different types of ionizing radiation, alone or mixed, in terms of likely biological effect.

Ionizing radiation is ubiquitous and cannot be avoided altogether, but exposure is to some extent controllable. All of us are exposed, all of the time, to cosmic rays from the sun and stars, terrestrial radiation from rocks, soil, and building materials, naturally occurring radioactive isotopes incorporated in our tissues (mainly potassium and carbon), and, by inhalation, radon and its decay products (Table 1). Radon itself results from the decay of radium in the soil and accumulates inside buildings and other closed spaces, especially if ventilation is poor. Levels of environmental radiation depend on altitude, geology, and how we construct our dwellings. For most organs, the average yearly environmental dose equivalent* is about 1 mSv; for the lung it is about 15 times as high due to alpha radiation from inhaled radon and its decay products (6).

Ionizing radiation is used extensively in medicine, for imaging and therapy. On the average, annual doses from diagnostic x ray are comparable to natural background radiation (Table 2) (7) Chest x-ray doses are very low, and breast tissue dose from a two-view film-screen mammography is somewhat higher than annual background. Therapeutic radiation, on the other hand, can reach dose levels thousands to tens of thousands of times higher than those from natural background to affected tissues, and can pose substantial risks of treatment-related cancer occurring years afterward. The trade-off is a chance of survival from the current cancer or disease, in

---

* "Dose" of ionizing radiation expresses the energy absorbed per unit volume of tissue. "Dose equivalent" is used when different types of ionizing radiation are quantified on a common scale in terms of biological effectiveness. Thus, in the present discussion, a dose of 100 mGy of neutrons is assumed to have the same carcinogenic effectiveness as 1000 mGy of gamma ray; both therefore correspond to a dose equivalent of 1000 mSv. In the present discussion, dose when expressed in millisieverts should be understood to mean dose equivalent.

Table 1 Annual Average Exposure to Ionizing Radiation from the Environment

Source	Average yearly dose equivalent (mSv)
Cosmic rays	0.3–0.5, depending on altitude
Rocks and soil	0.15–1.4
Naturally occurring radionuclides in the body	0.4
Inhaled radionuclides (radon, thoron, and their decay products)	15, to the lung

exchange for the possibility that, if successful, the treatment may produce another cancer later. That trade-off is also associated with treatment modalities other than radiation. Collimation, shielding, fractionation of exposure, and other protective measures often can be used to reduce subsequent risk without compromising on the therapeutic benefit.

3.1. Evaluation of Risk

Ionizing radiation is a proven and well-quantified cancer risk factor, but there is variation by organ site and histological subtype. The primary basis for risk assessment is epidemiological data from exposed populations. These include patient populations exposed to therapeutic and diagnostic radiation, occupationally defined cohorts like radiologists, uranium miners, and nuclear industry workers, and (notably) survivors of the atomic bombings of Hiroshima and Nagasaki, Japan. The last group is particularly important because it is a representative Japanese urban population in 1945, unselected for disease, and exposed at the same instant to acute doses of mixed gamma

Table 2 Organ-Specific Radiation Dose (X-ray) from Common Radiological Examinations

Examination	Dose (mGy)
Cervical spine	0.2
Lumbar spine	1.27
Upper gastrointestinal	2.44
Abdomen	0.56
Pelvis	0.44
Skull	0.22
Chest	0.08
Film screen mammogram, two films, with grid (breast dose)	2.7

and neutron radiation ranging from near zero to near lethal levels. Moreover, the population has been followed over time since 1950 for mortality at the level of death certificate diagnosis (8) and since 1958 for cancer morbidity as monitored by high-quality tumor registries in Hiroshima and Nagasaki (9,10). Evaluation of these data is influenced by a large body of experimental research in radiation biology.

The most informative data pertain to observations of cancer risk following exposure to radiation doses in the range 0.2–5 Gy (or neutron-weighted dose from mixed gamma–neutron radiation in the range 0.2–5 Sv), because at such levels the radiation-related excess risk can often (but not always) be distinguished statistically from the normal random variation in baseline cancer risk. Above 5 Gy (5 Sv), acute, whole-body exposures are usually lethal, whereas below 0.1 Sv, inferences may be severely constrained by lack of statistical power and by possible confounding from unknown or uncontrolled risk factors whose carcinogenic influences may be greater than those of low-dose radiation exposure. Moreover, radiation protection procedures already limit exposure [current International Commission on Radiation Protection (ICRP) recommendations (11) are no more than 20 mSv/year from occupational exposures and 2 mSv/year to the general public], and nontherapeutic exposures greater than 0.1 Sv are extremely rare in the general population. Thus, except for accidents and for medical procedures, the more controversial applications of risk estimates are to exposures that are considerably lower than those at which risk can be estimated directly.

Cancer risk can be expressed in absolute terms, as a rate or excess rate (e.g., cases per 10^5 persons per year), or in relative terms as a multiple of the baseline cancer rate. Figure 1 shows estimates of relative risk (RR) for solid cancer morbidity (all cancers except leukemia) during 1958–1987 among, members of the Life Span Study (LSS) population of atomic bomb survivors of both sexes and all ages combined, by interval of neutron-weighted whole-body dose (colon dose is assumed here to represent average dose to all tissues combined). Weighted dose is expressed in sieverts and reflects a 10-fold weight assigned to dose from neutrons compared to gamma rays, originally expressed in grays. Figure 1 also shows a fitted linear dose–response function with 90% confidence limits and a fitted quadratic function of dose which suggests a sub-linear dose–response at high dose levels ($p < 0.07$). The values in Figs. 1 and 2 were computed by the present author from LSS tumor registry data available from the Radiation Effects Research Foundation (RERF) website (12), using the AMFIT algorithm of the EPICURE statistical package (13).

Figure 2 illustrates the effect of fitting successive linear dose–responses based on data sets from which the higher-dose data have been progressively trimmed. Trimming observations at doses above 3 Sv increased the linear-model estimate, but there was no major change, except for a gradual widening of confidence bounds, until all the data above 0.2 Sv had been trimmed. The two estimates on the left, representing observations at 0–50 and

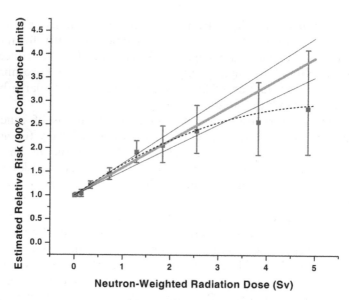

Figure 1 Dose-specific relative risk estimates, with dose <5 mSv as the referent. Exposed members of the RERF Life-Span Study population, all solid cancers combined. Error bars correspond to 90% confidence limits. The solid lines represent a fitted linear dose–response with 90% confidence limits; the dashed line represents a fitted quadratic dose–response function that does not fit significantly better than the linear dose–response ($p = 0.07$).

0–0.2 Sv, respectively, are substantially lower than the estimates based on higher-dose data, but the confidence limits of these estimates are very wide, and there is no lack of statistical consistency among the estimates. Excess risk clearly is proportional to dose over a wide dose range, and there is no clear *epidemiological or statistical* reason (although there may be other reasons) why the fitted, linear dose–response should not hold at lower as well as higher doses.

3.1.1. Statistical Evidence Concerning Radiation-Related Excess Risk

Cancer risk among atomic bomb survivors increases significantly with increasing radiation dose. This statement implies, and is implied by, the observation that the lower confidence bound for the fitted linear dose–response curve in Figure 1 increases with increasing dose. Another way of putting it is that it is unlikely that radiation exposure among atomic bomb survivors is *not* associated with increased cancer risk. The lower confidence bound on the dose–response in Figure 1 implies more than statistical significance. It also implies, for example, that a dose-related excess relative risk (ERR) less than 0.5 at 1 Sv is unlikely. Similarly, the upper confidence

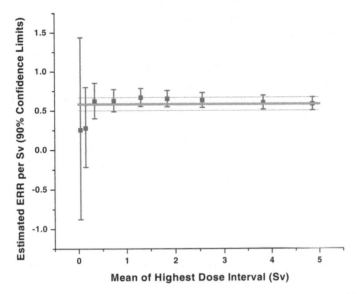

Figure 2 Effect on estimated dose–response of successively censoring high-dose data. The horizontal lines and the rightmost data point with error bars represent the slope of the fitted linear-model dose–response (excess relative risk per sievert, or ERR/Sv) in Fig. 1. The next data point to the left represents the slope based on data with doses in the 0–4.5 Sv range, the next 0–3 Sv, and so on.

bound implies that it is unlikely that the ERR at 1 Sv is greater than 0.7. If one should wish to argue that a certain radiation dose is "unsafe," in the sense that the risk is greater than some agreed, "tolerable" limit, an argument based on the lower confidence bound (e.g., "the lifetime cancer risk associated with a 0.1 Sv exposure is unlikely to be less than 2 per 100 exposed persons") would have more logical force than one based on the central estimate or on the upper bound. Conversely, an argument that another radiation dose is "safe," in the sense that risk is less than a presumably tolerable limit, would have more force if based on the upper confidence bound (e.g., "the lifetime risk associated with a 5 mSv exposure is unlikely to be greater than 1 per 1000").

3.1.2. Factors Affecting Radiation Dose–Response

The most thoroughly studied modifiers of radiation-related risk are factors that are almost always obtainable with information about exposure and disease incidence or mortality: sex, age at exposure, age at observation for risk, and time following exposure. Aside from cancers of gender-specific organs, age-specific baseline cancer rates of other organs often differ between men and women. Some of this may reflect differential exposure to cancer risk factors such as tobacco smoke, alcohol, and carcinogens in the workplace. Dose-specific ERR estimates for thyroid cancer and female breast cancer, among others, vary inversely with age at exposure, whereas age at observation appears to be a more important modifier of risk for cancers of the lung and colon (10). Leukemia risk [the combination of all types excluding chronic lymphoblastic leukemia (CLL)] clearly depends on both age at exposure and time following exposure (14).

Continuing with the data used to obtain Figures 1 and 2, excess relative risk of all solid cancers combined among atomic bomb survivors can be modeled as a linear function of neutron-weighted dose in sieverts times an exponential term that expresses modification by sex, exposure age, and attained age:

$$\mathrm{ERR}(D, s, e, a) = \alpha D \exp(\beta s + \gamma e + \delta a)$$

where α, β, γ, and δ are unknown parameters, D is the dose, $s = -1$ for males and $+1$ for females, $e =$ age at exposure minus 40 for exposure age < 40 and zero for exposure age ≥ 40, and $a = \log(\mathrm{age}/60)$ for age < 60 and zero for age ≥ 60. [This model, according to which estimated risk for a population equally distributed by sex does not vary by exposure age over 40 or attained age over 60, was chosen for this presentation in part because it gives a particularly simple description of risk at older ages, but in fact it fits these particular data somewhat better than a more conventional (in the radiation literature) model in which radiation-related risk continues to decline exponentially with exposure age >40 and as a power function of attained age >60, according to calculations carried out by the author for this report.] If we use E_1 to denote the estimated ERR per sievert for solid cancer risk at age 60 or older following an exposure at age 40 or older, in an exposed population with equal numbers of men and women, the statistical uncertainty of E_1 is obtained from the statistical likelihood function for the parameter α (Fig. 3, left-hand panel). That uncertainty distribution is approximately normal on the logarithmic scale and, therefore, on the arithmetic scale, approximately lognormal, with geometric mean (GM) 0.334 and geometric standard deviation (GSD) 1.167 (Fig. 3, right-hand panel). The arithmetic mean of this distribution is 0.34, and the 5th and 95th percentiles are 0.26 and 0.43, respectively.

3.1.3.   Risk Estimate Based on Statistical Information Only

According to the 1973–1996 SEER Cancer Statistics Review (15), the likelihood of eventually being diagnosed with a solid cancer, given that this has not occurred by age 50, is about 44.3% for U.S. males and 35.3% for U.S. females, or about 39.8% for a population composed of equal numbers of 50-year-old males and females (to simplify, we will ignore the uncertainties of this and other SEER estimates, and treat the estimated values as

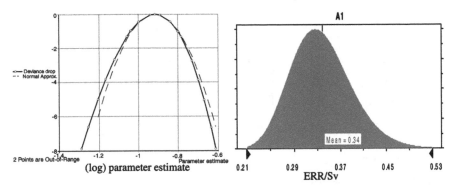

Figure 3 Estimated ERR/Sv after age 60 following radiation exposure at age 40 or older, for a population evenly distributed by sex, based on the model, $ERR(D,s,e,a) = \alpha D \exp(\beta s + \gamma e + \delta a)$. Here, α, β, γ, and δ are unknown parameters, D is the neutron-weighted radiation dose in sieverts, $s = -1$ for males and $+1$ for females, $e = $ age at exposure minus 40 for exposure age <40 and zero for exposure age ≥ 40, and $a = \log(\text{age}/60)$ for age < 60 and zero for age ≥ 60. The left-hand panel shows the statistical likelihood function, which corresponds closely to the lognormal uncertainty distribution shown in the right-hand panel.

known quantities). The values for a comparable population at age 60 are 35.3% for males and 31.9% for females. Because the rate of survival from age 50 to age 60 differs between males and females (92% and 95%, respectively) (16) the lifetime solid cancer rate from 60 onward for a 50-year-old population evenly distributed by sex would be $(0.92 \times 35.3\% + 0.95 \times 31.9\%)/2 = 31.4\%$. Assuming a whole-body radiation exposure at age 50, and allowing for a 10 year minimum latent period for radiation-related cancer (and ignoring the uncertainty of that assumption), the cancer consequence, per unit dose in sieverts, would be estimated as an increment in lifetime risk of about 31.4 times $0.34 = 11\%$ times dose in sieverts. For a dose of 0.01 Sv, that would be an excess lifetime risk of 0.11% or a total lifetime risk of about $39.8\% + 0.11\% = 39.9\%$ (the likelihood that an early death from a radiation-related cancer would preclude later diagnosis of a non-radiation-related cancer is sufficiently small, at 0.01 Sv, to be ignored). According to the statistical uncertainty distribution in Fig. 3, an excess risk less than 31.4% times 0.26 times $0.01 = 0.08\%$, or greater than 31.4% times 0.43 times $0.01 = 0.13\%$, is unlikely in the sense that such an excess is inconsistent with the statistical data.

3.1.4. Other Relevant Information

We know more about radiation-related cancer risk than is contained in the data used to obtain Figure 3. There is additional information on a number of other important factors that need to be taken into consideration when

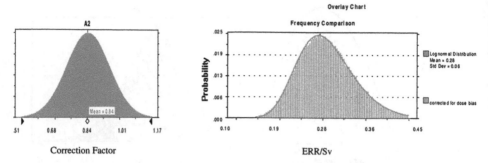

Figure 4 Effect of adjustment for uncertain error in dose reconstruction. The left-hand panel shows a normally distributed, subjective uncertainty distribution for a correction factor recommended by an expert panel of the National Council on Radiation Protection and Measurements (2) and the right-hand panel the simulated uncertainty distribution (*vertical lines*) of the uncertain ERR/Sv estimate represented on the right in Fig. 3, after multiplication by this correction factor. This distribution is well approximated by the lognormal distribution represented by the smooth outline drawn around the simulation results.

estimating radiation-related cancer risk in different populations and exposure situations, information which affects both estimated risk and its uncertainty. The information is objective in nature and is a part of a broad scientific consensus among investigators in this field, yet (unlike the statistical information summarized in Figure 4) its quantitative expression, particularly with respect to uncertainty, is largely subjective and, therefore, may vary by investigator. The important thing, however, is that the process is transparent: alternative subjective uncertainty distributions may be proposed, justified, and substituted into the calculations, and the results compared with those presented here.

3.1.5. Dosimetric Factors

Figure 3 and the related risk estimates discussed above apply to survivors of the atomic bombings of Hiroshima and Nagasaki. They depend on the data and algorithms used to estimate individual doses among A-bomb survivors, and possible biases and uncertainties in dose reconstruction for that population are sources of additional uncertainty for application of the estimates to other populations. The uncertain factors include source terms for the neutron and gamma-ray components of dose from the Hiroshima and Nagasaki bombs and information about the location of individual survivors and their shielding by buildings and terrain. An NCRP committee (2) evaluating this question judged that the effect of these factors might be to underestimate gamma-ray dose, and thus overestimate excess risk per unit dose by an uncertain amount. The committee developed a partly subjective, uncertain correction factor determined by Monte Carlo simulation to be approximately normally distributed with mean 0.84 and standard deviation 0.11 (Fig. 4, left-hand panel). The right-hand panel of Figure 4 shows the results of a Monte Carlo simulation to describe the effect, on the uncertainty distribution in Figure 3, of applying the uncertain correction factor represented in the left-hand panel of the figure. Since estimated risk is a multiple of dose, the correction involves multiplying an uncertain risk estimate by an uncertain dose correction factor. If we use E_2 to denote E_1 adjusted for dose reconstruction error, the uncertainty distribution of E_2 is approximately lognormal with GM $= 0.28$ and GSD $= 1.22$. The mean of that uncertainty distribution is 0.29 and the 5th and 95th percentiles are 0.20 and 0.39, respectively; thus, the adjusted central risk estimate is $31.4\% \times 0.29 \times 0.01 = 0.09\%$, with 90% probability limits 0.06% and 0.12%.

3.1.6. Transfer of Risk Coefficients Between Populations

According to statistics for the combined SEER tumor registries in the United States and the Hiroshima and Nagasaki tumor registries in Japan (17), age-standardized (world) cancer rates for all solid cancers combined, excluding skin, are about 30% higher in the United States than in the (present day) populations of Hiroshima and Nagasaki. For female breast cancer, U.S. rates are threefold higher, while for stomach cancer U.S. rates are only one-tenth as high as those in Japan. These differences complicate the problem of transferring estimates of radiation-related risk from the A-bomb survivors to a U.S. population, because different transfer rules give different results. Suppose, for example, that a certain radiation exposure at age 10 (say) is thought to increase breast cancer rates by 50% at all subsequent ages among the A-bomb survivors. Then the total (baseline plus excess) lifetime breast cancer risk would be 1.5 times the baseline, or about 6 (as against 4 in the absence of exposure) per 100 exposed, female A-bomb survivors. Applying the same multiplicative factor to U.S. rates would yield about 18 lifetime cases per 100, compared to 12 in the absence of exposure. If we knew that radiation acts primarily as an early-stage carcinogen and that the higher breast cancer rates in the U.S. population reflect greater exposure to later-stage factors that cause or allow cells affected by early-stage carcinogens to progress to cancer, a multiplicative transfer of risk would be logical. If, on the other hand, the U.S. population is more heavily exposed to other early-stage carcinogens that act much the same as radiation, we might just as logically assume that the differences, rather than the ratios, between breast cancer rates in exposed and nonexposed women should be the same in the United States and Japan and that the ERR per sievert for Americans would be one-third the value for the A-bomb survivors. In that case, the estimated lifetime rate among exposed American women would be about 14 per 100.

As it happens, combined analyses of breast cancer risks in A-bomb survivors and medically irradiated populations (18) suggest that the additive transfer model is more nearly correct for radiation-related breast cancer, but for most cancers we have very little guidance on the risk transfer problem. There are a number of cancer sites, notably stomach, liver, and prostate gland, for which age-specific baseline rates differ by an order of magnitude or more between the United States and Japan. With the possible exceptions of stomach (20) and liver (21), we have almost no information about which one, if either, of the two simple transfer models is correct. A reasonable presumption is that the truth is somewhere between them. Expert committees (2,3,5) have considered the problem and come up with different approaches involving subjectively weighted mixtures of additive and multiplicative transfer. The NCI/Centers for Disease Control and Prevention (CDC) committee (5) reasoned that, because of the almost total lack of information for the vast majority of cancer sites, on transfer of estimated radiation-related cancer risk between populations with different baseline cancer rates, equal allowance might be made for all linear combinations of additive and multiplicative transfer of the form, in this case multiplying estimated ERR/Sv by 1 for multiplicative transfer and (reflecting the 30% greater U.S. baseline) by $1/1.3 = 0.769$ for additive transfer: $T = u + (1 - u)/1.3$, for u between 0 and 1, with a very small weight given to u as low as -0.1 or as high as 1.1 (Fig. 5). The right-hand panel of Figure 5 shows the simulated uncertainty distribution of ERR per sievert for solid cancer morbidity risk after correction for both dose reconstruction error and transfer from the A-bomb survivors to a general U.S. population (call it E_3, or E_2 adjusted for transfer). The simulated distribution in Fig. 5 is approximately lognormal with $GM = 0.24$ and $GSD = 1.25$, with mean 0.25, and 5th and 95th percentiles

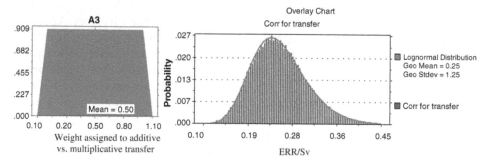

Figure 5   Effect of adjustment for uncertainty in transferring ERR/Sv from a Japanese to a U.S. population, given that age-standardized (world) solid cancer rates are 30% higher in the United States than in Japan. The uncertain transfer model is ERR/Sv(U.S.) = ERR/Sv(Japan) × $(1 - U + U/1.3)$, where the subjective uncertainty distribution of the random quantity U is given in the left-hand panel (5). The right-hand panel shows the simulated uncertainty distribution of ERR/Sv(U.S.) and its lognormal approximation.

0.17 and 0.35, respectively. The adjusted risk estimate is 0.08% with 90% probability limits 0.05% and 0.11%.

3.2. Extrapolation to Low Doses and Low Dose Rates

As mentioned earlier, one of the most difficult and controversial risk estimation problems is the extent to which estimates of ERR per unit dose based on high-dose data apply to low-dose exposures. Based on findings from experimental radiation biology, the ICRP (11) has recommended dividing linear-model risk estimates by a "dose and dose rate effectiveness factor" (DDREF) of 2 for sparsely ionizing radiation at acute doses under 200 mSv or chronic exposures at any dose level delivered at dose rates less than 6 mGy/h, and this recommendation was also accepted by the NCRP. In their most recent discussion of the application of DDREF, the United Nations Subcommittee on Effects of Atomic Radiation (22) recommended that the chosen DDREF be applied to chronic exposures (dose rates less than 6 mGy/h averaged over the first few hours) and to acute (high dose rate) exposures at total doses less than 0.2 Gy, a recommendation that was subsequently adopted by the Environmental Protection Agency (EPA, 1999). More recently, however, in quantitative uncertainty analyses by expert committees (2–5) subjective uncertainty distributions for DDREF have been used that place substantial probability on DDREF values between 1 and 5 and, in two instances (4,5) some probability on values less than 1. These new uncertainty distributions reflect new information from epidemiological studies, like that in Figs. 1 and 2, suggesting the possibility of DDREF values near 1. Figure 6 shows the discrete subjective uncertainty distribution for DDREF used by the NCI/CDC committee (5), and the

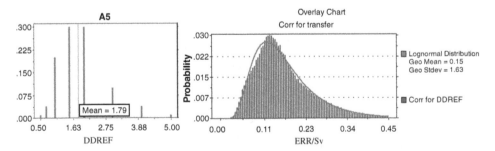

Figure 6 Effect of extrapolation to low doses and dose rates. The left-hand panel shows the subjective, discrete uncertainty distribution for DDREF used by an NCI/CDC working group to provide scientific guidance for the adjudication of compensation claims for cancer following exposure to ionizing radiation (5). The right-hand panel gives the simulated, approximately lognormal uncertainty distribution for ERR/Sv associated with high-energy photon irradiation at low doses and/or low dose rates.

right-hand panel shows the effect of the DDREF factor on the adjusted estimate (call it E_4) of ERR/Sv, and its uncertainty distribution, in Fig. 5. The new uncertainty distribution is roughly lognormal with GM = 0.15 and GSD = 1.63. The mean is 0.17 and the 5th and 95th percentiles are 0.07 and 0.34, corresponding to an adjusted risk estimate of 0.05%, with 90% probability limits 0.02%–0.11%.

3.2.1. Extrapolation from High-Energy to Lower-Energy Photons

It is well known, from experimental radiobiology, that different types of radiation vary in their effectiveness as agents for somatic damage to cellular DNA and therefore as contributors to carcinogenesis. Most uses of medical x-ray produce photons with energies in the 30–250 keV range. The biological effectiveness of such radiation per unit dose, at low doses and dose rates, is thought to be greater than that of higher-energy photons. The risk estimates, and their uncertainty distributions, discussed so far in the current example, pertain to fairly high-dose, acute exposures to sparsely ionizing radiation like that received from the atomic bombs, mainly photons at energy levels greater than 250 keV. In a report commissioned by the National Institute for Occupational Safety and Health, Kocher et al. (23) proposed an uncertainty distribution for the biological effectiveness of 30–250 keV photons, relative to higher-energy photons, that assigned 25% probability to 1 (identical effectiveness) and 75% to a lognormal distribution with 2.5% probability assigned to values less than 1 (i.e., less effective than higher-energy photons), 2.5% to values greater than 5, and the central 95% to values between 1 and 5 (GM = 2.236, GSD = 1.508; Fig. 7, left-hand panel). The resulting uncertainty distribution for E_5, denoting ERR per

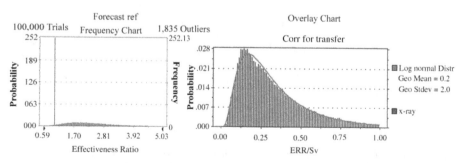

Figure 7 Effect of extrapolation from high-energy photon radiation to 30–250 keV photons (e.g., diagnostic X ray). Left-hand panel: subjective uncertainty distribution derived by Kocher et al. (23) for the relative effectiveness of this type of radiation compared to higher-energy photons, e.g., from the atomic bombings. The right-hand panel shows the simulated uncertainty distribution for ERR/Sv of 30–250 keV photons delivered at low doses and/or low dose rates.

sievert from low-dose or chronic medical x-ray exposure, is reasonably well approximated by a lognormal distribution with $GM = 0.28$ and $GSD = 2.01$ (Fig. 7, right-hand panel); the mean is 0.35, and the 5th and 95th percentiles 0.09 and 0.87. Thus, the estimated lifetime excess cancer risk associated with a 0.01 whole-body x-ray exposure at age 50 is 0.11% with 90% probability limits 0.03–0.27%, or a total solid cancer risk of 39.91% (39.83–40.07%) compared to a nominal risk of 39.8% in the absence of exposure.

4. SUMMARY AND CONCLUSIONS

Most of what we know about radiation-related cancer risk is based on follow-up studies of atomic bomb survivors who were exposed acutely, in 1945, predominantly to high-energy gamma-ray photons with an admixture of neutrons. The dosimetric basis for these studies is somewhat uncertain, and this uncertainty should be taken into account when applying risk estimates based on the A-bomb survivor studies to other populations; another source of uncertainty is how to adjust for differences in baseline cancer rates between the United States and Japan. The most informative data from the A-bomb survivor studies pertain to neutron-weighted whole-body doses in excess of 0.2 Sv. Annual background radiation from natural sources is on the order of 0.001 Sv to most tissues and 0.015 Sv to the lungs. Partial-body exposures from therapeutic radiation for cancer treatment can be tens of sieverts, but the vast majority of radiation exposures in excess of background are from diagnostic medical x-ray, at doses well under 0.1 Sv (24). Thus, additional uncertainty is attached to extrapolation of risk estimates to low doses and to types of radiation qualitatively different from that affecting A-bomb survivors. These (and other) additional sources of uncertainty can be factored into the risk estimation process through the use of largely subjective uncertainty distributions for correction factors and propagation of error through analytical or simulation methods. Thus, the validity of conclusions reached in this way can be evaluated in terms of the reasonableness of the algorithms and uncertainty distributions employed, and by comparison with plausible alternative formulations.

The results of the current exercise are summarized in Table 3. Beginning with the statistical dose–response coefficient estimate E_1, the amount of change and additional uncertainty introduced by adjustment for dose reconstruction error and (because baseline rates for all solid cancers combined are not very different between Japan and the United States) population transfer were relatively minor. More substantial changes were associated with low-dose extrapolation and, especially, extrapolation from high-energy photons to 30–250 keV photons from medical x-ray.

Low-dose extrapolation has long been considered one of the most important unresolved questions for radiation risk protection. Table 3

Table 3 Uncertain Estimates of Lifetime Excess Risk of Solid Cancer Following a Whole-Body, 10 mSv (0.01 Sv) Exposure to Sparsely Ionizing Radiation at Age 50, for a Population Evenly Distributed Between Males and Females

Estimate	Sources of uncertainty	Estimate, % (90% limits)
$E1$	Statistical uncertainty from dose–response analysis	0.10 (0.08–0.13)
$E2$	$E1$ and dose reconstruction error	0.09 (0.06–0.12)
$E3$	$E2$ and population transfer algorithm	0.10 (0.07–0.14)
$E4$	$E3$ and extrapolation to low doses and dose rates	0.07 (0.03–0.13)
$E5$	$E4$ and extrapolation to 30–250 keV photons	0.14 (0.03–0.36)

Results of a quantitative uncertainty analysis

suggests that a problem of equal importance is the relative effectiveness of medical x-ray vs. high-energy photons.

It should be kept in mind that the statistical risk estimates and the uncertain correction factors presented here are representative of information available at the time of writing, and can be expected to change as newer information is developed. The present document is an illustration of a particular approach, quantitative uncertainty analysis, as it is being increasingly applied to estimation of radiation-related risk, and is in no way a definitive presentation of radiation-related risk.

REFERENCES

1. National Council on Radiation Protection and Measurements. A Guide for Uncertainty Analysis in Dose and Risk Assessments Related to Environmental Contamination. NCRP Commentary No. 14. Bethesda, MD: National Council on Radiation Protection and Measurements, 1996.
2. National Council on Radiation Protection and Measurements. Uncertainties in Fatal Cancer Risk Estimates Used In Radiation Protection. NCRP Report No. 126. Bethesda, MD: National Council on Radiation Protection and Measurements, 1997.
3. EPA (Environmental Protection Agency). Estimating Radiogenic Cancer Risks. EPA Report 402-R-00-003. Washington, DC: EPA, 1999.
4. DOJ (Department of Justice). Final Report of the Radiation Exposure Compensation Act Committee. (Submitted to the Human Radiation Interagency Working Group), July 1996.
5. Land CE, Gilbert E, Smith J, Hoffman FO, Apostoaei I, Thomas B. Report of the NCI-CDC Working Group to Revise the 1985 NIH Radioepidemiological Tables. DHHS publication No. 03-5387, 2003, Washington, D.C. available on

request from Judi Patt (*pattj@mail.nih.gov*) or, in pdf format, from *http://www.irep.nci.gov/*.

6. National Council on Radiation Protection and Measurement. Exposure of the population in the United States and Canada from Natural Background Radiation. NCRP Report No. 94. Bethesda, MD: NCRP, 1987.

7. National Council on Radiation Protection and Measurement. Exposure of the U.S. Population from Diagnostic Medical Radiation. NCRP Report No. 100. Bethesda, MD: NCRP, 1989.

8. Pierce DA, Shimizu Y, Preston DL, Vaeth M, Mabuchi K. Studies of the mortality of atomic bomb survivors. Report 12, part I. Cancer: 1950–1990. Radiat Res 1996; 146:1–27.

9. Mabuchi K, Soda M, Ron E, Tokunaga M, Ochiubo S, Sugimoto S, Ikeda T, Terasaki M, Preston DL, Thompson DE. Cancer incidence in atomic bomb survivors. Part I: use of the tumor registries in Hiroshima and Nagasaki for incidence studies. Radiat Res 1994; 137:S1–S16.

10. Thompson DE, Mabuchi K, Ron E, Soda M, Tokunaga M, Ochikubo S, Sugimoto S, Ikeda T, Terasaki M, Izumi S, Preston DL. Cancer incidence in atomic bomb survivors. Part II: solid tumors, 1958–1987. Radiat Res 1994; 137:S17–S67.

11. ICRP (International Commission on Radiation Protection). 1990 recommendations of the International Commission on Radiological Protection. ICRP publication 60. Ann ICRP 1991; 21(1–3):1–193.

12. Radiation Effects Research Foundation. Cancer Incidence Dataset, tr87data.dat, and dose DS86 Organ Dose Adjustment File, ds86adjf.dat. (Downloadable computer files, www.rerf.or.jp. Hiroshima: RERF, 1994.

13. Preston DL, Lubin JH, Pierce DA. Epicure Users Guide. Seattle, WA: Hirosoft International, 1991.

14. Preston DL, Kusumi S, Tomonaga M, Izumu S, Ron E, Kuramoto A, Kamata N, Dohy H, Matsui T, Nonaka H, Thompson DE, Soda M, Mabuchi K. Cancer incidence in atomic bomb survivors, part III: leukemia, lymphoma, and multiple myeloma, 1950–87. Radiat Res 1994; 137:S68–S97.

15. Ries LAG, Kosary CL, Hankey BF, Miller BA, Clegg LX, Edwards BK, eds. SEER Cancer Statistics Review, 1973–1966, National Cancer Institute. NIH Pub. No. 99–2789. Bethesda, MD: National Institutes of Health, 1999.

16. Anderson RN, DeTurk PB. United States Life Tables, 1999. National Vital Statistics Reports. Vol. 50, No. 6. Hyattsville, MD: National Center for Health Statistics, 2002.

17. Parkin DM, Whelan SL, Ferlay J, Raymond L, Young J, eds. Cancer Incidence in Five Continents. Vol. VII. IARC Scientific Publications No. 143. Lyon: IARC, 1997.

18. Preston DL, Mattsson A, Holmberg E, Shore R, Hildreth NG, Boice JD. Radiation effects on breast cancer risk: a pooled analysis of eight cohorts. Radiat Res 2002; 158(2):220–235.

19. Land CE, Sinclair WK. The relative contributions of different cancer sites to the overall detriment associated with low-dose radiation exposure. Ann ICRP 1991; 22:31–57.

20. Carr ZA, Kleinerman RA, Weinstock R, Stovall M, Greim ML, Land CE. Malignant neoplasms after radiation therapy for peptic ulcer. Radiat Res 2002; 157:668–677.

21. Cologne JB, Tokuoka S, Beebe GW, Fukuhara T, Mabuchi K. Effects of radiation on incidence of primary liver cancer among atomic bomb survivors. Radiat Res 1999; 152:364–373.

22. United Nations Scientific Committee on the Effects of Atomic Radiation. Sources, Effects and Risks of Ionizing Radiation, No. E.94.IX.2. New York: United Nations, 1993.

23. Kocher DC, Apostoaei AI, Hoffman FO. Radiation Effectiveness Factors (REFs) for Use in Calculating Probability of Causation of Radiogenic Cancers. (draft report submitted to the National Institute of Occupational Safety and Health, June 17). Oak Ridge, TN: SENES Oak Ridge, Inc., 2002. Internet posting, http://www.cdc.gov/niosh/ocas/pdfs/irepref.pdf.

24. National Academy of Sciences/National Research Council, Committee on the Biological Effects of Ionizing Radiation. The Effects on Populations of Exposure to Low Levels of Ionizing Radiation. Washington, DC: BEIR V. National Academy Press, 1990.

14

Occupational Cancer

Robert J. McCunney

Department of Biological Engineering, Massachusetts Institute of Technology, Pulmonary Division, Massachusetts General Hospital, Boston, Massachusetts, U.S.A

Lee Okurowski

Department of Orthopedics, Occupational Health, New England Baptist Hospital, Boston, Massachusetts, U.S.A.

1. INTRODUCTION

This chapter is designed to provide an overview of occupational cancer, its causes, risks, and prevention. The subject is vast and extends into clinical, epidemiological, legal, toxicological, and ethical areas, among others. As a result, a complete discussion of this topic is beyond the scope of this chapter. It is intended, however, to be a basic resource on the subject for researchers, physicians, nurses, and other health professionals with a particular emphasis on biomarkers. The chapter includes a brief history of early occupational cancer, contemporary issues related to occupational cancer risks, and methods for determining such risks through epidemiological, animal and in vitro investigations. Sections on assessing risks of occupational cancer and its prevention follow, along with a discussion on addressing casual associations.

An occupational carcinogen can be any chemical, physical, or biologic agent that increases the risk of cancer associated with work. Although figures vary, approximately 2–8% of all human cancers may be due to exposure to occupational carcinogens (1–4). The proportion of cancers associated with certain occupations can be significantly higher (3–5). According to the National Occupational Research Agenda (NORA), about 10% of lung cancers, 21–27% of bladder cancers, and up to 80% of mesotheliomas in the United States are related to occupational exposure to carcinogens. In workers sufficiently exposed to specific carcinogens, such as vinyl chloride, the percentage of site-specific cancer (i.e., angiosarcoma of the liver) approaches 100%.

The assessment of risk associated with certain types of work and agents is not only challenging but also incomplete. As many as 6 million chemicals and approximately 4 million chemical mixtures are registered with the Chemical Abstracts Service and in commercial use. More than 50,000 chemicals are used regularly, but fewer than 1000 chemicals or work settings have been assessed in some way for their potential to cause cancer (3,6). An understanding of occupational cancer risk, however, has implications not only for the workplace but also for public and environmental health. In fact, public health policy is often based on occupational studies, despite limitations in extrapolations of the data. The workplace represents a unique environment in which a relatively large number of people may be exposed to relatively high concentrations of potential carcinogens. From these workplace exposures, adverse health effects can be assessed and extrapolated to larger populations.

Occupational cancers are theoretically *completely preventable* with appropriate engineering controls, personnel practices, and the use of protective equipment. In fact, exposure to potential carcinogens can be vigorously controlled and often eliminated in many work settings. Often, the efforts associated with reducing exposure to occupational carcinogens have resulted in efficient improvements in the process. Controls can be extraordinarily effective in preventing occupational cancer. Witness, for example, the vinyl chloride industry. As a result of measures taken to lower exposure levels below 1 ppm, no case of angiosarcoma has occurred in a worker hired in North America or Western Europe since 1974. Nonetheless, millions of workers may be exposed to potential carcinogens. Continued prevention of cancers that may result from certain jobs, however, will require refined assessments of risk. Clinicians, in particular, can make substantial contributions to assessing risk by keeping a keen awareness of potential links between work and illness and making note of them as appropriate.

2. HISTORY

A detailed history of occupational cancer is available in other sources (7,8). Although the association between work and ill health dates back to Ramazzini, an Italian physician in the early 18th century, the first clear link between cancer and a specific cause is attributed to Sir Percival Pott who in the late 18th century identified soot as responsible for scrotal cancer in young British chimney sweeps. It was not until the 1930s to the 1940s, however, that the probable causative agent was identified as benzo(a)pyrene (BAP), one of the many carcinogens found in soots, tars, and cigarette smoke (9,10). The work of Pott represents more than a historical highlight, because it illustrates that occupational cancers—then and now—were initially detected by astute physicians. In fact, nearly all occupational carcinogens were initially recognized in this manner (7,11).

The discovery of specific occupational carcinogens continued after Pott. In 1875, clinicians noted excess rates of skin cancer secondary to exposure to coal tar products, including mineral oils used in the Scottish shale and the English cotton industries (7). For centuries, miners suffered a multitude of breathing disorders associated with work. In 1879, Haerting and Hesse identified excess lung cancer among German uranium minors, although the potential contributions of arsenic and radioactive materials were yet to be recognized, until decades later. When large-scale uranium mining began in the United States in the late 1940s, it was finally recognized that radon caused lung cancer (7,10). The hazards of ionizing radiation were first reported in 1902, shortly after the discovery of x-rays when radiation-induced skin cancer was observed. Excess rates of leukemia occurred among radiologists and technicians, whereas excess rates of bone cancer (sarcomas) of the lower jaw were found among radium dial painters.

In 1948, Machle and Gregorius described an excess of lung cancer among chromate workers, and Hill and Fanning observed excess lung and skin cancer in a British arsenic factory (7). In 1955, Doll and Peto (12,13) published an epidemiological study associating asbestos with increased cancer of the lung; later, synergism between cigarette smoke and asbestos was reported.

In 1974, a cluster of angiosarcoma led to a proportional mortality study, a retrospective cohort study, and animal evaluations that uncovered vinyl chloride as a cause of liver cancer (14–16). In a similar fashion, exposure to bischloromethylether (BCME) was noted to increase risk of lung cancer among workers in the plexiglass industry.

By 1950, many occupational cancer risks recognized today had been discovered (Table 1), including bladder cancer among German dystuff workers (due to aniline dyes) and leukemia among Italian shoe workers exposed to benzene. Asbestos-related lung cancer was first reported in 1934; in 1947, Britains' Chief Factory Inspector reported lung cancer in 31 of 235 men with asbestosis who died between 1924 and 1946 (10). In 1932, the first reports associating arsenic with lung cancer and nickel with sinonasal carcinoma appeared.

Eventually, the recognition of occupational cancer underwent a transition from clinical case reporting to more formal quantitative epidemiological studies. Such studies included proportional mortality analyses of death certificates, retrospective follow-up studies among exposed workers, case–control evaluations, and prospective assessments. Their role in evaluating potential work place carcinogens will be described later in this chapter.

In the 1970s, a variety of Federal legislation was enacted, related to the formation of agencies charged with responsibilities for occupational and environmental health. The Occupational Safety and Health Administration (OSHA), the National Institute for Occupational Safety and Health (NIOSH), and the Environmental Protection Agency (EPA), are major examples.

Table 1   Established Occupational Carcinogens

Bladder	Benzidin, 2-naphthylamine, 4-aminobiphenyl (xenylamine), manufacture of certain dyes (e.g., auramine and magenta), gas retorts, rubber and cable making industries, coal tar pitch volatiles (aluminum reduction plant, chimney sweeps)
Blood (leukemia)	Benzene, X-radiation
Bone	Radium, mesothorium
Larynx	Mustard gas, sulfuric acid mist
Liver (angiosarcoma)	Arsenic (inorganic compounds), vinyl chloride
Lung, bronchus	Arsenic (inorganic compounds), asbestos, beryllium and beryllium compounds, bis-chloromethyl ether, cadmium and cadmium compounds, chromium compounds

Source: Adapted from Monson R. Occupational. In: Schottenfeld D, Fraumeni, JF, eds. Cancer Epidemiology and Preventive. New York: Oxford University Press, 1996.

3.   IDENTIFYING CARCINOGENS

Currently, the process of identifying substances and occupations associated with cancer is performed by a variety of state, national, and international organizations. The International Agency for Research on Cancer (IARC), the National Institute for Occupational Safety and Health, the U.S. Public Health Services' National Toxicology Program (NTP), the Environmental Protection Agency (EPA), the American Conference of Governmental Industrial Hygienists (ACGIH), and OSHA are noteworthy examples. These organizations establish lists of hazards and occupations with carcinogenic potential. Hazard identification tends to be based on assessments of epidemiological and clinical reports, as well as animal research and in vitro studies. Each agency classifies carcinogens differently, with criteria varying considerably. Some organizations simply identify a hazard, whereas others propose or require occupational exposure limits. Such variability underscores the complexity of occupational risk assessment. Case reports, epidemiology, and animal investigations form the basis of scientific information used to identify occupational carcinogens. Their scope, benefits, and limitations in the occupational setting are described below.

3.1.   Case Reports and Series

Case reports and case series describe the experience of a single patient (case report) or group of patients (case series). Usually, the case (or cases) represents a previously unrecognized health effect from exposure to a certain hazard or work in a particular industry. These types of reports often provide the first clue about potentially unrecognized effects of exposure to hazardous agents and may prompt the need for a formal epidemiological study. Once suspected exposures are identified by a case series, the potential causal link between the exposure and the disease outcome can be formally tested through cohort studies. Case reports, although inexpensive and straightforward to prepare, are limited in their usefulness for drawing causal inferences. One obvious shortcoming is that the risk of exposure identified by a case series lacks an appropriate comparison group (17). Nonetheless, case reports have played an important role in the identification of occupational carcinogens and will likely continue to be of value as early warning signals.

3.2. Cohort Studies

A cohort study refers to an epidemiologic assessment designed to evaluate a potential occupational cancer risk. In a classic cohort study, the investigator defines two or more groups of people (the cohorts) that are free of disease and which differ only according to the extent of their exposure to a potential agent (18) One group represents the exposed individuals; the other (the reference group) represents those unexposed. Workers from a common industry or plant process are identified as the exposure group, then compared to a nonexposed group, often workers from the same factory or members of the general population. The *vital status* (alive or deceased) or *disease status* (ill or not, depending on criteria) of each group is noted. Both groups can then be followed over time (*prospectively*) for the development of isease(s). In another approach, the exposed and unexposed cohorts are identified through historical records (a *retrospective study*) and then evaluated through a designated date in the past.

Retrospective cohort studies (in which defined records are used to characterize the exposure and disease status until a designated date) are most commonly found in the occupational literature (19). A useful type of retrospective study is the cohort *mortality* study, in which a group of exposed workers is identified and then followed to a designated date; the vital status of each cohort member is then determined from death certificates or disease registries. The rates of death, including specific types, among the work cohort are compared to national or local rates. Results are described in terms of the standardized mortality ratio (SMR), which is calculated by dividing the number of observed cases (deaths or new cancers) among the exposed population by the number (actual or expected based on standardized disease rates) in the unexposed (control) group. Calculated SMRs are usually adjusted for known confounders through stratification by age, sex, year of birth, and race (19). The major limitations of this type of study is the quality of available data used in both the health or mortality assessment of the cohort and the categorization of exposure. Inaccurate or missing information can limit the validity of certain results. Nonetheless, over the past 25 years, cohort mortality studies have identified many occupational carcinogens and have had a major impact on IARC's identification of carcinogens. From some studies, individual dose estimates have been calculated to enhance risk assessments and the establishment of effective control limits.

When death certificates are available, but the characterization of the exposure is incomplete, a *proportionate mortality ratio* (PMR) study may be valuable for an early assessment of potential occupational cancer risk. The PMR, which compares *distributions* of the causes of death among a group in comparison to the general population, can be used to test an hypothesis (7,19,20). The PMR is calculated by comparing the ratio of each type of cancer to the total number of cancer and noncancer deaths in the exposed population with similar ratios in the reference population (3). Although this method can provide valuable preliminary information, the method has distinct drawbacks. The PMR, for example, does not include information on years of exposure. Its critical flaw, however, is that an apparent excess of cancer may only be a reflection of a deficit in another cause of death (19).

The *prospective* cohort design is the ideal epidemiological study for occupational cancer risk assessment. This study design, however, is seldom used due to cost and long latency of most occupational cancers, which can be 5–30 years or longer. These studies have the major benefit in that *exposure* to suspected carcinogens can be accurately assessed, whereas in retrospective studies exposure may need to be approximated.

3.3. Case–Control Studies

In a case–control study, subjects are selected on the basis of whether they do (cases) or do not (controls) have a designated disease (17). They can be conducted de novo or following a retrospective or proportional mortality study in which an excess risk of disease is noted. In case–control studies, when a types of cancers are identified their occupational exposure histories are compared to matched control groups. Case–control studies are particularly suited for evaluating rare diseases, such as some types of occupational cancer. Diseases with long latency periods can be assessed, since the disease has already occurred at the time of the study. The proper definition of the disease under study and the selection of cases and controls is critical to the value of case–control studies. In any case–control study, the disease outcome of interest must be defined according to widely acknowledged diagnostic and histopathologic criteria. Cancer diagnoses affecting the same organ system often have different subtypes and separate etiologies and must be accounted for in the analysis.

Case–control studies are subject to a number of special issues that affect the interpretation of results. Since exposure information is obtained after the disease has occurred, the results can be affected by *recall bias*, which may occur if patients with a given disease report exposures differently than controls. In fact, people who have been diagnosed with a rare or life threatening disease tend to think about the possible "causes" of their illness and thus are likely to remember their exposure histories differently from those unaffected by the disease (17). Recall bias may be particularly acute when the disease is cancer and the cause may be related to work.

Case–control studies may also suffer from *selection bias* in that both exposure and disease have occurred prior to the time subjects are selected into the study. These studies can also be prone to *misclassification* and in some situations, the temporal relationship between exposure and disease is unclear, which limits interpretations of causality.

A "nested" case–control study is usually conducted as part of a large cohort evaluation. Although all case–control studies can be thought of as "nested" within a source population of exposed and unexposed people, the term *nested case–control study* refers to a case–control study where the population is obtained from a well-defined cohort. Such studies are usually performed after completion of a retrospective cohort study, which identifies an expected excess in cancer or other disease. Personnel and exposure records, where available, are reviewed in an attempt to identify agents suspected to be responsible for the excess in cancer mortality noted in the cohort study.

Similarly, a disease can be identified and then evaluated to determine specific risk factors. Employment records of those with a disease are analyzed by job and/or exposure or both and then compared to records of workers without disease. This effort is designed to identify the particular exposure or work process responsible for increased disease risk; confounding factors are addressed by interviews of the worker or next of kin. The nested case–control study focuses on interviews and examinations of records only on people with the disease of interest rather than on the entire original cohort.

4. SPECIAL ISSUES IN OCCUPATIONAL EPIDEMIOLOGY

4.1. Exposure Assessment

Occupational epidemiology is fundamentally concerned with the often-difficult task of relating exposure to outcomes. As a result, accurate exposure assessment has been described as the Achilles heel of the discipline. Limited or inaccurate information of a worker's exposure can lead to misclassification and weakening of the exposure–outcome assessment. This problem is exagerated in evaluating diseases of long latency. Clearly, as time passes, accurate retrospective exposure assessments can become increasingly problematic. As discussed earlier, the ideal epidemiologic study for assessing exposure–outcome relationships is the prospective cohort study, in which exposure is well categorized and health effects are properly assessed and followed into the future. Such ideal circumstances, however, are rarely present.

Several techniques have been developed to improve retrospective exposure assessments, because of their importance in assessing dose–

response relationships, latency, and combined effects of several exposures. Exposure reconstruction is frequently based on interviews with workers and others knowledgeable about historical events and procedures. Another approach is based on expert assessments, which, despite their value, are at their core only refined estimates. To address challenges of exposure reconstruction, job–exposure matrices (JEMs) evolved in the early 1980s to help quantify exposures and improve epidemiological analyses. A JEM is usually a two-entry data matrix with job depicted on one axis (including occupation, position, or task) and risk factors such as hazards, level of exposure, and time on the other axis. Numerous JEMs have been established for specific occupations, industries, and industrial processes (21). These matrices are relatively cost- and time-efficient. Nonetheless, the validity of JEMs can be weakened because of misclassification (13). More recent methods for conducting exposure assessment include the use of computer generated questionnaires (22).

4.1.1. Biomarkers

Genetic and molecular epidemiology methods have advanced the use of biomarkers, as indicators of exposure, risk and effect (23–26). In fact, biomarkers can be a significant component of medical surveillance protocols for many occupational exposures (27). Examples include blood lead levels, clara cell levels for silica, and urinary beta-2-microglobulin for cadmium, among numerous others. Genetic biomarkers offer particular promise for the detection of subtle preclinical effects of exposure to carcinogens.

Biomarkers are commonly divided into three categories: markers of exposure, markers of effect, and markers of susceptibility. Examples of biomarkers of exposure include DNA–protein adducts, which ideally can provide "an integrated measure of carcinogen exposure, uptake and absorption, and metabolism." They offer considerable value in providing an objective and relevant measure of exposure in contrast to questionnaires and nonspecific biological testing. The interpretation of DNA-adduct measurements in human tissues and body fluids, however, requires an understanding of a number of factors, including the sensitivity and specificity of the measurement, the temporal relationship between the exposure and the corresponding adduct levels, and the mechanistic role of adducts in carcinogenesis (28). Their use in occupational medical practice today remains limited but they remain a research focus with great potential (29).

Markers of *effect* indicate that the carcinogen has reached a cellular site and altered genetic material. Sister chromatid exchanges, micronuclei, abnormal genes, and gene products are notable examples. The interpretation of cytogenetic abnormalities and of abnormal gene products in relation to exposure remains problematic, despite their role in research initiatives. Cytogenic abnormalities and abnormal gene products have been studied in a variety of occupational settings involving benzene, vinyl chloride, asbestos, and ethylene oxide and in firefighters and hazardous materials workers.

Their use in routine settings, however, remains limited because they are in an early stage of validation.

Markers of *risk* offer promise in the prevention of occupational cancer. Although epidemiological studies have identified various exposure-related associations with cancer, the determination of *individual susceptibility* remains a considerable challenge. Recent advances in molecular biology have led to novel approaches in defining the role of genetic susceptibility in cancer etiology. Ongoing studies of the associations of inheritable polymorphisms and metabolic genes with specific carcinogen exposures reflect the most recent research. Future efforts will likely include examination of inherited variation in DNA repair, among other factors associated with cancer. Methods are also being developed to allow for analysis of gene–environment interaction in the development of cancer. These approaches hold considerable promise for defining the nature of genetic susceptibility in exposure related cancers (23).

An example of *markers of risk* is the relationship of polymorphic variants of cytochrome P450 in the metabolic activation of precarcinogens. Many Phase I P450 enzymes bioactivate carcinogens, whereas Phase II enzymes participate in the deactivation process. Both the CYP1A1 and CYP2E1 variants of Phase I P450 enzymes are involved in the metabolism of many suspected and established carcinogens. Since genetic polymorphisms have been identified for both Phase I and Phase II enzymes, risk assessments could be enhanced if polymorphisms in both enzyme categories are considered as biomarkers for susceptibility to cancer (30). Genetic and molecular epidemiology research involving the use of biomarkers also raises ethical questions, related to the potential for such information to be used for discriminatory purposes (31–33).

4.2. Outcome Assessment

Health outcome assessment is usually less of a problem than exposure assessment in occupational cancer epidemiology. Nonetheless, accurate determination of health end points presents challenges for many studies due to both the accuracy of diagnoses and underreporting of illnesses. Although most industrialized countries maintain cancer, occupational injury, and disease registries, the accuracy of these registries is questionable because many occupational diseases tend to be underreported. The Scandinavian countries, which are noted for their superior occupational illness and injury data collection systems, also showed limitations, when between 1983 and 1987, only 34% of occupationally related cancers were reported (1). Other industrialized countries have found similar results.

4.3. Combined Effects of Several Exposures

The combined effect of several exposures raises a number of challenges in occupational epidemiology, including accounting for confounding, synergy, interaction, and effect modification (9). In occupational epidemiological studies, age and smoking status are common confounders. Interaction has a number of connotations depending on the literature, whether statistical, epidemiological, chemical, biological, or public health. For risk assessment, the concept of "mechanical interaction" that can occur between chemicals and biological systems encompasses the notion of direct physical or chemical reactions among exposures, their metabolites, or their reaction products (34). Mechanical interaction occurs when the combined effect of two or more carcinogens is greater than what would have been anticipated based on individual exposures. The exposure effect may change depending on the presence, or level, of other chemicals involved. *Synergistic* interactions occur when the combined effects of certain hazards exceed their individual effects. In contrast, *antagonism* results when the combined effects are less than individual effects. Notable synergistic effects include those of asbestos and smoking, whose coexposure results in much higher risks of lung.

4.4. Healthy Worker Effect

When the mortality and disease patterns of a group of workers are compared to those of the general population, the working group is generally found to be healthier. This phenomenon—termed the healthy worker effect—has particular importance in the assessment of epidemiological studies. The basis of the healthy worker effect is multifactorial. First, working populations are generally more physically and emotionally fit than the general population, which includes persons unable to work due to a variety of restrictions. The healthy worker effect is also affected by healthy survival, in that those more physically and emotionally fit are less likely to need to leave work. Workers also tend to have improved access to healthcare services and a higher standard of living, other factors contributing to the healthy worker effect. Some studies have demonstrated that the healthy worker effect plays a role in some occupational epidemiology studies, whereas others urge caution in applying it to the assessment of cancer, since its development is not strongly associated to "fitness" for employment.

5. IN VITRO STUDIES

Occupational epidemiology studies assess exposure–disease associations in human populations under actual conditions. The long latency periods, however, between initial exposure and the onset of cancers, render the timely epidemiologic evaluation of potential carcinogens in the workplace pressingly difficult (19). Moreover, epidemiological studies tend to be inefficient in detecting low-level cancer risks since relatively large sample sizes are needed to uncover true increases of disease. In vivo and in vitro studies can be valuable supplements to epidemiology in assessing occupational cancer risk. These studies, extensively used over the past 30 years, have also yielded advances in understanding *mechanisms* of cancer (4).

In vitro studies refer to short-term assays used to evaluate the mutagenicity of a substance as a surrogate for carcinogenicity. Historically, such assays screen potential carcinogens to set priorities for other methods of carcinogen risk assessment. More recently, several cell lines and animal strains have been developed to assess classes of carcinogens (35). Short-term assays can shed light on mechanisms and tend to be time-efficient and inexpensive to perform.

The most widely used in vitro study in cancer risk assessment is the mutagenicity assay, developed by Bruce Ames and colleagues in 1973 (36). The Ames test involves testing a substances' ability to mutate a strain of *Salmonella typhimurium*. This strain is a mutant form that is deficient in DNA repair, and in its ability to synthesize the amino acid histidine. As a result, the bacteria cannot grow in culture media that lacks histidine. In the assay, *S. typhimurium* is treated with several doses of the compound of interest, plated on histidine deficient medium, and then examined later for growth. Growth represents a back mutation of the defective gene into revertants that synthesize histidine and multiply. In humans and mammals, many chemicals are only activated into mutagens and/or carcinogens after metabolism in the body. Furthermore, bacteria and mammals differ in the metabolic capabilities. Therefore, in the Ames test, a mixture of rat liver enzymes that includes multiple P-450s is used in conjunction with an NADPH regenerating system. Several lines of *Salmonella* have been created for the detection of point and frameshift mutations. Certain carcinogens cannot be detected by these bacterial assays such as metals, hormonal agents, and nongenotoxic hazards (35).

A variety of other in vitro tests is available for carcinogen identification, including: (1) gene mutation assays, (2) chromosome aberration, and (3) primary DNA damage assays. The scope of this chapter precludes a detailed discussion of the specific tests in each of these groups; however, some of the more common tests for each group are described. Gene mutation assays include the Ames test and the mammalian mouse lymphoma thymidine kinase assay. Chromosome aberration assays include assays of specific cell lines, mouse micronuclei, and rat bone marrow cytogenic studies. Primary DNA breakage assays include examination of animal cell lines for DNA adducts through ^{32}P postlabelling, assays of DNA strand breakage, sister chromatid exchange assays, and assays assessing DNA repair.

The application of short-term assays in occupational risk assessment has limitations; as a result their use is regarded by some as controversial. Although most short-term assays for mutagenicity are considered a proxy for assessing carcinogenicity, a mutagenic substance, per se, is not necessarily carcinogenic. Although almost half of the known carcinogens are mutagenic, not all substances that test positive in 2-year in vivo animal assays are mutagenic in short-term assays (21). The sensitivity, specificity, and positive predictive value of many in vitro tests are unclear in their implications to humans (37,38). Nonetheless, in vitro studies will likely continue to play a role in the investigation of occupational carcinogens as screening tests.

6. IN VIVO EXPERIMENTS

In vivo experiments refer to animal bioassays used to test the carcinogenicity of substances under controlled conditions. Animal bioassays, an essential component of occupational cancer risk assessment, are particularly effective in screening suspected carcinogens for which epidemiological studies are not practical or impossible.

The controlled nature of in vivo assays allows investigators to manipulate experimental conditions to evaluate many biological responses to chemical exposures. Standard cancer animal bioassays commonly involve testing two species of animals, typically rats and mice. Testing of both sexes, using 50 animals per dose group, and using near-lifetime exposures prior to assessing cancer endpoints are routine (37). Individual studies usually vary by the strains of rats and mice selected, and the number and concentration of doses of the suspected carcinogen administered. Most animal bioassays involve incidence studies with 2 years of follow-up. The National Cancer Institute and the National Toxicology Program have established guidelines for the conduction of animal bioassays for the purposes of evaluating carcinogens (35). Dose levels given to animals under study are most often percentages of the maximum tolerated dose (MTD). In addition to the carcinogen tested in the exposed group, there is frequently a solvent treated control group and an untreated control group. Exposed animals are subjected to 90, 50, and 10–25% of the MTD, and then sacrificed after 2 years to assess designated cancer endpoints (35).

Cancer endpoints in animal studies can vary, especially as to how cancer (or lack thereof) is defined histopathologically. Carcinogenicity in animal studies is confirmed by an increase in the number of tumors at a given site as compared to controls, the induction of atypical tumors, earlier induction of common tumors, and/or increases in the absolute number of tumors (37).

Most often, chemicals that consistently cause tumors in animals are presumed to be human carcinogens, since all known human carcinogens are carcinogenic when tested in animals (4,37). On the interpretation of animal carcinogens as applied to humans, IARC states: "in the absence of adequate data on humans, it is biologically plausible and prudent to regard agents and mixtures for which there is sufficient evidence of carcinogenicity in experimental animals as if they presented a carcinogenic risk to humans" (37,39). Ideally, the animal bioassays should simulate the exposure pathways that are applicable to humans.

The use of animal bioassays to determine human carcinogenicity has certain limitations, including the extrapolation of high exposures in animal studies to the lower exposures experienced by people at work (40). Tumors in animals are often only increased at the highest dose tested, which is often just below the dose that causes systemic toxicity (41). Furthermore, high doses of a potential carcinogen may produce entirely different effects than the lower doses human workers might encounter. High exposure concentrations in animal bioassays may saturate "detoxification" pathways and produce different effects than those at lower concentrations, when such pathways are not saturated. A notable example is the particle overload phenomenon associated with inorganic particles and lung cancer in rodents (42).

Interspecies extrapolation is complicated by factors such as the greater homogeneity of animal species as compared to humans, well-regulated living conditions including diet of lab animals, and genetic differences between animals and humans, among others. Rats and mice, for example, often demonstrate differences in animal bioassays of carcinogens. Similar results between rats and mice occur only 70% of the time and even when the results are similar, differences in dose–response relationships are usually noted between species. Despite the limitations of animal bioassays, they provide useful information in the assessment of occupational cancer risk. The vast majority of chemical exposures that are carcinogenic in animals have not been evaluated in humans. As a result, new methods are needed to strengthen the scientific basis for extrapolations of animal bioassays to human populations. Of increasing importance are methods that serve to validate risk in animals as predictive of risks in workers (4).

7. REGULATED CARCINOGENS

In the United States, the Occupational Safety and Health Administration (OSHA), under the U.S. Department of Labor, is the regulatory agency responsible for enacting standards regarding carcinogens. OSHA recognizes that in industry there are many potential exposures to carcinogens and that workplace exposures are generally higher than public settings. OSHA also maintains that carcinogen exposure at the workplace should be controlled primarily through the use of engineering and process controls and that personal protective equipment should only be used as an extension to these other measures. Specifically, OSHA in its *Identification, Classification, and Regulation of Carcinogens* standard establishes criteria and procedures for the identification, classification, and regulation of potential occupational carcinogens found in the U.S. workplace (OSHA;1990.101). According to OSHA, the term carcinogen applies to individual substances, groups of substances, or combinations or mixtures of substances. In establishing the criteria and procedures for which substances will be regulated, the agency relies on an extensive review of the scientific data and opinions of the National Toxicology Program, NIOSH, and IARC. Substances with OSHA

Table 2   Carcinogens Regulated by OSHA Standard 1910.1003

Carcinogen	CAS number	Related standard CFR
4-Nitrobiphenyl	92933	
Alpha-naphthylamine	134327	1910.1004
Methyl chloromethyl ether	107302	1910.1006
3,3'-Dichlorobenzidine	91941	1910.1007
Bis-chloromethyl ether	542881	1910.1008
Beta-naphthylamine	91598	1910.1009
Benzidine	92875	1910.1010
4-Aminodiphenyl	92671	1910.1011
Ethyleneimine	151564	1910.1012
Beta-propiolactone	57578	1910.1013
2-Acetylaminofluorene	53963	1910.1014
4-Dimethylaminoazobenzene	60117	1910.1015
N-Nitrosodimethylamine	62759	1910.1016

standards are classified into two groups as "carcinogens" or "potential carcinogens" as established by the National Toxicology Program. Such substances require medical surveillance and/or screening to protect human health.

OSHA Standard 1910.1003 (4-nitrobiphenyl, etc.) addresses the regulation of 13 carcinogens as listed in Table 2 with regard to their manufacturing, processing, repackaging, releasing, handling, and storage. Under OSHA standard 1910.1003, medical surveillance shall be established and implemented for employees considered for assignment in regulated areas of the workplace where such carcinogens are present. Before an employee can be assigned to a regulated area, a preassignment physical examination by a physician shall be provided and include the personal history of the employee, and the family and occupational background, including genetic and environmental factors [1910.1003 (g) (1) (i)]. Authorized employees shall also be provided with periodic physical examinations, no less often than annually, following the preassignment examination [1910.1003 (g) (1) (ii)]. In all examinations, the examining physician is required to consider whether there exist conditions of increased risk, including reduced immunological competence, those undergoing treatment with steroids or cytotoxic agents, pregnancy, and cigarette smoking [1910.1003 (g) (1) (iii)].

The scope of this chapter prohibits a detailed discussion of the medical surveillance and/or screening of the other carcinogens or suspected carcinogens.

8. CLINICAL ISSUES

The foregoing sections have included a historical overview of occupational cancer and a discussion of the major methods used today to evaluate substances and work processes regarding risk for causing cancer. This section is designed for the clinician asked to make recommendations for the prevention and diagnosis of cancers related to work. Guidance is also provided on determining whether a particular cancer may be related to work. Clinicians can participate in programs designed for the prevention of occupational cancer and in monitoring workers potentially exposed to carcinogenic substances and processes. Formulating a diagnosis and evaluating potential occupational causal connections may also be necessary.

Prevention of occupational cancer requires not only a firm understanding of agents that can cause malignancies but also an awareness of the critical importance of exposure control methods. Ideally, one should strive to reduce exposure to carcinogens as much as feasible. Carcinogens tend to follow a straightforward dose–response pattern, in that higher exposures (both in concentration and duration) tend to be associated with the highest risk. From a public policy perspective, however, control of occupational cancer has focused on eliminating exposure to agents that can cause cancer. Future preventive methods are likely to address genetic risk factors such as polymorphisms that predict people at higher risk of developing cancer (Table 3). Work resulting from the human genome project may prove beneficially for identifying people at particularly high risk of developing all sorts of illnesses, including cancer. In turn, considerations of privacy, discrimination, and other ethical challenges will surface. At the time of the preparation of this chapter, the use of genetic screening to predict those at risk of occupational cancer is not routinely used outside of research settings. At this time, the prevention of occupational cancer rests not only on the recognition

Table 3 Cancer Susceptibility Genes

Gene	Metabolic pathway	Cancer sites
GSTM1	Conjugation of organic epoxides with reduced glutathione	Lung, bladder, colon, stomach, breast, liver
CYP2S6	Hydroxylation of lipoophilic xenobiotics, possibly NNK	Lung, bladder, breast
NAT2	*N*-acetylation of arylamines and N-hydroxylated heterocyclicaryl amines	Bladder, lung, colorectal, breast
CA1A1	Metabolism of polycyclic aromatic hydrocarbons, TCDD, and estrogens	Lung, stomach, colon, breast
CYP2E1	Oxidation of *N*-nitrosamines, alcohol	Lung, bladder, colon

Source: Adapted from Garte SJ. Environmental carcinogenesis. In: Rom WN, ed. Environmental and Occupational Medicine. Philadelphia: Lippincott-Raven, 1998.

of potential hazards, but also and more importantly on their corresponding control.

Clinicians may also monitor people exposed to potential carcinogenic processes and agents in the course of their work. A variety of standards established by Occupational Safety Health Administration focus on carcinogens and specify monitoring protocols to ensure that work does not cause early effects of cancer (Table 2). Although valuable research has been performed on studies that have employed DNA adducts as early indicators of cancer, their use in clinical settings is not routine. Future efforts of monitoring workers exposed to carcinogens are likely to include assessments of early effects on DNA because of the role of genetic mutations in carcinogenesis.

The *diagnosis* of occupational cancer is conducted in a manner similar to the diagnosis of any other of cancer. Occupational illnesses, in general, are diagnosed and treated the same way as any other type of illness. In fact, cancer and other illnesses due to work have similar manifestations and prognoses, and differ primarily in their cause, not in their diagnosis. Through the occupational exposure assessment, a refined determination can be conducted regarding the contribution that work may have played in the development of the illness.

Determining the contribution that work or a specific agent may have played in the development of cancer is a complicated exercise. In some cases, such as an evaluating angiosarcoma in association with vinyl chloride monomer, the exercise can be straightforward. Similarly, determining the cause of mesothelioma in an asbestos worker is an uncomplicated challenge. On the other hand, determining the contribution that work played in the development of lung cancer in an individual who has a long history of cigarette smoking and work in chromate plating operations can be a daunting task. Fundamental principles related to evaluating dose–response effects, confounders, biological plausibility, latency, and the temporal relationship between exposure and disease must be considered.

An astute causality assessment considers both human and animal literature, with particular attention to the epidemiological studies described earlier in this chapter. Evaluations of animal studies regarding their applicability to humans must be undertaken with great care. Although all human carcinogens are animal carcinogens, not all animal carcinogens have been shown to cause cancer in humans. In some animal studies, exposure to the agent under study is often extraordinarily higher than can conceivable be anticipated to occur in humans.

In evaluating the contribution that work may have played in the development of any cancer, a firm review of major epidemiological studies, especially those that controlled for confounding factors, is essential. Limitations of the studies such as selection bias and dose–response assessments should also be addressed. Ultimately, judgment based on a review of the literature and the individual's medical and occupational history is required.

9. FUTURE EFFORTS

The National Cancer Institute's Occupational Epidemiology (OE) Branch (43) is currently conducting extensive research in occupational cancer risk assessment and prevention. Specifically, the OE Branch conducts studies to identify groups at high risk of cancer. This goal is accomplished through the execution of case–control and cohort studies to identify occupational and environmental exposures that are carcinogenic as well as conducting interdisciplinary studies using biomarkers, environmental measurements, and genetic susceptibility. The epidemiology branch also performs methodological studies to evaluate the reliability and validity of occupational and environmental assessment methods and techniques.

Current work of the branch includes research in agriculture, pesticide applicators, and farming. New research examining chronic diseases such as cancer among migrant and seasonal farm workers is also underway. In women's health, several studies are examining the role of occupational factors in the origin of breast cancer. The NCI is conducting a case–control study of breast cancer and benign breast disease in Michigan, in relation to exposure to polybrominated biphenyls. Case–control studies are in place to evaluate the hypothesized relationship between DDT and risk of breast cancer.

The NCI and NIOSH are currently conducting a number of studies examining cancer and the use of organic solvents and other industrial chemicals. A large retrospective cohort mortality and nested case–control study is underway investigating the risk of lung cancer in relation to quantitative measures of exposure to diesel exhaust among miners. In China, a cohort of approximately 75,000 benzene-exposed workers is being compared to 35,000 unexposed workers in order to obtain exposure–response and biological data. Studies are also underway examining the risk of lung cancer among workers employed in the production of acrylonitrile and among dry cleaners to evaluate the cancer risk of exposure to perchloroethylene and other petroleum solvents.

APPENDIX
International Agency for Research on Cancer (IARC)*

In 1969, the International Agency for Research on Cancer (IARC) began its program to formally evaluate carcinogenic risks of chemicals to humans and to produce monographs outlining the identification of individual hazards and work processes. Subsequently, the monograph program has expanded to consider human exposures to mixtures of chemicals, certain occupations,

---

* IARC web site; October 3, 2000.

radiation, viruses, and medications. Criteria for the determination of carcinogenic risk that were first established in 1971 have subsequently been
updated by the agency (IARC, 1977, 1978, 1979, 1982, 1983, 1987b,
1991a; Vainio et al., 1992).

The objective of the IARC Monograph Program is to provide national
and international authorities and agencies with scientific and qualitative
information on the evidence for or against carcinogenicity for the purposes
of cancer risk assessments and in formulating decisions regarding cancer
prevention. Regulations and exposure limits are delegated to individual governments, international organizations, or other agencies.

The monographs include biological and epidemiological data published in openly available scientific literature. IARC also considers government reports if they have been peer reviewed. In making cancer risk
determinations, IARC working groups rely principally on cohort, case–
control, and correlation studies (ecological) studies but they also consider
randomized trial data when available and on rare occasion consider results
from case series and case reports of cancer in humans. IARC pays particular
attention to the quality of studies, taking into account the possibility of bias,
chance, confounding, and inferences about mechanism of action.

IARC also examines studies of cancer in experimental animals. This
task is based on the fact that all known human carcinogens that have been
studied adequately in experimental animals have produced positive results in
one or more animal species. (Wilbourn et al., 1986; Tomatis et al., 1989).
IARC recognizes, however, that not all agents and mixtures that cause
cancer in experimental animals cause cancer in humans. Nonetheless, in
the absence of adequate data on humans, it is biologically plausible and prudent to consider agents and mixtures for which there is sufficient evidence of
carcinogenicity and experimental animals as if they presented a carcinogenic
risk to humans. IARC, in examining studies of cancer in experimental
animals, considers numerous qualitative and quantitative aspects of such
studies.

Once an overall valuation of the carcinogenicity to humans of the
agent, mixture, or circumstance of exposure has been completed, IARC
assigns the agent, mixture, and exposure circumstance to a designated
group. The group designation "is a matter of scientific judgment, reflecting
the strength of the evidence derived from studies in humans and experimental animals and from other relevant data." IARC assigns an agent, mixture,
or circumstance of exposure to Group 1, Group 2A, Group 2B, Group 3, or
Group 4 under the criteria outlined below.

- Group 1: The agent (mixture) is carcinogenic to humans. The exposure circumstance entails exposures that are carcinogenic to humans. This category is used when there is sufficient evidence of carcinogenicity in
  humans. Exceptionally, an agent (mixture) may be placed in this category
  when evidence of carcinogenicity in humans is less than sufficient but there

is sufficient evidence of carcinogenicity in experimental animals and strong evidence in exposed humans that the agent (mixture) acts through a relevant mechanism of carcinogenicity.

- Group 2: This category includes agents, mixtures and exposure circumstances for which, at one extreme, the degree of evidence of carcinogenicity in humans is almost sufficient, as well as those for which, at the other extreme, there are no human data but for which there is evidence of carcinogenicity in experimental animals. Agents, mixtures and exposure circumstances are assigned to either group 2A (probably carcinogenic to humans) or group 2B (possibly carcinogenic to humans) on the basis of epidemiological and experimental evidence of carcinogenicity and other relevant data.

- Group 2A: The agent (mixture) is probably carcinogenic to humans. The exposure circumstance entails exposures that are probably carcinogenic to humans. This category is used when there is limited evidence of carcinogenicity in humans and sufficient evidence of carcinogenicity in experimental animals. In some cases, an agent (mixture) may be classified in this category when there is inadequate evidence of carcinogenicity in humans and sufficient evidence of carcinogenicity in experimental animals and strong evidence that the carcinogenesis is mediated by a mechanism that also operates in humans. Exceptionally, an agent, mixture or exposure circumstance may be classified in this category solely on the basis of limited evidence of carcinogenicity in humans.

- Group 2B: The agent (mixture) is possibly carcinogenic to humans. The exposure circumstance entails exposures that are possibly carcinogenic to humans. This category is used for agents, mixtures and exposure circumstances for which there is limited evidence of carcinogenicity in humans and less than sufficient evidence of carcinogenicity in experimental animals. It may also be used when there is inadequate evidence of carcinogenicity in humans but there is sufficient evidence of carcinogenicity in experimental animals. In some instances, an agent, mixture or exposure circumstance for which there is inadequate evidence of carcinogenicity in humans but limited evidence of carcinogenicity in experimental animals together with supporting evidence from other relevant data may be placed in this group.

- Group 3: The agent (mixture or exposure circumstance) is not classifiable as to its carcinogenicity to humans. This category is used most commonly for agents, mixtures and exposure circumstances for which the evidence of carcinogenicity is inadequate in humans and inadequate or limited in experimental animals. Exceptionally, agents (mixtures) for which the evidence of carcinogenicity is inadequate in humans but sufficient in experimental animals may be placed in this category when there is strong evidence that the mechanism of carcinogenicity in experimental animals does not operate in humans. Agents, mixtures and exposure circumstances that do not fall into any other group are also placed in this category.

- Group 4: The agent (mixture) is probably not carcinogenic to humans. This category is used for agents or mixtures for which there is evidence suggesting lack of carcinogenicity in humans and in experimental animals. In some instances, agents or mixtures for which there is inadequate evidence of carcinogenicity in humans but evidence suggesting lack of carcinogenicity in experimental animals, consistently and— strongly supported by a broad range of other relevant data, may be classified in this group

REFERENCES

1. Agency for Toxic Substance and Disease Registry (ATSDR). Annual Report. Atlanta: United States Public Health Service, 1993.
2. Bouyer J. Performance of odds ratio obtained with a job–exposure matrix and individual exposure assessment with special reference to misclassification errors. Scand J Work Environ Health 1995; 21:265–271.
3. Beck B, Rude R, Calabrese E. The use of toxicology in the regulatory rocess. In: Hayes A, ed. Principles and Methods of Toxicology. 3rd ed. New York: Raven Press, 1994:19–58.
4. Lerchen ML, Samet JM. An assessement of the validity of questionnaire responses provided by a surviving spouse. Am J Epidemiol 1986; 123:481–489.
5. Breslow NE, Day NE. Statistical methods in cancer research. In: The Design and Analysis of Cohort Studies. Lyon, France: International Agency for Research on Cancer, 1987.
6. Siemiatycki J, Dewar R, Richardson L. Costs and statistical power associated with five methods of collecting exposure information for population-based case–control studies. Am J Epidemiol 1989; 130:1236–1246.
7. Schulte P, Perera F, eds. Molecular Epidemiology. New York: Academic Press.
8. Steliman J, Steliman S. Cancer and the workplace. CA Cancer J Clin 1996; 70–96.
9. NORA. National Occupational Research Agenda—Cancer Research Methods. http://www.cdc.gov./niosh/nrcan.html (12/15/1999).
10. Thriault G, Infante-Rivard C, Armonstrong B, Ernst P. Occupational neoplasia. In: Zenz C, Dickerson OB, Horvath EP, eds. Occupational Neoplasia. St. Louis: Mosby, 1994:813–823.
11. Wright W. The case report. In: McCunney RJ, ed. A practical Approach to Occupational and Environmental Medicine. 3rd ed. Baltimore: Lippincott, Williams and Wilcox, 2003. In press.
12. Doll R, Peto R. The causes of cancer: quantitative estimates avoidable risks of cancer in the United States today. J Natl Cancer Inst 1981; 66: 1191–1308.
13. Doll R, Peto R. The Causes of Cancer. Quannitative Estimates of Avoidable Risks of Cancer in the United States Today. New York: Oxford University Press, 1981.
14. Van Damme K, Casteleyn L, Heseltine E, et al. Individual susceptibility and prevention of occupation diseases: scientific and ethical issues. JOEM 1995; 137:91–99.
15. Waxweiler RJ, Stringer W, Wagoner JK. Neoplastic risk among workers exposed to vinyl chloride. Ann NY Acad Sci 1976; 271:40–48.
16. Wild C. Carcinogen–DNA and carcinogen–protein adducts in molecular epidemiology. IARC Sci Publ 1997; 142:143–158.
17. Rothman KJ, Greenland S. Case–control studies. In: Rothman KJ, Greenland S, eds. Moderm Epidemiology. 2nd ed. Philadelphia: Lippincott Williams and Wilkins, 1998:67–78.

18. Schaftenfeld D, Hass J. Carcinogens in the workplace. CA Cancer J Clin 1979; 29:144–168.
19. Khoury M. Genetic epidemiology. In: Rothman K, Greenland S, eds. Modern Epidemiology. 2nd ed. Philadelphia: Lippicott Williams and Wilkins, 1998:609–621.
20. Schulte, Hunter, Rothman. Ethical and social issues in the use of biomarkers in epidemiologic research. IARC Sci Publ 1997; 142:313–318.
21. Pitot HC, Dragan YP. Chemical Carcinogenesis. In: Klaassen CD, ed. Casarett & Doull's, The Basic Science of Poisons. 5th ed. New York: McGraw-Hill, 1996:201–267.
22. Faustman E, Omenn G. Risk assessment. In: Klaassen C, ed. Casarett & Doull's Toxicology. The Basic Science of Poisons. New York: McGraw-Hill, 1996:75–88.
23. Frumkin H. Cancer epidemiology and the workplace. Salud Publica Mex 1997;139.
24. Greenland S, Rothman KJ. Concepts of interaction. In: Rothman KJ, Greenland S, eds. Modern Epidemiology. Philadelphia: Lippincott Williams and Wilkins, 1998:329–342.
25. Harber P, Merz B, Lam I, Yuan M, Parker J, Chen W. Intelligent database generated occupational questionnaire system. J Occup Environ Med 2000; 42:483.
26. Hennekens CH, Buring JE. Epidemiology in Medicine. Boston: Little, Brown and Company, 1987.
27. Grandjean P. Ethical aspects of genetic predisposition to disease. In: Grandjean P, ed. Ecogenetics. London: Chapman & Hall, 1991:237–251.
28. Frumkin H. Occupational cancers. In: McCunney R, ed. A Practical Approach to Occupational and Environmental Medicine. 2nd ed. Boston: Little, Brown and Company, 1994:187–198.
29. McCunney RJ. The use of biomarkers in occupational medical practice. In: Mendelsohn M, Mohr L, Peeters P, eds. Biomarkers. John Henry Press, 1998: 377–386.
30. Golden AL, Markowitz SB, Landrigan PL. The risk of cancer in firefighters. In: Orris P, Melius J, Duffy M, eds. Occupational Medicine State of the Art Reviews—Firefighters' Safety and Health. Vol. 10. 1995:803–827.
31. Pott P. Cancer scroti. In: The Chirugical Works. Vol. 1. London, 1779.
32. Rannug A, Alexandrie A, Persson I, Ingelman-Sundberg M. Genetic polymorphism of cytochromes P450 1Al, 2D6 and 2El: regulation and toxocological significance. JOEM 1995;137.
33. Rothman KJ, Greenland S. Types of epidemiologic studies. In: Rothman KJ, Greenland S, eds. Modem Epidemiology. 2nd ed. Philadelphia: Lippincott Williams & Wilkins, 1998:67–78.
34. Rugo HS, Fischman ML. Occupational cancer. In: LaDou J, ed. Occupational and Environmental Medicine. 2nd ed. Stamford: Appleton & Lange, 1997.
35. McLaughlin J, Brookmeyer R. Epidemiology and biostatistics. In: McCunney R, ed. A Practical Approach to Occupational and Environmental Medicine. 2nd ed. Boston: Little, Brown and Company, 1994:346–357.
36. Monson RR. Analysis of relative survival and proportional mortality. Comput Biomed Res 1974; 7:325–332.
37. Husgafvel-Pursiainen K, Ridanpaa M, Sisko A, Vainio H. P53 and ras gene mutations in lung cancer: implications for smoking and occupational exposures. JOEM 1995;37.

38. Monson RR. Occupation. In: Monson RR, ed. Occupational Epidemiology. 2nd ed. Boca Raton, FL: CRC Press, 1990:373–405.

39. IARC. IARC Monographs on the Evaluation of Carcinogenic Risks to Humans, Suppl. 7, Overall Evaluations of Carcinogenicity. An Updating of IARC Monographs. Vols 1 to 42. Lyon: World Health Organization/Interna-International Agency for Research on Cancer, 1987.

40. IARC. IARC Monographs on the Evaluation of Carcinogenic Risks to Humans. Lyon: World Health Organization, 1994.

41. Ishibe N. Genetic susceptibility to environmental and occupational cancers. Cancer Causes Control 1997; 8:504–513.

42. Mauderly JL, McCunney RJ. Particle overload in the rat lung and lung cancer: the role in human risk assessment. Inhal Taxicol 1996.

43. National Cancer Institute. Occupational Epidemiology Branch—Major Research Areas. http://www.dceg.ims.nci.nih.gov/ebp/oeb/MRA.html (06/06/2000).

44. Ames BN, Durston WE, Yamasaki E, Lee FD. Carcinogens are mutagens. A simple test system combining liver homogenates for activation and bacteria for detection. Proc Natl Acad Sci USA 1973; 70:2281–2285.

45. Ames B, Gold L. Too many rodent carcinogens: mitogenesis increases mutagenesis. Science 1990; 1249:970–971.

46. Checkoway H, Pearce N, Crawford-Brown DJ. Research Methods in Occupational Epidemiology. New York: Oxford Univerisity Press, 1989.

47. Creech JL, Johnson MN. Angiosarcoma of the liver in the manufacture of polyvinyl chloride. J Occup Med 1974; 16:150–151.

48. Dano H, Skov T, Lynge E. Underreporting of occupational cancers in denmark. Scand J Work Environ Health 1996; 22:55–57.

49. Gilles T, Infante-Rivard C, Ernst P. Occupational neoplasia. In: Zenz C, ed. Occupational Medicine. St. Louis: Mosby, 1994:813–823.

50. Jaffe M. Validity of exposure data derived from a structured questionnaire. Am J Epidemiol 1992; 135:564–570.

51. Morabia A, Markowitz S, Garibaldi K, Wynder E. Lung cancer and occupation—results of a multicentre case–control study. Sr J Ind Med 1992; 49: 721–727.

52. Morton N. Outline of Genetic Epidemiology. Basel: S Karger, 1982.

53. NORA. NORA Posters/Cancer Research Methods. http:// www.cdc.gov/ niosh/pscanc.html (12/15/1999).

54. NORA. NORA Posters—Cancer Research Methods, 1999.

55. Omenn GS, Lave LB. Scientific and cost-effectiveness criteria in selecting batteries of short-term tests. Mutat Res 1988; 205:41–49.

56. Selikoff IJ, Hammond EC, Seidman H. Mortality experience of insulation workers in the United States and Canada, 1943–1976. Ann NY Acad Sci 1979;330.

57. Sieber WK, Sundin DS, Frazier TM. Development, use, and availability of a job exposure matrix based on national occupational hazard survey data. Am J Ind Med 1991; 20:163–174.

58. Vainio H, Husgafvel-Pursiainen K. Elimination of environmental factors or elimination of individuals: biomarkers and prevention. JOEM 1995; 37.

15

Quantification of Occupational and Environmental Exposures in Epidemiological Studies

Mustafa Dosemeci

Occupational and Enviromental Epidemiology Branch, Division of Cancer Epidemiology and Genetic, National Cancer Institute, Rockville, Maryland, U.S.A.

1. BACKGROUND

Accurate assessment of exposure to occupational and environmental risk factors is needed to ensure that epidemiological studies meet their objectives in investigating the exposure–disease relationship. The basic principle of exposure assessment for epidemiological studies is to identify the determinants of exposure variability within the study population and to classify study subjects accurately with respect to their level of exposure to the risk factor of interest. In the last 20 years or so, the quantification of exposure to occupational and environmental risk factors in the evaluation of dose–response relationships has been improved significantly in various epidemiological studies, including cohort follow-up, case–control and cross-sectional epidemiological studies. In this chapter, improvements in quantifying exposure to occupational and environmental risk factors, starting from very crude assessment by occupation or industries to detailed subject-specific biological effective dose, are presented. In addition, exposure related methodological issues, such as effects of misclassification of exposure on risk estimates, selection of appropriate exposure indices in the evaluation of exposure–disease relationship, and issues that need to be considered when an epidemiological study is used in risk management or a standard setting, are also covered in this chapter.

2. EXPOSURE ASSESSMENT METHODS USED IN EPIDEMIOLOGICAL STUDIES

2.1. Exposure Assessment by Occupation and Industry Title

In early occupational epidemiological studies on chronic diseases, job or industry titles have been used as surrogates of exposure to occupational risk factors, assuming that every study subject with the same job or industry title has the same level of exposure to all the risk factors in that occupation or industry. Epidemiological analyses usually have been carried out by evaluating the risk of disease in either a single or a group of occupations [e.g., leukemia among farmers (1,2) or bladder cancer among truck drivers (3,4)], or industries [e.g., liver cancer in the paint manufacturing industry (5,6), and in some cases occupation/industry combinations (7)]. This approach is still being used particularly in cross-sectional surveillance and case–control studies for hypothesis generating and screening purposes (8–12). For example, a death certificate-based mortality study from 24 states of the United States showed excess risk of prostate cancer among power plant operators and stationary engineers, brick masons, machinery maintenance workers, airplane pilots, longshoreman, and railroad industry workers (12). In this crude assessment approach, the variability of exposure among different work places, departments, and study subjects has been ignored and this omission caused a great deal of exposure misclassification in the evaluation of associations between exposures and diseases. Although these type of associations do not give us direct information on specific exposures and may suffer from potential exposure misclassification due to the neglected variability, they still provide us with some clues about potential risk factors. For example, based on associations between various occupations and prostate cancer risk observed in the above study (12), the authors suggested that polycyclic aromatic hydrocarbons (PAHs) may play an etiological role in prostate cancer risk. Evaluation of cancer risk by occupation or industry may not be an appropriate approach to hypothesis testing studies, but they may be very useful for screening or hypothesis generating studies.

2.2. Exposure Assessment by Application of Job Exposure Matrices

Job exposure matrices (JEMs) are designed to assign a priori exposure levels for study subjects based on their job and industry titles obtained from their work histories in case–control and surveillance studies. In applications of JEMs to occupational epidemiological studies, job and industry titles are coded using one of the standard occupational and industrial coding schemes, such as Standardized Occupational Classification codes (SOC) and Standardized Industrial Classification codes (SOC) or Census Occupational and Industrial Coding Schemes. Then, a priori exposure levels are merged with those job and industry titles using the same standardized coding scheme. In earlier applications of JEMs, exposure levels have been usually assigned directly on job title/industry combinations and they were limited to the specific study and were not applicable for other studies (13–16). However, in recent JEM applications (17,18), assignments of exposure levels have been carried out separately for job titles and industries and then integrated to specific occupation/industry combinations using an algorithm (19) to be applicable to any data set having work histories with the same coding scheme. The new JEMs are generic, can be applied to any occupational study, and have assignments of exposure levels (i.e., level of intensity), exposure probabilities (i.e., likelihood of occurrence of exposure), confidence in the assignments (i.e., accuracy of the estimates), and source indicators (i.e., whether the origin of exposure is based on the occupation or the industry). Some of these generic JEMs, such as the one for solvents and chlorinated aliphatic hydrocarbons, also have decade indicators that determine the existence of exposure by decades since 1920 (17). Although JEMs provide us with semiquantitative evaluations, assessing exposure by JEMs is a very practical approach in the evaluation of dose–response relationships. For example, JEMs for methylene chloride and other aliphatic chlorinated hydrocarbons have been applied in a case–control study of astrocytic brain cancer (20). Three new features (i.e., probability of exposure, more specific five-digit occupational and industrial codes, and changes in exposure status over decades) have been introduced to reduce the misclassification of exposure (17). Risk estimates with and without these features in the assessment of exposure to methylene chloride were compared. The introduction of each feature had a striking effect on the estimate of risk, from OR = 1.5 with intensity only and without any of these new features, to 2.5 with the high probability feature, to 4.2 with high probability and more specific occupational coding features, and to 6.1 with all three features, suggesting that the degree of exposure misclassification was significantly reduced by the introduction of these three features into these new job exposure matrices (21).

Another application of JEMs has been carried out recently in a renal cell cancer; case–control study in Minnesota (22). In earlier studies, organic solvents have been associated with renal cell cancer, however, the risk by gender and type of solvents was unclear (23–26). A priori JEMs for all organic solvents combined, all chlorinated aliphatic hydrocarbons combined, and nine individual chlorinated aliphatic hydrocarbons were developed to evaluate the risk of renal cell carcinoma among men and women in a population-based case–control study in Minnesota, USA. Work histories were collected for 438 renal cell cancer cases (273 men and 165 women) and 687 controls (462 men and 225 women) through a self-administered interview. Overall, 34% of male cases and 21% of female cases were exposed to organic solvents in general. Both intensity level and probability of exposure to these chlorinated hydrocarbons were assigned using JEMs similar to those used in the earlier study (17,18). The risk of renal cell carcinoma was significantly elevated among women exposed to all organic solvents combined [odds ratio (OR) = 2.3; 95% CI = 1.3–4.2)], to chlorinated aliphatic hydrocarbons combined (OR = 2.1; 95% CI = 1.1–3.9), and to trichloroethylene (TCE) (OR = 2.0; 95% CI = 1.0–4.0). In the case of men, no significant excess risk was observed among men exposed to any of these nine individual chlorinated aliphatic hydrocarbons, all chlorinated aliphatic hydrocarbons combined, or all organic solvents combined. These observed gender differences in the risk of renal cell carcinoma in relation to exposure to organic solvents may be explained by the differences in body fat contents (27), the metabolic activity (28,29), the rate of elimination of xenobiotics from the body (27), or the differences in the level of exposure between men and women, even though they have the same job title (30–32).

Job exposure matrices are very useful tools for investigations of an occupational or environmental agent and cancer risk. They provide us with an opportunity to group several occupations and industries by common exposures. However, they have some limitations compared to the workplace or subject-specific exposure evaluation. For example, even though JEMs consider the exposure variability for a given job title in various industrial classifications, they do not provide us with a variability of information among different workplaces. They still assume that the level of exposure for the same job title/industry combination is the same regardless of the variability among different workplaces in the same industry, which we know, from most of the previous studies, is not the case (33–36). Even though some JEMs have information on the time-dependent exposure variability (17), they are still not as accurate as the workplace-/calendar time-specific exposure assessment, which is usually used in cohort or nested case-control studies. Job exposure matrices also have a potential for exposure misclassification by ignoring the variability of exposure among study subjects who held the same job title/industry combination and assuming that every worker with the same job title/industry combination has the same level of exposure, whereas earlier studies show significant variability among subjects and even within subjects (37,38). If that level of quantification is needed, as in some risk assessment studies, then either work place/department/job title/calendar year- or subject-specific exposure assessment approaches would be preferable.

2.3. Exposure Assessment by the Facility/Department/Job Title/Calendar Year Approach

In most occupational cohort studies, work histories and historical exposure information are collected from written records existing in the workplace. In contrast to case-control and cross-sectional surveillance studies, cohort studies usually have facility-specific exposure information that allows the exposure assessor to consider the variability of exposure for the same job titles in different workplaces, and even in different departments within the same facility. In this approach, jobs in work histories are usually categorized in facility/department/job title combinations using the study-specific occupational coding schemes. Historical exposure information is collected for each standardized facility/department/job title combination, starting from the beginning of cohort enrollment. For example, a study has been conducted to develop an exposure assessment method to be used in a cohort follow-up study of workers exposed to benzene (34). Assessment of exposure to benzene was carried out in 672 factories in 12 Chinese cities. Historical exposure data were collected for 3179 unique facility/department/job title combinations over seven time periods between 1949 and 1987. A total of 18,435 exposure estimates was developed for 75,000 benzene exposed subjects, using all available historical information, including 8477 monitoring data, work activities, amount of benzene use, control measures in the departments, and personal protective equipment use. Levels of exposure for each combination are then merged with subject-specific work histories to calculate various exposure indices, such as cumulative exposure, life-time average exposure, or peak exposures. Overall, 38% of the estimates were based on benzene monitoring data. The highest time-weighted average exposures occurred in the rubber industry (30.7 ppm), particularly for rubber glue applicators (52.6 ppm) (34).

n the follow-up study, because of its recognized link with benzene exposure, the association between a clinical diagnosis of benzene poisoning (hematotoxicity) and benzene exposure was evaluated (412 cases and 614,509 person-years) to validate the exposure assessment method (39). Relative risks of benzene hematotoxicity increased very sharply with increasing estimated intensity of benzene exposure. Odds ratios were 1.0, 2.2, 4.7, and 7.2 for the intensity levels of <5, 5–19, 20–39, and 40+ ppm, respectively (Table 1). This sharp trend between benzene hematotoxicity and estimated exposure to benzene indicated that the consideration of variability of exposure among facilities and departments provides us with an important tool in reducing misclassification of exposure.

Table 1 Odds Ratios for Benzene Poisoning by Duration and Intensity of Benzene

Exposure years	< 5 years	5–9 years	10–19 years	20+ years
Duration of exposure	1.0[a] (—)	1.3 (1.0–1.8)[b]	1.6 (1.2–2.1)	2.7 (1.9–3.9)
Concentration	<5 ppm	5–19 ppm	20–39 ppm	40+ ppm
Intensity of exposure	1.0[a] (—)	2.2 (1.7–2.9)[b]	4.7 (3.4–6.5)	7.2 (5.3–9.8)

Another facility-specific exposure assessment procedure has been carried out among workers exposed to acrylonitrile (40). The study comprised over 25,000 workers in eight monomer, fiber, and resin companies from 1952 to 1983. Multiple visits to the companies were made and over 100 interviews of workers with more than 10 years of employment were conducted at the companies. Historical records, including data on over 18,000 measurements taken by the companies since 1977 and over 400 measurements, were collected by the study investigators. Three thousand six hundred exposure groups were formed from 127,000 job entries noted in personnel records, based on similar tasks, locations, and other exposures, and a similar distribution of exposures to acrylonitrile. Special procedures were used to reduce the exposure misclassification that may occur with maintenance workers, engineers, and other workers who may perform specialized tasks that vary in time and are not adequately reflected by a job title. Names of workers in these jobs were sent to the companies and unions to quantify the time each worker spent in acrylonitrile areas. A software program developed specifically for this study (Job Exposure Profiles), was used to organize and retain all the information available by exposure group. Quantitative estimates of acrylonitrile exposure were developed using a second software program that documented the derivation of each estimate and facilitated data review. Four methods were used to estimate exposures in a hierarchical fashion: arithmetic means; a time-weighting method, which weighted acrylonitrile concentrations in different areas by the time spent in those areas; a deterministic method that estimated the impact of changes in the workplace on exposures; and professional judgment. Over 85% of the estimates based on professional judgment were for jobs in areas without acrylonitrile exposure. Only a qualitative assessment was performed for exposures other than acrylonitrile. To evaluate the ability of the time-weighting and deterministic methods to predict actual measurement data, estimates derived from these two methods were developed independently of the study and compared to actual measurement data. The estimates from the time-weighting method underestimated the measurements by 24% and had a standard deviation relative to the measurement mean of 166%. The estimates from the deterministic method had a positive bias of 1% and a relative standard deviation of 236%. The methodologies developed for this study have pragmatic and theoretical applications.

Although this approach provides us with a great deal of advancement in accuracy of assessing exposure to occupational risk factors compared to previous approaches such as JEMs or the occupational and industrial title approach, it still has potential misclassification of exposure due to the assumption that every subject in the same facility/department/job title/ calendar year combination has the same exposure levels, which may not be a valid assumption based on our previous studies (35,41).

2.4. Subject-Specific Exposure Assessment

Because of the high exposure variability between workers within the same job title, subject-specific exposure information can play a significant role in reducing the potential exposure misclassification by considering the between-individual variability. One of the efficient ways of collecting subject-specific exposure information is the administration of the interview to study subjects. Questions related to the determinants of subject-specific exposures provide us with a great opportunity to calculate the overall exposure level for each study subject. For example, a quantitative method was developed to estimate pesticide exposures in a large cohort study of over 58,000 pesticide applicators in North Carolina and Iowa (42). An enrolment questionnaire was administered to applicators to collect basic time- and intensity-related information on pesticide exposure such as duration and frequency of application, specific chemicals used, mixing condition, application methods, and personal protective equipment used. In addition, a detailed take-home questionnaire was administered to collect further intensity-related exposure information such as maintenance or repair of mixing and application equipment, work practices, and personal hygiene.

Two algorithms were developed to estimate the intensity level of exposure for applicators, using the responses from the questionnaires and the information from the literature. The first algorithm was based on the enrollment questionnaire and included variables of the mixing status (Mix, with exposure scores ranging from 3 to 9), application method (Appl, with scores ranging from 1 to 9), status of repairing of mixing and/or application equipment (Repair, with score of 2), and personal protective equipment use (PPE, 0.1 to 1.0).

The algorithm based on the enrollment questionnaire

$$\text{Intensity score(IS)} = (\text{Mix} + \text{Appl} + \text{Repair}) * \text{PPE}$$

The scores assigned to each of these exposure variables were derived from the published pesticide exposure literature, the Pesticide Handlers Exposure Database (PHED), and the Environmental protection Agency's pilot monitoring survey conducted as part of the AHS.

The second algorithm was based on the take-home questionnaire, and included additional exposure variables, such as types of enclosed mixing system [Enclosed], having a tractor with an enclosed cab and/or charcoal filter (Cab), status of equipment washed after application (Wash), personal hygiene (Hyg) (e.g., changing into clean clothes and washing hands or taking a bath/shower), status of changing clothes after a spill (Spill), and frequency of replacing old gloves (Gloves-life).

The algorithm based on the enrollment questionnaire

IS = {(Mix * Enclosed) + (Appl * Cab) + Repair

+ *Wash*}* *Hyg* Spill** Gloves-life

The exposure levels associated with these variables were estimated using primarily measurement data from the published pesticide exposure literature and professional judgments. For each study subject, a pesticide-specific lifetime cumulative exposure level was estimated by merging the intensity scores calculated from algorithms and the duration and frequency of pesticide use identified in the questionnaire. Although this approach provides us with an opportunity to consider the variability among subjects with the same job titles, it takes into account only the level of external exposure and does not consider the variability in host factors for subjects with the same level of external exposure. Due to the differences in genetical susceptibility markers among study subjects, their biologically effective doses (i.e., the internal doses that may have an impact on disease development) may be totally different, even though they may have the same external exposure.

2.5. Exposure Assessment by Biologically Effective Dose

The main goal of the exposure assessment for epidemiological studies is to identify the variability of an exposure in the study population and then classify study subjects accurately with respect to their variability of exposure. In traditional exposure assessment approaches, we usually limit ourselves to dealing with the variability of external risk factors either in their concentrations in the ambient air or their intake into the body without considering the variability of host factors that determine the amount of the internal dose from the external exposure. Because our main goal is to reduce the exposure misclassification in the evaluation of dose–response relationships between occupational/environmental exposures and cancer risks, there is also a need to consider the variability of genetical susceptibility factors that eventually determine the internal dose, the biologically effective dose, or in the case of evaluating cancer risk, the cancer-causing dose of the external risk factors. The evaluation of gene–environment interactions has power limitations when the prevalence of environmental risk factors and/or genetical susceptibility markers is low in the study population and multiple genetical markers interact with the exposure of interest. Recently, a method for estimating the biologically effective dose has been developed by integrating levels of external exposure with the protective ability of genetical susceptibility markers. In this process, the level of external occupational or environmental exposure may either be reduced or increased depending on the capacity of phase I (activation), phase II (detoxification), and DNA repair enzymes. In this approach, genetical susceptibility markers (e.g., CYP1A1, CYP2E1,

NAT1, NAT2, GSTM1, GSTT1, or DNA repair capacity) are used as if they were internal personal protective equipment. For example, low capacity of activation enzymes (e.g., CYP1A1), and high capacity of detoxification (e.g., NAT2) and DNA repair enzymes would have higher protective functions than high capacity of activation enzymes, and low capacity of detoxification and DNA repair enzymes, which may result in reducing cancer-causing doses of xenobiotics. This approach allows us to evaluate relationships between an unlimited number of genetic susceptibility markers and the exposure under investigation, without losing power. For example, in the application of this approach to the effects of interactions between NAT2, GSTM1, and CYP1A1 genetical polymorphisms and exposure to smoking on breast cancer risk (43), the smoking status of each study subject was reclassified based on the protective effects of a wild-type gene against its mutant type. Subjects with NAT2 wild-type gene had 60% protection from smoking in the development breast cancer compared to subjects with mutant NAT2 genotype. Similarly, subjects with wild-type CYP1A1 genotype showed 76% protection, while subjects with GSTM1 showed only 6% protection compared to subjects with mutant genotypes. Depending on the subject's genotype status (i.e., wild type or mutant type), we either reduced or increased the amount of smoking based on the protection factor of each genotype. After recalculation of the smoking status, the odds ratios for the high smoking category increased from 1.3 to 2.2, indicating that the estimated biologically effective dose of cigarette smoking has less misclassification than the reported amount of cigarette smoking.

3. SELECTION OF THE OPTIMAL INDEX OF EXPOSURE IN OCCUPATIONAL EPIDEMIOLOGY

A wide variety of exposure indices, ranging from very simple ones (e.g., ever/never exposed or duration of exposure) to complex ones (e.g., time-weighted cumulative exposure or biologically effective dose), have been developed and are used in occupational epidemiological analyses. They can be classified into three major categories according to their associations with disease outcomes. The first group consists of the time-dependent exposure indices, such as duration of exposure, frequency of exposure, latency of exposure, and recency of exposure. The second category is the intensity-dependent exposure indices, such as average intensity, highest intensity, longest intensity, and peak exposure. The last category is the combination of the first and the second, the time-and-intensity-dependent indices, such as cumulative exposure, time-weighted cumulative exposure, intensity by duration, intensity by latency, intensity by recency, cumulative exposure by latency, cumulative exposure by recency, internal dose, or biologically effective dose. The selection of the optimum exposure index is based on the mechanism of the exposure–disease relationship. An exposure index may be an optimum one for certain relationships, an acceptable one for others, or a totally inappropriate one for some other relationships. For example, duration of benzene exposure would be an acceptable index for the benzene–lymphoma relationship, but it is an inappropriate index for the benzene–leukemia relationship. The optimum benzene exposure index for lymphomas would be cumulative exposure, while for leukemia, it would be the intensity of benzene exposure. For silicosis, the optimum silica exposure index would be time-weighted respirable cumulative silica dust exposure, while the average intensity of respirable silica dust would be a poor exposure index. Before deciding which index would be optimal, it is important to know about the characteristics of the metabolism of the agent of interest, such as the level of metabolic saturation, half-life in the body, and activity of metabolic enzymes. The other important clue may come from the epidemiological observations. For example, a cross-tabulation of the risk of the disease by a time-dependent exposure, such as duration of exposure, and by an intensity-dependent exposure index, such as average intensity, could give us useful information for the selection of an optimum exposure index. If both the duration of exposure at various intensity levels and the intensity of exposure at various duration levels do not show associations with the disease risk, then it is unlikely that cumulative exposure would be an optimum index for that association. Because the role of exposure in the disease process is the key factor for the selection of the optimum exposure index, and because the biologically effective does requires an understanding of the mechanism, it is recommended to consider the use of either of these indices as a potential optimal index of exposure in the evaluation of an exposure–disease relationship.

4. RECOMMENDATION TO EXPOSURE ASSESSORS TO MINIMIZE THE EFFECTS OF EXPOSURE MISCLASSIFICATION ON RISK ESTIMATES

Misclassification of exposure can severely affect estimates of disease risks, and even in some extreme situations, cause misleading interpretations about exposure–disease associations. Although several studies have evaluated the effects of misclassification on risk estimates (44–48), no recommendation to exposure assessors is available to reduce these adverse effects of misclassification of exposure. There are four major determinants of exposure misclassification which are usually observed in epidemiological studies. These determinants are: (1) the size of the true risk, (2) the amount of misclassification, (3) the exposure prevalence of the true distribution, and (4) the direction of misclassification. For cohort-type distributions, where the exposure prevalence is high, extreme distortions are observed when misclassification occurred from the exposed categories to the unexposed category (49). Little effect is observed when the misclassification occurred from the unexposed to the exposed categories. For the type of distributions seen in case–control studies, where the exposure prevalence is low, greater effects are observed when misclassification occurred from the unexposed category to the exposed categories, while little effect was observed when the misclassification occurred from the unexposed category to the exposed ones or occurred between the exposed categories.

5. ISSUES TO BE CONSIDERED IN USING RETROSPECTIVE EPIDEMIOLOGICAL STUDIES FOR RISK ASSESSMENT

The majority of established occupational and environmental exposure limits (e.g., TLV, MAK, PEL, PDK, REL, or BEI) are based on available information from industrial or environmental experiences; from experimental human and animal studies; and, when possible, from a combination of the two. Although, the use of information from retrospective epidemiological studies for the development of exposure limits has been limited in the past, there has been a growing interest in the use of these studies among the institutions responsible for the occupational and environmental regulations. Exposure limits are defined as airborne concentrations of substances to which nearly all workers or general population may be exposed on a daily basis without adverse health effects. There are various issues that need to be taken into account when data from retrospective epidemiological studies are used by regulatory institutions to develop these exposure limits:

1. *Selection of an appropriate exposure index:* Almost all exposure limits represent an "intensity of exposure" (in ppm, mg/M^3, or fiber/cc, etc.). However, epidemiological studies use a variety of exposure indices, such as duration of exposure, intensity of exposure, or cumulative exposure, in the evaluation of the exposure–disease relationship. The optimum index depends on the mechanism by which the exposure affects the disease. For some exposure–disease relationships, intensity of exposure is the best index, while for others, duration of exposure or lifetime cumulative exposure may be more appropriate. Use of an inappropriate exposure index may result in the development of unrealistic exposure limits.

2. *Mechanistic considerations:* The mechanisms underlying the exposure–disease relationships need to be taken into account when interpreting epidemiological studies. For example, if there are saturation effects at a certain concentration level, extrapolating risk estimates from high doses to low doses may lead to an underestimate of true risk at low-level exposures. Similarly, if there is a

threshold effect in the relationship, extrapolating risk from high
to low doses may lead to an overestimate of risk at low levels.
There has been some concern about the relevance of risk estimates
obtained at very high exposure levels. For example, the validity of
the linear extrapolation of risk from high to lower doses has been
questioned, with the argument that at low exposure levels, risk
might be overestimated if there is a threshold level in the dose–
response relationship (50). However, it was also argued that,
linear extrapolation from high to low doses might actually underestimate risk in some circumstances (51). Indeed, it has been
showed that metabolic saturations exist for some chemicals, and
calculated distortion from linearity for benzene, tetrachloroethy-
lene, and trichloroethylene starts at levels of 63, 22, and 178 mg/m^3,
respectively, indicating that the risks of solvent-related outcomes
do not necessarily rise linearly with increasing dose above the
saturation point (52). Because of metabolic saturation at high
levels of exposure, the actual risk at such exposures would
be below the dose–response line, and linear extrapolation of
risk from high to low doses could underestimate the risk at low
levels (53).

3. *Estimating effective durations and doses:* In most exposure–disease
    relationships, we do not know the exact time at which the expo-
    sure of interest induces the disease. Therefore, it may be quite dif-
    ficult to estimate the effective duration of exposure and effective
    dose that has induced the disease in an epidemiological study.
    For example, a disease might be initiated in the early stage of expo-
    sure and the remaining duration of exposure may not be relevant
    for the disease development, or the disease might be initiated in the
    later stage of the exposure duration, and at that time, effective
    duration should be calculated from the beginning of the exposure.

4. *Absoluteness of the quantitative estimates:* In most retrospective
    occupational epidemiological studies, quantitative assessments
    of exposures are based on a few historical measurements for a
    few job titles. Because of this limitation, exposure assessors often
    extrapolate or interpolate from the available exposure informa-
    tion to estimate the quantitative level of exposure. Even though
    these estimates may be quite accurate on a relative scale, they
    may not be accurate on an absolute scale. This may not be an
    important issue for etiological studies, but it may be crucial when
    the studies are used as a basis for developing exposure limits.
    Carefully designed prospective epidemiological studies may solve
    most of the issues associated with retrospective epidemiological
    studies.

REFERENCES

1. Blair A, Thomas TL. Leukemia among Nebraska farmers: a death certificate study. Am J Epidemiol 1979; 110:264–273.
2. Delzell E, Grufferman S. Mortality among white and nonwhite farmers in North Carolina, 1976–1978. Am J Epidemiol 1985; 121:392–402.
3. Silverman DT, Hoover RN, Albert S, Graff KM. Occupation and cancer of the lower urinary tract in Detroit. J Natl Cancer Inst 1983; 70:237–245.
4. Hoar SK, Hoover R. Truck driving and bladder cancer mortality in rural New England. J Natl Cancer Inst 1985; 74:771–774.
5. Englund A. Cancer incidence among painters and some allied trades. J Toxicol Environ Health 1980; 6:1267–1273.
6. Matanoski GM, Stockwell HG, Diamond EL, Haring-Sweeney M, Joffe RD, Mele LM, Johnson ML. A cohort mortality study of painters and allied tradesmen. Scand J Work Environ Health 1986; 12:16–21.
7. Zahm SH, Hartge P, Hoover R. The National Bladder Cancer Study: employment in the chemical industry. J Natl Cancer Inst 1987; 79:217–222.
8. Ward MH, Dosemeci M, Cocco P. Mortality from gastric cardia and lower esophagus cancer and occupation. J Occup Med 1994; 36:1222–1227.
9. Figgs LW, Dosemeci M, Blair A. United States non-Hodgkin's lymphoma surveillance by occupation 1984–1989: twenty-four state death certificate study. Am J Ind Med 1995; 27:817–835.
10. Heineman EF, Gao YT, Dosemeci M, McLaughlin JK. Occupational risk factors for brain tumors among women in Shanghai, China. J Occup Environ Med 1995; 37:288–293.
11. Chow WH, Ji BT, Dosemeci M, McLaughlin JK, Gao YT, Fraumeni JF Jr. Biliary tract cancers among textile and other workers in Shanghai, China. Am J Ind Med 1996; 30:36–40.
12. Krstev S, Baris D, Stewart PA, Hayes RB, Blair A, Dosemeci M. Risk of prostate cancer by occupation and industry: a 24-state death certificate study. Am J Ind Med 1998; 34:413–420.
13. Hoar SK, Morrison AS, Cole P, Silverman D. An occupation and exposure linkage system for the study of occupational arcinogenesis. J Occup Med 1980; 22:722–726.
14. Acheson ED. What Are JEM's? In: Acheson ED, ed. Job-exposure matrices. Proceedings of a conference held in April 1982 at the University of Southampton, Southampton, U.K., 1983.
15. Hinds MW, Kolonel LN, Lee J. Application of a job-exposure matrix to a case-control study of lung cancer. J Natl Cancer Inst 1985; 75:193–197.
16. Pannett B, Coggon D, Acheson ED. A job-exposure matrix for use in population-based studies in England and Wales. Br J Ind Med 1985; 42:777–783.
17. Dosemeci M, Cocco P, Gomez M, Stewart PA, Heineman EF. Effects of three features of a job-exposure matrix on risk estimates. Epidemiology 1994; 5: 124–127.
18. Gomez MR, Cocco P, Dosemeci M, Stewart PA. Occupational exposure to chlorinated aliphatic hydrocarbons: job-exposure matrix. Am J Ind Med 1994; 26:171–183.

19. Dosemeci M, Stewart PA, Blair A. Evaluating occupation and industry separately to assess exposure in case-control studies. Appl Ind Hyg 1989; 4: 256–259.

20. Heineman EF, Cocco P, Gomez MR, Dosemeci M, Stewart PA, Hayes RB, Zahm SH, Thomas TL, Blair A. Occupational exposure to chlorinated aliphatic hydrocarbons and risk of astrocytic brain cancer. Am J Ind Med 1994; 26: 155–169.

21. Greenland S, Robins JM. Confounding and misclassification. Am J Epidemiol 1985; 122:495–506.

22. Dosemeci M, Cocco P, Chow WH. Gender differences in risk of renal cell carcinoma and occupational exposures to chlorinated aliphatic hydrocarbons. Am J Ind Med 1999; 36:54–59.

23. Katz RM, Jowett D. Female laundry and dry cleaning workers in Wisconsin: a mortality analysis. Am J Public Health 1981; 71:305–307.

24. Duh RW, Asal NR. Mortality among laundry and dry cleaning workers in Oklahoma. Am J Public Health 1984; 74:1278–1280.

25. Lynge E, Andersen O, Carstensen B. Primary liver cancer and renal cell carcinoma in laundry and dry-cleaning workers in Denmark. Scand J Work Environ Health 1995; 21:293–295.

26. McCredie M, Stewart JH. Risk factors for kidney cancer in New South Wales. IV. Occupation. Br J Ind Med 1993; 50:349–354.

27. Silvaggio T, Mattison DR. Setting occupational health standards: toxicokinetic differences among and between men and women. J Occup Med 1994; 36: 849–854.

28. Kihara M, Kihara M, Noda K. Distribution of GSTM1 null genotype in relation to gender, age and smoking status in Japanese lung cancer patients. Pharmacogenetics 1995; 5:74–79.

29. Rodilla V, Hawksworth GM, Benzie AA. Glutathione S-transferase of human kidney: are there gender-related quantitative differences? BiochemSoc Trans 1996; 24:322.

30. Hernberg S, Kauppinen T, Riala R, Korkala ML, Asikainen U. Increased risk for primary liver cancer among women exposed to solvents. Scand J Work Environ Health 1988; 14:356–365.

31. Greenberg GN, Dement JM. Exposure assessment and gender differences. J Occup Med 1994; 36:907–912.

32. Roxburgh S. Gender differences in work and well-being: effects of exposure and vulnerability. Health Soc Behav 1996; 37:265–277.

33. Stewart PA, Blair A, Cubit DA, Bales RE, Kaplan SA, Ward J, Gaffey W, O'Berg MT, Walrath J. Estimating historical exposures to formaldehyde in a retrospective mortality study. Appl Ind Hyg 1986; 1:34–41.

34. Dosemeci M, Li GL, Hayes RB, Yin SN, Linet M, Chow WH, Wang YZ, Jiang ZL, Dai TR, Zhang WU, Chao XJ, Zhang XJ, Ye PZ, Kou QR, Fan YH, Zhang XC, Lin XF, Meng JF, Zho JS, Wacholder S, Kneller R, Blot WJ. Cohort study among workers exposed to benzene in China: II. Exposure assessment. Am J Ind Med 1994; 26:401–411.

35. Dosemeci M, McLaughlin JK, Chen JQ, Hearl FJ, Chen RG, McCawley MA, Wu Z, Peng KL, Chen AL, Rexing SH, Blot WJ. Historical total and respirable

silica dust exposure levels in mines and pottery factories in China. Scand J Work Environ Health 1995; 21:39–43.

36. Stewart PA, Zaebst D, Zey JN, Herrick R, Dosemeci M, Hornung R, Bloom T, Pottern L, Miller B, Blair A. Exposure assessment for a study of workers exposed to acrylonitrile. Scand J Work Environ Health 1998; 24:42–53.

37. Rappaport SM, Kromhout H, Symanski E. Variation of exposure between workers in homogeneous exposure groups. Am Ind Hyg Assoc J 1993; 54: 654–662.

38. Kromhout H, Symanski E, Rappaport SM. A comprehensive evaluation of within- and between-worker components of occupational exposure to chemical agents. Ann Occup Hyg 1993; 37:253–270.

39. Dosemeci M, Yin SN, Linet M, Wacholder S, Rothman N, Li GL, Chow WH, Wang YZ, Jiang ZL, Dai TR, Zhang WU, Chao XJ, Ye PZ, Kou QR, Fan YH, Zhang XC, Lin XF, Meng JF, Zho JS, Blot WJ, Hayes RB. Indirect validation of benzene exposure assessment by association with benzene poisoning. Environ Health Perspect 1996; 104:1343–1347.

40. Stewart PA, Zey J, Hornung R, Herrick RF, Dosemeci M, Zaebst D, Pottern L. Exposure assessment for a study of workers exposed to acrylonitrile. III. Evaluation of exposure assessment methods. Appl Occup Environ Hyg 1996; 11:1312–1321.

41. Stewart WF, Stewart PA, Heineman EF, White D, Dosemeci M, Ward MH. A method for collecting work history information in occupational community-based case-control studies. Occup Hyg 1996; 3:145–152.

42. Alavanja MC, Akland G, Baird D, Blair A, Bond A, Dosemeci M, Kamel F, Lewis R, Lubin J, Lynch C, McMaster SB, Moore M, Pennybacker M, Ritz L, Rothman N, Rowland A, Sandler DP, Sinha R, Swanson C, Tarone R, Weinberg C, Zahm SH. Cancer and noncancer risk to women in agriculture and pest control: the agriculture health study. J Occup Med 1994; 36: 1247–1250.

43. Ambrosone CB, Freudenheim JL, Graham S, Marshall JR, Vena JE, Brasure JR, Michalek AM, Laughlin R, Nemoto T, Gillenwater KA, Shields PG. Cigarette smoking N-acetyltransferase 2 genetic polymorphisms breast cancer risk. J Am Med Assoc 1996; 13(276):1494–1501.

44. Dosemeci M, Wacholder S, Lubin JH. Does non-differential misclassification of exposure always bias a true effect toward the null value? AmJ Epidemiol 1990; 132:746–748.

45. Wacholder S, Dosemeci M, Lubin JH. Blind assignment of exposure does not always prevent differential misclassification. Am J Epidemiol 1991; 134: 433–437.

46. Lundberg M, Hallqvist J, Diderichsen F. Exposure-dependent misclassification of exposure in interaction analyses. Epidemiology 1999; 10:545–549.

47. Marshall RJ. Assessment of exposure misclassification bias in case-control studies using validation data. J Clin Epidemiol 1997; 50:15–19.

48. Sorahan T, Gilthorpe MS. Non-differential misclassification of exposure always leads to an underestimate of risk: an incorrect conclusion. Occup Environ Med 1994; 51:839–840.

49. Dosemeci M, Stewart PA. Recommendation to occupational hygienists to minimize the effects of exposure misclassification on risk estimates. Occup Hyg 1996; 3:169–176.
50. Abelson PH. Risk assessments of low-level exposures. Science 1994; 265:1507.
51. Portier CJ, Lucier GW, Edler L. Risk from low-dose exposures. Science 1994; 266:1141–1142.
52. Rappaport SM. Biological considerations in assessing exposures to genotoxic and carcinogenic agents. Int Arch Occup Environ Health 1993; 65:29–35.
53. Dosemeci M. Invited editorial: retrospective exposure assessment in large cohort studies in China: advantages and concerns. Ann Occup Hyg 1999; 43:377–379.

16

Cancer Risk for Tobacco and Alcohol Use

Peter G. Shields

Cancer Genetics and Epidemiology Program, Department of Medicine and Oncology, Lombardi Comprehensive Cancer Center, Georgetown University, Washington, D.C., U.S.A.

1. INTRODUCTION

In the 1960s, the first Surgeon General's Report (1) clearly demonstrated that lung cancer was caused by smoking. Since then, we have recognized that smoking contributes to many other cancers, such as leukemia, bladder, oral cavity, and cervical cancers. Tobacco smoke contains more than 100 carcinogens and mutagens, many of which are classified as carcinogens based on human and animal studies. The effect on people has been obvious. Before the widespread use of cigarettes in this century, lung cancer was a rare illness. Over the last 40 years, the type of cigarettes most frequently used has been changing, namely the increased use of low-tar and low-nicotine yield cigarettes. While initially thought to confer some decreased risk compared with higher-tar cigarettes, a benefit has not been realized. The use of low-tar and low-nicotine yield cigarettes has been paradoxically accompanied by an increased risk of lung cancer due to increased tobacco use and exposure to cigarette yields with higher mutagen and carcinogen content. This higher consumption has been due to a smoker's need to maintain blood nicotine levels, which in turn causes the need for smoking more cigarettes per day and deeper inhalation. This phenomenon has led to the increasing rates of lung adenocarcinoma, compared to squamous cell carcinoma. It also probably explains, in part, the greater risk of lung cancer in women compared to men (in addition to some biological differences).

The study of tobacco-related cancer involves many types of biomarkers, including those that measure exposure, the biologically effective dose, and harm. Genetic susceptibilities for smoking behavior, carcinogen metabolism, DNA repair, and others likely also play a large role in cancer risk.

Alcoholic beverages clearly increase the risk of oral cavity, liver, esophageal, breast, and other cancers. However, the actual mechanisms that alcohol drinking contributes to carcinogenesis have not been well defined. It is clear that ethanol has mutagenic metabolites, that free radicals are generated during ethanol metabolism, that there is an interaction and under-utilization with vitamins (e.g., folic acid), and that there is an effect on steroid hormones. Also, various alcoholic beverages contain contaminants that might contribute to cancer risk, such as urethane in wines and *n*-nitrosamines in beer. The increased risk from alcohol drinking must be weighed against the reduction in mortality and heart disease risk from lower levels of drinking. Thus, there are data to indicate that taking one drink per day confers some benefit, but taking more than that might be offset by increased cancer risks. How this risk changes by genetic susceptibilities is unknown. But, some people might get more benefits, and some might be more easily harmed, from alcohol use.

2. TOBACCO

2.1. Tobacco Mutagens and Carcinogens

The use of tobacco products, as they are intended to be used, results in the exposure to more than 100 mutagens and carcinogens (2,3). A partial list of these constituents is provided in Table 1. It is thought that tobacco-specific nitrosamines (TSNs) and polycyclic aromatic hydrocarbons (PAHs) are classes of compounds that most affect human cancer risk (4). Tobacco and tobacco products have changed over time, with resultant differences in predicted exposure using the Federal Trade Commission (FTC) method for the measurement of "tar" and "nicotine" (2). It is known that the FTC method for estimating tar exposure provides substantial underestimates of actual human exposure because it does not sufficiently mimic human smoking behavior (2).

Prior to the 1950s, most manufactured cigarettes did not have filters, but now, almost all cigarettes are filtered and fall into the category of low tar and nicotine (2,5). Tar yield actually has declined since the 1950s, from about 37 mg to less than 15 mg (2,5). Because of similar decreases in nicotine, and increased quitting among lighter smokers, the actual number of cigarettes smoked per person has increased (5). The introduction of low-tar and low-nicotine cigarettes was conceptualized to make cigarettes "safer," but currently available scientific data suggest that potential benefits may not be realized for some or most persons, and in fact these products are probably more dangerous. Many persons who smoke low-tar and

Table 1 List of Selected Tobacco Mutagens and Carcinogens[a]

Constituent class	Phase	IARC evaluation[b]	Examples
N-nitrosamines	Particulate	Sufficient in animals	Tobacco-specific nitrosamines (NNK, NNN), dimethylnitrosamine, diethylnitrosamine
Polycyclic aromatic hydrocarbons	Particulate	Probable in humans	Benzo(a)pyrene, benzo(a)anthracene, benzo(b) flouranthene, 5-methylchrysene
Aryl aromatic amines	Particulate	Sufficient in humans	4-Aminobiphenyl, 2-toluidine, 2-napthylamine
Heterocyclic amines	Particulate	Probable in humans	2-Amino-3-methylimmidzzo[4,5-b]quinolone(IQ)
Organic solvents	Vapor	Sufficient in humans	Benzene, methanol, toluene, styrene
Aldehydes	Vapor	Limited in humans	Acetaldehyde, formaldehyde
Volatile organic compounds	Vapor	Probable	1,3-Butadiene, isoprene
Inorganic compounds	Vapor	Sufficient in humans	Arsenic, nickel, chromium, polonium-210

[a]This list is intended to provide a conceptual overview of the complexity of tobacco product exposures. It is not all-inclusive, but is included to allow the reader to understand the number of considerations that must be made in assessing harm reduction strategies.
[b]IARC classification is from the International Agency for Research on Cancer. The classifications here refer to evaluations of the compound from any exposure, and not just tobacco. Not all chemicals within the class have been considered to be carcinogenic in humans. There is no consideration given in this table to delivered dose or route of exposure.

low-nicotine cigarettes compensate for lower nicotine delivery by smoking more (6–10). But also, the tar from "light" cigarettes is more mutagenic and levels of TSNs and benzo(a)pyrene in tobacco smoke can be similar for low- and high-tar cigarettes when people oversmoke their cigarettes (11,12).

PAHs are formed from the incomplete pyrolysis of tobacco leaves, and many types of PAHs are present in tobacco smoke. Parent PAHs can be detected in human lung tissue (13,14). As a class, they are mutagenic and carcinogenic in experimental animals (including the lung) and human (2,15,16). PAHs are metabolically activated in humans through cytochrome P450 (CYP) 1A1, CYP1B1, and CYP3A4 (17,18). They are conjugated for excretion by glutathione-S-transferases, sulfuronyl transferases, and glucuronyl transferases (19), and the lack of such activity increases mutagenic potential (20). PAH-related DNA adducts have been demonstrated in human lung (21), while the presence of hemoglobin and albumen adducts also show that these compounds circulate in human blood (22,23). In vitro studies indicate that PAHs can cause the same types of p53 mutations observed in human tumors (24,25).

N-nitrosamines (26–29) are among the most potent rodent carcinogens (30). There are some N-nitrosamines that are only found in tobacco smoke (TSNs). N-nitrosamines cause cancer in more than 40 animal species and there is target organ specificity, including for TSNs and lung tumors (30,31). Experimental animal studies show that higher doses of exposure cause tumors in less time, suggesting that intensity and duration are equally important (30,32). Mutations in K-*Ras* have been found in the lung tumors of experimentally exposed animals. TSNs can transform human bronchial epithelial cells (33). The same type of adducts that occur from TSNs in experimental animals also have been detected in humans, including in lung tissue (34). Different types of tobacco have different TSN yields (29). In humans, metabolites of TSNs are found in urine (35) and adducts are detected in blood, so TSNs circulate through the body, including in persons who are passively exposed (36–38). N-nitrosamines undergo metabolic activation by human CYPs located in the lung, buccal mucosa, and other tissues (e.g., CYP2E1 and CYP2A6) (39–41). The metabolic activation of TSNs and other tobacco N-nitrosamines leads to the formation of DNA adducts in target tissues associated with specific cancers (32,42–46). Different tobacco products contain widely differing amounts of TSNs (28), and changing smoking patterns can result in higher delivery of TSNs (47). For example, Swedish snuff products contain substantially less TSNs than snuff sold in the United States. Lower-tar and -nicotine cigarettes result in greater exposure to TSNs than high-tar and -nicotine cigarettes (2,29).

Both the gaseous and the particulate phases of cigarette smoke contain free radicals (such as nitric oxides in the gaseous phase) which induce oxidative damage (2,48). Many components of cigarette smoke can individually cause oxidative damage (49). While free radicals cause DNA damage in experimental systems and are suspected to be involved in carcinogenesis (50), a direct relationship to human carcinogenesis has been suspected but not proven (51,52). It is difficult to measure free radicals and oxidative damage in humans from tobacco smoke or any other source (endogenous or exogenous), because it is impossible to distinguish sources of free radicals and biomarker methods can artifactually induce oxidative damage (51,53). Nonetheless, levels are generally higher in leucocytes excreted in the urine of smokers than in nonsmokers (54,55).

2.2. Biomarkers for Assessing Risks in Humans

Different types of methods for assessing tobacco-related cancer risk in humans are available. External exposure markers attempt to predict exposure without regard to interindividual differences in smoking behavior and cellular processes. Biomarker assays can assess internal exposure, the biologically effective dose, and harm. Biomarkers of exposure represent an internal dose, of a tobacco smoke or tobacco product constituent that is either the parent compound or its metabolite (e.g., exhaled carbon monoxide, nicotine boosts, carboxyhemoglobin, urinary TSNs or PAH metabolites, and urine mutagenicity). These markers have been the most extensively studied of biomarkers, because they better estimate exposure to individual cigarettes, are technically feasible, and can provide information about short-term (e.g., from a single cigarette) and long-term exposure.

The biologically effective dose (56) is the amount of tobacco smoke or tobacco toxin that binds to a macromolecule in a cell. The biologically effective dose represents the net effect of toxic metabolic activation, lack of detoxification, lack of repair or control mechanisms, and lack of cell death. One measure of the biologically effective dose are the carcinogen–DNA adduct levels. In humans, tobacco smoking leads to increased adduct formation in target tissues such as the lung (57–59) and in surrogate tissues such as the blood (58,60,61). Evidence exists that carcinogen–DNA adduct levels in target and nontarget organs are modulated by genetics (21,62,63–67). In humans, a link between carcinogen–DNA adducts and tobacco-related cancer risk has been reported using different study designs (69,68–70).

Biomarkers of harm can range from isolated early changes with or without effects on function to events that clearly lead to carcinogenesis and can be observed in cancer cells. Several types of assays are available. Chromosomal damage can be measured using classical cytogenetic methods, micronuclei formation (71,82), COMET (73,74), fluorescent in situ hybridization, and PCR methods assessing loss of heterozygosity (using tandem repeats or comparative genomic hybridization). Mutations in reporter genes, such as *HPRT* (75,76) or *GPA*, have been used, but it is better to identify mutation rates in cancer susceptibility genes such as *p53* (77,78) or K-*Ras* (77,79–81).

Biomarkers of harm that reflect later stages of carcinogenesis include morphological markers of preneoplastic lesions (e.g., dysplasia), altered phenotypic expression of normal cellular functions (e.g., overexpression of the proto-oncogene *Erb-B2*), and mutations in cancer-related genes, such as the *p53* tumor suppressor gene. It is possible to measure *p53* mutation rates in normal tissues (82–84) of persons without cancer, and to measure mutations in sputum for persons with cancer (85). It also has been found that measuring loss of heterozygosity (86) or hypermethylation of genes involved in neoplasia (87) might be useful for assessing the effects of tobacco smoke.

2.3. Lung Cancer

In this country, there were about 171,000 newly diagnosed lung cancer cases in 1999; 92.6% of these are in curable (88). A dose–response relationship for cigarette smoking and lung cancer is consistently shown in cohort studies of both men and women (89–91).

Lung cancer consists of four major histological types, namely squamous cell cancer (SCC), small cell lung cancer (SCLC), adenocarcinoma (AD) and large cell carcinoma (LCC) (90). There has been a shift in the prevalence of histology types over time, where AD has been increasing relative to SCC (90–94). Associations between cigarette smoking and death from AD vs. SCC in Connecticut increased nearly 17-fold in women and nearly 10-fold in men from 1959 through 1991, while smoking-related lung cancer risk increased from 4.6 to 19 in men and from 1.5 to 8.1 in women (93). This is likely due to the use of lower-nicotine cigarettes, increased exposures to TSNs, and greater depths of inhalation.

Less women tend to smoke than men and consequently there are lower rates of lung cancer (95) and preneoplastic lesions (96) in women. Lung cancer rates have been decreasing for men but not for women (97). Women more commonly have AD than SCC, even after controlling for smoking status (98). In a study of 1108 males and 781 females with lung cancer, compared with 1122 male and 948 female controls, women were found to have a 1.2- to 1.7-fold higher risk, which was limited to AD and SCLC, rather than SCC (99). Other studies have provided similar findings (100–104), although some have not (91,105). While some might hypothesize that the differences in cancer risks between men and women are due to differing baseline non-smoking rates (106), this was found not to be the case using summary statistics from several large cohort studies (107). An increased risk in women is also evidenced by data showing that there is a higher risk for lung cancer in women at similar ages of initiation, and the risks are the same in women over the age of 25 years compared to men over the age of 20 years (108). There are several plausible explanations for the increased risk that relate to the fact that women tend to smoke "light" cigarettes and also that biological differences might also be a factor. Women more commonly have estrogen or progesterone receptors in their lung cancers (109) [one study found such a high abundance in both males and females that a difference between the two could not be discerned (110)], or by estrogens that can induce metabolizing enzymes carcinogen activation. Women have higher levels of carcinogen–DNA adducts in lung tissues, even though they have the same or lower levels of smoking (111), which supports the latter hypothesis. Women might also be more susceptible if they have particular metabolic polymorphisms affecting carcinogen detoxification (63,112–115).

The risk of lung cancer in former smokers is less than in current smokers, as demonstrated by both case–control and prospective studies (91,105,115).

Heritable susceptibilities can affect tobacco-related cancer risks (116–118,119). Evidence for familial transmission of risk has been reported (120,121). Specific genes that have been studied include the glutathione-*S*-transferase M1 (*GSTM1*) (118,122–128), *CYP1A1* (129,130), glutathione-*S*-transferase Pi72, and others (125,131,132). These genetic polymorphisms, and others, are believed to affect biomarker levels, such as DNA adducts (21,63,67,133). Also, several biomarker phenotypes representing carcinogen metabolism and DNA repair also have been shown to modify the effects of smoking-related risks (134–136).

Environmental tobacco smoke (ETS), also termed passive smoking or exposure to second-hand smoke, has been estimated to cause 2600–7400 lung cancer deaths per year among nonsmokers in the United States, according to a review of nine studies of lung cancer mortality (137). The conclusion that ETS is a cause of lung cancer has been opined by several reviewers and persons conducting meta-analysis (138–142). Until recently, it was not possible to show that ETS affects biomarkers of cancer risk (143). But, improved methodologies now show that ETS-exposed persons have elevated levels of TSN metabolites in their urine (4). Other studies have reported an increase in aryl aromatic amine-related adducts (144).

2.4. Oropharyngeal Cancers

Almost all oropharyngeal cancers are SCCs. Their annual incidence is about 40,000 cases, of whom about 12,000 will eventually die from their disease (145). The major risk factors for oropharyngeal cancers are tobacco (cigarettes and smokeless tobacco products) and alcohol use. There is a dose–response for both smoking and alcohol use; together the two agents act synergistically (146–159). Some studies suggest that tobacco consumption is more likely than alcohol consumption to give rise to precursor lesions (160,161) and to cancer (149,162). Talamini and coworkers (151) studied 60 nonsmoking drinkers and 32 nondrinking smokers and compared them to controls. Depending on the amount of drinks per week, the OR reached 5.3 (95% CI = 1.1–24.8) in the nonsmokers and 7.2 (95% CI = 1.1–46) in the smokers. Three published studies indicate that there is an increased risk for women compared to men, especially at the highest levels of smoking (147,152,156).

Cessation of smoking decreases the risk of oropharyngeal cancers (159). In one study, cancer of the larynx was found to be markedly less likely among ex-smokers than among current cigarette smokers (1).

Smokeless tobacco is consumed in a variety of different ways in various cultures around the world. Examples of smokeless tobacco products include chewing tobacco, dry snuff (used in the nasal cavity), wet snuff (a moist wad of tobacco, usually placed between the lips and gums), and nass (a mixture of tobacco, lime, ash, and cotton oil), with many local variations in Asia and Africa. Large geographical differences in the prevalence of smokeless tobacco consumption are evident, with particularly high consumption in Scandinavia (where a popular form of snuff is known as snus), India, southeastern Asia, Sudan, and parts of the United States. Smokeless tobacco products from these different regions are produced differently and have different levels of carcinogens (163–165). Smokeless tobacco products are associated with cancers of the head and neck, depending on the type of tobacco used (166–172). In some of these studies it is difficult to separate the effects of chewing tobacco from alcohol drinking because of few nondrinkers. In the United States, Winn and coworkers (170) reported a 4.2-fold increased risk (95% CI = 2.6–6.7) in Southern white women who exclusively use snuff. In contrast, an analysis of the relationship between smokeless tobacco and cancer of the oral cavity in the National Mortality Followback Study did not detect increased risk (173). Evidence for an elevated risk of nasal cancer in association with the use of snuff was reported in a case–control study in North Carolina and Virginia (171).

Oropharyngeal tissues clearly have the capacity to metabolically activate tobacco smoke carcinogens and cause DNA damage (174,175). Several studies have indicated that there is increased risk of oropharyngeal cancers in those who have a heritable trait demonstrated by genetical polymorphisms, although which markers play the greatest role is not yet known (122,124,129,176,177), and there is some evidence for a greater effect in persons with lower levels of smoking (127). In one study, heritable traits in carcinogen metabolism increased the frequency of *p53* mutations (178). When cultured lymphocytes are exposed to mutagens and the resultant chromosomal breaks are counted, there is a greater mutagen sensitivity in cases, especially in smokers (179–182). This trait also predicts the risk of secondary cancers in persons with oropharyngeal cancers (183).

2.5. Bladder Cancer

Over 53,000 cases of bladder cancer occured in the United States in the year 2000, and approximately 12,000 will eventually die from their disease (145).

The male to female ratio is about 2.6:1. Many studies have shown a dose–response effect of smoking on bladder cancer risk, and a decreased risk with cessation (184–188). Doll and Peto (91) found that among male British physicians followed for 20 years since an initial survey on smoking habits the annual age-adjusted rate of bladder cancer deaths was 11 per 100,000 among men who had quit smoking, compared to 9 among nonsmokers and 19 among men who smoked cigarettes exclusively (189). There is a higher risk with black tobaccos compared with blond tobaccos (184,186,190).

Studies have shown that smoking-related bladder cancer risk increases with genetical susceptibilities for carcinogen metabolism and detoxification, mostly for *GSTM1* and *NAT2* (118,122,126,191–196). Persons with low activity of *CYP3A* were associated with higher *p53* overexpression (197). There is only one study that relates adduct levels to bladder cancer risk (70), but because this was a case–control study, conclusions are limited. However, in a small group of patients ($n = 45$), adduct levels were not related to *p53* mutations in the tumors, but this was not a prospective study (198).

2.6. Studies of Nicotine Mutagenicity and Carcinogenicity

Several studies have been conducted to determine if nicotine is genotoxic. Almost all studies that could be identified failed to find increased genotoxicity (199–204), although there are conflicting data about the potential for nicotine to have mutagenic activity (200,201). Urine from rats exposed to nicotine was not mutagenic (199). The effects of coculture of nicotine and known genotoxic substances indicated an increased rate of mutations for some compounds and a decrease for others (200). Experimental animal studies using nicotine alone have not found that nicotine is carcinogenic (205–207), or in offspring of animals treated with nicotine (207). However, in experimental animals, nicotine can increase the frequency of tumors induced by other agents such as 7,12-dimethylbenz(*a*) anthracene (208), *N*-nitrosamines (209), and *N*-[4-(5-nitro-2-furyl)-2-thiazolyl]formamide (210), although there was no effect for other *N*-nitrosamines (211) and there was an antitumor effect in some cases (212). Nicotine also is reported to reduce apoptosis (213).

Long-term studies of persons treated with nicotine replacement therapy are not yet possible because of the short time that such products have been available. Even though it is possible that nicotine might be increasing tumor occurrence due to other agents (e.g., a promotional effect), the risk from cotreatment with nicotine replacement therapy in persons who continue to smoke is likely to be small compared to continued use of tobacco products at a higher rate. The amount of nicotine replaced is less than that available from cigarettes and it does not have the spectrum of carcinogens present in tobacco products. Human studies have shown that the use of nicotine replacement products do not result in the formation of TSNs such as NNK (214).

3. ALCOHOL DRINKING

Alcohol beverages are known risk factors for several cancers. However, the etiological mechanism remains obscure. Given that all types of alcoholic beverages have been associated with cancers, it is reasonable to assume that ethanol is the carcinogenic agent. However, animal models have not demonstrated that ethanol causes cancer. Still, there are ways in which ethanol may cause cancer in humans that can be inferred from experimental animal studies. It is known that ethanol causes cell damage and inflammation, oxidative damage, mutations via acetaldehyde, pertubations in estrogen metabolism and response, and alterations in folic acid utilization. Also, there are contaminants that might have contribute to cancer risk, such as urethane in wine, and *N*-nitrosamines in beer.

Ethanol metabolism occurs in the liver, breast, and other tissues (215–221). Ethanol is initially oxidized to acetaldehyde, which is then converted to acetate. This first step is catalyzed mostly by alcohol dehydrogenase (ADH), and to a lesser extent by CYP2E1. ADH is constitutively expressed, while CYP2E1 is induced with chronic high-level exposure (222,223). There are seven ADH genes among five classes, although not all metabolize ethanol. In the last few years, the nomenclature for *ADH* has changed (224). Acetaldehyde is mostly catalyzed by aldehyde dehydrogenase to form acetate (225). This reaction also is catalyzed by oxoreductase and aldehyde oxidase.

Acetaldehyde is a highly reactive compound, binding protein and DNA (226–229), and causes DNA cross-linking (230,231), micronuclei (231), aneuploidy (232,233), and chromosomal aberrations (227,231,233–238). The interaction of acetaldehyde with DNA bases results in different types of adducts, especially N^2-ethyl-2'-deoxyguanosine. Acetaldehyde also induces hypoxanthine phosphoribosyl transferase mutations, including large deletions (239), and G → A transitions, also seen in esophageal cancer (240). The DNA damage caused by acetaldehyde is repaired through nucleotide excision repair pathways (241). Acetaldehyde toxicity occurs, in part, through the formation of protein adducts, which are measurable in both experimental animals and humans (222,242–246). Acetaldehyde is a weak carcinogen (237,238). DNA repair is inhibited by acetaldehyde in vitro and in vivo (235,236,247), including the repair of induced double-stranded breaks (248).

There are several *ADH* polymorphisms that affect functional activity (249). There is a polymorphism in *ADH1B* (*ADH2*, old nomenclature) that encodes a high-activity *3 isozyme subunit, which is present only in African

Americans (250,251). Another polymorphism exists in *ADH1C* (*ADH3*, old nomenclature), where the *2 allele increases ethanol oxidation two fold (252). For this polymorphism, we found that fast oxidizers have an increased risk of premenopausal breast and oral cavity cancers (253,254). While another study of breast cancer did not replicate our positive association, it was reported that the high-risk variant was associated with increased endogenous estrogen levels (255). *ADH2* (*ADH4*, old nomenclature) has a polymorphism at position −75 of the promoter region that has been shown to increase the activity two fold (−75A is greater than −75C) (256). There is a second polymorphism in the *ADH2* in exon 7 at position 925 (257). This results in an Ile to Val substitution at amino acid 308, which decreases protein stability. While there are several known polymorphisms that have been identified in *CYP2E1*, such as in the promoter region, the functional significance has not been clearly elucidated (258). However, a common allele in African Americans, consisting of a 96 bp insertion in the regulatory region, has been identified that increases activity in drinkers (259,260).

The mitochondria respiratory chain is probably the most important source of superoxide anions (246), and is clearly affected by alcohol (261). Superoxide dismutase (SOD) catalyzes the dismutation of superoxide to hydrogen peroxide and oxygen. Thus, it both clears and creates free radicals (262,263). Importantly, SOD blocks the formation of free radicals by acetaldehyde (264). 17-β-Estradiol-related increases of 8-OH-dG can be inhibited by SOD (265,268).

Mitochondrial DNA (mtDNA) is a target for ethanol-induced oxidative stress (261,267,268), which can affect functions such as apoptosis. mtDNA mutations are present in about 40% of breast tumors (269–277). Chronic ethanol exposure in animal models shows a cumulative effect of oxidative damage and mtDNA strand breaks (261). The cycle of ROS formation and mtDNA damage can be synergistic and exponential (278). In the mitochondria, base excision, mismatch, recombination, and OGG1 repair occur (261). Ethanol decreases glutathione peroxidase activity, which increases mitochondrial structural and functional disturbances (246,261,279,280).

3.1. Liver Cancer

Almost all liver cancer (80%) is associated with cirrhosis (281,282). Even in noncirrhotic liver cancers, the risk factors are typically the same. Ethanol induces chronic hepatitis, which in turn results in liver cell necrosis, inflammation, regeneration, and fibrosis. This results in a proliferative process prone to development of clonal evolution.

Ethanol causes liver cirrhosis in regular drinkers. The resulting alcohol-related damage includes liver cell necrosis, inflammation, regeneration, and fibrosis. The local inflammation results in excessive oxidative damage.

Alcohol is considered to be responsible for about 15% of liver cancers, but this can be much higher in regions of low hepatitis virus prevalence (283). There also are several reports that alcohol and hepatitis viruses interact to increase liver cancer risk (283), but this is due to an interaction for liver cirrhosis risk (281). There has been limited study on the role of alcohol metabolizing genetical polymorphisms in liver cancer risk (284), but null studies exist (285).

3.2. Gastrointestinal Cancers

Esophageal cancer is relatively rare in the United States. The most common risk factors are alcohol drinking and tobacco. The effects are considered multiplicative. Almost a 100-fold risk has been reported for heavy smokers and drinkers (229). The association is more commonly reported for SCC of the esophagus, compared with ADs. There is some evidence that genetical polymorphisms in alcohol metabolizing genes can affect risk (286), including in persons who develop a new esophageal primary after the diagnosis of oropharyngeal cancer (287).

Overall, alcohol does not appear to be a risk factor for stomach cancer, although several studies indicate that when examined by site, there is an association with ADs of the gastric cardia (288).

Alcohol drinking is a reported risk factor for colon cancer, even at low levels (289). There are changes in normal colon morphology in alcoholics (290). Acetaldehyde correlates with colon crypt cell production in animals (291). While only a few studies have been reported, there is no effect of *ADH* polymorphisms on colon cancer risk (292), although there are some reported interactions with polymorphisms in the methylene tetrahydrofolate reductase (293).

3.3. Oropharyngeal Cancer

About 75% of oropharyngeal cancers are attributable to smoking and drinking (147,229). Heavy drinkers can have up to a 15-fold risk of cancer (147, 294), and a multiplicative effect has been reported (295,296). More than 95% of persons with oropharyngeal cancer who smoke also consume alcohol (296). *ADH* polymorphisms have been investigated for effects on alcohol-related oral cavity cancer. There is evidence of effect modification on the dose–response curve (254,297), although there are some conflicting data (298–301).

3.4. Breast Cancer

Epidemiological evidence indicates that alcohol drinking is associated with a moderate increase in breast cancer risk (302–304). Singletary and Gapstur (305) summarized the relationship of alcohol to breast cancer in a recent review. They cited more than 5 separate meta-analyses, 2 major reviews, 5 prospective studies, and 33 other reports. There is a dose–response relationship between drinking and risk (306). Although some studies only identify a statistical increase for the highest levels of drinking, there is evidence that one to two drinks per day also contribute to breast cancer risk (307–309), and threshold values between 5 and 60 g per day have been suggested (310,311). Overall, there is about a 9% incremental increase in risk for 10 g of alcohol consumed per day (equivalent to less than one drink per day) (302,303,312). While ethanol generally is not an animal carcinogen, there are supportive models for breast cancer (313,314). In animal models, ethanol initiates mammary tumors (315) and dimethylbenzathracene (DMBA) followed by ethanol caused SD rat tumors (305).

There are several lines of evidence showing that alcohol affects estrogen pathways. It is associated with decreased menstrual cycle variability and more frequent long cycles (316). In premenopausal women mostly, but also in postmenopausal women, drinking is associated with increased serum and urinary estrogen metabolites, and decreased sex-hormone binding globulin, follicle stimulating hormone, and luteinizing hormone levels (317–322). In drinkers, the half-life of transdermal estrogen replacement is longer (323,324), and some studies indicate an increased breast cancer risk in postmenopausal women who use HRT (59). [There are some studies that do not support the effect of alcohol on hormone replacement therapy related breast cancer risk (325)]. Alcohol use is associated with decreased bone loss and osteoporosis (326). Alcohol stimulates the transcriptional activity of ER-α, upregulates ER-α expression (327,328), and is associated with estrogen-negative tumors (329–331).

Increased breast density is associated with a 4–6 fold increased breast cancer risk (332–338). There are many epidemiological studies that have shown that alcohol drinking is associated with increased breast density (305). Other risk factors are nulliparity, late age at first birth, younger age, and low body mass (339). HRT also increases density (341), although there is some inconsistency (339,341–343). Animal studies with the DMBA rat model show that alcohol increases mammary terminal end bud density and reduces the density of differentiated lobules (344). Interestingly, urinary malondialdehyde is associated with increased breast density, suggesting a role for oxidative stress (342).

REFERENCES

1. Public Health Service. Smoking and Health. Report of the Advisory Committee to the Surgeon General of the Public Health Service. PHS publication No. 1103. 1964. Ref. Type: Report.
2. Hoffmann D, Hoffmann I. The changing cigarette, 1950–1995. J Toxicol Environ Health 1997; 50:307–364.

3. Zaridze DG, Safaev RD, Belitsky GA, Brunnemann KD, Hoffmann D. Carcinogenic substances in Soviet tobacco products. IARC Sci Publ 1991:485–488.

4. Hecht SS. Tobacco smoke carcinogens and lung cancer. J Natl Cancer Inst 1999; 91:1194–1210.

5. Ebert RV, McNabb ME, McCusker KT, Snow SL. Amount of nicotine and carbon monoxide inhaled by smokers of low-tar, low-nicotine cigarettes. JAMA 1983; 250:2840–2842.

6. Gritz ER, Rose JE, Jarvik ME. Regulation of tobacco smoke intake with paced cigarette presentation. Pharmacol Biochem Behav 1983; 18:457–462.

7. Benowitz NL, Jacob P, Yu L, Talcott R, Hall S, Jones RT. Reduced tar, nicotine, and carbon monoxide exposure while smoking ultralow- but not low-yield cigarettes. JAMA 1986; 256:241–246.

8. Benowitz NL, Hall SM, Herning RI, Jacob P, Jones RT, Osman AL. Smokers of low-yield cigarettes do not consume less nicotine. N Engl J Med 1983; 309:139–142.

9. Djordjevic MV, Fan J, Ferguson S, Hoffmann D. Self-regulation of smoking intensity. Smoke yields of the low-nicotine, low 'tar' cigarettes. Carcinogenesis 1995; 16:2015–2021.

10. Djordjevic MV, Hoffmann D, Hoffmann I. Nicotine regulates smoking patterns. Prev Med 1997; 26:435–440.

11. Seto H, Ohkubo T, Kanoh T, Koike M, Nakamura K, Kawahara Y. Determination of polycyclic aromatic hydrocarbons in the lung. Arch Environ Contam Toxicol 1993; 24:498–503.

12. Lodovici M, Akpan V, Giovannini L, Migliani F, Dolara P. Benzo[a]pyrene diol-epoxide DNA adducts and levels of polycyclic aromatic hydrocarbons in autoptic samples from human lungs. Chem Biol Interact 1998; 116:199–212.

13. van Delft JH, Baan RA, Roza L. Biological effect markers for exposure to carcinogenic compound and their relevance for risk assessment. Crit Rev Toxicol 1998; 28:477–510.

14. International Agency on the Research of Cancer. IARC Monographs on the Evaluation of the Carcinogenic Risk of Chemicals of Humans: Tobacco Smoking. Vol.38. Lyon: IARC, 1986.

15. Shimada T, Hayes CL, Yamazaki H, Amin S, Hecht SS, Guengerich FP, Sutter TR. Activation of chemically diverse procarcinogens by human cytochrome P-450 1B1. Cancer Res 1996; 56:2979–2984.

16. Kim JH, Stansbury KH, Walker NJ, Trush MA, Strickland PT, Sutter TR. Metabolism of benzo[a]pyrene and benzo[a]pyrene-7,8-diol by human cytochrome P450 1B1. Carcinogenesis 1998; 19:1847–1853.

17. Robertson IGC, Guthenberg C, Mannervik B, Jernstrom B. The glutathione conjugation of benzo(a)pyrene diol-epoxide by human glutathione transferases. In: Cooke M, Dennis AJ, eds. Polynuclear Aromatic Hydrocarbons: A Decade of Progress. Columbus, Ohio: Battelle Press, 1988:799–808.

18. Romert L, Dock L, Jenssen D, Jernstrom B. Effects of glutathione transferase activity on benzo[a]pyrene 7,8- dihydrodiol metabolism and mutagenesis studied in a mammalian cell co-cultivation assay. Carcinogenesis 1989; 10: 1701–1707.

19. Kato S, Bowman ED, Harrington AM, Blomeke B, Shields PG. Human lung carcinogen-DNA adduct levels mediated by genetic polymorphisms in vivo. J Natl Cancer Inst 1995; 87:902–907.
20. Day BW, Naylor S, Gan LS, Sahali Y, Nguyen TT, Skipper PL, Wishnok JS, Tannenbaum SR. Molecular dosimetry of polycyclic aromatic hydrocarbon epoxides and diol epoxides via hemoglobin adducts. Cancer Res 1990; 50:4611–4618.
21. Kriek E, Rojas M, Alexandrov K, Bartsch H. Polycyclic aromatic hydrocarbon-DNA adducts in humans: relevance as biomarkers for exposure and cancer risk. Mutat Res 1998; 400:215–231.
22. Smith LE, Denissenko MF, Bennett WP, Li H, Amin S, Tang M, Pfeifer GP. Targeting of lung cancer mutational hotspots by polycyclic aromatic hydrocarbons (see comments). J Natl Cancer Inst 2000; 92:803–811.
23. Denissenko MF, Pao A, Tang M, Pfeifer GP. Preferential formation of benzo[a]pyrene adducts at lung cancer mutational hotspots in P53. Science 1996; 274:430–432.
24. Fischer S, Spiegelhalder B, Eisenbarth J, Preussmann R. Investigations on the origin of tobacco-specific nitrosamines in mainstream smoke of cigarettes. Carcinogenesis 1990; 11:723–730.
25. Tricker AR, Ditrich C, Preussmann R. N-nitroso compounds in cigarette tobacco and their occurrence in mainstream tobacco smoke. Carcinogenesis 1991; 12:257–261.
26. Fischer S, Spiegelhalder B, Preussmann R. Preformed tobacco-specific nitrosamines in tobacco—role of nitrate and influence of tobacco type. Carcinogenesis 1989; 10:1511–1517.
27. Brunnemann KD, Prokopczyk B, Djordjevic MV, Hoffmann D. Formation and analysis of tobacco-specific *N*-nitrosamines. Crit Rev Toxicol 1996; 26:121–137.
28. Lewis DF, Brantom PG, Ioannides C, Walker R, Parke DV. Nitrosamine carcinogenesis: rodent assays, quantitative structure–activity relationships, and human risk assessment. Drug Metab Rev 1997; 29:1055–1078.
29. Belinsky SA, Foley JF, White CM, Anderson MW, Maronpot RR. Dose–response relationship between O6-methylguanine formation in Clara cells and induction of pulmonary neoplasia in the rat by 4-(methylnitrosamino)-1-(3-pyridyl)-1-butanone. Cancer Res 1990; 50:3772–3780.
30. La DK, Swenberg JA. DNA adducts: biological markers of exposure and potential applications to risk assessment. Mutat Res 1996; 365:129–146.
31. Klein-Szanto AJ, Iizasa T, Momiki S, Garcia-Palazzo I, Caamano J, Metcalf R, Welsh J, Harris CC. A tobacco-specific *N*-nitrosamine or cigarette smoke condensate causes neoplastic transformation of xenotransplanted human bronchial epithelial cells. Proc Natl Acad Sci USA 1992; 89:6693–6697.
32. Hecht SS. DNA adduct formation from tobacco-specific *N*-nitrosamines. Mutat Res 1999; 424:127–142.
33. Benowitz NL, Zevin S, Jacob P. Suppression of nicotine intake during ad libitum cigarette smoking by high-dose transdermal nicotine. J Pharmacol Exp Ther 1998; 287:958–962.

34. Carmella SG, Akerkar SA, Richie JP Jr, Hecht SS. Intraindividual and inter-individual differences in metabolites of the tobacco-specific lung carcinogen 4-(methylnitrosamino)-1- (3-pyridyl)-1-butanone (NNK) in smokers' urine. Cancer Epidemiol Biomarkers Prev 1995; 4:635–642.

35. Atawodi SE, Lea S, Nyberg F, Mukeria A, Constantinescu V, Ahrens W, Brueske-Hohlfeld I, Fortes C, Boffetta P, Friesen MD. 4-Hydroxy-1-(3-pyridyl)-1-butanone-hemoglobin adducts as biomarkers of exposure to tobacco smoke: validation of a method to be used in multicenter studies. Cancer Epidemiol Biomarkers Prev 1998; 7:817–821.

36. Hecht SS, Carmella SG, Murphy SE, Akerkar S, Brunnemann KD, Hoffmann D. A tobacco-specific lung carcinogen in the urine of men exposed to cigarette smoke (see comments). N Engl J Med 1993; 329:1543–1546.

37. Parsons WD, Carmella SG, Akerkar S, Bonilla LE, Hecht SS. A metabolite of the tobacco-specific lung carcinogen 4- (methylnitrosamino)-1-(3-pyridyl)-1-butanone in the urine of hospital workers exposed to environmental tobacco smoke. Cancer Epidemiol Biomarkers Prev 1998; 7:257–260.

38. Hecht SS. Biochemistry, biology, and carcinogenicity of tobacco-specific *N*-nitrosamines. Chem Res Toxicol 1998; 11:559–603.

39. Smith TJ, Stoner GD, Yang CS. Activation of 4-(methylnitrosamino)-1-(3-pyridyl)-1-butanone (NNK) in human lung microsomes by cytochromes P450, lipoxygenase, and hydroperoxides. Cancer Res 1995; 55:5566–5573.

40. Smith TJ, Guo Z, Gonzalez FJ, Guengerich FP, Stoner GD, Yang CS. Metabolism of 4-(methylnitrosamino)-1-(3-pyridyl)-1-butanone in human lung and liver microsomes and cytochromes P-450 expressed in hepatoma cells. Cancer Res 1992; 52:1757–1763.

41. Yang CS, Yoo JS, Ishizaki H, Hong JY. Cytochrome P450IIE1: roles in nitrosamine metabolism and mechanisms of regulation. Drug Metab Rev 1990; 22:147–159.

42. Tiano HF, Hosokawa M, Chulada PC, Smith PB, Wang RL, Gonzalez FJ, Crespi CL, Langenbach R. Retroviral mediated expression of human cytochrome P450 2A6 in C3H/10T1/2 cells confers transformability by 4-(methylnitrosamino)-1-(3-pyridyl)-1-butanone (NNK). Carcinogenesis 1993; 14:1421–1427.

43. Nesnow S, Beck S, Rosenblum S, Lasley J, Tiano HF, Hosokawa M, Crespi CL, Langenbach R. *N*-nitrosodiethylamine and 4-(methylnitrosamino)-1-(3-pyridyl)-1-butanone induced morphological transformation of C3H/10T1/2CL8 cells expressing human cytochrome P450 2A6. Mutat Res 1994; 324: 93–102.

44. Zhang Y-J, Chen C-J, Lee C-S, Haghighi B, Yang G-Y, Wang L-W, Feitelson M, Santella R. Aflatoxin B1-DNA adducts and hepatitis B virus antigens in hepatocellular carcinoma and nontumorous liver tissue. Carcinogenesis 1991; 12:2247–2252.

45. Chang F, Syrjanen SM, Shen Q, Ji H, Syrjanen KJ. Human papillomavirus (HPV) DNA in esophageal precancer lesions and squamous cell carcinomas from China. Int J Cancer 1990; 45:21–25.

46. Fischer S, Spiegelhalder B, Preussmann R. Influence of smoking parameters on the delivery of tobacco-specific nitrosamines in cigarette smoke—a contribution to relative risk evaluation. Carcinogenesis 1989; 10:1059–1066.
47. Pryor WA, Stone K, Zang LY, Bermudez E. Fractionation of aqueous cigarette tar extracts: fractions that contain the tar radical cause DNA damage. Chem Res Toxicol 1998; 11:441–448.
48. Wiencke JK, Kelsey KT, Varkonyi A, Semey K, Wain JC, Mark E, Christiani DC. Correlation of DNA adducts in blood mononuclear cells with tobacco carcinogene-induced damage in human lung. Cancer Res 1995; 55:4910–4914.
49. Phillips DH, Hewer A, Martin CN, Garner RC, King MM. Correlation of DNA adduct levels in human lung with cigarette smoking. Nature 1988; 336:790–792.
50. Vineis P, Bartsch H, Caporaso N, Harrington AM, Kadlubar FF, Landi MT, Malaveille C, Shields PG, Skipper P, Talaska G, et al. Genetically based N-acetyltransferase metabolic polymorphism and low-level environmental exposure to carcinogens. Nature 1994; 369:154–156.
51. Tang D, Santella RM, Blackwood AM, Young TL, Mayer J, Jaretzki A, Grantham S, Tsai WY, Perera FP. A molecular epidemiological case-control study of lung cancer. Cancer Epidemiol Biomarkers Prev 1995; 4:341–346.
52. Ryberg D, Skaug V, Hewer A, Phillips DH, Harries LW, Wolf CR, Ogreid D, Ulvik A, Vu P, Haugen A. Genotypes of glutathione transferase M1 and P1 and their significance for lung DNA adduct levels and cancer risk. Carcinogenesis 1997; 18:1285–1289.
53. Rojas M, Alexandrov K, Cascorbi I, Brockmoller J, Likhachev A, Pozharisski K, Bouvier G, Auburtin G, Mayer L, Kopp-Schneider A, Roots I, Bartsch H. High benz[a]pyrene diol-epoxide DNA adduct levels in lung and blood cells from individuals with combined CYP1A1 MspI/MspI-GSTM1*0/*0 genotypes. Pharmacogen 1998; 8:109–118.
54. Badawi AF, Hirvonen A, Bell DA, Lang NP, Kadlubar FF. Role of aromatic amine acetyltransferases, NAT1 and NAT2, in carcinogen-DNA adduct formation in the human urinary bladder. Cancer Res 1995; 55:5230–5237.
55. Stern SJ, Degawa M, Martin MV, Guengerich FP, Kaderlik RK, Ilett KF, Breau R, McGhee M, Montague D, Lyn-Cook B. Metabolic activation, DNA adducts, and H-ras mutations in human neoplastic and non-neoplastic laryngeal tissue. J Cell Biochem Suppl 1993; 17F:129–137.
56. Grinberg-Funes RA, Singh VN, Perera FP, Bell DA, Young TL, Dickey C, Wang LW, Santella RM. Polycyclic aromatic hydrocarbon-DNA adducts in smokers and their relationship to micronutrient levels and the glutathione-S-transferase M1 genotype. Carcinogenesis 1994; 15:2449–2454.
57. Pastorelli R, Guanci M, Cerri A, Negri E, La Vecchia C, Fumagalli F, Mezzetti M, Cappelli R, Panigalli T, Fanelli R, Airoldi L. Impact of inherited polymorphisms in glutathione S-transferase M1, microsomal epoxide hydrolase, cytochrome P450 enzymes on DNA, and blood protein adducts of benzo(a)pyrene-diolepoxide. Cancer Epidemiol Biomarkers Prev 1998; 7:703–709.
58. Dunn BP, Vedal S, San RH, Kwan WF, Nelems B, Enarson DA, Stich HF. DNA adducts in bronchial biopsies. Int J Cancer 1991; 48:485–492.

59. Van Schooten FJ, Hillebrand MJ, Van Leeuwen FE, Lutgerink JT, van Zandwijk N, Jansen HM, Kriek E. Polycyclic aromatic hydrocarbon-DNA adducts in lung tissue from lung cancer patients. Carcinogenesis 1990; 11:1677–1681.

60. Peluso M, Airoldi L, Armelle M, Martone T, Coda R, Malaveille C, Giacomelli G, Terrone C, Casetta G, Vineis P. White blood cell DNA adducts, smoking, and NAT2 and GSTM1 genotypes in bladder cancer: a case-control study. Cancer Epidemiol Biomarkers Prev 1998; 7:341–346.

61. Schmid W. The micronucleus test. Mutation Research. Amsterdam: Elsevier Scientific Publishing Co., 1975:9–15.

62. Czerwinski M, McLemore TL, Gelboin HV, Gonzalez FJ. Quantification of CYP2B7, CYP4B1, and CYPOR messenger RNAs in normal human lung and lung tumors. Cancer Res 1994; 54:1085–1091.

63. Xue KX, Wang S, Ma GJ, Zhou P, Wu PQ, Zhang RF, Xu Z, Chen WS, Wang YQ. Micronucleus formation in peripheral-blood lymphocytes from smokers and the influence of alc. Int J Cancer 1992; 50:702–705.

64. Speit G, Hartmann A. The comet assay (single-cell gel test). A sensitive genotoxicity test for the detection of DNA damage and repair. Methods Mol Biol 1999; 113:203–212.

65. Poli P, Buschini A, Spaggiari A, Rizzoli V, Carlo-Stella C, Rossi C. DNA damage by tobacco smoke and some antiblastic drugs evaluated using the Comet assay. Toxicol Lett 1999; 108:267–276.

66. Hou SM, Yang K, Nyberg F, Hemminki K, Pershagen G, Lambert B. Hprt mutant frequency and aromatic DNA adduct level in non-smoking and smoking lung cancer patients and population controls. Carcinogenesis 1999; 20:437–444.

67. Bailar JC III. Passive smoking, coronary heart disease, and meta-analysis (editorial; comment) (see comments). N Engl J Med 1999; 340:958–959.

68. Valkonen M, Kuusi T. Passive smoking induces atherogenic changes in low-density lipoprotein. Circulation 1998; 97:2012–2016.

69. Brennan JA, Boyle JO, Koch WM, Goodman SN, Hruban RH, Eby YJ, Couch MJ, Forastiere AA, Sidransky D. Association between cigarette smoking and mutation of the p53 gene in squamous-cell carcinoma of the head and neck. N Engl J Med 1995; 332:712–717.

70. Slebos RJ, Hruban RH, Dalesio O, Mooi WJ, Offerhaus GJ, Rodenhuis S. Relationship between K-ras oncogene activation and smoking in adenocarcinoma of the human lung. J Natl Cancer Inst 1991; 83:1024–1027.

71. Yakubovskaya MS, Spiegelman V, Luo FC, Malaev S, Salnev A, Zborovskaya I, Gasparyan A, Polotsky B, Machaladze Z, Trachtenberg AC. High frequency of K-ras mutations in normal appearing lung tissues and sputum of patients with lung cancer. Int J Cancer 1995; 63:810–814.

72. Scott FM, Modali R, Lehman TA, Seddon M, Kelly K, Dempsey EC, Wilson V, Tockman MS, Mulshine JL. High frequency of K-ras codon 12 mutations in bronchoalveolar lavage fluid of patients at high risk for second primary lung cancer. Clin Cancer Res 1997; 3:479–482.

73. Hussain SP, Harris CC. p53 mutation spectrum and load: the generation of hypotheses linking the exposure of endogenous or exogenous carcinogens to human cancer. Mutat Res 1999; 428:23–32.
74. Greiner JW, Malan-Shibley LB, Janss DH. Detection of aryl hydrocarbon hydroxylase activity in normal and neoplastic human breast epithelium. Life Sci 1980; 26:313–319.
75. Hasdai D, Garratt KN, Grill DE, Lerman A, Holmes DR Jr. Effect of smoking status on the long-term outcome after successful percutaneous coronary revascularization (see comments). N Engl J Med 1997; 336:755–761.
76. Sidransky D. Nucleic acid-based methods for the detection of cancer. Science 1997; 278:1054–1059.
77. Mao L, Lee JS, Kurie JM, Fan YH, Lippman SM, Lee JJ, Ro JY, Broxson A, Yu R, Morice RC, Kemp BL, Khuri FR, Walsh GL, Hittelman WN, Hong WK. Clonal genetic alterations in the lungs of current and former smokers (see comments). J Natl Cancer Inst 1997; 89:857–862.
78. Belinsky SA, Nikula KJ, Palmisano WA, Michels R, Saccomanno G, Gabrielson E, Baylin SB, Herman JG. Aberrant methylation of p16(INK4a) is an early event in lung cancer and a potential biomarker for early diagnosis. Proc Natl Acad Sci USA 1998; 95:11891–11896.
79. Landis SH, Murray T, Bolden S, Wingo PA. Cancer statistics, 1999 (see comments). CA Cancer J Clin 1999; 49:8–31, 1.
80. Nordlund LA, Carstensen JM, Pershagen G. Cancer incidence in female smokers: a 26-year follow-up. Int J Cancer 1997; 73:625–628.
81. Winter E, Yamamoto F, Almoguera C, Perucho M. A method to detect and characterize point mutations in transcribed genes: amplification and overexpression of the mutant c-Ki-ras allele in human tumor cells. Proc Natl Acad Sci USA 1985; 82:7575–7579.
82. Doll R, Peto R. Mortality in relation to smoking: 20 years' observations on male British doctors. Br Med J 1976; 2:1525–1536.
83. Travis WD, Travis LB, Devesa SS. Lung cancer. Cancer 1995; 75:191–202.
84. Thun MJ, Lally CA, Flannery JT, Calle EE, Flanders WD, Heath CW Jr. Cigarette smoking and changes in the histopathology of lung cancer (see comments). J Natl Cancer Inst 1997; 89:1580–1586.
85. Charloux A, Quoix E, Wolkove N, Small D, Pauli G, Kreisman H. The increasing incidence of lung adenocarcinoma: reality or artefact? A review of the epidemiology of lung adenocarcinoma. Int J Epidemiol 1997; 26:14–23.
86. Shopland DR, Eyre HJ, Pechacek TF. Smoking-attributable cancer mortality in 1991: is lung cancer now the leading cause of death among smokers in the United States? J Natl Cancer Inst 1991; 83:1142–1148
87. Lam S, leRiche JC, Zheng Y, Coldman A, MacAulay C, Hawk E, Kelloff G, Gazdar AF. Sex-related differences in bronchial epithelial changes associated with tobacco smoking. J Natl Cancer Inst 1999; 91:691–696.
88. Lubin JH, Blot WJ. Assessment of lung cancer risk factors by histologic category. J Natl Cancer Inst 1984; 73:383–389.
89. Osann KE, Anton-Culver H, Kurosaki T, Taylor T. Sex differences in lung-cancer risk associated with cigarette smoking. Int J Cancer 1993; 54:44–48.

90. Brownson RC, Chang JC, Davis JR. Gender and histologic type variations in smoking-related risk of lung cancer. Epidemiology 1992; 3:61–64.
91. Cohn BA, Wingard DL, Cirillo PM, Cohen RD, Reynolds P, Kaplan GA. Re: Differences in lung cancer risk between men and women: examination of the evidence (letter; comment). J Natl Cancer Inst 1996; 88:1867–1868.
92. Halpern MT, Gillespie BW, Warner KE. Patterns of absolute risk of lung cancer mortality in former smokers (see comments). J Natl Cancer Inst 1993; 85:457–464.
93. Prescott E, Osler M, Andersen PK, Hein HO, Borch–Johnsen K, Lange P, Schnohr P, Vestbo J. Mortality in women and men in relation to smoking. Int J Epidemiol 1998; 27:27–32.
94. Risch HA, Howe GR, Jain M, Burch JD, Holowaty EJ, Miller AB. Lung cancer risk for female smokers (letter; comment). Science 1994; 263: 1206–1208.
95. Hegmann KT, Fraser AM, Keaney RP, Moser SE, Nilasena DS, Sedlars M, Higham-Gren L, Lyon JL. The effect of age at smoking initiation on lung cancer risk (see comments). Epidemiology 1993; 4:444–448.
96. Kaiser U, Hofmann J, Schilli M, Wegmann B, Klotz U, Wedel S, Virmani AK, Wollmer E, Branscheid D, Gazdar AF, Havemann K. Steroid-hormone receptors in cell lines and tumor biopsies of human lung cancer. Int J Cancer 1996; 67:357–364.
97. Canver CC, Memoli VA, Vanderveer PL, Dingivan CA, Mentzer RM Jr. Sex hormone receptors in non-small-cell lung cancer in human beings. J Thorac Cardiovasc Surg 1994; 108:153–157.
98. Ryberg D, Hewer A, Phillips DH, Haugen A. Different susceptibility to smoking-induced DNA damage among male and female lung cancer patients. Cancer Res 1994; 54:5801–5803.
99. Mollerup S, Ryberg D, Hewer A, Phillips DH, Haugen A. Sex differences in lung CYP1A1 expression and DNA adduct levels among lung cancer patients. Cancer Res 1999; 59:3317–3320.
100. Tang DL, Rundle A, Warburton D, Santella RM, Tsai WY, Chiamprasert S, Hsu YZ, Perera FP. Associations between both genetic and environmental biomarkers and lung cancer: evidence of a greater risk of lung cancer in women smokers. Carcinogenesis 1998; 19:1949–1953.
101. Rennard SI, Daughton D, Fujita J, Oehlerking MB, Dobson JR, Stahl MG, Robbins RA, Thompson AB. Short-term smoking reduction is associated with reduction in measures of lower respiratory tract inflammation in heavy smokers. Eur Respir J 1990; 3:752–759.
102. Kuller LH, Ockene JK, Meilahn E, Wentworth DN, Svendsen KH, Neaton JD. Cigarette smoking and mortality. MRFIT Research Group. Prev Med 1991; 20:638–654.
103. Shields PG, Harris CC. Cancer risk and low penetrance susceptibility genes in gene-environment interactions. J Clin Oncol 2000; 18:2309–2315.
104. Shields PG. Epidemiology of tobacco carcinogenesis. Curr Oncol Rep 2000; 2:257–262.

105. Brockmoller J, Cascorbi I, Kerb R, Sachse C, Roots I. Polymorphisms in xenobiotic conjugation and disease predisposition. Toxicol Lett 1998; 102–103:173–183.
106. Khoury MJ, Wagener DK. Epidemiological evaluation of the use of genetics to improve the predictive value of disease risk factors (see comments) (published erratum appears in Am J Hum Genet 1996 58(1):253). Am J Hum Genet 1995; 56:835–844.
107. Sellers TA, Bailey-Wilson JE, Potter JD, Rich SS, Rothschild H, Elston RC. Effect of cohort differences in smoking prevalence on models of lung cancer susceptibility. Genet Epidemiol 1992; 9:261–271.
108. Amos CI, Xu W, Spitz MR. Is there a genetic basis for lung cancer susceptibility? Recent Results Cancer Res 1999; 151:3–12.
109. Rebbeck TR. Molecular epidemiology of the human glutathione S-transferase genotypes GSTM1 and GSTT1 in cancer susceptibility. Cancer Epidemiol Biomarkers Prev 1997; 6:733–743.
110. Lehman TA, Scott F, Seddon M, Kelly K, Dempsey EC, Wilson VL, Mulshine JL, Modali R. Detection of K-ras oncogene mutations by polymerase chain reaction–based ligase chain reaction. Anal Biochem 1996; 239: 153–159.
111. Cullen P, Schulte H, Assmann G. The Munster Heart Study (PROCAM): total mortality in middle-aged men is increased at low total and LDL cholesterol concentrations in smokers but not in nonsmokers. Circulation 1997; 96:2128–2136.
112. Jourenkova-Mironova N, Voho A, Bouchardy C, Wikman H, Dayer P, Benhamou S, Hirvonen A. Glutathione S-transferase GSTM1, GSTM3, GSTP1 and GSTT1 genotypes and the risk of smoking-related oral and pharyngeal cancers. Int J Cancer 1999; 81:44–48.
113. Brockmoller J, Cascorbi I, Kerb R, Roots I. Combined analysis of inherited polymorphisms in arylamine N-acetyltransferase 2, glutathione S-transferases M1 and T1, microsomal epoxide hydrolase, and cytochrome P450 enzymes as modulators of bladder cancer risk. Cancer Res 1996; 56:3915–3925.
114. Jourenkova N, Reinikainen M, Bouchardy C, Dayer P, Benhamou S, Hirvonen A. Larynx cancer risk in relation to glutathione S-transferase M1 and T1 genotypes and tobacco smoking. Cancer Epidemiol Biomarkers Prev 1998; 7:19–23.
115. Bell DA, Taylor JA, Paulson DF, Robertson CN, Mohler JL, Lucier GW. Genetic risk and carcinogen exposure: a common inherited defect of the carcinogen-metabolism gene glutathione S-transferase M1 (GSTM1) that increases susceptibility to bladder cancer. J Natl Cancer Inst 1993; 85: 1159–1164.
116. LeVois MF. Environmental tobacco smoke and coronary heart disease (letter; comment). Circulation 1997; 96:2086–2089.
117. Ishibe N, Wiencke JK, Zuo ZF, McMillan A, Spitz M, Kelsey KT. Susceptibility to lung cancer in light smokers associated with CYP1A1 polymorphisms in Mexican- and African-Americans. Cancer Epidemiol Biomarkers Prev 1997; 6:1075–1080.

118. Wiencke JK, Spitz MR, McMillan A, Kelsey KT. Lung cancer in Mexican-Americans and African-Americans is associated with the wild-type genotype of the NAD(P)H: quinone oxidoreductase polymorphism. Cancer Epidemiol Biomarkers Prev 1997; 6:87–92.

119. Rosvold EA, McGlynn KA, Lustbader ED, Buetow KH. Identification of an NAD(P)H:quinone oxidoreductase polymorphism and its association with lung cancer and smoking. Pharmacogenom 1995; 5:199–206.

120. Yu MC, Ross RK, Chan KK, Henderson BE, Skipper PL, Tannenbaum SR, Coetzee GA. Glutathione S-transferase M1 genotype affects aminobiphenyl-hemoglobin adduct levels in white, black and Asian smokers and nonsmokers. Cancer Epidemiol Biomarkers Prev 1995; 4:861–864.

121. Li D, Wang M, Cheng L, Spitz MR, Hittelman WN, Wei Q. In vitro induction of benzo(a)pyrene diol epoxide-DNA adducts in peripheral lymphocytes as a susceptibility marker for human lung cancer. Cancer Res 1996; 56:3638–3641.

122. Spitz MR, Hsu TC, Wu X, Fueger JJ, Amos CI, Roth JA. Mutagen sensitivity as a biological marker of lung cancer risk in African Americans. Cancer Epidemiol Biomarkers Prev 1995; 4:99–103.

123. Wei Q, Gu J, Cheng L, Bondy ML, Jiang H, Hong WK, Spitz MR. Benzo(a)-pyrene diol epoxide-induced chromosomal aberrations and risk of lung cancer. Cancer Res 1996; 56:3975–3979.

124. Repace JL, Lowrey AH. Risk assessment methodologies for passive smoking-induced lung cancer. Risk Anal 1990; 10:27–37.

125. Brownson RC, Alavanja MC, Caporaso N, Simoes EJ, Chang JC. Epidemiology and prevention of lung cancer in nonsmokers. Epidemiol Rev 1998; 20:218–236.

126. Zeise L, Dunn A, Haroun L, Ting D, Windham G, Golub M, Waller K, Lipsett M, Shusterman D, Mann J, Wu A. Health Effects of Exposure to Environmental Tobacco Smoke. Office of Health and Environmental Health Hazard Assessment. California: Environmental Protection Agency, 1997; Ref Type: Report.

127. Brownson RC, Eriksen MP, Davis RM, Warner KE. Environmental tobacco smoke: health effects and policies to reduce exposure. Annu Rev Public Health 1997; 18:163–185.

128. Sunyer J, Munoz A, Peng Y, Margolick J, Chmiel JS, Oishi J, Kingsley L, Samet JM. Longitudinal relation between smoking and white blood cells. Am J Epidemiol 1996; 144:734–741.

129. NCI Expert Committee. The FTC Cogarette Test Method for Determining Tar, Nicotine, and Carbon Monoxide Yields of U.S. Cigarettes. Number 7:238–247. Bethesda, MD: U.S. Department of Health and Human Services, NIH. Smoking and Tobacco Control Monograph. 2000 Ref Type: Report.

130. Scherer G, Conze C, Tricker AR, Adlkofer F. Uptake of tobacco smoke constituents on exposure to environmental tobacco smoke (ETS). Clin Investig 1992; 70:352–367.

131. Maclure M, Katz RB, Bryant MS, Skipper PL, Tannenbaum SR. Elevated blood levels of carcinogens in passive smokers. Am J Public Health 1989; 79:1381–1384.

132. Greenlee RT, Murray T, Bolden S, Wingo PA. Cancer statistics, 2000. CA Cancer J Clin 2000; 50:7–33.
133. Keller AZ, Terris M. The association of alcohol and tobacco with cancer of the mouth and pharynx. Am J Public Health Nations Health 1965; 55: 1578–1585.
134. Blot WJ, McLaughlin JK, Winn DM, Austin DF, Greenberg RS, Preston-Martin S, Bernstein L, Schoenberg JB, Stemhagen A, Fraumeni JF Jr. Smoking and drinking in relation to oral and pharyngeal cancer. Cancer Res 1988; 48:3282–3287.
135. Sanderson RJ, de Boer MF, Damhuis RA, Meeuwis CA, Knegt PP. The influence of alcohol and smoking on the incidence of oral and oropharyngeal cancer in women. Clin Otolaryngol 1997; 22:444–448.
136. Macfarlane GJ, Zheng T, Marshall JR, Boffetta P, Niu S, Brasure J, Merletti F, Boyle P. Alcohol, tobacco, diet and the risk of oral cancer: a pooled analysis of three case-control studies. Eur J Cancer B Oral Oncol 1995; 31B: 181–187.
137. Schildt EB, Eriksson M, Hardell L, Magnuson A. Oral snuff, smoking habits and alcohol consumption in relation to oral cancer in a Swedish case-control study. Int J Cancer 1998; 77:341–346.
138. Talamini R, La Vecchia C, Levi F, Conti E, Favero A, Franceschi, S. Cancer of the oral cavity and pharynx in nonsmokers who drink alcohol and in nondrinkers who smoke tobacco. J Natl Cancer Inst 1998; 90:1901–1903.
139. Hayes RB, Bravo-Otero E, Kleinman DV, Brown LM, Fraumeni JF Jr. Harty LC, Winn DM. Tobacco and alcohol use and oral cancer in Puerto Rico. Cancer Causes Control 1999; 10:27–33.
140. Takezaki T, Hirose K, Inoue M, Hamajima N, Kuroishi T, Nakamura S, Koshikawa T, Matsuura H, Tajima K. Tobacco, alcohol and dietary factors associated with the risk of oral cancer among Japanese. Jpn J Cancer Res 1996; 87:555–562.
141. Mashberg A, Boffetta P, Winkelman R, Garfinkel L. Tobacco smoking, alcohol drinking, and cancer of the oral cavity and oropharynx among U.S. veterans. Cancer 1993; 72:1369–1375.
142. La Vecchia C, Bidoli E, Barra S, D'Avanzo B, Negri E, Talamini R, Franceschi S. Type of cigarettes and cancers of the upper digestive and respiratory tract. Cancer Causes Control 1990; 1:69–74.
143. Muscat JE, Richie JP Jr, Thompson S, Wynder EL. Gender differences in smoking and risk for oral cancer. Cancer Res 1996; 56:5192–5197.
144. Iribarren C, Tekawa IS, Sidney S, Friedman GD. Effect of cigar smoking on the risk of cardiovascular disease, chronic obstructive pulmonary disease, and cancer in men (see comments). N Engl J Med 1999; 340:1773–1780.
145. Lewin F, Norell SE, Johansson H, Gustavsson P, Wennerberg J, Biorklund A, Rutqvist LE. Smoking tobacco, oral snuff, alcohol in the etiology of squamous cell carcinoma of the head and neck: a population-based case-referent study in Sweden. Cancer 1998; 82:1367–1375.
146. Schlecht NF, Franco EL, Pintos J, Negassa A, Kowalski LP, Oliveira BV, Curado MP. Interaction between tobacco and alcohol consumption and the

risk of cancers of the upper aero-digestive tract in Brazil (see comments). Am J Epidemiol 1999; 150:1129–1137.

147. Jaber MA, Porter SR, Gilthorpe MS, Bedi R, Scully C. Risk factors for oral epithelial dysplasia–the role of smoking and alcohol. Oral Oncol 1999; 35: 151–156.

148. Kulasegaram R, Downer MC, Jullien JA, Zakrzewska JM, Speight PM. Case-control study of oral dysplasia and risk habits among patients of a dental hospital. Eur J Cancer B Oral Oncol 1995; 31B:227–231.

149. Elwood JM, Pearson JC, Skippen DH, Jackson SM. Alcohol, smoking, social and occupational factors in the aetiology of cancer of the oral cavity, pharynx and larynx. Int J Cancer 1984; 34:603–612.

150. Hoffmann D, Djordjevic MV. Chemical composition and carcinogenicity of smokeless tobacco. Adv Dent Res 1997; 11:322–329.

151. Gupta PC, Murti PR, Bhonsle RB. Epidemiology of cancer by tobacco products and the significance of TSNA. Crit Rev Toxicol 1996; 26:183–198.

152. Campisi R, Czernin J, Schoder H, Sayre JW, Schelbert HR. L-Arginine normalizes coronary vasomotion in long-term smokers. Circulation 1999; 99: 491–497.

153. Wynder EL, Bross IJ, Feldman RM. A study of the etiological factors in cancer of the mouth. Cancer 1957; 10:1300–1323.

154. Rao DN, Ganesh B, Rao RS, Desai PB. Risk assessment of tobacco, alcohol and diet in oral cancer–a case-control study. Int J Cancer 1994; 58:469–473.

155. Carpenter CL, Jarvik ME, Morgenstern H, McCarthy WJ, London SJ. Mentholated cigarette smoking and lung-cancer risk. Ann Epidemiol 1999; 9:114–120.

156. Jacob P III, Yu L, Shulgin AT, Benowitz NL. Minor tobacco alkaloids as biomarkers for tobacco use: comparison of users of cigarettes, smokeless tobacco, cigars, pipes. Am J Public Health 1999; 89:731–736.

157. Winn DM, Blot WJ, Shy CM, Pickle LW, Toledo A, Fraumeni JF Jr. Snuff dipping and oral cancer among women in the southern United States. N Engl J Med 1981; 304:745–749.

158. Brinton LA, Blot WJ, Becker JA, Winn DM, Browder JP, Farmer JC Jr, Fraumeni JF Jr. A case-control study of cancers of the nasal cavity and paranasal sinuses. Am J Epidemiol 1984; 119:896–906.

159. Winn DM. Epidemiology of cancer and other systemic effects associated with the use of smokeless tobacco. Adv Dent Res 1997; 11:313–321.

160. Ruengsakulrach P, Sinclair R, Komeda M, Raman J, Gordon I, Buxton B. Comparative histopathology of radial artery versus internal thoracic artery and risk factors for development of intimal hyperplasia and atherosclerosis. Circulation 1999; 100:II139–II144.

161. Badawi AF, Stern SJ, Lang NP, Kadlubar FF. Cytochrome P-450 and acetyltransferase expression as biomarkers of carcinogen-DNA adduct levels and human cancer susceptibility. Prog Clin Biol Res 1996; 395:109–140.

162. Kabat GC, Morabia A, Wynder EL. Comparison of smoking habits of blacks and whites in a case- control study. Am J Public Health 1991; 81:1483–1486.

163. Helbock HJ, Beckman KB, Shigenaga MK, Walter PB, Woodall AA, Yeo HC, Ames BN. DNA oxidation matters: the HPLC-electrochemical detection assay

of 8-oxo-deoxyguanosine and 8-oxo-guanine. Proc Natl Acad Sci USA 1998; 95:288–293.

164. Sumida H, Watanabe H, Kugiyama K, Ohgushi M, Matsumura T, Yasue, H. Does passive smoking impair endothelium-dependent coronary artery dilation in women? J Am Coll Cardiol 1998; 31:811–815.

165. Lazarus P, Sheikh SN, Ren Q, Schantz SP, Stern JC, Richie JP Jr, Park JY. p53, but not p16 mutations in oral squamous cell carcinomas are associated with specific CYP1A1 and GSTM1 polymorphic genotypes and patient tobacco use. Carcinogenesis 1998; 19:509–514.

166. Cheng L, Eicher SA, Guo Z, Hong WK, Spitz MR, Wei Q. Reduced DNA repair capacity in head and neck cancer patients. Cancer Epidemiol Biomarkers Prev 1998; 7:465–468.

167. Cloos J, Spitz MR, Schantz SP, Hsu TC, Zhang ZF, Tobi H, Braakhuis BJ, Snow GB. Genetic susceptibility to head and neck squamous cell carcinoma. J Natl Cancer Inst 1996; 88:530–535.

168. Schantz SP, Zhang ZF, Spitz MS, Sun M, Hsu TC. Genetic susceptibility to head and neck cancer: interaction between nutrition and mutagen sensitivity. Laryngoscope 1997; 107:765–781.

169. Spitz MR, Fueger JJ, Halabi S, Schantz SP, Sample D, Hsu TC. Mutagen sensitivity in upper aerodigestive tract cancer: a case- control analysis. Cancer Epidemiol Biomarkers Prev 1993; 2:329–333.

170. Spitz MR, Hoque A, Trizna Z, Schantz SP, Amos CI, King TM, Bondy ML, Hong WK, Hsu TC. Mutagen sensitivity as a risk factor for second malignant tumors following malignancies of the upper aerodigestive tract (see comments). J Natl Cancer Inst 1994; 86:1681–1684.

171. Vineis P, Esteve J, Terracini B. Bladder cancer and smoking in males: types of cigarettes, age at start, effect of stopping and interaction with occupation. Int J Cancer 1984; 34:165–170.

172. Brennan P, Bogillot O, Cordier S, Greiser E, Schill W, Vineis P, Lopez-Abente G, Tzonou A, Chang-Claude J, Bolm-Audorff U, Jockel KH, Donato F, Serra C, Wahrendorf J, Hours M, T'Mannetje A, Kogevinas M, Boffetta, P. Cigarette smoking and bladder cancer in men: a pooled analysis of 11 case-control studies. Int J Cancer 2000; 86:289–294.

173. D'Avanzo B, Negri E, La Vecchia C, Gramenzi A, Bianchi C, Franceschi S, Boyle P. Cigarette smoking and bladder cancer. Eur J Cancer 1990; 26: 714–718.

174. Loft S, Vistisen K, Ewertz M, Tjonneland A, Overvad K, Poulsen HE. Oxidative DNA damage estimated by 8-hydroxydeoxyguanosine excretion in humans: influence of smoking, gender and body mass index. Carcinogenesis 1992; 13:2241–2247.

175. Augustine A, Hebert JR, Kabat GC, Wynder EL. Bladder cancer in relation to cigarette smoking. Cancer Res 1988; 48:4405–4408.

176. Slattery ML, Schumacher MC, West DW, Robison LM. Smoking and bladder cancer. The modifying effect of cigarettes on other factors. Cancer 1988; 61:402–408.

177. Stevens RG, Moolgavkar SH. Estimation of relative risk from vital data: smoking and cancers of the lung and bladder. J Natl Cancer Inst 1979; 63:1351–1357.

178. Vineis P, Martone T. Molecular epidemiology of bladder cancer. Ann Ist Super Sanita 1996; 32:21–27.

179. Harris CC, Yoakum GH, Lechner JF, Willey JC, Gerwin BI, Banks-Schlegel SP, Masui T, Mark GE. Growth, differentiation, and neoplastic transformation of human bronchial epithelial cells. In: Harris CC, ed. Biochemical and Molecular Epidemiology of Cancer. New York: Alan R Liss, Inc, 1986:213–226.

180. Katoh T, Kaneko S, Boissy R, Watson M, Ikemura K, Bell DA. A pilot study testing the association between N-acetyltransferases 1 and 2 and risk of oral squamous cell carcinoma in Japanese people. Carcinogenesis 1998; 19:1803–1807.

181. Mommsen S, Aagaard J. Susceptibility in urinary bladder cancer: acetyltransferase phenotypes and related risk factors. Cancer Lett 1986; 32:199–205.

182. Risch A, Wallace DM, Bathers S, Sim E. Slow N-acetylation genotype is a susceptibility factor in occupational and smoking related bladder cancer. Hum Mol Genet 1995; 4:231–236.

183. Taylor JA, Umbach DM, Stephens E, Paulson D, Robertson C, Mohler JL, Bell DA. The role of N-acetylation polymorphisms at NAT1 and NAT2 is smoking-associated bladder cancer. Proc Am Assoc Cancer Res 36, 282. 1995. Ref Type: Abstract.

184. Yim SH, Hee SS. Genotoxicity of nicotine and cotinine in the bacterial luminescence test. Mutat Res 1995; 335:275–283.

185. Doolittle DJ, Winegar R, Lee CK, Caldwell WS, Hayes AW, de Bethizy JD. The genotoxic potential of nicotine and its major metabolites. Mutat Res 1995; 344:95–102.

186. Trivedi AH, Dave BJ, Adhvaryu SG. Assessment of genotoxicity of nicotine employing in vitro mammalian test system. Cancer Lett 1990; 54:89–94.

187. Trivedi AH, Dave BJ, Adhvaryu SC. Genotoxic effects of nicotine in combination with arecoline on CHO cells. Cancer Lett 1993; 74:105–110.

188. Mizusaki S, Okamoto H, Akiyama A, Fukuhara, Y. Relation between chemical constituents of tobacco and mutagenic activity of cigarette smoke condensate. Mutat Res 1977; 48:319–325.

189. Toth B. Effects of lifelong administration of beta-phenylisopropylhydrazine hydrochloride and thiocarbamylhydrazine in mice. Fundam Appl Toxicol 1982; 2:173–176.

190. Waldum HL, Nilsen OG, Nilsen T, Rorvik H, Syversen V, Sanvik AK, Haugen OA, Torp SH, Brenna E. Long-term effects of inhaled nicotine. Life Sci 1996; 58:1339–1346.

191. Martin JC, Martin DD, Radow B, Day HE. Life span and pathology in offspring following nicotine and methamphetamine exposure. Exp Aging Res 1979; 5:509–522.

192. Chen YP, Squier CA. Effect of nicotine on 7,12-dimethylbenz[a]anthracene carcinogenesis in hamster cheek pouch. J Natl Cancer Inst 1990; 82:861–864.

193. Gurkalo VK, Volfson NI. Nicotine influence upon the development of experimental stomach tumors. Arch Geschwulstforsch 1982; 52:259–265.

194. LaVoie EJ, Shigematsu A, Rivenson A, Mu B, Hoffmann D. Evaluation of the effects of cotinine and nicotine-N′-oxides on the development of tumors in rats initiated with N-[4-(5-nitro-2-furyl)-2-thiazolyl]formamide. J Natl Cancer Inst 1985; 75:1075–1081.
195. Habs M, Schmahl D. Influence of nicotine on N-nitrosomethylurea-induced mammary tumors in rats. Klin Wochenschr 1984; 62(suppl 2):105–108.
196. Zeller WJ, Berger MR. Nicotine and estrogen metabolism—possible implications of smoking for growth and outcome of treatment of hormone-dependent cancer? Discussion of experimental results. J Cancer Res Clin Oncol 1989; 115:601–603.
197. Wright SC, Zhong J, Zheng H, Larrick JW. Nicotine inhibition of apoptosis suggests a role in tumor promotion. FASEB J 1993; 7:1045–1051.
198. Hecht SS, Carmella SG, Chen M, Dor Koch JF, Miller AT, Murphy SE, Jensen JA, Zimmerman CL, Hatsukami DK. Quantitation of urinary metabolites of a tobacco-specific lung carcinogen after smoking cessation. Cancer Res 1999; 59:590–596.
199. Wright RM, McManaman JL, Repine JE. Alcohol-induced breast cancer: a proposed mechanism. Free Radic Biol Med 1999; 26:348–354.
200. Yin SJ, Han CL, Lee AI, Wu CW. Human alcohol dehydrogenase family. Functional classification, ethanol/retinol metabolism, medical implications. Adv Exp Med Biol 1999; 463:265–274.
201. Sreerama L, Sladek NE. Identification of the class-3 aldehyde dehydrogenases present in human MCF-7/0 breast adenocarcinoma cells and normal human breast tissue. Biochem Pharmacol 1994; 48:617–620.
202. Castro GD, Delgado de Layno AM, Costantini MH, Castro JA. Cytosolic xanthine oxidoreductase mediated bioactivation of ethanol to acetaldehyde and free radicals in rat breast tissue. Its potential role in alcohol-promoted mammary cancer. Toxicology 2001; 160:11–18.
203. Saleem MM, Al Tamer YY, Skursky L, Al Habbal Z. Alcohol dehydrogenase activity in the human tissues. Biochem Med 1984; 31:1–9.
204. Powell D, Benboutra M, Newey S, Harrison R. Xanthine oxidase activity and subscellular localization in human mammary epithelial cells. Biochem Soc Trans 1995:616S.
205. Hellmold H, Rylander T, Magnusson M, Reihner E, Warner M, Gustafsson JA. Characterization of cytochrome P450 enzymes in human breast tissue from reduction mammaplasties. J Clin Endocrinol Metab 1998; 83:886–895.
206. Jeong KS, Soh Y, Jeng J, Felder MR, Hardwick JP, Song BJ. Cytochrome P450 2E1 (CYP2E1)-dependent production of a 37-kDa acetaldehyde-protein adduct in the rat liver. Arch Biochem Biophys 2000; 384:81–87.
207. Roberts BJ, Shoaf SE, Song BJ. Rapid changes in cytochrome P4502E1 (CYP2E1) activity and other P450 isozymes following ethanol withdrawal in rats. Biochem Pharmacol 1995; 49:1665–1673.
208. Hardell L, Hallquist A, Mild KH, Carlberg M, Pahlson A, Lilja A. Cellular and cordless telephones and the risk for brain tumours. Eur J Cancer Prev 2002; 11:377–386.

209. Kitson KE. Regulation of alcohol and aldehyde dehydrogenase activity: a metabolic balancing act with important social consequences. Alcohol Clin Exp Res 1999; 23:955–957.

210. Dellarco VL. A mutagenicity assessment of acetaldehyde. Mutat Res 1988; 195:1–20.

211. Ristow H, Seyfarth A, Lochmann ER. Chromosomal damages by ethanol and acetaldehyde in *Saccharomyces cerevisiae* as studied by pulsed field gel electrophoresis. Mutat Res 1995; 326:165–170.

212. International Agency for Research on Cancer. IARC Monographs on the Evaluation of the Carcinogenic Risk of Chemicals to Man: Allyl Compounds, Aldehydes, Epoxides, Peroxides. Vol. 36. Lyon: IARC, 1985; 189–226. Ref Type: Report.

213. International Agency for Research on Cancer. Alchohol Drinking. Biological Data Relevant to the Evaluation of Carcinogenic Risk to Humans. Vol. 44. Lyon, France: IARC Monographs on the Evaluation of Carcinogenic Risks to Humans, 1988: 101–152. Ref Type: Report.

214. Kuykendall JR, Bogdanffy MS. Formation and stability of acetaldehyde-induced crosslinks between poly-lysine and poly-deoxyguanosine. Mutat Res 1994; 311:49–56.

215. Bird RP, Draper HH, Basrur PK. Effect of malonaldehyde and acetaldehyde on cultured mammalian cells. Production of micronuclei and chromosomal aberrations. Mutat Res 1982; 101:237–246.

216. Dulout FN, Furnus CC. Acetaldehyde-induced aneuploidy in cultured Chinese hamster cells. Mutagenesis 1988; 3:207–211.

217. Migliore L, Cocchi L, Scarpato R. Detection of the centromere in micronuclei by fluorescence in situ hybridization:its application to the human lymphocyte micronucleus assay after treatment with four suspected aneugens. Mutagenesis 1996; 11:285–290.

218. Blasiak J, Trzeciak A, Malecka-Panas E, Drzewoski J, Wojewodzka M. In vitro genotoxicity of ethanol and acetaldehyde in human lymphocytes and the gastrointestinal tract mucosa cells. Toxicol In Vitro ; 14:287–295.

219. Singh NP, Khan A. Acetaldehyde: genotoxicity and cytotoxicity in human lymphocytes. Mutat Res 1995; 337:9–17.

220. Grafstrom RC, Dypbukt JM, Sundqvist K, Atzori L, Nielsen I, Curren RD, Harris CC. Pathobiological effects of acetaldehyde in cultured human epithelial cells and fibroblasts. Carcinogenesis 1994; 15:985–990.

221. Woutersen RA, Appelman LM, Garderen-Hoetmer A, Feron VJ. Inhalation toxicity of acetaldehyde in rats. III. Carcinogenicity study. Toxicology 1986; 41:213–231.

222. Feron VJ, Kruysse A, Woutersen RA. Respiratory tract tumours in hamsters exposed to acetaldehyde vapour alone or simultaneously to benzo(a)pyrene or diethylnitrosamine. Eur J Cancer Clin Oncol 1982; 18:13–31.

223. Lambert B, Andersson B, Bastlova T, Hou SM, Hellgren D, Kolman A. Mutations induced in the hypoxanthine phosphoribosyl transferase gene by three urban air pollutants: acetaldehyde, benzo[a]pyrene diolepoxide, and ethylene oxide. Environ Health Perspect 1994; 102(suppl 4):135–138.

224. Noori P, Hou SM. Mutational spectrum induced by acetaldehyde in the HPRT gene of human T lymphocytes resembles that in the p53 gene of esophageal cancers. Carcinogenesis 2001; 22:1825–1830.
225. Matsuda T, Kawanishi M, Yagi T, Matsui S, Takebe H. Specific tandem GG to TT base substitutions induced by acetaldehyde are due to intra-strand crosslinks between adjacent guanine bases. Nucleic Acids Res 1998; 26: 1769–1774.
226. Worrall S, De Jersey J, Shanely B, Wilce P. Ethanol induces the production of antibodies to acetaldehyde-modified epitopes in rats. Alcohol Alochol 1989; 24:217–233.
227. Lin RC, Smith RS, Lumeng L. Detection of a protein-acetaldehyde adduct in the liver of rats fed alcohol chronically. J Clin Invest 1988; 81:615–619.
228. Niemela O, Klajner F, Orrego H, Vidnis E, Blendis L, Israel Y. Antibodies against acetaldehyde-modified proteins epitopes in human alcoholics. Hepatology 1987; 7:1210–1214.
229. Svengliati-Baroni G, Baraoana E, Rosman E, Lieber C. Collagen-acetaldehyde adducts in alcoholic and non-alcoholic liver disease. Hepatology 1994; 20: 111–118.
230. Ishii H, Kurose I, Kato S. Pathogenesis of alcoholic liver disease with particular emphasis on oxidative stress. J Gastroenterol Hepatol 1997; 12:S272–S282.
231. Espina N, Lima V, Lieber CS, Garro AJ. In vitro and in vivo inhibitory effect of ethanol and acetaldehyde on O6-methylguanine transferase. Carcinogenesis 1988; 9:761–766.
232. Blasiak J. Ethanol and acetaldehyde impair the repair of bleomycin-damaged DNA in human lymphocytes. Cytobios 2001; 106:141–149.
233. Pastino GM, Flynn EJ, Sultatos LG. Genetic polymorphisms in ethanol metabolism: issues and goals for physiologically based pharmacokinetic modeling. Drug Chem Toxicol 2000; 23:179–201.
234. Thomasson HR, Beard JD, Li TK. ADH2 gene polymorphisms are determinants of alcohol pharmacokinetics. Alcohol Clin Exp Res 1995; 19:1494–1499.
235. Bosron WF, Li TK. Catalytic properties of human liver alcohol dehydrogenase isoenzymes. Enzyme 1987; 37:19–28.
236. Groppi A, Begueret J, Iron A. Improved methods for genotype determination of human alcohol dehydrogenase (ADH) at ADH 2 and ADH 3 loci by using polymerase chain reaction–directed mutagenesis. Physiol Rev 1990; 36: 1765–1768.
237. Freudenheim JL, Ambrosone CB, Moysich KB, Vena JE, Graham S, Marshall JR, Muti P, Laughlin R, Nemoto T, Harty LC, Crits GA, Chan AW, Shields PG. Alcohol dehydrogenase 3 genotype modification of the association of alcohol consumption with breast cancer risk. Cancer Causes Control 1999; 10:369–377.
238. Harty LC, Caporaso NE, Hayes RB, Winn DM, Bravo-Otero E, Blot WJ, Kleinman DV, Brown LM, Armenian HK, Fraumeni JF Jr, Shields PG. Alcohol dehydrogenase 3 genotype and risk of oral cavity and pharyngeal cancers (see comments). J Natl Cancer Inst 1997; 89:1698–1705.
239. Hines LM, Hankinson SE, Smith-Warner SA, Spiegelman D, Kelsey KT, Colditz GA, Willett WC, Hunter DJ. A prospective study of the effect of

alcohol consumption and ADH3 genotype on plasma steroid hormone levels and breast cancer risk. Cancer Epidemiol Biomarkers Prev 2000; 9:1099–1105.

240. Edenberg HJ, Jerome RE, Li M. Polymorphism of the human alcohol dehydrogenase 4 (ADH4) promoter affects gene expression. Pharmacogenom 2000; 9:25–30.

241. Stromberg P, Svensson S, Hedberg JJ, Nordling E, Hoog JO. Identification and characterisation of two allelic forms of human alcohol dehydrogenase 2. Cell Mol Life Sci 2002; 59:552–559.

242. Uematsu F, Kikuchi H, Motomiya M, Abe T, Sagami I, Ohmachi T, Wakui A, Kanamaru R, Watanabe M. Association between restriction fragment length polymorphism of the human cytochrome P450IIE1 gene and susceptibility to lung cancer. Jpn J Cancer Res 1991; 82:254–256.

243. McCarver DG, Byun R, Hines RN, Hichme M, Wegenek W. A genetic polymorphism in the regulatory sequences of human CYP2E1: association with increased chlorzoxazone hydroxylation in the presence of obesity and ethanol intake. Toxicol Appl Pharmacol 1998; 152:276–281.

244. McCarver DG. ADH2 and CYP2E1 genetic polymorphisms: risk factors for alcohol-related birth defects. Drug Metab Dispos 2001; 29:562–565.

245. Hoek JB, Cahill A, Pastorino JG. Alcohol and mitochondria: a dysfunctional relationship. Gastroenterology 2002; 122:2049–2063.

246. Lindau-Shepard B, Shaffer JB, Del Vecchio PJ. Overexpression of manganous superoxide dismutase (MnSOD) in pulmonary endothelial cells confers resistance to hyperoxia. J Cell Physiol 1994; 161:237–242.

247. Stephanz GB, Gwinner W, Cannon JK, Tisher CC, Nick HS. Heat-aggregated IgG and interleukin-1-beta stimulate manganese superoxide dismutase in mesangial cells. Exp Nephrol 1996; 4:151–158.

248. Albano E, Clot P, Comoglio A, Dianzani MU, Tomasi, A. Free radical activation of acetaldehyde and its role in protein alkylation. FEBS Lett 1998; 348:65–69.

249. Mobley JA, Bhat AS, Brueggemeier RW. Measurement of oxidative DNA damage by catechol estrogens and analogues in vitro. Chem Res Toxicol 1999; 12:270–277.

250. Ambrosone CB. Oxidants and antioxidants in breast cancer. Antioxid Redox Signal 2000; 2:903–917.

251. Straif K, Weiland SK, Werner B, Chambless L, Mundt KA, Keil, U. Workplace risk factors for cancer in the German rubber industry: Part 2. Mortality from non-respiratory cancers. Occup Environ Med 1998; 55:325–332.

252. Johansen C, Boice J Jr, McLaughlin J, Olsen J. Cellular telephones and cancer—a nationwide cohort study in Denmark. J Natl Cancer Inst 2001; 93: 203–207.

253. Penta JS, Johnson FM, Wachsman JT, Copeland WC. Mitochondrial DNA in human malignancy. Mutat Res-Rev Mutat Res 2001; 488:119–133.

254. Fliss MS, Usadel H, Cabellero OL, Wu L, Buta MR, Eleff SM, Jen J, Sidransky D. Facile detection of mitochondrial DNA mutations in tumors and bodily fluids. Science 2000; 287:2017–2019.

255. Habano W, Sugai T, Yoshida T, Nakamura S. Mitochondrial gene mutation, but not large-scale deletion, is a feature of colorectal carcinomas with mitochondrial microsatellite instability. Int J Cancer 1999; 83:625–629.
256. Kirches E, Krause G, Warich-Kirches M, Weis S, Schneider T, Meyer-Puttlitz B, Mawrin C, Dietzmann K. High frequency of mitochondrial DNA mutations in glioblastoma multiforme identified by direct sequence comparison to blook samples. Int J Cancer 2001; 93:534–538.
257. Liu VWS, Shi HH, Cheung ANY, Chiu PM, Leung TW, Nagley P, Wong LC, Ngan HYS. High incidence of somatic mitochondrial DNA mutations in human ovarian carcinomas. Cancer Res 2001; 61:5998–6001.
258. Polyak K, Li YB, Zhu H, Lengauer C, Willson JKV, Markowitz SD, Trush MA, Kinzler KW, Vogelstein B. Somatic mutations of the mitochondrial genome in human colorectal tumours. Nature Genet 1998; 20:291–293.
259. Tamura G, Nishizuka S, Maesawa C, Suzuki Y, Iwaya T, Sakata K, Endoh Y, Motoyama T. Mutations in mitochondrial control region DNA in gastric tumours of Japanese patients. Eur J Cancer 1999; 35:316–319.
260. Tan DJ, Bai R, Wong LJ. Comprehensive scanning of somatic mitochondrial DNA mutations in breast cancer. 2002; 62:972–976. Ref Type: Generic.
261. Yeh JJ, Lunetta KL, van Orsouw NJ, Moore FD, Mutter GL, Vijg J, Dahia PLM, Eng C. Somatic mitochondrial DNA (mtDNA) mutations in papillary thyroid carcinomas and differential mtDNA sequence variatns in cases with thyroid tumours. Oncogene 2000; 19:2060–2066.
262. Hayakawa M, Katsumata K, Yoneda M, Tanaka M, Sugiyama S, Ozawa T. Age-related extensive fragmentation of mitochondrial DNA into minicircles. Biochem Biophys Res Commun 1996; 226:369–377.
263. Kohno T, Shinmura K, Tosaka M, Tani M, Kim SR, Sugimura H, Nohmi T, Kasai H, Yokota J. Genetic polymorphisms and alternative splicing of the hOGG1 gene, that is involved in the repair of 8-hydroxyguanine in damaged DNA. Oncogene 1998; 16:3219–3225.
264. Dherin C, Radicella JP, Dizdaroglu M, Boiteux S. Excision of oxidatively damaged DNA bases by the human alpha-hOgg1 protein and the polymorphic alpha-hOgg1(Ser326Cys) protein which is frequently found in human populations. Nucleic Acids Res 1999; 27:4001–4007.
265. Inoue H, Seitz HK. Viruses and alcohol in the pathogenesis of primary hepatic carcinoma. Eur J Cancer Prev 2001; 10:107–110.
266. Rocken C, Carl-McGrath S. Pathology and pathogenesis of hepatocellular carcinoma. Dig Dis 2001; 19:269–278.
267. Monto A, Wright TL. The epidemiology and prevention of hepatocellular carcinoma. Semin Oncol 2001; 28:441–449.
268. Hori H, Kawano T, Endo M, Yuasa Y. Genetic polymorphisms of tobacco- and alcohol-related metabolizing enzymes and human esophageal squamous cell carcinoma susceptibility. J Clin Gastroenterol 1997; 25:568–575.
269. Takeshita T, Yang X, Inoue Y, Sato S, Morimoto K. Relationship between alcohol drinking, ADH2 and ALDH2 genotypes, risk for hepatocellular carcinoma in Japanese. Cancer Lett 2000; 149:69–76.
270. Yokoyama A, Muramatsu T, Ohmori T, Yokoyama T, Okuyama K, Takahashi H, Hasegawa Y, Higuchi S, Maruyama K, Shirakura K, Ishii H.

Alcohol-related cancers and aldehyde dehydrogenase-2 in Japanese alcoholics. Carcinogenesis 1998; 19:1383–1387.

271. Muto M, Nakane M, Hitomi Y, Yoshida S, Sasaki S, Ohtsu A, Yoshida S, Ebihara S, Esumi H. Association between aldehyde dehydrogenase gene polymorphisms and the phenomenon of field cancerization in patients with head and neck cancer. Carcinogenesis 2002; 23:1759–1765.

272. Terry MB, Gaudet MM, Gammon MD. The epidemiology of gastric cancer. Semin Radiat Oncol 2002; 12:111–127.

273. Scheppach W, Bingham S, Boutron-Ruault MC, Gerhardssond V, Moreno V, Nagengast FM, Reifen R, Riboli E, Seitz HK, Wahrendorf J. WHO consensus statement on the role of nutrition in colorectal cancer. Eur J Cancer Prev 1999; 8:57–62.

274. Seitz HK, Poschl G, Simanowski UA. Alcohol and cancer. Recent Dev Alcohol 1998; 14:67–95.

275. Simanowski UA, Suter P, Russell RM, Heller M, Waldherr R, Ward R, Peters TJ, Smith D, Seitz HK. Enhancement of ethanol induced rectal mucosal hyper regeneration with age in F344 rats. Gut 1994; 35:1102–1106.

276. Chen J, Ma J, Stampfer MJ, Hines LM, Selhub J, Hunter DJ. Alcohol dehydrogenase 3 genotype is not predictive for risk of colorectal cancer. Cancer Epidemiol Biomarkers Prev 2001; 10:1303–1304.

277. Chen J, Giovannucci E, Kelsey K, Rimm EB, Stampfer MJ, Colditz GA, Spiegelman D, Willett WC, Hunter DJ. A methylenetetrahydrofolate reductase polymorphism and the risk of colorectal cancer. Cancer Res 1996; 56: 4862–4864.

278. Marshall JR, Graham S, Haughey BP, Shedd D, O'Shea R, Brasure J, Wilkinson GS, West D. Smoking, alcohol, dentition and diet in the epidemiology of oral cancer. Eur J Cancer B Oral Oncol 1992; 28B:9–15.

279. Licitra L, Bernier J, Grandi C, Merlano M, Bruzzi P, Lefebvre JL. Cancer of the oropharynx. Crit Rev Oncol Hematol 2002; 41:107–122.

280. Casiglia J, Woo SB. A comprehensive review of oral cancer. Gen Dent 2001; 49:72–82.

281. Coutelle C, Ward PJ, Fleury B, Quattrocchi P, Chambrin H, Iron A, Couzigou P, Cassaigne A. Laryngeal and oropharyngeal cancer, alcohol dehydrogenase 3 and glutathione S-transferase M1 polymorphisms. Hum Genet 1997; 99:319–325.

282. Bouchardy C, Hirvonen A, Coutelle C, Ward PJ, Dayer P, Benhamou S. Role of alcohol dehydrogenase 3 and cytochrome P-4502E1 genotypes in susceptibility to cancers of the upper aerodigestive tract. Int J Cancer 2000; 87: 734–740.

283. Zavras AI, Wu T, Laskaris G, Wang YF, Cartsos V, Segas J, Lefantzis D, Joshipura K, Douglass CW, Diehl SR. Interaction between a single nucleotide polymorphism in the alcohol dehydrogenase 3 gene, alcohol consumption and oral cancer risk. Int J Cancer 2002; 97:526–530.

284. Schwartz SM, Doody DR, Fitzgibbons ED, Ricks S, Porter PL, Chen C. Oral squamous cell cancer risk in relation to alcohol consumption and alcohol dehydrogenase-3 genotypes. Cancer Epidemiol Biomarkers Prev 2001; 10: 1137–1144.

285. Olshan AF, Weissler MC, Watson MA, Bell DA. Risk of head and neck cancer and the alcohol dehydrogenase 3 genotype. Carcinogenesis 2001; 22:57–61.
286. Smith-Warner SA, Spiegelman D, Yaun SS, van den Brandt PA, Folsom AR, Goldbohm RA, Graham S, Holmberg L, Howe GR, Marshall JR, Miller AB, Potter JD, Speizer FE, Willett WC, Wolk A, Hunter DJ. Alcohol and breast cancer in women: a pooled analysis of cohort studies. JAMA 1998; 279: 535–540.
287. Longnecker MP. Alcoholic beverage consumption in relation to risk of breast cancer: meta-analysis and review. Cancer Causes Control 1994; 5:73–82.
288. Howe GR, Hirohata T, Hislop TG, Iscovich JM, Yuan JM, Katsouyanni K, Lubin F, Marubini E, Modan B, Rohan T. Dietary factors and risk of breast cancer: combined analysis of 12 case-control studies. J Natl Cancer Inst 1990; 82:561–569.
289. Singletary KW, Gapstur SM. Alcohol and breast cancer – Review of epidemiologic and experimental evidence and potential mechanisms. JAMA 2001; 286:2143–2151.
290. Howe G, Rohan T, Decarli A, Iscovich J, Kaldor J, Katsouyanni K, Marubini E, Miller A, Riboli E, Toniolo P. The association between alcohol and breast cancer risk: evidence from the combined analysis of six dietary case-control studies. Int J Cancer 1991; 47:707–710.
291. Harvey EB, Schairer C, Brinton LA, Hoover RN, Fraumeni JF Jr. Alcohol consumption and breast cancer. J Natl Cancer Inst 1987; 78:657–661.
292. Longnecker MP, Newcomb PA, Mittendorf R, Greenberg ER, Clapp RW, Bogdan GF, Baron J, MacMahon B, Willett WC. Risk of breast cancer in relation to lifetime alcohol consumption. J Natl Cancer Inst 1995; 87:923–929.
293. O'Connell DL, Hulka BS, Chambless LE, Wilkinson WE, Deubner DC. Cigarette smoking, alcohol consumption, breast cancer risk. J Natl Cancer Inst 1987; 78:229–234.
294. Willett WC, Stampfer MJ, Colditz GA, Bosner BA, Hennekens CH, Speizer FE. Moderate alcohol consumption and the risk of breast cancer. N Engl J Med 1987; 316:1174–1180.
295. Garfinkel L, Boffeta P, Stellman SD. Alcohol and breast cancer: a cohort study. Prev Med 1988; 17:686–693.
296. Ellison RC, Zhang YQ, McLennan CE, Rothman KJ. Exploring the relation of alcohol consumption to risk of breast cancer. Am J Epidemiol 2001; 154:740–747.
297. Watabiki T, Okii Y, Tokiyasu T, Yoshimura S, Yoshida M, Akane A, Shikata N, Tsubura A. Long-term ethanol consumption in ICR mice causes mammary tumor in females and liver fibrosis in males. Alcohol Clin Exp Res 2000; 24:117S–122S.
298. Singletary K, Nelshoppen J, Wallig M. Enhancement by chronic ethanol intake of N-methyl-N-nitrosourea-induced rat mammary tumorigenesis. Carcinogenesis 1995; 16:959–964.
299. Holmberg B, Ekstrom T. The effects of long-term oral-administration of ethanol on Sprague–dawley rats—a condensed report. Toxicology 1995; 96:133–145.

300. Cooper G, Sandler D, Whelan E, Smith K. Association of physical and behavioral characteristics with menstrual cycle patterns in women 29–31 years of age. Epidemiology 2002; 7:624–628. Ref Type: Generic.

301. Verkasalo PK, Thomas HV, Appleby PN, Davey GK, Key TJ. Circulating levels of sex hormones and their relation to risk factors for breast cancer: a cross-sectional study in 1092 pre- and postmenopausal women (United Kingdom). Cancer Causes Control 2001; 12:47–59.

302. Muti P, Trevisan M, Micheli A, Krogh V, Bolelli G, Sciajno R, Schunemann HJ, Berrino F. Alcohol consumption and total estradiol in premenopausal women. Cancer Epidemiol Biomarkers Prev 1998; 7:189–193.

303. Ginsburg ES. Estrogen, alcohol and breast cancer risk. J Steroid Biochem Mol Biol 1999; 69:299–306.

304. Reichman ME, Judd JT, Longcope C, Schatzkin A, Clevidence BA, Nair PP, Campbell WS, Taylor PR. Effects of alcohol consumption on plasma and urinary hormone concentrations in premenopausal women. J Natl Cancer Inst 1993; 85:722–727.

305. Dorgan JF, Reichman ME, Judd JT, Brown C, Longcope C, Schatzkin A, Campbell WS, Franz C, Kahle L, Taylor PR. The relation of reported alcohol ingestion to plasma levels of estrogens and androgens in premenopausal women (Maryland, United States). Cancer Causes Control 1994; 5: 53–60.

306. Martin CA, Mainous AG III, Curry T, Martin D. Alcohol use in adolescent females: correlates with estradiol and testosterone. Am J Addict 1999; 8: 9–14.

307. Purohit V. Moderate alcohol consumption and estrogen levels in postmenopausal women: a review. Alcohol Clin Exp Res 1998; 22:994–997.

308. Ginsburg ES, Walsh BW, Shea BF, Gao X, Gleason RE, Barbieri RL. The effects of ethanol on the clearance of estradiol in postmenopausal women. Fertil Steril 1995; 63:1227–1230.

309. Ursin G, Tseng CC, Paganini-Hill A, Enger S, Wan PC, Formenti S, Pike MC, Ross RK. Does menopausal hormone replacement therapy interact with known factors to increase risk of breast cancer? J Clin Oncol 2002; 20: 699–706.

310. Turner RT, Sibonga JD. Effects of alcohol use and estrogen on bone. Alcohol Res Health 2001; 25:276–281.

311. Fan S, Meng Q, Gao B, Grossman J, Yadegari M, Goldberg ID, Rosen EM. Alcohol stimulates estrogen receptor signaling in human breast cancer cell lines. Cancer Res 2000; 60:5635–5639.

312. Singletary KW, Frey RS, Yan W. Effect of ethanol on proliferation and estrogen receptor-alpha expression in human breast cancer cells. Cancer Lett 2001; 165:131–137.

313. Enger SM, Ross RK, Paganini-Hill A, Longnecker MP, Bernstein L. Alcohol consumption and breast cancer oestrogen and progesterone receptor status. Br J Cancer 1999; 79:1308–1314.

314. Fornace AJ Jr, Lechner JF, Grafstrom RC, Harris CC. DNA repair in human bronchial epithelial cells. Carcinogenesis 1982; 3:1373–1377.

315. Gapstur SM, Potter JD, Drinkard C, Folsom AR. Synergistic effect between alcohol and estrogen replacement therapy on risk of breast cancer differs by estrogen/progesterone receptor status in the Iowa Women's Health Study. Cancer Epidemiol Biomarkers Prev 1995; 4:313–318.

316. Wolfe JN. Risk for breast cancer development determined by mammographic parenchymal pattern. Cancer 1976; 37:2486–2492.

317. Boyd NF, Byng JW, Jong RA, Fishell EK, Little LE, Miller AB, Lockwood GA, Tritchler DL, Yaffe MJ. Quantitative classification of mammographic densities and breast cancer risk: results from the Canadian National Breast Screening Study. J Natl Cancer Inst 1995; 87:670–675.

318. Hilakivi-Clarke L, Cho E, deAssis S, Olivo S, Ealley E, Bouker KB, Welch JN, Khan G, Clarke R, Cabanes A. Maternal and prepubertal diet, mammary development and breast cancer risk. J Nutr 2001; 131:154S–157S.

319. Brisson J, Verreault R, Morrison AS, Tennina A, Meyer F. Diet, mammographic features of breast tissue, and breast cancer risk. Am J Epidemiol 1989; 130:14–24.

320. Wolfe JN, Saftlas AF, Salane M. Mammographic parenchymal patterns and quantitative evaluation of mammographic densities: a case-control study. AJR Am J Roentgenol 1987; 148:1087–1092.

321. Saftlas AF, Hoover RN, Brinton LA, Szklo M, Olson DR, Salane M, Wolfe JN. Mammographic densities and risk of breast cancer. Cancer 1991; 67:2833–2838.

322. Byrne C, Schairer C, Wolfe J, Parekh N, Salane M, Brinton LA, Hoover R, Haile R. Mammographic features and breast cancer risk: effects with time, age, menopause status. J Natl Cancer Inst 1995; 87:1622–1629.

323. Vachon CM, Kuni CC, Anderson K, Anderson VE, Sellers TA. Association of mammographically defined percent breast density with epidemiologic risk factors for breast cancer (United States). Cancer Causes Control 2000; 11:653–662.

324. Freedman M, San Martin J, O'Gorman J, Eckert S, Lippman ME, Lo SC, Walls EL, Zeng J. Digitized mammography: a clinical trial of postmenopausal women randomly assigned to receive raloxifene, estrogen, or placebo. J Natl Cancer Inst 2001; 93:51–56.

325. Herrinton LJ, Saftlas AF, Stanford JL, Brinton LA, Wolfe JN. Do alcohol intake and mammographic densities interact in regard to the risk of breast cancer? Cancer 1993; 71:3029–3035.

326. Boyd NF, Connelly P, Byng J, Yaffe M, Draper H, Little L, Jones D, Martin LJ, Lockwood G, Tritchler D. Plasma lipids, lipoproteins, mammographic densities. Cancer Epidemiol Biomarkers Prev 1995; 4:727–733.

327. Vachon CM, Kushi LH, Cerhan JR, Kuni CC, Sellers TA. Association of diet and mammographic breast density in the Minnesota breast cancer family cohort. Cancer Epidemiol Biomarkers Prev 2000; 9:151–160.

328. Singletary KW, McNary MQ. Influence of ethanol intake on mammary gland morphology and cell proliferation in normal and carcinogen-treated rats. Alcohol Clin Exp Res 1994; 18:1261–1266.

329. Cummings KM. Changes in the Smoking habits of adults in the United States and recent trends in lung cancer mortality. Cancer Detect Prev 1984; 7: 125–134.

330. Leanderson P, Tagesson C. Cigarette smoke-induced DNA-damage: role of hydroquinone and catechol in the formation of the oxidative DNA-adduct, 8-hydroxyguanosine. Chem Biol Interact 1990; 75:71–81.

331. Floyd RA. The role of 8-hydroxydeoxyguanosine in carcinogenesis. Carcinogenesis 1990; 11:1447–1450.

332. Marnett LJ. Oxyradicals and DNA damage. Carcinogenesis 2000; 21:361–370.

333. Poulsen HE, Prieme H, Loft S. Role of oxidative DNA damage in cancer initiation and promotion. Eur J Cancer Prev 1998; 7:9–16.

334. Asami S, Hirano T, Yamaguchi R, Tomioka Y, Itoh H, Kasai H. Increase of a type of oxidative DNA damage, 8-hydroxyguanine and its repair activity in human leukocytes by cigarette smoking. Cancer Res 1996; 56:2546–2549.

335. Perera FP. Molecular cancer epidemiology. a new tool in cancer prevention. J Natl Cancer Inst 1987; 78:887–898.

336. Schoket B, Phillips DH, Kostic S, Vincze I. Smoking-associated bulky DNA adducts in bronchial tissue related to CYP1A1 MspI and GSTM1 genotypes in lung patients. Carginogenesis. 1998; 19:841–846.

337. Wingo PA, Ries LA, Giovino GA, Miller DS, Rosenberg HM, Shopland DR, Thun MJ, Edwards BK. Annual report to the nation on the status of cancer, 1973–1996, with a special section on lung cancer and tobacco smoking (see comments). J Natl Cancer Inst 1999; 91:675–690.

338. Ernster VL. Female lung cancer. Annu Rev Public Health 1996; 17:97–114.

339. Zang EA, Wynder EL. Differences in lung cancer risk between men and women: examination of the evidence. J Natl Cancer Inst 1996; 88:183–192.

340. Risch HA, Howe GR, Jain M, Burch JD, Holowaty EJ, Miller AB. Are female smokers at higher risk for lung cancer than male smokers? A case-control analysis by histologic type. Am J Epidemiol 1993; 138:281–293.

341. Bell DA, Taylor JA, Paulson DF, Robertson CN, Mohler JL, Miller CR, Lucier GW. Glutathione transferase u gene deletion is associated with increased risk for bladder cancer. Proc Am Assoc Cancer Res 1992; 33:291 Ref Type: Abstract.

342. Romkes M, Chern HD, Lesnick TG, Becich MJ, Persad R, Smith P, Branch RA. Association of low CYP3A activity with p53 mutation and CYP2D6 activity with Rb mutation in human bladder cancer. Carcinogenesis 1996; 17:1057–1062.

343. Martone T, Airoldi L, Magagnotti C, Coda R, Randone D, Malaveille C, Avanzi G, Merletti F, Hautefeuille A, Vineis P. 4-Aminobiphenyl-DNA adducts and p53 mutations in bladder cancer. Int J Cancer 1998; 75:512–516.

344. Doolittle DJ, Rahn CA, Lee CK. The effect of exposure to nicotine, carbon monoxide, cigarette smoke or cigarette smoke condensate on the mutagenicity of rat urine. Mutat Res 1991; 260:9–18.

17

Hormones and Cancer

Heather Spencer Feigelson

Department of Epidemiology and Surveillance Research,
American Cancer Society, Atlanta, Georgia, U.S.A.

Roberta McKean-Cowdin

Norris Comprehensive Cancer Center, Keck School of Medicine,
Los Angeles, California, U.S.A.

Neoplasia of hormone-responsive tissues currently accounts for more that 35% of all newly diagnosed cancers in men, and more than 40% of all newly diagnosed cancers in women in the United States (1). Bittner (2) first proposed the idea that hormones may play a role in the formation of cancer in studies of estrogens and mammary tumors in mice. Since that time, that theory has been refined and expanded with substantial and convincing evidence from experimental, clinical, and epidemiological studies. It is now generally recognized that hormones play an etiological role in cancers of the breast, prostate, ovary, endometrium, testis, thyroid, and bone.

This chapter will focus primarily on endogenous and exogenous sources of steroid hormones and their role in carcinogenesis of hormone-responsive tissue. Further, the chapter will review multigenic models that are being used to understand the etiology of breast and prostate cancers and that may serve as examples to establish new models for other hormone-dependent cancers.

1. MODEL OF CARCINOGENESIS

How do hormones fit into the traditional model of carcinogenesis? The normal growth and function of hormone-responsive organs is controlled by one or more steroid or polypeptide hormones. The underlying mechanism proposed for all of these cancers is that neoplasia is a consequence of prolonged hormonal stimulation of the particular target organ, which may occur from endogenous sources produced in the body, or through exogenous sources such as oral contraceptives or hormone replacement therapy (HRT).

The major carcinogenic consequence of hormonal exposure at the end organ is cellular proliferation. The emergence of a malignant phenotype depends on a series of somatic mutations that occur during cell division, but the specific genes involved in progression are unknown at this time. Candidate genes include those in the endocrine pathway (3,4), as well as DNA repair genes, tumor suppressor genes, and oncogenes (5–7). *BRCA1* and *BRCA2* are two such tumor suppressor genes that have been associated with susceptibility to breast, ovarian, and possibly other cancers in certain kindreds (8,9). Germline mutations in *TP53* are also associated with an increased risk of breast cancer in certain families (10). However, mutations in these genes do not appear to be involved in the majority of sporadic breast cancer. The *HER2* oncogene is overexpressed in advanced breast cancer and probably represents one critical event in the later part of breast cancer progression (11).

Although there is evidence that hormonal secretion and metabolism can be environmentally influenced, for example, through diet and physical activity, the control of hormonal patterns is largely genetically regulated. We must begin to characterize the complex genetic arrays that contribute to carcinogenesis in hormone-responsive tissue and identify alleles responsible for interindividual differences in steroid hormone levels. High-risk alleles will likely be variants in genes involved in steroid hormone metabolism and transport. These allelic variants may alter the encoded protein structure, function, interaction with other proteins, or half-life and stability within the cell. Research toward identifying alleles using the candidate gene approach will be discussed later in this chapter in relation to breast and prostate cancer.

2. ENDOGENOUS HORMONES

2.1. Steroid Hormone Synthesis

The primary sex steroid hormones are estrogens and progestins for women and androgens for men. Steroid hormones, including estrogens, androgens, progestins, mineralocorticoids, and glucorticoids, are synthesized in a tightly controlled system involving cytochrome P450 enzymes and dehydrogenases (12) (Fig. 1). The process begins with the conversion of acetate into cholesterol, which may occur in the liver, skin, adrenals, ovaries, testes, brain, or intestine (13). Over 25 enzymes are involved in this initial step. Cholesterol is then converted into pregnenolone by the p450 side chain clea-

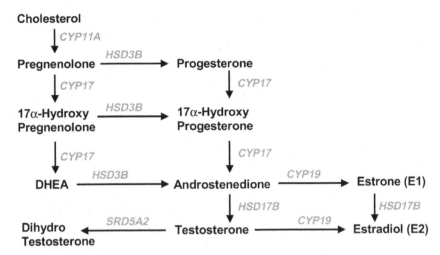

Figure 1 Steroid hormone biosynthesis pathway showing the genes involved in biosynthesis.

vage enzyme (p450scc, also known as CYP11A1) in the mitochondrion of the adrenals, ovaries, or testes. The rate-limiting step of steroid biosynthesis is the diffusion of cholesterol across the mitochondrial membrane (14,15). At this point of steroidogenesis, pregnenolone may be converted into 17OH-pregnenolone by the p450c17 (CYP17) enzyme or into progesterone by hydroxysteroid dehydrogenase-3-beta-1 (HSD3B1); both products may then be converted into estrogens or androgens.

The production of estrogen is accomplished through the conversion of progesterone or 17OH-pregnenolone into androstenedione in the adrenals or ovaries. CYP17 is required for both reactions, while HSD3B1 must additionally be present for the conversion of 17OH-pregnenolone. The reaction proceeds with the aromatization of androstenedione into estrone (E1) through CYP19, which occurs primarily in the ovaries of premenopausal women and in the adipose tissue of postmenopausal women. E1 is then converted to a more biologically active form, 17-beta-estradiol (E2), through the mediation of 17-beta-hydroxysteroid dehydrogenases (HSD17B1). The reverse reaction (conversion of E2 back to E1) is catalyzed by HSD17B2.

There are two androgen synthesis pathways that occur in the adrenals and the testes. The 5-delta pathway is most common in humans, whereas the 4-delta pathway is common in rodents. Both pathways begin with the rate-limiting conversion of cholesterol to prenenolone through the action of CYP11A1, as previously described. The 5-delta pathway consists of the conversion of pregnenolone to 17-alpha hydroxy-pregnenolone and subsequently dehydroepiandrosterone (DHEA) through the action of CYP17 in either the testes or the adrenals. Dehydroepiandrosterone is then converted to androstenediol in the testes by HSD17B3. The final step of the 5-delta pathway, also limited to the testes, is the metabolism of androstenediol to testosterone by the enzyme HSD3B2.

To exert an effect, steroids must find their way from the cytoplasmic organelles in the ovarian or testes cells into the cells of the hormone-responsive tissues where they can bind with steroid receptors in the nucleus. Roughly 95% of total circulating hormones reach the appropriate cells bound to "carrier" proteins such as sex-hormone binding globulin (SHBG) and albumin. Steroids enter the cell by diffusion or by interaction between serum proteins and recognition sites on the cell surface (16). Once the steroid reaches the appropriate cells, the steroid may bind to its associated receptor, resulting in a conformational change in the receptor that enhances its affinity for specific hormone response elements (HRE) in the DNA. The steroid receptor complex, made of a hormone, a receptor dimer, and various nonreceptor proteins, interacts with specific sights in the preinitiation complex and proximal promoter (TATA) box to signal the activation of transcription of target genes. The precise mechanism of how steroid receptors regulate gene expression, however, remains elusive.

3. EXOGENOUS HORMONES

External sources of steroid hormones also influence cell proliferation and, therefore, risk of hormone-dependent cancers. Hormone replacement therapy and oral contraceptives are two forms of exogenous hormones that have been studied extensively. One or both of these agents play a role in the risk of breast, ovary, cervical, endometrial, and colorectal cancers. More recently, environmental estrogens and dietary phytoestrogens, plant substances that are structurally or functionally similar to estrogen, have been suggested to be important in the etiology of hormone related cancers.

3.1. Oral Contraceptives

Combination oral contraceptives (COC), which include an estrogen and high-dose progesterone, reduce the risk of ovarian and endometrial cancers. The relationship of OC use to breast cancer has been the topic of many review articles (17). A recent meta-analysis of 54 studies, including over 150,000 women, provided important information about the risk of breast cancer among COC users (18). Results from the meta-analysis indicate that a modest increase in relative risk (RR) of breast cancer was associated with current (RR = 1.24; $p < 0.00001$) and recent (RR = 1.16; $p < 0.00001$) COC use. There is no evidence that this excess in risk continues to persist 10 or more years after cessation of COC use. However, the degree of the association was modified by age at first use of COCs. For recent users, risk was greatest for those who began COCs before the age of 20, and tended to decline with increasing age at diagnosis. Total duration of COC use was not associated with increased risk of breast cancer once recency of use was taken into account. Although the scope of this meta-analysis was broad, there is little information about cancer risk 10 years after cessation of COC use. Moreover, most women who stopped use 10 or more years ago had used COCs for only short periods of time. In the next decade, women who began use as teenagers will reach their late 40s and early 50s. At that time, it will be important to reexamine the effects of long-term and early use of COCs.

3.2. Hormone Replacement Therapy

Hormone replacement therapy use is associated with endometrial, breast, colorectal, and possibly ovarian cancers. When the use of HRT to provide short-term relief of menopausal symptoms was introduced, prescriptions were for estrogen-only replacement therapy (ERT). What resulted was an epidemic of endometrial cancers in the 1960s and 1970s that was related to both dose and duration of therapy (19). Subsequently, progestogens were added to the estrogen in various doses and schedules and the incidence of endometrial cancer once again declined. Combination hormone replacement therapy (CHRT), in which a progestin is given sequentially or continuously with estrogen during a monthly cycle, has grown rapidly in popularity in the past three decades.

Until recently, the vast majority of epidemiological studies of HRT and breast cancer had sufficient data to examine ERT use only. The accumulated evidence suggested that postmenopausal hormone use imparts a relatively small increased risk of breast cancer. In a meta-analysis including over 160,000 women, current or recent use of postmenopausal hormones increased the risk of breast cancer in relation to increasing duration of use (20). For women whose last use of HRT was less than 5 years before diagnosis, risk increased by 2.3% ($p = 0.0002$) for each year of use. However, women who stopped using HRT 5 or more years before diagnosis had no increased risk, regardless of duration of use. After taking these timing factors into account, no other index of timing was important, including age at first use or time between menopause and first use. Although this meta-analysis suggested that risk of breast cancer associated with CHRT might be greater than for ERT, there were few long-term users of CHRT available for analysis so the risk estimates are statistically imprecise (20).

The first observational studies specifically examining the breast cancer risk associated with CHRT use appeared in 2000. Ross et al. (21) reported that for every 5 years of use, risk was four times greater for CHRT users than for ERT users; specifically, the odd ratio (OR) per 5 years of use for CHRT was 1.24 [95% confidence interval (CI): 1.07–1.45] and the OR per 5 years of use for ERT was 1.06 (95% CI: 0.97–1.15). Schairer et al. (22) observed similar risks among a cohort of 46,355 women in the Breast Cancer Detection

Demonstration Project (BCDDP). The relative risk increased by 1% per year of estrogen-only use and by 8% per year of CHRT use.

In May 2002 the Women's Health Initiative (WHI), a set of randomized clinical trials designed to determine the efficacy of several strategies to reduce the incidence of breast cancer, heart disease, colorectal cancer, and fractures in postmenopausal women, stopped the study arm that was testing the use of CHRT vs. placebo among 16,600 women (23). The trial was stopped after a mean of 5.2 years of follow-up when the test statistic for invasive breast cancer exceeded the stopping boundary. The estimated hazard ratio (HR) for breast cancer was 1.29 (95% CI: 1.00–1.59) among women who had taken CHRT vs. placebo. The trial also found that women in the CHRT group were at increased risk of heart disease and stroke, and decreased risk of colorectal cancer, endometrial cancer, and hip fractures. The HR for colorectal cancer was 0.63 (95% CI: 0.43–0.92), and 0.83 (95% CI: 0.48–1.47) for endometrial cancer. Although randomized trials are considered the gold standard of epidemiological research, controversy around the use of CHRT remains. A similar trial under way in the United Kingdom, called the WISDOM study, will continue to study the long-term health effects of CHRT (24).

Emerging evidence suggests that ERT may also increase the risk of ovarian cancer (25). In a large prospective study including over 900 cases of ovarian cancer, Rodriguez et al. found that ERT users had higher ovarian cancer death rates than nonusers (RR = 1.51, 95% CI: 1.16–1.96). Risk was also slightly increased among former ERT users, and more than doubled among women who had used ERT for 10 or more years (RR = 2.20, 95% CI: 1.53–3.17). Although lifetime risk of ovarian cancer is low (1.7%) (26), these data add to concerns about the safety of long-term HRT use. Further studies are needed to confirm these findings and to examine whether effects are similar for CHRT use.

3.3. Xenobiotic Pesticides and Phytoestrogens

Both natural and man-made environmental estrogens have been shown to mimic the estrogenic activity of steroid hormones. Dietary phytoestrogens, plant substances that are structurally or functionally similar to estrogen, have been proposed to act as estrogen antagonists in breast, prostate, and endometrial cells, potentially protecting these tissues from cancer formation. In contrast, xenobiotics, environmental estrogens such as pesticides, have been proposed to act as estrogen agonists, possibly increasing the risk of cancer formation. Although we would expect that a weak estrogen, whether from natural or synthetic sources, would act in a similar manner when applied to the same system, the effect is difficult to predict due to variable characteristics of the estrogen-like substances and the test systems. The size, structure, and concentration of the chemicals, the presence of other natural or synthetic estrogens, the type of cell or animal model being tested, and the concentration of estrogen receptors (ER) will all influence the effect of the estrogen-like substance. Further, interpretation of findings may be influenced by prior beliefs that natural chemicals are beneficial, while synthetic agents are harmful.

There are several proposed mechanisms by which environmental estrogens may act. They may competitively bind with the ER to prevent the more potent mammalian form of estrogen (17β-estradiol, E2) from binding to the ER, or act synergistically by increasing the total concentration of estrogen and estrogen-like substances. Alternatively, environmental estrogens may interfere with the release of gonadotropins and, therefore, disrupt the feedback loop of the hypothalamic–pituitary gonadal axis. It also has been proposed that environmental estrogens may decrease free estrogen concentrations via stimulation of SHBG synthesis in the liver, which is one of the primary estrogen transport proteins in humans. In cell studies, it was shown that low concentrations ($1–10\,\mu M$) of the phytoestrogen enterolactone increased SHBG synthesis by HepG2 cells (27). However, higher production of SHBG has not been shown among humans consuming phytoestrogen-rich diets (28). Several nonhormonal actions of environmental estrogens also have been proposed. Phytoestrogens have been shown to suppress angiogenesis (29) and inhibit protein tyrosine kinases involved in tumor cell signal transduction and proliferation (30). Finally, it has been suggested that phytoestrogens may act as antioxidants, have inhibitory effects on apoptosis (31), and inhibit the activity of topoisomerases (32).

3.4. Phytoestrogens and Breast Cancer

Epidemiological studies of dietary phytoestrogens and breast cancer indicate that soy intake may reduce a woman's risk of premenopausal breast cancer (33–35), however at least one study found no association between dietary soy and breast cancer (36). Soy is the most significant source of dietary phytoestrogen (37–39), but phytoestrogens also are found in fruits, vegetables, whole grains, clover, and alfalfa sprouts (28). Of the studies that reported an association between premenopausal breast cancer and soy intake, one reported a decrease in risk of postmenopausal breast cancer (35). However, the postmenopausal finding was restricted largely to non-U.S. born Asians, suggesting that some other correlate of traditional Asian lifestyle may explain the association. Ingram et al. (40), re-examined the association between phytoestrogens and breast cancer by measuring urinary excretion rates of two classes of phytochemicals (lignans and isoflavonoids). An inverse relation was found between the risk of both premenopausal and postmenopausal breast cancer and urinary excretion of daidzein, equol, and enterolactone (40) and in a subsequent study, of daidzein, glycitein, and total isoflavonoids (41). It remains untested whether the measured phytochemicals actually serve as markers of other correlated dietary components such as fiber, which also has been postulated to reduce breast cancer risk (42).

While epidemiological data indicate that dietary phytoestrogens may decrease a woman's risk of breast cancer, the results of dietary intervention studies are less clear. The reported associations between dietary soy and circulating estrogens are inconsistent (43–45). Dietary studies did find that premenopausal women on soy-rich diets had lower levels of leutinizing hormone, follicular stimulating hormone, and progesterone, with longer menstrual cycles (43,44). Of potential concern are two reports that found that women on soy-rich diets had elevated numbers of hyperplastic epithelial cells in their breast fluid (46) and significantly increased rates of breast lobular epithelial proliferation (47).

Experimental studies show that phytoestrogens can exhibit both an estrogenic and an antiestrogenic effect, depending on the study conditions. For example, several types of phytoestrogens were shown to stimulate DNA synthesis and growth of human estrogen-dependent MCF-7 breast cancer cells at low concentrations (1–10 µM) (48–51), while inhibiting DNA synthesis at higher concentrations (20–90 µM) (50). Phytoestrogens also have been shown to inhibit the growth of estrogen receptor-negative human breast cancer cell lines (52). Animal studies indicate that soy administered by injection can reduce the incidence (53–55) or multiplicity (54–57) of chemically induced rat mammary tumors (58) and that they can be inhibited by soy-based diets as well (59). It is hypothesized that short-term feedings of dietary phytoestrogens to young rats may decrease carcinogen-induced breast cancer by increasing the proportion of differentiated cells in the mammary gland (55).

3.5. Xenobiotic Pesticides and Breast Cancer

Concern over environmental contaminants with estrogenic potential became an issue in the 1990s when an unusual number of wild animals, including fish (60–62), reptiles (63,64), and birds, were discovered with developmental abnormalities. Furthermore, there was concern that if environmental contaminants were responsible, humans also would be at increased risk. Fueling these concerns, a number of studies reported associations between environmental estrogens and increased risks of human breast cancer (65–67) and a decrease in sperm quality (67,68). Although, the activity level of most environmental pesticides is at least 1000 times less than that of the endogenous E2, there was uncertainty whether combinations of pesticides found in the environment could act in concert to produce stronger effects. This was supported by findings that a panel of chemical pesticides acted synergistically in competitive estrogen receptor binding and estrogen-responsive yeast assays. Specifically, a mixture of the insecticides dieldrin and endosulfan produced a 1000-fold higher combined activity level than either chemical alone (69). However, the findings were not supported by subsequent studies using over 10 different estrogen-responsive assays (70,71). More recent studies of turtles showed that endogenous steroid hormones with differing activity levels (estradiol, estrone, estriol) act synergistically, suggesting that weak environmental estrogens also may synergize with endogenous steroidal estrogens (72).

Rigorous, systematic study is needed to determine if a relationship exists between weak environmental estrogens and cancer risk. If the mechanism of action of environmental estrogens on cancer risk is strictly hormonal, it is unlikely that estrogenic pesticides and dietary phytoestrogens would exclusively produce opposite effects. Evaluation of in vitro and in vivo work for both phytoestrogens and xenobiotics as a whole may lead to a more objective interpretation of the current data and assessment of what questions remain unanswered.

4. EPIDEMIOLOGICAL REVIEW OF HORMONE-DEPENDENT CANCERS

4.1. Breast Cancer

A large and compelling body of epidemiological and experimental data implicate estrogens in the etiology of human breast cancer (73). Animal studies repeatedly demonstrated that estrogens can induce and promote mammary tumors in rodents and that removing the animals' ovaries or administering an antiestrogenic drug had the opposite effect (74).

4.1.1. Risk Factors

The most widely accepted risk factors for breast cancer, shown in Table 1, can be thought of as measures of the cumulative "dose" of estrogen that breast epithelium is exposed to over time. Early menarche and late

Table 1 Summary of Established Risk and Protective Factors for Breast Cancer

Risk factors (increased hormone exposure)
   Early menarche
   Late menopause
   Alcohol consumption
   Postmenopausal obesity
   Hormone replacement therapy
Protective factors (decreased hormone exposure)
   Young age at first full-term pregnancy
   Prolonged lactation
   Exercise

menopause maximize the number of ovulatory cycles experienced over time, during which a woman is exposed to high levels of estrogen and progesterone. Prolonged lactation, and more importantly, physical activity can reduce the number of ovulatory cycles. Both occupational and recreational types of physical activity have been shown to reduce risk (75–77). Exercise may decrease the risk of breast cancer by delaying the age of onset of regular ovulatory cycles, decreasing the frequency of those cycles, and reducing circulating levels of endogenous steroid hormones and insulin-like growth factors (IGFs) (78–81). Alcohol appears to increase breast cancer risk by increasing plasma estrogen and IGF levels (82). In a recent study, alcohol consumption was associated with a linear increase in breast cancer incidence for women who drank up to 60 g of alcohol per day (two to five drinks) (83). The primary source of estrogen in postmenopausal women is from the conversion of androstenedione to E1 in adipose tissue; thus, postmenopausal obesity increases the risk of breast cancer through increased production of estrogen. Obesity also is associated with decreased SHBG production and increased proportions of free and albumin-bound estrogens. The protective effect of early age at first birth is complex. During the first trimester of pregnancy, the level of free E2 rises rapidly. However, as the pregnancy progresses, prolactin and free E2 levels lower and SHBG levels rise yielding a net overall benefit with respect to the endogenous estrogen profile. Perhaps more importantly, the effect of a first pregnancy may be to cause some premalignant cells to terminally differentiate, thereby losing their malignant potential.

4.1.2. Endogenous Hormones

The most carefully conducted international studies comparing estrogen levels in populations at differing risk of breast cancer support the role of estrogens, especially E2, in the pathogenesis of breast cancer. Most studies have focused on women from China and Japan, because Asian women have experienced lower breast cancer rates than women from North America. In the early 1970s, MacMahon et al. (84) conducted a series of studies on teenagers and young women in Asia and North America. They found that in overnight urine samples collected on the morning of day 21 of the menstrual cycle, total urinary estrogen was 36% higher in the North American teenagers than in Asian teenagers. Similar differences were found among women aged 20–39. In two more recent studies, the relationship between serum estradiol and breast cancer risk was re-examined in Asian and North American populations (85,86). In one study, E2 levels were 20% higher in Los Angeles compared to premenopausal controls from Shanghai (85). In a comparison of postmenopausal women, E2 was 36% higher in Los Angeles than in age-matched Japanese women (86). The reasons for these differences remain poorly defined, but part of the explanation may be that there are genetic differences that affect steroid hormone biosynthesis.

A recent reanalysis of nine prospective studies of endogenous hormones and postmenopausal breast cancer has clearly demonstrated the strong association between elevated sex hormones and breast cancer risk (87). The risk of breast cancer increased statistically significantly with increasing concentrations of all the hormones examined: total E2, free E2, non-SHBG bound E2, E1, estrone sulfate, androstenedione, DHEA, DHEA-S, and testosterone. Women in the highest quintile of E2 were at twofold increased risk of breast cancer compared to those in the lowest quintile (RR = 2.0, 95% CI: 1.47–2.71, p for trend <0.001). High levels of free E2 (the form of estrogen that is most bioavailable) were even more strongly associated with risk (RR = 2.58, 95% CI: 1.76–3.78, p for trend <0.001, highest compared to lowest quintile). Increasing SHBG was associated with decreasing breast cancer risk (p for trend = 0.04). This study did not measure progesterone, and the role of elevated progesterone levels in breast cancer etiology remains controversial (89). Recent experimental data suggest that progestins are breast mitogens and, as such, are likely to increase breast cancer risk (90).

4.1.3. Genetic Models of Breast Cancer Susceptibility

It has been hypothesized that a multigenic model of breast cancer predisposition can be developed that includes polymorphisms in genes involved in estrogen biosynthesis and intracellular binding (3). This model would include functionally relevant polymorphisms that would act together, and in combination with established risk factors, to define a high-risk profile for breast cancer. Although many candidate genes for such a model exist, the genes originally proposed included three genes of interest: the 17-beta-hydroxysteroid dehydrogenase 1 (*HSD17B1*) gene, the cytochrome P459c17α (*CYP17*) gene, and the estrogen receptor alpha (*ESR1*) gene. Data have been published supporting the joint effect of *CYP17* and *HSD17B1* on breast cancer risk (91). Huang et al. (92) have also published findings of a similar model with the estrogen metabolizing genes *CYP17*, *CYP1A1*, which participates in estrogen hydroxylation, and the catechol-*O*-methyltransferase (*COMT*) gene, which encodes the enzyme responsible for *O*-methylation leading to inactivation of catechol estrogen (CE). Association studies of genes in the steroid hormone pathway are being published with increasing frequency, but little consistency. Several reviews appear elsewhere (92a,94b–d). As an example of one candidate gene, *CYP17* is discussed below.

4.1.3.1. CYP17: At present, data suggest that variation in *CYP17* may influence endocrine function. As summarized below, it has been shown to be associated with the risk of breast cancer, serum hormone levels in pre- and postmenopausal women, estrogen metabolites measured in urine, age at menarche, and use of HRT.

The *CYP17* gene codes for the cytochrome P450c17α enzyme, which mediates both steroid 17α-hydroxylase and 17,20-lyase activities, and functions at key branch points in human steroidogenesis (93). The 5' untranslated region (UTR) of *CYP17* contains a single base-pair polymorphism 34 bp upstream from the initiation of translation, and 27 bp downstream from the transcription start site (T27C) (94) and has been used to designate two alleles, *A*1 (the published sequence) and *A*2.

An association between risk of breast cancer and this *CYP17* polymorphism was first reported in 1997 (95). In a case–control study of incident breast cancer among Asian, African-American, and Latina women, a 2.5-fold increased risk of advanced breast cancer was observed among women who carried the *CYP17 A*2 allele. This study also presented preliminary evidence suggesting that *CYP17* may be associated with age at menarche.

These results suggested that serum hormone levels may differ by *CYP17* genotype. In a follow-up study, it was reported that *CYP17* genotype was associated with E2 and progesterone levels among young nulliparous women (96). As shown in Fig. 2, serum E2 measured around day 11 of the menstrual cycle was 11% and 57% higher ($p = 0.04$), respectively, among women hetero- and homozygous for the *CYP17 A*2 allele compared to *A*1/*A*1 women. Similarly, around cycle day 22 (Fig. 3), E2 was 7% and 28% higher ($p = 0.06$) and progesterone was 24% and 30% higher ($p = 0.04$). These data provided direct evidence of genetic control of serum hormone levels.

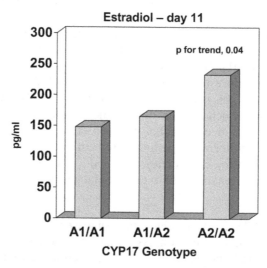

Figure 2 Geometric mean serum estradial concentration (pg/ml) among young nulliparous women on day 11 of the menstrual cycle by CYP17 genotype.

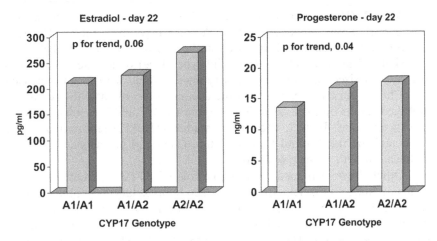

Figure 3 Geometric mean serum estradiol concentration (pg/ml) and progesterone concentration (ng/ml) among young nulliparous women on day 22 of the menstrual cycle by CYP17 genotype.

Since this original study of *CYP17* was published, at least 11 other studies have reported on *CYP17* and breast cancer (97–103). The results of these studies are largely negative and suggest heterogeneity by ethnicity. Although the two of the largest studies conducted to date found no association (97,98), several of the smaller studies (99,100,102) found a modest, but nonsignificant, elevation in breast cancer risk with the *CYP17 A2* allele in some subgroups. Others have shown an association between *CYP17* and breast cancer only among specific age groups of women. Kristensen et al. (103) and Miyoshi et al. (104) suggest that the effect of *CYP17* may be limited to older cases (i.e. over 55 years of age at diagnosis) while Bergman-Jungestrom et al. (102) and Spurdle et al. (105) found increased risk among premenopausal women.

More consistent data are accumulating to suggest that *CYP17* is a modifier of other breast cancer risk factors, such as age at menarche and parity (106,92). At least three studies have shown that the protective effect of later onset of menarche was limited to women with the *A*1/*A*1 genotype (95,97,106). One study has shown that *CYP17* genotype was associated with estrogen metabolites measured in urine (107). The ratio between 2-hydroxyestrone (2OHE) and 16α-hydroxyestrone (16αOHE) demonstrated a dose–response relationship by which women with the *A*1/*A*1 genotype had the highest urinary ratio of 2OHE to 16αOHE (median = 1.47) and women with the A2/A2 genotype had the lowest ratio (median = 1.21, p = 0.01. Lower 2OHE:16αOHE ratios may be associated with increased risk of breast cancer (108,109). Thus, this observation is compatible with the hypothesis that the *CYP17 A2* allele confers a higher risk of breast cancer.

4.1.3.2. Other Candidate Genes: Work is emerging on other candidate genes that may fit into this model. A polymorphism in the *COMT* gene has been investigated in at least three studies (110–112). *COMT* alleles can be designated as high activity (the wild-type allele) or low activity. It has been hypothesized that the low-activity alleles would lead to an increased risk of breast cancer, secondary to the accumulation of catechol estrogens. Published results on the association between *COMT* and breast cancer have been inconsistent. In fact, two of the studies (110,112) reported opposite effects and the third found no association (111) and no evidence of effect modification with other risk factors.

Others have examined the possible role of *CYP1A1*, which is among the major enzymes participating in estrogen hydroxylation, in breast cancer etiology (113–116). Several polymorphisms in *CYP1A1* have been described and two of these polymorphisms have been associated with breast cancer risk in some (113,114,116) but not all (115) studies. The strongest associations for *CYP1A1* and breast cancer are limited to women who smoke.

4.2. Prostate Cancer

The two most important risk factors for prostate cancer are age and ethnicity. Prostate cancer is rare before age 40, but the rate of increase with age is greater than for any other cancer (4). African–American men have the highest incidence in prostate cancer in the world. In the United States, prostate cancer rates among African–Americans are about 50–70% higher compared to whites (117). Unfortunately, adequate data does not exist on prostate cancer rates among blacks in Africa. Lowest rates of prostate cancer are seen among Asian populations (Native Japanese and Chinese men). Japanese- and Chinese-American men have rates higher than men in their respective homelands; however, their rates still remain much lower than U.S. whites (4). Years of epidemiological research has failed to uncover any environmental agents or lifestyle risk factors that can explain these pronounced differences found across different ethnic groups. Like breast cancer, risk of prostate cancer appears to be explained by endogenous hormone levels.

Among participants of the Physician's Health Study, a strong trend of increasing prostate cancer risk was observed with increasing levels of plasma testosterone after simultaneous adjustment for SHBG and other endogenous hormones (118). In the highest quartile of testosterone, risk of prostate cancer was more than 2.5 times the risk in the lowest quartile (*p* for trend = 0.004). Further, the study found an inverse trend with increasing levels of SHBG and with estradiol.

In a comparison of healthy young U.S. white and black men, testosterone levels were 19% higher on average among the African–Americans (119). This study was later extended to include young men from rural Japan (120).

Although the expectation was that these Asian men would have the lowest levels of testosterone, they, in fact, had levels that were intermediate between the black and white U.S. men and did not differ significantly from either group. However, circulating levels of androstanediol glucuronide, a reliable index of 5α reductase activity, were 25–35% lower than in either African-American or U.S. white men. Chinese men have also been shown to have low androstanediol glucuronide levels (121a).

4.2.1. Genetic Models of Prostate Cancer Susceptibility

These studies suggest that differences in prostate cancer risk among ethnic groups are a result of differences in hormone biosynthesis and metabolism. Thus, a multigenic model (similar to the model for breast cancer) has been proposed to explain the occurrence of prostate cancer (4). In developing a model of prostate carcinogenesis, genes involved in androgen biosynthesis, activation, inactivation, and transport are all of interest. Four genes were initially specified: the androgen receptor gene (*AR*), steroid 5α-reductase type II (*SRD5A2*), *CYP17*, and 3β-hydroxysteroid dehydrogenase (*HSD3B2*). AR is responsible for androgen binding and activation, *SRD5A2* encodes the enzyme responsible for converting testosterone to the metabolically more active dihydrotestosterone (DHT), and *CYP17* (as described above) encodes an enzyme that functions at key branch points in human steroidogenesis. *HSD3B2* has a dual role: it encodes an enzyme that catalyzes a critical reaction in testosterone biosynthesis, and it is involved in the metabolism of dihydrotestosterone in the prostate (possibly different isozymes). As with genetic susceptibility to breast cancer, the search for genetic polymorphisms involved in prostate carcinogenesis is an area of great interest. The *AR* and *SRD5A2* genes provide examples of work in this field.

4.2.1.1. Androgen Receptor (AR):   Within exon 1 of *AR*, two polymorphic polyamino acid tracts (trinucleotide repeats) have been studied: a poly-glutamine $(CAG)_n$ and a poly-glycine $(GGC)_n$. Androgen receptor activity has been shown to be negatively correlated with the number of CAG repeats and the association been prostate cancer and this microsatellite polymorphism has been the focus of over 20 epidemiological publications and review articles, but a consistent and reproducible association has yet to be confirmed (Refs. 105–109) and (123b).

Other polymorphic markers at the *AR* locus have also been evaluated (4,123b). A *StuI* single-nucleotide polymorphism at codon 211, which designates two alleles, *S1* and *S2*, is located roughly half-way between the two trinucleotide repeats. Among African–American men the *S1* allele was associated with a statistically significant threefold increased risk of prostate cancer among men under the age of 65. An excess proportion of this allele was also found among prostate cancer cases with an affected brother. The *StuI* polymorphism did not seem to simply reflect short CAG repeats as a function of linkage disequilibrium. These preliminary data suggested that among African-American men, non-CAG repeat variation at the *AR* locus might contribute to hereditary prostate cancer. However, a systematic evaluation and haplotype analysis of generic variation in AR in a multiethnic population failed to show evidence that common genetic variation in AR influences risk of prostate cancer (123b).

4.2.1.2. SRD5A2:   Investigation of the *SRD5A2* gene began with a polymorphic dinucleotide repeat $(TA)_n$ in the 3' untranslated region of the gene. Analysis of this marker suggested that a series of alleles with a relatively high number of repeats (17 or greater) was unique to African-Americans and somewhat more common in African-American men with prostate cancer compared to healthy African-American men (127). Subsequent sequencing of *SRD5A2* in a sample of men with either high or low levels of circulating androstanediol glucoronide (AAG—the biochemical serological correlate of prostatic 5α-reductase activity in vivo) identified numerous sequence variants. Two of these variants, V89L (valine to leucine at codon 89) and A49T (alanine to threonine at codon 49), have been proven to be strong candidates for conferring risk of prostate cancer (128,129). The V89L substitution showed marked differences among ethnic groups. The *VV* genotype is most common in African-Americans, Latinos, and whites, but relatively rare among Chinese and Japanese. Among Asian men, V89L shows a strong correlation with AAG levels. Although the A49T mutation is uncommon in healthy men, it confers a very high risk, especially for advanced prostate cancer. In African-American men, the RR = 7.22 ($p = 0.001$) for advanced disease and in Latino men the OR = 3.60 ($p = 0.04$). These epidemiological findings are supported by in vitro data that show that the A49T mutation has a fivefold higher V_{max} for testosterone conversion than the normal enzyme and the V89L has approximately 33% reduced activity compared to the wild type.

These molecular models that are being developed for prostate and breast cancer illustrate the importance of collaborative efforts between multiple specialties, such as molecular biology and epidemiology, in determining the etiology of cancer. We must begin thinking of these hormonally based cancers as being complex genetic traits and begin to both expand these models and develop similar multigenic models for the other hormone-related cancers. In Table 2, we provide a summary of likely candidate genes for such models.

4.3.   Ovarian Cancer

Like other cancers of hormonal etiology, ovarian cancer is driven by stimulation of cell division. The ovulation hypothesis posits that each cycle of

Table 2 Selected Candidate Genes in Hormone-Related Cancers

Cancer site	Hormones	Potentially important genes
Breast	Estrogen, progesterone	*CYP17, CYP19, HSD17B1, ESR1, PGR*
Prostate	Dihydrotestosterone	*CYP17, HSD17B3, SRD5A2, AR*
Ovary	FSH, progesterone	*FSH, FSHR, PGR*
Endometrium	Estrogen	*CYP17, HSD17B1, HSD17B2, ESR1*
Testis	In utero estrogen	*CYP17, HSD17B1*
Thyroid	TSH, estrogen	*TSH, CYP17, HSD17B1*

ovulation, which includes follicle development and repair of ovarian surface epithelium, increases the risk of ovarian cancer (130). Actions that suppress ovulation, such as pregnancy or the use of oral contraceptives, permanently decrease the risk of ovarian cancer. An important paper appearing in 1983 (131) suggested that ovarian cancer risk resulted from excessive gonadotropin secretion. Under this model, excessive stimulation by gonadotropins (namely FSH or LH) would result in stimulation of the ovarian stroma from estrogen and estrogen precursors. This, in turn, would lead to proliferation (and malignant transformation) of the epithelium.

Progesterone may also play a role in ovarian cancer. Risch (132) suggests that the protective aspect of pregnancy is due not only to the suppression of ovulation, but also to the 8–9 months of elevated progesterone. Further, a previous finding that increased physical activity leads to an increased risk of ovarian cancer may be explained by endogenous progesterone levels. Physical activity may result in a shortened luteal phase and lower luteal progesterone levels in premenopausal women.

A multigenic model, like we have described for breast and prostate cancers, may be emerging to support this hypothesis. Recent evidence suggests that a common variation in the progesterone receptor may be associated with increased risk of ovarian cancer (123b). The development of such a model for ovarian cancer may be able to provide important genetical markers that could improve early detection and survival of ovarian cancer.

4.4. Endometrial Cancer

The established risk factors for endometrial cancer (Table 3) show that exposure to estrogens unopposed to progestins can predict the risk of endometrial cancer (133,135). During the premenopausal period, risk of endometrial cancer can be attributed to mitotic activity during the first half of the menstrual cycle when estrogen in unopposed by progesterone (135).

Table 3 Summary of Established Risk and Protective Factors for
Endometrial Cancer

Risk factors (increased "unopposed" estrogen exposure)
  Late menopause
  Sequential oral contraceptives
  Obesity
  Estrogen replacement therapy
Protective factors (decreased unopposed estrogen exposure)
  Pregnancy
  Combined oral contraceptives

Use of sequential oral contraceptives doubled the risk of endometrial cancer
among women who used them prior to their removal from the market in
1976 (136). In contrast, combination oral contraceptives, which deliver
estrogen and a high-dose progesterone for 21 days of a 28 day cycle,
decrease the risk of endometrial cancer (137–139). As discussed above, an
alarming increase in endometrial cancer occurred in the 1960s and 1970s,
resulting from widespread use of ERT for menopausal symptoms. The
incidence of endometrial cancer once again declined after progestogens were
added to the estrogen in various doses and schedules.

Obesity is also an important risk factor for endometrial cancer. In
postmenopausal women, it is postulated that the conversion of androstenedione to estrone in adipose tissue results in the increased risk. In premenopausal women, obesity is thought to operate through increased anovulatory
cycles and associated progesterone insufficiency (140).

The protective effect of parity can also be explained by the unopposed
estrogen hypothesis (135). The highest risk of endometrial cancer occurs
in nulliparous women and risk decreases with each pregnancy. This is
explained by the fact that no mitotic activity occurs during pregnancy due
to the persistently high progesterone levels.

4.5. Testicular Cancer

Experimental and epidemiological evidence indicates that hormonally
influenced prenatal events are important risk factors for testicular cancer
(141). Excess maternal nausea and vomiting in the prenatal period, prenatal
exposure to diethylstilbestrol, and maternal obesity have been associated
with testes cancer and with cryptorchidism, the most important risk factor
for testes cancer (141–145). It has been hypothesized that in utero exposure
to endogenous and exogenous estrogen could be the common denominator
in these risk factors (141). Consistent with this hypothesis is the observation
that a major determinant of the risk of excessive nausea and vomiting

during pregnancy is an early age at first pregnancy (146). Free estradiol levels are higher in the first pregnancy.

Several lines of evidence suggest that the risk of testicular cancer has strong genetical influence. Normal descent of the testes is under hormonal control (147). Interestingly, surgical correction of cryptorchidism does not appear to reduce this risk (148). Further, the contralateral testicle which is normally decended is also at increased risk for the development of cancer, although the risk is not as high as for the cryptorchid testis (149,150). Individuals with an affected first-degree relative are themselves at increased risk, with some studies suggesting the relative risk to be between 2 and 12 (151–154). The risk appears to be higher in brothers of cases than in fathers of cases. Westergaard et al. (154) found a twofold increased risk in fathers of cases and a 12.3 (95% CI: 3.3–31.5) times increased risk for brothers of cases. Swerdlow et al. (155) also reports increased risk for the twin of a testicular cancer case. Twins of cases were 37.5 times more likely to have testicular cancer than twins of noncases (OR = 37.5, 95% CI: 12.3–115.6). Finally, a recent segregation analysis suggested that testis cancer follows a recessive major gene model of inheritance (156). Although these data suggest a role for genetic factors in the etiology of testis cancer, they also are compatible with the hypothesis that the in utero hormonal environment is responsible for increased cancer risk.

Several candidate genes have been studied with regard to risk of testicular cancer. The Wilms' tumor 1 suppressor gene (*WT1*) was evaluated because of the belief that this gene plays a role in urogenital fetal development (157). Although the researchers found no overall association between *WT1* and testicular cancer, one allele was more frequently found in patients with either bilateral or metastatic disease. The *ESR* gene and several *GST* genes have also been studied with little success (158,159). Based on the existing epidemiological data, genes involved in determining the in utero hormonal environment, including *CYP17* and *HSD17B1*, may be more promising candidates to study.

4.6. Thyroid Cancer

The principal hormone regulating the growth and function of the thyroid gland is the pituitary hormone thyroid-stimulating hormone (TSH). Excess TSH may be of etiological relevance in the development of thyroid cancer (160). This is supported by the fact that the growth of some thyroid cancers is TSH secretion dependent, so that suppression of TSH by administration of thyroxin is frequently an effective treatment for thyroid carcinomas (161). Experimental studies show that sustained elevation of TSH levels induces thyroid tumors in rodents (162,163), which has been achieved by a number of mechanisms including iodine-deficient diets, blocking thyroid hormone synthesis, direct administration of TSH, and chemical goitrogens (164).

A notable trend in thyroid cancer incidence is the dramatic increase in rates over the past three decades. Although the incidence of thyroid cancer in men appears to have stabilized by the early 1990s, the incidence in women has continued to increase, averaging 1.8% per year from 1991 to 1995. In general, incidence rates for women increase sharply from childhood to age 30 and then plateau; whereas in men, incidence rates increase gradually between the ages of 20 and 35, during which women have four to five times the risk of men. This ratio remains above 3 until menopause, when it begins to level off around 1.5. The differential change in rates by gender and the high rate of thyroid cancer in women overall compared to men (165), suggest a probable role of hormones in thyroid cancer etiology.

A number of epidemiological studies have shown a strong association between select reproductive factors and thyroid cancer risk. A history of pregnancy has been associated with elevated risk of thyroid cancer in several case–control studies and risk was especially elevated among women with pregnancies terminated by spontaneous or induced abortions (166–170). Diffuse enlargement of the thyroid gland occurs during pregnancy, as a compensatory response to the increased requirement for thyroid hormone production (171). This alteration in normal thyroid activity occurs primarily during the first trimester and seems to plateau by 20 weeks of gestation, suggesting that changes in thyroid cells may occur early in pregnancy (172). It is possible that some of these cellular changes during the first few weeks of a pregnancy may alter thyroid cancer risk and that these changes may be mitigated by full-term pregnancy, but persist following early termination of a pregnancy.

The normal level of thyroid binding globulin (TBG) in females is 10–20% higher than in males. During pregnancy, there is a 50% increase in the level of TBG due to increasing estrogen concentrations (173), which produces an increase in TSH of similar magnitude (174–176). It is likely that TSH levels of nonpregnant, normal females also may vary and be elevated above the level of males at some point during the menstrual cycle.

5. CONCLUSIONS

Our knowledge of the relationship between relevant circulating hormones and cancer is now contributing to the prevention and treatment of the disease. Hormonal chemoprevention trials for breast and prostate cancers are currently under way and hormonal chemoprevention of ovarian and endometrial cancers has been in process for years with the prescription of oral contraceptives and in the case of endometrial cancer, CHRT. Further work is needed to determine the individual risk and benefits from use of these products. The development of multigene models for hormone related cancers should help to better define individual susceptibility and determine who would benefit from specific prevention and treatment programs.

REFERENCES

1. Wingo PA, Tong T, Bolden S. Cancer statistics. CA Cancer J Clin 1995; 45(1):8–30.
2. Bittner JJ. The causes and control of mammary cancer in mice. Harvey Lect 1947; 42:221–246.
3. HS, Ross RK, Yu MC, Coetzee GA, Reichardt JKV, Henderson BE. Genetic susceptibility to cancer from exogenous and endogenous exposures. J Cell Biochem 1996; 25S:15–22.
4. Ross RK, Pike MC, Coetzee GA, Reichardt JKV, Yu MC, Feigelson H, Stanczyk FZ, Kolonel LN, Henderson BE. Androgen metabolism and prostate cancer: establishing a model of genetic susceptibility. Cancer Res 1998; 58:4497–4504.
5. Sager R. Tumor-suppressor genes: the puzzle and the promise. Science 1989; 246:1406.
6. Stanbridge E. Identifying tumor-suppressor genes in human colorectal cancer. Science 1990; 247:12.
7. Knudson A. Mutation and cancer: statistical study of retinoblastoma. Proc Natl Acad Sci USA 1971; 68:820.
8. Miki Y, Swensen J, Shattuck-Eidens D, Futreal PA, Harshman K, Tavtigian S, Liu Q, Cochran C, Benett LM, Ding W, et al., A strong candidate for the breast and ovarian cancer susceptibility gene BRCA1. Science 1994; 266(5182): 66–71.
9. Wooster R, Bignell G, Lancaster J, Swift S, Seal S, Mangion J, Collins N, Gregory S, Gumbs C, Micklem G. Identification of the breast cancer susceptibility gene BRCA2. Nature 1995; 378:789–792.
10. Li FP. Familial aggregation. In: Schottenfeld D, Fraumeni JF, eds. Cancer Epidemiology and Prevention. 2nd ed. New York: Oxford Univeristy Press, 1996:546–558.
11. Pietras RJ, Pegram MD. Oncogene activation and breast cancer progression. In: Manni A, ed. Endocrinology of Breast Cancer. Totowa, NJ: Humana Press, 1999:133–154.
12. Simpson ER. Estrogens. In: Adashi EY, Rock JA, Rosenwaks Z, eds. Reproductive Endocrinology, Surgery, and Technology. Philadelphia: Lippincott-Raven Publishers, 1996:477–492.
13. Mahley RW, Weisgraber KH, Farese JV Jr. Disorders of lipid metabolism. In: Wilson JD, Foster DW, Kronenberg HM, Larsen PR, eds. Williams Textbook of Endocrinology. 9th ed. Philadephia: WB Saunders Company, 1998:1099–1153.
14. Lambeth JD, Xu XX, Glover M. Cholesterol sulfate inhibits adrenal mitochondrial cholesterol side chain cleavage at a site distinct from cytochrome P-450scc. Evidence for an intramitochondrial cholesterol translocator. J Biol Chem 1987; 262:9181–9188.
15. Jefcoate CR, DiBartolomeis MJ, Williams CA, McNamara BC. ACTH regulation of cholesterol movement in isolated adrenal cells. J Steroid Biochem 1987; 27:721–729.

16. Maclusky NJ. Sex steroid receptors. In: Adashi EY, Rock JA, Rosenwaks Z, eds. Reproductive Endocrinology, Surgery, and Technology. Philadelphia: Lippincott-Raven Publishers, 1996:627–664.

17. Feigelson HS, Henderson BE. Estrogens and breast cancer. Carcinogenesis 1996; 17:2279–2284.

18. Collaborative Group on Hormonal Factors in Breast Cancer. Breast cancer and hormonal contraceptives: collaborative reanalysis of individual data on 53,297 women with breast cancer and 100,239 women without breast cancer from 54 epidemiological studies. Lancet 1996; 347:1713–1727.

19. Bernstein L, Ross R, Henderson B. Cancer prevention: hormones. In: DeVita VT Jr, Rosenburg SA, eds. Cancer: Principles and practice of oncology, 5th ed. Philadelphia: Lippincott-Raven, 1997:609–617.

20. Collaborative Group on Hormonal Factors in Breast Cancer. Breast cancer and hormone replacement therapy: collaborative reanalysis of data from 51 epidemiological studies of 52,705 women with breast cancer and 108,411 women without breast cancer. Lancet 1997; 350:1047–1059.

21. Ross RK, Paganini-Hill A, Wan PC, Pike MC. Effect of hormone replacement therapy on breast cancer risk: estrogen versus estrogen plus progestin. J Nat Cancer Inst 2000; 92:328–332.

22. Schairer C, Lubin J, Troisi R, Sturgeon S, Brinton L, Hoover R. Menopausal estrogen and estrogen-progestin replacement therapy and breast cancer risk. JAMA 2000; 283:485–491.

23. Writing Group for the Women's Health Initiative Investigators. Risk and benefits of estrogen plus progestin in healthy postmenopausal women. J Am Med Assoc 2002; 288:321–333.

24. Enserink M. Despite safety concerns, U.K. hormone study to proceed. Science 2002; 297:492.

25. Rodriguez C, Patel E, Calle E, Jacobs E, Thun M. Estrogen replacement therapy and ovarian cancer mortality in a large prospective study of US women. JAMA 2001; 285(11):1460–1465.

26. Ries L, Kosary C, Hankey B, Miller B, Edwards B. SEER Cancer Statistics Review, 1973–1996. Bethesda, MD: National Cancer Institute, 1999.

27. Adlercreutz H, Mousavi Y, Clark J, Hockerstedt K, Hamalainen E, Wahala K, Makela T, Hase T. Dietary phytoestrogens and cancer: in vitro and in vivo studies. J Steroid Biochem Mol Biol 1992; 41(3–8):331–337.

28. Kurzer MS, Xu X. Dietary phytoestrogens. Annu Rev Nutri 1997; 17: 353–381.

29. Fotsis T, Pepper M, Adlercreutz H, Fleischmann G, Hase T, Montesano R, Schweigerer L. Genistein, a dietary-derived inhibitor of in vitro angiogenesis. Proceedings of the National Academy of Sciences of the United States of America 1993; 907(7):2690–2694.

30. Hunter T, Cooper JA. Protein-tyrosine kinases. Annu Rev Biochem 1985; 54:897–930.

31. Kyle E, Neckers L, Takimoto C, Curt G, Bergan R. Genistein-induced apoptosis of prostate cancer cells is preceded by a specific decrease in focal adhesion kinase activity. Mol Pharmacol 1997; 51:193–200.

32. Constantinou A, Huberman E. Genistein as an inducer of tumor cell differentiation: possible mechanisms of action. Proc Soc Exp Biol Med 1995; 208: 109–115.
33. Lee HP, Gourley L, Duffy SW, Esteve J, Lee J, Day NE. Dietary effects on breast-cancer risk in Singapore. Lancet 1991; 337:1197–1200.
34. Hirose K, Tajima K, Hamajima N, Inoue M, Takezaki T, Kuroisha T, Yoshida M, Tokudome S. A large-scale, hospital-based case–control study of risk factors of breast cancers according to menopausal status. Jpn J Cancer Res 1995; 86:146–154.
35. Wu AH, Ziegler RG, Horn-Ross PL, Nomura AMY, West DW, Kolonel LN, Rosenthal JF, Hoover RN, Pike MC. Tofu and risk of breast cancer in Asian–Americans. Cancer Epidemiol Biomarkers Prev 1996; 5:901–906.
36. Yuan JM, Wang QS, Ros RK, Henderson BE, Yu MC. Diet and breast cancer in Shanghai Tianjin, China. Br J Cancer 1995; 71:1353–1358.
37. Coward L, Barnes NC, Setchell KDR, Barnes S. Genistein, daidzein, and their B-glycoside conjugates: antitumor isoflavones in soybean foods from American and Asian diets. J Agric Food Chem 1993; 41:1961–1967.
38. Murphy PA. Phytoestrogen content of processed soybean products. Food Technol 1982; 36:62–64.
39. Wang HJ, Murphy PA. Isoflavone content in commercial soybean foods. J Agric Food Chem 1994; 42:1666–1673.
40. Ingram D, Sanders K, Kolybaba M, Lopez D. Case–control study of phyto-oestrogens and breast cancer. Lancet 1997; 350(9083):990–994.
41. Zheng W, Dai Q, Custer LJ, Shu XO, Wen WQ, Jin F, Franke AA. Urinary excretion of isoflavonoids and the risk of breast cancer. Cancer Epidemiol Biomarkers Prev 1999; 8(1):35–40.
42. De Stefani E, Correa P, Ronco A, Mendilaharsu M, Guidobono M, Denco-Pellegrini H. Dietary fiber and risk of breast cancer: a case–control study in Uruguay. Nutr Cancer 1997; 28:14–19.
43. Cassidy A, Bingham S, Setchell KDR. Biological effects of a diet of soy protein rich in isoflavones on the menstrual cycle of premenopausal women. Am J Clin Nutr 1994; 60:333–340.
44. Lu LJW, Anderson KE, Grady JJ, Nagamani M. Effects of soya consumption for one month on steroid hormones in premenopausal women: implications for breast cancer risk reduction. Cancer Epidemiol Biomarkers Prev 1996; 5:63–70.
45. Baird DD, Umbach DM, Lansdell L, Hughes CL, Setchell KDR, Weinberg CR, Haney AF, Wilcox AJ, McLachlan JA. Dietary intervention study to assess estrogenicity of dietary soy among postmenopausal women. J Clin Endocrinol Metab 1995; 80:1685–1690.
46. Petrakis NL, Barnes S, King EB, Lowenstein J, Wiencke J, Lee MM, Miike R, Kirk M, Coward L. Stimulatory influence of soy protein isolate on breast secretion in pre- and postmenopausal women. Cancer Epidemiol Biomarkers Prev 1996; 5:785–794.
47. McMichael-Phillips DE, Harding C, Morton M, Potten CS, Bundred NJ. Effects of soy-protein supplementation on epithelial proliferation in the histo-

logically normal human breast. Am J Clin Nutr 1998; 68(suppl 6): 1431S–1435S.

48. Makela S, Davis VL, Tally WC, Korkman J, Salo L. Dietary estrogens act through estrogen receptor-mediated processes and show no antiestrogenicity in cultured breast cancer cells. Environmental Health Perspectives 1994(102):572–578.

49. Martin PM, Horwitz KB, Ryan DS, McGuire WL. Phytoestrogen interaction with estrogen receptors in human breast cancer cells. Endocrinology 1978; 103:1860–1867.

50. Welshons WV, Rottinghaus GE, Nonneman DJ, Dolan-Timpe M, Ross PF. A sensitive bioassay for detection of dietary estrogens in animal feeds. J Vet Diagn Invest 1990; 2:268–273.

51. Wang C, Kurzer MS. Phytoestrogen concentration determines effects on DNA synthesis in human breast cancer cells. Nutr Cancer 1997; 28(3):236–247.

52. Peterson G, Barnes S. Genistein inhibition of the growth of human breast cancer cells: independence from estrogen receptors and the multi-drug resistance gene. Biochem Biophys Res Commun 1991; 179:661–667.

53. Constantinou AI, Mehta RG, Vaughan A. Inhibition of N-methyl-N-nitrosourea-induced mammary tumors in rats by the soybean isoflavones. Anticancer Res 1996; 16:3293–3298.

54. Lamartiniere CA, Moore JB, Brown NM, Thompson R, Hardin MJ, Barnes S. Genistein suppresses mammary cancer in rats. Carcinogenesis 1995; 16:2833–2840.

55. Murrill WB, Brown NM, Zhang JX, Manxolillo PA, Barnes S, Lamartiniere CA. Prepubertal genistein exposure suppresses mammary cancer and enhances gland diferentiation in rats. Carcinogenesis 1996; 7:1451–1457.

56. Ito A, Goto T, Okamoto T, Yamada K, Roy G. A combined effect of tamoxifen (Tam) and miso for the development of mammary tumors induced with MNU in SD rats. Proc Am Assoc Cancer Res 1996; 37:271.

57. Constantinou A, Thomas C, Mehta RG, Runyan C, Moon R. The effect of genistein and daidzein on MNU-induced mammary tumors in rats. Proc Am Assoc Cancer Res 1995; 36:109–115.

58. Fournier DB, Erdman JW Jr, Gordon GB. Soy, its components, and cancer prevention: a review of the in vitro, animal, and human data. Cancer Epidemiol Biomarkers Prev 1998; 7:1055–1065.

59. Barnes S, Grubbs C, Setchell KD, Carlson J. Soybeans inhibit mammary tumors in models of breast cancer. Clin Biol Res 1990; 347:329–353.

60. White R, Jobling SA, Hoare JP, Sumpter M, Parker G. Environmentally persistent alkylphenolic compounds are estrogenic. Endocrinology 1994; 135(1):175–182.

61. Jobling S, Sumpter JP. Detergent components in sewage effluent are weakly oestrogenic to fish: an in vitro study using rainbow trout (*Oncorhynchus mykiss*) hepatocytes. Aquat Toxicol 1993; 27:361.

62. Jobling S, Reynolds T, White R, Parker MG, Sumpter JP. A variety of environmentally persistent chemicals, including some phthalate plasticizers are weakly estrogenic. Environ Health Perspect 1995; 103(6):582–587.

63. Guillette LJ Jr, Gross TS, Masson GR, Matter JM, Percival HF, Woodward AR. Developmental abnormalities of the gonad and abnormal sex hormone concentrations in juvenile alligators from contaminated and control lakes in Florida. Environ Health Perspect 1994; 102(8):680–688.
64. Guillette LJ Jr, Gross TS, Gross DA, Rooney AA, Percival HF. Gonadal steroidogenesis in vitro from juvenile alligators obtained from contaminated or control lakes. Environ Health Perspect 1992; 47(2):143–146.
65. Falck F Jr, Ricci A Jr, Wolff MS, Godbold J, Deckers P. Pesticides and polychlorinated biphenyl residues in human breast lipids and their relation to breast cancer. Arch Environ Health 1992; 47(2):143–146.
66. Wolff MS, Toniolo PG, Lee EW, Rivera M, Dubin N. Blood levels of organochlorine residues and risk of breast cancer. J Natl Cancer Inst 1993; 85(8): 648–652.
67. Carlsen E, Giwercman A, Keiding N, Skakkebaek NE. Evidence of decreasing quality of semen during past 50 years. Br Med J 1992; 305(6854):609–613.
68. Auger J, Kunstmann JM, Czyglik F, Jouannet P. Decline in semen quality among fertile men in Paris during the past 20 years. N Engl J Med 1995; 332:281–285.
69. Arnold SF, Klotz DM, Collins BM, Vonier PM, Guillette LJ Jr, McLachlan JA. Synergistic activation of estrogen receptor with combinations of environmental chemicals. Science 1996; 272:1489–1492.
70. Ashby J, Lefevre PA, Odum J, Harris CA, Routledge EJ, Sumpter JP. Synergy between synthetic oestrogens? Nature 1997; 385:494.
71. Ramamoorthy K, Wang F, Chen IC, Safe S, Norris JD, McDonnell DP, Gaido KW, Bocchinfuso WP, Korach KS. Potency of combined estrogenic pesticides. Science 1997; 275:405.
72. Bergeron JM, Willingham E, Osborn CT III, Rhen T, Crews D. Developmental synergism of steroidal estrogens in sex determination. Environ Health Perspect 1999; 107(2):93–97.
73. Henderson BE, Ross RK, Pike MC, Cassagrande JT. Endogenous hormones as a major factor in human cancer. Cancer Res 1982; 24:3232–3239.
74. Dao TL. The role of ovarian steroid hormones in mammary carcinogenesis. In: Pike MC, Siiteri PK, Welsch CW, eds. Hormones and Breast Cancer. Banbury Report No. 8. Cold Spring Harbor, NY: Cold Spring Harbor Laboratory, 1981:281–295.
75. Friedenreich CM, Bryant HE, Courneya KS. Case–control study of lifetime physical activity and breast cancer risk. Am J Epidemiol 2001; 154:336–347.
76. Bernstein L, Henderson BE, Hanisch R, Sullivan-Halley J, Ross RK. Physical exercise and reduced risk of breast cancer in young women. J Natl Cancer Inst 1994; 86:1403–1408.
77. Thune I, Brenn T, Lunde E, Gaard M. Physical activity and the risk of breast cancer. N Engl J Med 1997; 336:1269–1275.
78. Broocks A, Pirke KM, Schweiger U, Tuschl RJ, Laessle RG, Strowitzki T, Horl E, Horl T, Horl E, Haas W, Jeschke D. Cyclic ovarian function in recreational athletes. J Appl Physiol 1990; 68(5):2083–2086.

79. Bullen BA, Skrinar GS, Beitins IZ, von Mering G, Turnbull BA, McArthur JW. Induction of menstrual disorders by strenuous exercise in untrained women. N Engl J Med 1985; 312:1349–1353.

80. Feicht CB, Johnson TS, Martin BJ, Sparkes KE, Wagner WW Jr. Secondary amenorrhoea in athletes. Lancet 1978; 2:1145–1146.

81. Frisch RE, Wyshak G, Vincent L. Delayed menarche and amenorrhea in ballet dancers. N Engl J Med 1980; 303:17–19.

82. Yu H. Alcohol consumption and breast cancer risk. J Am Med Assoc 1998; 280(13):1138–1139.

83. Smith-Warner S, Spiegelman D, Yaun SS, van den Brandt PA, Folsom AR, Goldbohm RA, Graham S, Holmberg L, Howe GR, Marshall JR, Miller AB, Potter JD, Speizer FE, Willet WC, Wolk A, Hunter DJ. Alcohol and breast cancer in women. A pooled analysis of cohort studies. J Am Med Assoc 1998; 279(7):535–540.

84. MacMahon B, Cole P, Brown JB, Aoki K, Lin TM, Morgan RW, Woo NC. Urine oestrogen profiles of Asian and North American women. Int J Cancer 1974; 14(2):161–167.

85. Bernstein L, Yuan JM, Ross RK, Pike MC, Hanisch R, Lobo R, Stanczyk F, Gao YT, Henderson BE. Serum hormone levels in pre-menopausal Chinese women in Shanghai and white women in Los Angeles: results form two breast cancer case–control studies. Cancer Causes Control 1990; 1(1):51–58.

86. Shimizu H, Ross RK, Bernstein L, Pike MC, Henderson BE. Serum oestrogen levels in postmenopausal women: comparison of American whites and Japanese in Japan. Br J Cancer 1990; 62:451–453.

87. The Endogenous Hormones and Breast Cancer Collaborative Group. Endogenous sex hormones and breast cancer in postmenopausal women: reanalysis of nine prospective studies. J Nat Cancer Inst 2002; 94:606–616.

88. Pike MC, Spicer DV, Dahmoush L, Press MF. Estrogens, progestogens, normal breast cell proliferation, and breast cancer risk. Epidemiol Rev 1993; 15:17–35.

89. Cline JM, Soderqvist G, von Schoultz E, Skoog L, von Schoultz B. Effects of hormone replacement therapy on the mammary gland of surgically postmenopausal macaques. Am J Obstet Gynecol 1996; 174:93–100.

90. Feigelson H, McKean-Cowdin R, Coetzee G, Stram D, Kolonel L, Henderson B. Building a multigenic model of breast cancer susceptibility: CYP17 and HSD17B1 are two important candidates. Cancer Res 2001; 61:785–789.

91. Huang CS , Chern HD, Chang K-J, Cheng C-W, Hsu S-M, Shen C-Y. Breast cancer risk associated with genotype polymorphisms of the estrogen-metabolizing genes CYP17, CYP1A1, and COMT: a multigenic study on cancer susceptibility. Cancer Res 1999; 59:4870–4875.

92a. Thompson P, Ambrosone C. Molecular epidemiology of genetic polymorphisms in estrogen metabolizing enzymes in human breast cancer. J Natl Cancer Inst Monogr 2000; 27:125–134.

92b. Wu A, Seow A, Arakawa K, Berg DVD, Lee H-P, MC Y. HSD17B1 and CYP17 polymorphisms and breast cancer risk among Chinese women in Singapore, Int J Cancer. 104: 450-457, 2003.

93. Brentano ST, Picado-Leonard J, Mellon SH, Moore CCD, Miller WL. Tissue-specific cyclic adenosine 3′,5′-monophosphate-induced, and phorbol ester-repressed transcription from the human P450c17 promoter in mouse cells. Mol Endocrinol 1990; 4:1972–1979.

94a. Carey AH, Waterworth D, Patel K, White D, Little J, Novelli P, Franks S, Williamson R. Polycystic ovaries and premature male pattern baldness are associated with one allele of the steroid metabolism gene CYP17. Hum Mol Genet 1994; 3:1873–1876.

94b. Hirschhorn J, Lohmueller K, Byrne E, Hirschhorn K. A comprehensive review of genetic association studies. Genet Med. 2: 45–61, 2002.

94c. Lohmueller K, Pearce C, Pike M, Lander E, and Hirschhorn J. Meta-analysis of genetic association studies supports a contribution of common variants to susceptibility to common disease. Nature Genetics. 33: 177–182, 2003.

94d. Dunning AM, Healey CS, Pharoah PDP, Teare MD, Ponder BAJ, and Easton DF. A systematic review of genetic polymorphisms and breast cancer risk, Cancer Epidemiol, Biomarkers, Prev. 8: 843-854, 1999.

95. Feigelson HS, Coetzee GA, Kolonel LN, Ross RK, Henderson BE. A polymorphism in the CYP17 gene increases the risk of breast cancer. Cancer Res 1997; 57:1063–1065.

96. Feigelson HS, Shames LS, Pike MC, Coetzee GA, Stanczyk FZ, Henderson BE. CYP17 polymorphism is associated with serum estrogen and progesterone concentrations. Cancer Res 1998; 58:585–587.

97. Haiman CA, Hankinson SE, Spiegelman D, Colditz GA, Willett WC, Speizer FE, Kelsey KT, Hunter DJ. The relationship between a polymorphism in CYP17 with plasma hormone levels and breast cancer. Cancer Res 1999; 59: 1015–1020.

98. Dunning AM, Healey CS, Pharoah PDP, Foster NA, Lipscombe JM, Redman KL, Easton DF, Day NE, Ponder BAJ. No association between a polymorphism in the steroid metabolism gene CYP17 and risk of breast cancer. Br J Cancer 1998; 77(11):2045–2047.

99. Chern HD, Huang CS, Shen CY, Cheng CW, Yang SY, Chang KJ. Association of CYP17 with the susceptibility of breast cancer in Taiwan. Proceedings of the Eighty-Ninth Annual Meeting of the American Association for Cancer Research in Cooperation With the Center for Continuing Education at Tulane University Medical Center Vol. 39. 1998:393.

100. Weston A, Pan C, Bleiweiss IJ, Ksieski HB, Roy N, Maloney N, Wolff MS. CYP17 genotype and breast cancer risk. Cancer Epidemiol Biomarkers Prev 1998; 7:941–944.

101. Helzlsouer KJ, Huang HY, Strickland PT, Hoffman S, Alberg AJ, Comstock GW, Bell DA. Association between CYP17 polymorphism and the development of breast cancer. Cancer Epidemiol Biomarkers Prev 1998; 7:945–949.

102. Bergman-Jungestrom M, Gentile M, Lundin A-C, Group S-EBC, Wingren S. Association between CYP17 gene polymorphism and risk of breast cancer in young women. Int J Cancer 1999; 84:350–353.

103. Kristensen VN, Haraldsen EK, Anderson KB, Lonning PE, Erikstein B, Karesen R, Gabrielsen OS, Borresen-Dale A-L. CYP17 and breast cancer risk:

the polymorphism in the 5′ flanking area of the gene does not influence binding to Sp-1. Cancer Res 1999; 59:2825–2828.

104. Miyoshi Y, Iwao K, Ikeda N, Egawa C, Noguchi S. Genetic polymorphism in CYP17 and breast cancer risk in Japanese women. Eur J Cancer 2000; 36(18):2375–2379.

105. Spurdle A, Hopper J, Dite G, Chen X, Cui J, McCredie M, Giles G, Southey M, Venter D, Easton D, Chenevix-Trench G. CYP17 promoter polymorphism and breast cancer in Australian women under age forty years. J Natl Cancer Inst 2000; 92 2000; 92:1674–1681.

106. Mitrunen K, Jourenkova N, Kataja V, Eskelinen M, Kosma VM, Benhamou S, Vainio H, Uusitupa M, Hirvonen A. Steroid metabolism gene CYP17 polymorphism and the development of breast cancer. Cancer Epidemiol Biomarkers Prev 2000; 9(12):1343–1348.

107. Jernstrom H, Vesprini D, Bradlow H, Narod S. Re: CYP17 promoter polymorphism and breast cancer in Australian women under age forty years. J Natl Cancer Inst 2001; 93(7):554–555.

108. Meilahn E, DeStavola B, Allen D, Fentiman I, Bradlow H, Sepkovic D, Kuller L. Do urinary oestrogen metabolites predict breast cancer? Guernsey III cohort follow-up. Br J Cancer 1998; 78:1250–1255.

109. Muti P, Bradlow H, Micheli A, Krogh V, Freudenheim J, Schunemann H, Stanulla M, Yang J, Sepkovic D, Trevisan M, Berrino F. Estrogen metabolism and risk of breast cancer: a prospective study of the 2:16alpha-hydroxyestrone ratio in premenopausal and postmenopausal women. Epidemiology 2000; 11:635–640.

110. Lavigne JA, Helzlsouer KJ, Huang HY, Strickland PT, Bell DA, Selmin O, Watson S, Hoffman S, Comstock GW, Yager JD. An association between the allele coding for a low activity variant of catechol-O-methyltransferase and the risk for breast cancer. Cancer Res 1997; 57(24):5493–5497.

111. Millikan RC, Pittman GS, Tse CK, Duell E, Newman B, Savitz PG Boissy RJ, Bell DA. Catechol-O-methyltransferase and breast cancer risk. Carcinogenesis 1947; 19(11):1943–1947.

112. Thompson PA, Shields PG, Freudenheim JL, et al. Genetic polymorphisms in catechol-O-methyltransferase, menopausal status, and breast cancer risk. Cancer Res 1998; 58: 2107–2110.

113. Ambrosone CB, Freudenheim JL, Graham S, et al. Cytochrome P4501A1 and glutathione S-transferase (M1) genetic polymorphisms and postmenopausal breast cancer risk. Cancer Res 1995; 55:3483–3485.

114. Taioli E, Trachman J, Chen X, Toniolo P, Garte SJ. A CYP1A1 restriction fragment length polymorphism is associated with breast cancer in African-American women. Cancer Res 1995; 55:3757–3758.

115. Bailey LR, Roodi N, Verrier CS, Yee CJ, Dupont WD, Parl FF. Breast cancer and CYPIA1, GSTM1, and GSTT1 polymorphisms: evidence of a lack of association in Caucasians and African Americans. Cancer Res 1998; 58(1):65–70.

116. Ishibe N, Hankinson SE, Colditz GA, Spiegelman D, Willett WC, Speizer FE, Kelsey KT, Hunter DJ. Cigarette smoking, cytochrome P450 1A1 polymorphisms, and breast cancer risk in the Nurses' Health Study. Cancer Res 1998; 58(4):667–671.

117. Ross RK, Schottenfeld D. Prostate cancer. In: Shottenfeld D, Fraumeni JF, eds. Cancer Epidemiology and Prevention. New York: Oxford University Press, 1996:1180–1206.

118. Gann PH, Hennekens CH, Ma J, Longcope C, Stampfer MJ. Prospective study of sex hormone levels and risk of prostate cancer. J Natl Cancer Inst 1996; 88:1118–1126.

119. Ross RK, Bernstein L, Judd H, Hanisch R, Pike M, Henderson B. Serum testosterone levels in healthy young black and white men. J Natl Cancer Inst 1986; 76(1):45–48.

120. Ross RK, Bernstein L, Lobo RA, Shimizu H, Stanczyk FZ, Pike MC, Henderson BE. 5-Alpha-reductase activity and risk of prostate cancer among Japanese and U.S. white and black males. Lancet 1992; 339:887–889.

121. Lookingbill DP, Demers LM, Wang C, Leung A, Rittmaster RS, Santen RJ. Clinical and biochemical parameters of androgen action in normal healthy Caucasian versus Chinese subjects. J Clin Endocrinol Metab 1991; 72: 1242–1248.

122. Ingles SA, Ross RK, Yu MC, Irvine RA, LaPera G, Haile RW, Coetzee GA. Association of prostate cancer risk with genetic polymorphism in vitamin D receptor and androgen receptor. J Natl Cancer Inst 1997; 89:166–170.

123a. Stanford JL, Just JJ, Gibbs M, Wicklund KG, Neal CL, Blumenstein BA, Ostrander EA. Polymorphic repeats in the androgen receptor gene: molecular markers of prostate cancer risk. Cancer Res 1997; 57:1194–1198.

123b. Freedman M, Pearce C, Pennet K, Hirschhorn J, Kolonel L, Henderson B, and Altshuler, D. Systematic evaluation of genetic variation at the androgen receptor locus and risk of prostate cancer in a multicenter cohort study, Am J Hum Genet. 76:82–90, 2005.

124. Giovannucci E, Stampfer MJ, Krithivas K, Brown M, Brufsky A, Talcott J, Hennekens CH, Kantoff PW. The CAG repeat within the androgen receptor gene and its relationship to prostate cancer. Proc Natl Acad Sci USA 1997; 94:3320–3323.

125. Hardy DO, Scher HI, Bogenreider T, Sabbatini P, Zhang ZF, Nanus DM, Catterall JF. Androgen receptor CAG repeat lengths in prostate cancer: correlation with age of onset. J Clin Endocrinol Metab 1996; 81:4400–4405.

126. Hakimi JM, Schoenberg MP, Rodinelli RH, Piantadosi S, Barrack ER. Androgen receptor variants with short glutamine or glycine repeats identify unique subpopulations of men with prostate cancer. Clin Cancer Res 1993; 3:1599–1608.

127. Ross RK, Coetzee GA, Reichardt J, Skinner E, Henderson BE. Does the racial-ethnic variation in prostate cancer risk have a harmonal basis? Cancer (Philadelphia) 1995; 75:1778–1782.

128. Makridakis N, Ross RK, Mike MC, Chang L, Stanczyk FZ, Kolonel LN, Shi C-Y, Yu MC, Henderson BE, Reichardt JKV. A prevalent missense substitution that modulates activity of prostatic steroid 5-reductase. Cancer Res 1997; 57:1020–1022.

129. Makridakis N, Ross RK, Pike MC, Crocitto LE, Kolonel LN, Pearce CL, Henderson BE, Reichardt JKV. A missense substitution in the SRD5A2 gene

is associated with prostate cancer in African-American and Latino men in Los Angeles. Lancet 1999; 354:975–978.

130. Henderson BE, Bernstein L, Ross RK. Hormones and the etiology of cancer. In: Holland JF, et al., eds. Cancer and Medicine. 3rd ed. Philadelphia: Lea & Febiger, 1993:223–232.

131. Cramer DW, Welch WR. Determinants of ovarian cancer risk. II. Inferences regarding pathogenesis. J Natl Cancer Inst 1983; 71:717–721.

132. Risch HA. Hormonal etiology of epithelial ovarian cancer, with a hypothesis concerning the role of androgens and progesterone. J Natl Cancer Inst 1998; 23:1774–1786.

133. Henderson BE, Ross RK, Pike MC, Casagrande JT. Endogenous hormones as a major factor in human cancer. Cancer Res 1982; 42:3232.

134. Key TJA, Pike MC. The dose-effect relationship between "unopposed" estrogens and endometrial mitotic rate: its central role in explaining and predicting endometrial cancer risk. Br J Cancer 1988; 57:205.

135. Henderson BE, Bernstein L, Ross R. Etiology of cancer: hormonal factors. In: DeVita VT, Hellman S, Rosenberg SA, eds. Cancer: Principles and Practice of Oncology. 5th ed. Philadephia: Lippincott-Raven, 1997:219–229.

136. Weiss NS, Szekely DR, Austin DF. Increasing incidence of endometrial cancer in the United States. N Engl J Med 1976; 294(23):1259–1262.

137. The Centers for Disease Control Cancer and Steriod Hormone Study. Oral Contraceptive use and the risk of endometrial cancer. J Am Med Assoc 1983; 249:1600–1604.

138. Henderson BE, Casagrande JT, Pike MC, Mack T, Rosario I, Duke A. The epidemiology of endometrial cancer in young women. Br J Cancer 1983; 47(6):749–756.

139. Weiss NS, Sayvetz TA. Incidence of endometrial cancer in relation to the use of oral contraceptives. N Engl J Med 1980; 302(10):551–554.

140. Potischman N, Hoover RN, Brinton LA, Siiteri P, Dorgan JF, Swanson CA, Berman ML, Mortel R, Twiggs LB, Barrett RJ, Wilbanks GD, Persky V, Lurain JR. Case-control study of endogenous hormones and endometrial cancer. J Natl Cancer Inst 1996; 88(16):1127–1135.

141. Depue RH, Pike MC, Henderson BE. Estrogen exposure during gestation and risk of testicular cancer. J Natl Cancer Inst 1983; 71:1151–1155.

142. Henderson BE, Benton B, Jing J, Yu MC, Bernstein L. Risk factors for cancer of testis in young men. Int J Cancer 1997; 23:598–602.

143. Petridou E, Roukas KI, Dessypris N, Aravantinos G, Bafaloukos D, Efraimidis A, Papacharalambous A, Pektasidis D, Rigatos G, Trichopoulos D. Baldness and other correlates of sex hormones in relation to testicular cancer. Int J Cancer 1997; 71(6):982–985.

144. Leary FJ, Ressenguie LJ, Kurland LT, Brien PC, Emslander RF, Noller KL. Males exposed to utero to diethlystilbestrol. J Am Med Assoc 1984; 252:2984–2989.

145. Depue RH, Bernstein L, Ross RK, Judd HL, Henderson BE. Hyperemesis gravidarum in relation to estradiol levels, pregnancy outcome, and other maternal factors: a seroepidemiologic study. Am J Obstet Gynecol 1987; 156:1137–1141.

146. Henderson BE, Ross RK, Yu MC, Bernstein L. An explanation for the increasing incidence of testis cancer: decreasing age at first full-term pregnancy. J Natl Cancer Inst 1997; 89:818–819.

147. Goodman LS, Gilman A. eds. The Pharmacological Basis of Therapeutics. London: Macmillan, 1970:1528.

148. Prener A, Engholm G, Jensen OM. Genital anomalies and risk for testicular cancer in Danish men. Epidemiology 1996; 7:14–19.

149. Strader CH, Weiss NS, Daling JR. Vasectomy and the incidence of testicular cancer. Am J Epidemiol 1988; 128:56–63.

150. United Kingdom Testicular Cancer Study Group. Aetiology of testicular cancer: association with congenital abnormalities, age at puberty, infertility, and exercise. Br Med J 1994; 308:1393–1399.

151. Tollerud DJ, Blattner WA, Fraser MC, Brown LM, Pottern L, Shapiro E, Kirkemo A, Shawker TH, Javadpour N, O'Connell K, Stutzman RE, Fraumeni JF. Familial testicular cancer and urogenital developmental anomalies. Cancer 1985; 55:1849–1854.

152. Dieckmann KP, Pichlmeier U. The prevalence of familial testicular cancer—an analysis of two patient populations and a review of the literature. Cancer 1997; 80:1954–1960.

153. Forman D, Oliver RTD, Brett AR, Marsh SGE, Moses JH, Bodmer JG, Chilvers CED, Pike MC. Familial testicular cancer: a report of UK family register, estimation of risk and an HLA class 1 sib-pair analysis. Br J Cancer 1992; 65:255–262.

154. Westergaard T, Olsen JH, Frisch M, Kroman N, Nielsen JW, Melbye M. Cancer risk in fathers and brothers of testicular cancer patients in Denmark. A population-based study. Int J Cancer 1996; 66:627–631.

155. Swerdlow AJ, De Stavola BL, Swanwick MA, Maconochie NES. Risks of breast and testicular cancers in young adult twins in England and Wales: evidence on prenatal and genetic aetiology. Lancet 1997; 350(9093):1723–1728.

156. Heimdal K, Olsson H, Tretli S, Fossa SD, Borresen AL, Bishop DT. A segregation analysis of testicular cancer based on Norwegian and Swedish families. Br J Cancer 1997; 75:1084–1087.

157. Heimdal kR, Lothe RA, Fossa SD, Borresen AL. Association studies of a polymorphism in the Wilms' tumor 1 locus in Norwegian patients with testicular cancer. Int J Cancer 1994; 58:523–526.

158. Heimdal K, Andersen TI, Skrede M, Fossa SD, Berg K, Borresen AL. Association studies of estrogen receptor polymorphism in a Norwegian testicular cancer population. Cancer Epidemiol Biomarkers Prev 1995; 4:123–126.

159. Vistisen K, Prieme H, Okkels H, Vallentin S, Loft S, Olsen JH, Poulsen HE. Genotype and phenotype of glutathione S-transferase mu in testicular cancer patients. Pharmacogenetics 1997; 7:21–25.

160. Ingbar SH, Woeber KA. The thyroid gland. In: Williams RH, ed. Textbook of Endocrinology. Philiadelphia: WB Saunders Company, 1974:95.

161. Crile G. Endocrine dependency of papillary carcinomas of the thyroid. J Am Med Assoc 1966; 195:721.

162. Axelrad AA, Leblond CP. Induction of thyroid tumors in rats by a low iodine diet. Cancer 1955; 8:339.

163. Griesback WE, Kennedy TH, Purves HD. Studies on experimental goitre. III. The effect of goitrogenic diet of hypophysectomized rats. Br J Exp Pathol 1941; 22:249.

164. Morris HP. Experimental thyroid tumors. Brookhaven Symp Biol 1954; 7:192.

165. Ron E. Thyroid cancer. In: Schottenfeld D, Fraumeni JF, eds. Cancer Epidemiology and Prevention. 2nd ed. New York: Oxford Univeristy Press, 1996:546–558.

166. McTiernan AM, Weiss NS, Daling JR. Incidence of thyroid cancer in women in relation to reproductive and hormonal factors. Am J Epidemiol 1984; 120:423.

167. Preston-Martin S, Bernstein L, Pike MC, Maldonado AA, Henderson BE. Thyroid cancer among young women related to prior thyroid disease and pregnancy history. Br J Cancer. 1987; 55:191.

168. Ron E, Kleinerman RA, Boice JD, LiVolsi VA, Flannery JT, Fraumeni JF. A population-based case–control study of thyroid cancer. J Natl Cancer Inst 1987; 79:1.

169. Paoff K, Preston-Martin S, Mack WJ, Monroe K. A case–control study of maternal risk factors for thyroid cancer in young women (California, United States). Cancer Causes Control 1995; 6:389–397.

170. Preston-Martin S, Jin F, Duda MJ, Mack WJ. A case–control study of thyroid cancer in women under age 55 in Shanghai (People's Republic of China). Cancer Causes Control 1993; 4:431–440.

171. Rabin D, McKenna TJ. Thyrotoxicosis. In: Dietschy JM, ed. Clinical Endocrinology and Metabolism Principles and Practice. New York: Grune & Stratton, Inc, 1982:265.

172. Mestman JH, Goodwin M, Montoro MM. Thyroid disorders of pregnancy. Endocrinol Metabol Clin North Am 1995; 24(1):41–71.

173. Burrow GN. Thyroid function in relation to age and pregnancy. In: DeVisscher M, ed. The Thyroid Gland. New York: Raven, 1980:215.

174. Gershengorn MC, Glinoer D, Robbins J. Transport and metabolism of thyroid hormones. In: DeVisscher M, ed. The Thyroid Gland. New York: Raven, 1980:81.

175. Malkasian GD, Mayberry WE. Serum total and free thyroxine and thyrotropin in normal and pregnant women, neonates, and women receiving progestogens. Am J Obstet Gynecol 1970; 108:1234.

176. Pacchiarotti A, Martino E, Bartalena L, Buratti L, Mammoli C, Strigini F, Fruzzetti F, Melis GB, Pinchera A. Serum thyrotropin by ultrasensitive immunoradiometric assay and serum free thyroid hormones in pregnancy. J Endocrinol Invest 1986; 9:185.

18

Cancer in Multiracial and Multiethnic Populations

Carrie P. Hunter

North Potomac, Maryland, U.S.A.

1. INTRODUCTION

Cancer, a disease of altered cellular growth, is the second most common cause of death in the United States. It is no respecter of persons and affects individuals of all ages, sexes, socioeconomic strata, and racial and ethnic populations. In 2002, the American Cancer Society estimated that approximately 1,284,900 new cancer cases will be diagnosed and 555,500 deaths will occur in the United States (1). Cancer increases with advancing age. In year 2000, over 60% of all new cancer cases occurred in men and women age 65 years and older. And, within the next three decades the cancer burden will increase as the absolute number of cancers in persons 65 years and older is expected to double (2). A large part of the increasing cancer burden will occur in multiracial and multiethnic subgroups of the United States who in year 2000 comprised nearly 30% of the U.S. population and are projected to increase to 42% by year 2030 (3).

The burden of cancer is not borne equally by all population subgroups in the United States. Marked variations in cancer incidence, mortality, and survival rates exits among multiracial and multiethnic populations, and cancer-related health disparities account for much of the excess morbidity and mortality observed. A complex spectrum of diseases constitutes what is defined as "cancer." Subgroup variations in cancer incidence rates reflect the dynamics of culture on health, the diversity of host experiences, the impact of environmental conditions on health, and the degree of genetic susceptibility of individuals to cancer. Etiologic or causative factors are associated with cancer risk, yet may differ in their biological effect and disease expression within subgroups of the American population. Inherited genetic susceptibility and environmental exposures to carcinogens that predispose an individual to cancer may also be different across these groups.

Scientific knowledge of the cellular and molecular basis of disease is advanced through the examination of diverse relationships and interactions. The study of molecular and genetic markers of cancer risk in multiracial and multiethnic populations provides opportunities to identify individuals at risk, to enhance screening and detection capabilities, to determine markers of cancer prognosis, and to potentially effect treatment outcomes. In this report, disparities in cancer incidence rates among multiracial and multiethnic populations of the United States are presented. Risk factors and biological markers that may be related to breast cancer risk or prognosis, and which may contribute to differential rates of disease expression, are discussed.

2. CANCER INCIDENCE

There is considerable variation in cancer incidence rates across racial and ethnic groups in the United States. The overall cancer incidence rate is higher in Blacks (444.6 per 100,000) and non-Hispanic Whites (402.1 per 100,000), intermediate in Asian/Pacific Islanders (279.3 per 100,000) and Hispanics [272.9 per 100,000], and lowest in American Indians (152.8 per 100,000) (Table 1). Rates for all cancers combined in women are 22–26% lower than in men of the same racial/ethnic group, except for African Americans where the rate in men is 44% higher than in women. African-Americans also are 1.6 times more likely than Hispanics or Asian/Pacific Islanders to develop cancer, and three times more likely to develop cancer than American Indians (Fig. 1) (4)

Between 1973 and 1997, the age-adjusted cancer incidence rate for all sites combined and all races increased 25.0% in men and 19.9% in women (5). During this quarter century, trend data of cancer incidence for all sites combined, both sexes, and all races show that rates increased from 1973 through 1982, accelerated from 1982 through 1992, and declined from 1992 through 1998 (Table 2) (6). Following several decades of rising incidence of prostate and lung cancer in men, the incidence rates leveled or declined between 1992 and 1998 with a decrease of 2.9% per year in white males and 3.1% per year in black males. Among females, the overall cancer incidence rate between 1992 and 1998 increased 0.3% per year compared to rate increases of 1.6% per year from 1980 to 1987. The current lower rate in females is related to a leveling off of the high breast cancer incidence rate

Table 1   Cancer Incidence Rates[a] by Site, Race, and Ethnicity (U.S., 1990–1997)

	White	Black	Asian/PI	Am. Indian	Hispanic[b]
All sites					
Total	402.1	444.6	279.3	152.8	272.9
Males	476.3	597.9	323.5	175.9	323.2
Females	352.4	337.4	246.9	137.3	240.9
Breast (females)	114.0	100.2	74.6	33.4	68.9
Colon and rectum					
Total	43.6	50.7	38.1	16.3	28.8
Males	52.7	58.3	47.2	20.4	35.7
Females	36.6	45.2	30.9	13.1	23.6
Lung and bronchus					
Total	55.4	73.3	35.5	18.4	27.1
Males	71.9	111.1	51.9	25.1	38.0
Females	43.3	45.8	22.5	13.3	19.4
Prostate	145.8	225.0	80.4	45.8	101.6

[a]Rates are per 100,000 and are age-adjusted to the 1970 standard population.
[b]Hispanic is not mutually exclusive from white, black, Asian/Pacific Islander, or American Indian.
Source: Data from Surveillance, Epidemiology, and End Results Program, NCI, 2000. Ref. 4, Table 11, p. 33.

due to more screened–detected cancers during the 1980s, and some stabilization of lung rates in females since 1991(4,6). These changes in rates reflect a number of events: advancements in our understanding of tumor biology and the role of risk factors in cancer development, resulting in better strategies to modulate exposures and reduce risk; improved medical diagnostic capabilities and screening and early detection practices; and the impact of targeted prevention efforts and behavioral change strategies related to more effective public health educational campaigns.

Breast, prostate, lung, and colon and rectum are the most frequent sites of cancer in all American population subgroups and they account for approximately 56% of all new cases. Figures 2 and 3 show racial and ethnic differences in cancer incidence rates for each site (5). Population variations are most pronounced in breast and prostate cancer, two tumors also strongly influenced by the intrinsic hormonal environment. Within population subgroups (for example: Hispanics and Asian/Pacific Islanders), cancer-specific incidence rates may also vary according to ancestral origin of different cultural groups, geographic location, and the phase of epidemiologic transition of a particular population subgroup from its native country of origin to full acculturation in its adopted homeland. Rates also differ widely among indigenous Native American populations (Table 3) (1,4). While incidence

Table 2   Cancer Incidence Trends: Join-Point Analyses for 1973–1998, Selected Cancers by Sex and Race

	Trend 1		Trend 2		Trend 3		Trend 4	
	Range of years	APC	Range of years	APC	Range of years	APC	Range of years	APC
All sites	1973–1982	0.8	1982–1992	1.7	1992–1998	−1.0		
Males	1973–1989	1.4	1982–1992	5.2	1992–1995	−4.3	1995–1998	−0.8
White	1973–1989	1.4	1989–1992	5.2	1992–1995	−4.8	1995–1998	−0.8
Black	1973–1981	2.6	1981–1989	0.8	1989–1993	5.4	1993–1998	−4.2
Females	1973–1980	0.1	1980–1987	1.6	1987–1998	0.3		
White	1973–1980	0.2	1980–1987	1.7	1987–1998	0.3		
Black	1973–1991	1.2	1991–1998	−0.2	1992–1998	−1.0		
Prostate	1973–1988	2.9	1988–1992	17.5	1992–1995	−10.0	1995–1998	0.3
White	1973–1988	3.1	1988–1992	17.4	1992–1995	−11.3	1995–1998	0.4
Black	1973–1989	2.2	1989–1992	12.0	1992–1998	−4.0		
Breast (females)	1973–1980	−0.7	1980–1987	3.8	1987–1998	0.5		
White	1973–1980	−0.6	1980–1987	3.9	1987–1998	0.4		
Black	1973–1979	−0.8	1979–1986	4.0	1986–1998	0.9		
Lung	1973–1981	3.0	1981–1991	0.9	1991–1998	−1.2		
Male	1973–1981	1.9	1981–1991	−0.4	1991–1998	−2.4		
White	1973–1981	1.7	1981–1991	−0.4	1991–1998	−2.5		
Black	1973–1984	3.0	1984–1998	−1.8				
Female	1973–1976	9.1	1976–1983	5.2	1983–1991	3.1	1991–1998	0.2
White	1973–1982	6.5	1982–1991	3.2	1991–1998	0.4		
Black	1973–1990	4.7	1990–1998	−0.7				
Colon-rectum	1973–1985	0.8	1985–1995	−1.8	1995–1998	0.5		

APC, annual percentage change cancer incidence rate, age-adjusted to 1970 U.S. population. Join-point analyses (1973–1998) for selected cancers.
Source: Surveillance, Epidemiology, & End Results Program, NCI. Ref. 6, Table 1, p. 828.

Table 3 Cancer Incidence Rates[a] by Selected Sites in American Indians & Alaska Natives (United States, SEER, 1990–1997)

	American Indian 1990–1997[b]	American Indian & Alaska Native 1992–1998[c]
All Sites		
Total	152.8	202.7
Males	175.9	227.7
Females	137.3	186.3
Breast (females)	33.4	50.4
Colon and Rectum		
Total	16.3	28.6
Males	20.4	33.5
Females	13.1	24.6
Lung and Bronchus		
Total	18.4	31.0
Males	25.1	44.3
Females	13.3	20.6
Prostate	45.8	47.8

[a]Rates are per 100,000 and are age-adjusted to the 1970 standard population.
[b]Ref. 1
[c]Ref. 11

rates for prostate cancer are similar in American Indians and Alaska Natives, the rates for total cancers, breast, colon and rectum, and lung and bronchus cancers are greatly increased when aggregate data are presented for American Indians and Alaska Natives combined. Differential expressions of incidence rates among population subgroups suggest that different levels of etiological factors (for example, environmental exposures, diet, smoking), host experiences (for example, hormonal milieu, reproductive factors), and genetic susceptibility, as well as different rates of disease detection may contribute to variations in incidence rates observed.

There are limitations in the trend statistics for some racial and ethnic subgroups due to the lack of available cancer data for these groups. Difficulties in case ascertainment by race/ethnicity and the misreporting of race or ethnicity on basic records (medical records, census reports) from which information is collected are just a few of the issues that need to be resolved (2). In addition, the cancer incidence rates presented in this paper are taken from published articles and reports of data derived from the National Cancer Institute's Surveillance, Epidemiology, and End Results Program (SEER) and the rates utilized are age-adjusted to the 1970 U.S. standard population. SEER has recently shifted from the 1970 U.S. standard population to the 2000 standard population, which will increase cancer incidence rates and death rates by 20–50% compared to the 1970 standard. This is largely due to an increased representation of the older age group in the 2000 standard calculation (2). While rates age-adjusted to the 2000 standard population are not used in this report, caution must be taken in comparing and interpreting data using these two standard population reference sources.

3. BREAST CANCER

Breast cancer is the most frequent cancer in all subgroups of American women, except for Vietnamese American women who have higher rates of cervical cancer. A comprehensive review of SEER data from 1988 to 1992 shows that rates are highest in non-Hispanic white, Native Hawaiian, and African-American women; intermediate in Hispanic women; and lowest among Filipino American, Korean American, Japanese-American, Chinese American, and American Indian women (Table 4). Differences in cancer rates must be interpreted with some caution because of less precise rates in smaller population groups (7). Also aggregate subgroup rates may not reflect the condition of all populations included in a category. For example, breast cancer incidence rate for Asian/Pacific Islanders is approximately 30% lower than in whites. However, the Native Hawaiians

Table 4   Breast Cancer Incidence Rate by Race and Ethnicity (Females) (SEER[a])

Race/ethnicity	1988–1992[b]	1992–1998[c]	Trend 1992–1998
All races		111.2	1.2
White		115.5	1.1
White Hispanic	73.5	72.9	0.4
White Non-Hispanic	115.7	120.5	1.3
Black	95.4	101.5	0.1
Asian/Pacific Islander		78.1	3.9
Chinese American	55.0		
Filipino American	73.1		
Native Hawaiian	105.6		
Japanese American	82.3		
Korean American	28.5		
Vietnamese American	37.5		
Amer. Indian/Alaska Native		50.5	−0.1
Alaska Native	78.9		
Amer. Indian (N.M.)	31.6		
Hispanic	69.8	68.5	0.3

[a]Rates are age-adjusted per 100,000 to 1970 U.S. population.
[b]Ref. 7.
[c]From Cancer Statistics Review (2001).

have the second highest rate of any subgroup. The significance of this observation is obscured when data are combined into the broader category of Asian/Pacific Islander. Similar disparities in rates are also found among American Indians and Alaska Natives who live in different geographic regions and among the diverse groups within the Hispanic category. Such differences in rates reflect—in large part—the diversities of culture and environmental exposures, dietary habits, and behavioral characteristics of the population subgroups.

3.1. Risk Factors

A number of factors may increase the risk of breast cancer. They include factors that: (1) change the macro-environment by creating or augmenting conditions that contribute to the risk of disease (e.g., migration from low-risk to high-risk areas, acculturation within adopted country) (2) modulate or alter conditions of cellular growth (e.g., exposures to environmental carcinogens, smoking, diet, reproductive experiences and hormone replacement therapy), and (3) are intrinsic to the host (e.g., age, family history of breast cancer, and BRCA1/BRCA2 susceptibility genes). Racial and ethnic differences in risk factor profiles may provide clues to possible genetic and environmental changes in tumor biology.

The "migration effect" on cancer is well established. Descents of women of Japanese origin who migrated to Hawaii or mainland America develop within two to three generations a higher rate of breast cancer than that observed in native Japanese women. A similar pattern has been observed in women who migrated from Italy to Australia, Poland to the United States (8) and from Puerto Rico to Long Island, New York (9). Age at migration affects risks. Asian and Hispanic women who migrated to the United States at an early age had much higher incidence rates than those who migrated in adulthood, suggesting that either some exposure early in life or total years since migration is of etiologic importance (10). Diet and other environmental exposures have been implicated as major causative factors for generational changes in incidence rates. Also different rates of acculturation may explain the continued lower rise in breast cancer rates among descendents of Japanese, Chinese, and Mexican women who migrated to the United States (11).

The level of breast cancer risk attributable to a particular factor may differ in younger and older women (12). Overall, the breast cancer incidence rate in African-American women is lower than in whites. However, for African-American women under age 45 years the rate is higher than in whites, a paradox unexplained by present studies. Reproductive experiences and intrinsic and exogenous hormone exposures are known to influence breast cancer development and a number of epidemiological studies show the magnitude of risk in blacks and whites to be similar (13–15). Pathak et al.

reviewed the literature on the effects and distribution of reproductive and hormonal risk factors in black and white populations. They also examined whether the distribution of reproductive risk factors could explain, in part, this paradoxical phenomena. They postulated that the crossover in incidence rates between the races may be expected based on Pike's "breast tissue age" model, and given the effects and distribution of early age at first full-term pregnancy and high parity (16). In a case–control study of black and white breast cancer patients, Brinton et al. observed that whites (age 40–54) had a higher population-attributable risk (62%) than blacks (54%) that appeared to account for the observed differences in incidence between the groups. A large part of the difference in population attributable risks between older whites and blacks was accounted for by whites having fewer births, later age at first birth, and slightly higher risks associated with reproductive and menstrual factors. Among younger women (ages 20–39) there was little association with the factors studied, but numbers were small. However, the data suggest that the difference in breast cancer incidence rate between younger blacks and whites was not due to established risk factors, but possibly to some other yet unidentified predictors (17).

Selected dietary factors (e.g., fat, specific fatty acids, heterocyclic amines, and alcohol) are hypothesized to increase the risk of breast cancer. Alternatively, a protective role on breast cancer risk of nutrients in fruits and vegetables and of phytoestrogens has been postulated. Multiracial/ ethnic populations have a wide range of food intakes and great diversity in food sources of fat and fiber as well as caloric intake. Newell et al. observed-that the mean caloric intake was highest for whites, followed by Mexican-Americans, and by African-Americans—a group which also had lower mean fiber than whites or Mexican-Americans. Hispanics had higher dietary fiber intake than other groups, and lower breast cancer rates (18).

Well-established differences between racial/ethnic groups in the intake of specific vegetables, fruits, legunes, and soy have been reported. Zang et al. studied dietary habits and observed that Hispanic and African-Americans have a greater consumption of vegetables, citrus fruit, and fish than whites. Hispanics also consume a greater intake of beans. Carotenoid-containing fruits and vegetables were substantially higher in African-Americans than in whites or Hispanics. No significant differences were seen in total fat or fiber intake in this study (19). Wu et al. examined the diets of multiethnic populations using data from the 1992 National Health Interview Survey. In this study, the intake of fiber, carotene, vitamin C, and folate were higher among African-Americans and Latino women compared to whites. Hawaiian-Americans had higher intakes of micronutrients whereas Japanese-American women showed comparable intakes of carotene and vitamin C but lower intakes of fiber and folate. The intake of legunes was twice as high among Latino women compared to white women and the intake of tofu (a main source of isoflavones) was at least four times higher among Japanese-

American women compared to white women (20). Isoflavonoids in soy, genistein, and diadzein have been shown to possess agonist and antagonist estrogenic activity similar to that of tamoxifen. They also mimic estrogens. Soy consumption in the form of tofu was more than twice as high among Asian-American women born in Asia than among Chinese women born in the United States (21). These reports strongly suggest that differences in dietary patterns among racial/ethnic groups may account, in part, for the variations in incidence rates of breast cancers observed in these subgroups. More definitive results are needed. The NIH Women's Health Initiative clinical trial on dietary patterns in postmenopausal women may provide new and important information on breast cancer risk in multiethnic populations, when it is available.

Environmental exposures to pesticides, organochlorines, and other industrial products and carcinogens are postulated to contribute to cancer development. Epidemiological studies have implicated exposure to organochlorines such as, dichlorodiphenyltrichloroethane (DDT) and its metabolite, DDE, as possible risk factors for breast cancer. Dichlorodiphenyltrichloroethane was widely used in the United States for insect control in forestry, agriculture, and building protection between 1940s and 1960s until it was banned in 1972. A large proportion of the U.S. population, including large segments of African-American, Hispanic subgroups, were exposed as workers in the farming industry. Only a few studies of environmental exposures and breast cancer risk in multiethnic populations have been done and they are inconclusive. Krieger et al. found ethnic differences in both the prevalence of organochlorines and the associated breast cancer risk. However, the differences in levels among whites, African-American, and Asian women were not significant (22). Overall, the body of evidence does not support an association between these chemicals and breast cancer risk (23,24).

3.2. Biological Markers, Genetic Polymorphisms, and Breast Cancer Risk

Breast cancer in African-American women is a biologically more aggressive tumor than that observed in whites (25–30) or Hispanics (26,27). It is well established that African-American women with breast cancer have less estrogen receptor positive tumors than Caucasian women. This is especially true for premenopausal women. Chen et al. examined the histological features of breast cancer in 573 black and 492 white patients recruited in the population-based, National Cancer Institute Black/White Cancer Survival Study. African-American women had more poorly differentiated tumors, higher grade of nuclear atypia, less estrogen receptor positive tumors, and lesser tubular formation or marked fibrosis when compared to white women. These differences remained after controlling for socioeconomic status, body mass index, use of alcohol or tobacco, reproductive experiences, and health care access and utilization (25). Elledge et al. examined breast cancer prognostic factors among 777 Hispanic, 1016 black, and 4885 white patients with breast cancer. Whites had a lower S-phase fraction than Hispanics or blacks. The estrogen receptor and progesterone receptor levels in Hispanics were intermediate to the level of the other two ethnic groups. There were no clinically significant differences in DNA ploidy, HER-2/neu, or p53 expression among the three groups (26). In another study of prognostic biomarkers among 43 Asian, 48 white, and 44 black patients with breast cancer, Kreiger et al. observed no differences in distributions of estrogen, progesterone, and epithelial growth factor receptors, in HER-2/neu and p53, in cytoplasmic proteins cathepsin D and pS2, and two indices of cell growth, Ki67 and DNA ploidy after adjusting for age at diagnosis, menopausal status, or place of birth (31). Weiss et al.'s study of risk and prognostic factors in multiethnic populations (172 white, 32 black, 49 Hispanic) did not reveal significant differences in molecular indices including estrogen and progesterone receptor, ploidy status, S-phase, Ki-67, Her-2/neu expression, tumor grade, and epidermal growth factor receptor. However, small sample size is a limitation in this study (29).

Mutations of the p53 tumor suppressor gene are common in breast cancer and are associated with poor prognosis and reduced survival (30). Elledge et al. observed no difference in the nuclear accumulation of p53 protein in tumors of black, white, or Hispanic patients (26). In a subset of 45 black and 47 white breast cancer patients with stage I and Ii disease from the New Orleans component of the NCI Black/White Cancer Survival Study, Shioa et al. observed that blacks with p53 alterations had a four- to five fold excess risk of dying from breast cancer than those without p53 alterations. An adjustment for stage, age, tumor histopathology, receptor status and adjuvant treatment did not change the excess risk. This observation was not seen in whites (32). In addition, further study showed that blacks more often had p53 mutations without protein accumulation and whites commonly had p53 protein accumulations without mutations (33).

Her-2 gene amplification and protein overexpression is an important predictor of disease progression and has been observed in 20–30% of breast cancers. A polymorphism at codon 655 (Val655Ile) in the transmembrane domain-coding region of the HER2 gene has been identified and may be associated with breast cancer risk in young women under age 45 years. Xie et al. examined the Val(655)Ile polymorphism in a population-based, case–control study of breast cancer in women of Shanghai, China. They observed that women with the Ile/Val or Val/Val genotype had an elevated risk of breast cancer [OR=1.4 (95% CI 1.0–2.0; $p = 0.05$)] after adjusting for age, education, study period, history of breast fibroadenoma, leisure physical activity, and age at first live birth. The risk was highest in younger women <45 years (OR = 14.1; 95% CI = 1.8–113.4) than in older women (34). A few studies have examined this potential etiological marker and prognostic predictor of disease in racial/ethnic groups. Ameyaw et al. studied this polymorphism in a multiethnic population of 257 Caucasians, 90 African-American, and 200 African (Ghanaian) healthy blood donors. The Val allele was not detected in the African population. There was no difference in the HER2 allele frequency between African-Americans and Caucasians. The Val allele was detected in 20% of Caucasian alleles, 24% of African-American alleles, and 11% of Chinese alleles. The homozygous Val/Val genotype that is associated with an increased risk of breast cancer was observed in 5.4% Caucasians, 4.4% African-Americans, and 0.3% Chinese (35). In another study of postmenopausal breast cancer patients participating in the Hawaii and Los Angeles Multiethnic Cohort, McKean-Cowdin et al. observed that women with at least one copy of the Valine variant were approximately one-half as likely to have high-stage as low-stage breast cancer. This effect was present across racial/ethnic groups (36).

Cyclin D1 overexpression occurs in 60–80% of female breast cancers. In a study of 139 female breast cancer patients from multiethnic population, Joe et al. reported that 77% of non-Caucasians (African-American, $N=19$; Hispanic, $N=24$; Asian, $N=5$) vs. 59% of Caucasians ($N=86$) had cyclin D1 overexpression ($p=0.051$). Although sample sizes were small, when non-Caucasians were analyzed separately by ethnicity, there was no significant difference (37).

Overall, about 5–10% of women have an inherited predisposition to develop breast cancer. Genetic and molecular epidemiology studies indicate that carriers of the BRCA1 gene have a lifetime risk of developing breast cancer that is approximately 80%. For BRCA2 mutation carriers, the lifetime risk is approximately 50%. In the general Ashkenazi population, the carrier frequency of mutation is estimated to be $\sim$0.9% for 185delAG (Struewing et al. 1995a), $\sim$0.9–1.5% for 6174delT, and $\sim$0.13% for 5382ins (Benjamin, 1996; and Oddour, 1996) (38). Identifying women at risk for BRCA1 and BRCA2 may provide opportunities for earlier diagnosis and preventive intervention.

Most studies of BRCA1 and BRCA2 mutations to date have been performed in white populations. Only a few studies of BRCA1 susceptibility genes have being reported in other racial/ethnic groups, and, samples have been small. In one of the first preliminary reports on familial aggregation of BRCA1 mutations in an African-American population, Gao et al. concluded that genetic susceptibility to breast cancer could be explained by the BRCA1 mutations in nearly half of the high-risk families ascertained through young African-American breast cancer patients (39). Panguluri et al. examined germline mutations in 45 African-American families at high risk for breast cancer. The entire coding region and flanking introns were analyzed by single-stranded conformation polymorphism analysis followed by sequencing of variant bands. Eleven different BRCA1 germline mutations/variations in seven patients from the 45 high-risk families were observed: two pathogenic, protein-truncating mutations; four amino acid substitutions; one amino acid polymorphism; and four substitutions in noncoding regions (introns). These findings along with reports from other investigators suggest that a large number of distinct pathological mutations and variations exist among African-Americans that have not been reported in Caucasians (39–42). Two mutations (943ins10 and 1832del5) have been reported to be recurrent in African-American families (39–42). Meffort et al. also reported finding a 943ins10 mutation in five different families who may have a common distant African ancestry (43).

In another study, Whittemore et al. examined the prevalence and contribution of BRCA1 mutations in breast and ovarian cancer using data from three case–control studies of ovarian cancer. Ethnicity of the women were: white non-Hispanic, 823; black, 40; Hispanic, 35; and Asian or other ethnicity, 24. Although data were sparse for non-white and Hispanic women, there was no difference in familial aggregation by ethnicity of the probands. Among women < 40 years at diagnosis, it was estimated that 11% of breast cancer and 18% of ovarian cancers are due to BRCA1. They observed that families with non-white and Hispanic probands had more cancer clustering at young ages and postulated that this may reflect higher mutation prevalence in these ethnic groups than in non-Hispanic white women (44). The Carolina Breast Cancer Study, a population-based, case–control study, evaluated BRCA1 mutations among women not selected on the basis of family history of breast cancer or age at diagnosis. A variant in the 3′ untranslated region was observed to be more common in black cases than in black controls. After adjusting for sampling probabilities, they found that the prevalence of BRCA1 mutations among breast cancer patients was 3.3% in whites and 0.0% in blacks (45).

A number of genetic polymorphisms that are involved in the metabolism of estrogen and carcinogens have been studied. Dunning et al. recently completed a comprehensive reviewed of genetic polymorphisms and breast cancer risk. Among 46 studies involving 18 genes, 12 studies reported statistically significant associations. Racial and ethnic groups were described in only 6 of the 21 American studies. Analyses revealed that genotype frequencies were statistically significant in case-control comparisons for three genes: the CYP19 (TTTA) n polymorphism, the GSTP1 Ile105Val polymorphism, and the TP53 Arg72Pro polymorphism. The GSTM1 gene deletion was significant in postmenopausal women only (46). Of the six studies that described racial and ethnic subgroups, only one reported statistically significant observations. Taioli et al. evaluated the role of estradiol metabolism and CYP1A1 polymorphisms in breast cancer risk of Caucasian and African-American women. They observed that African-American women with the wild type CYP1A1 gene showed a significant increase in the 2-OHE1/16-OHE ratio following a 5-day treatment with a 2-OHE inducer.

In a case–control study of 57 women with breast cancer and 312 female controls, the frequency of the homozygous Msp1 polymorphism was 4.2% in African-American controls and 16% in African-American breast cancer cases. The odds ratio of breast cancer with the Msp1 homozygous variant was 8.4 (95% CI: 1.7–41.7), and was not observed in Caucasian women (47,48).

Studies of other genetic polymorphisms have been less conclusive. CYP1B1 is a cytochrome P450 enzyme that is involved in the production of potentially carcinogenic estrogen metabolites and the activation of environmental carcinogens. Bailey et al. examined the role of CYP1B1 in normal breast tissue and breast cancer of 59 African-American and 164 Caucasian women. There was no association between the CYP1B1 genotype and breast cancer risk (49). In addition, a study of GSTM1 polymorphism revealed no association with breast cancer risk, even in environments low in antioxidants (50).

The UDP-glucuronosyltransferase (UGT) plays a major role in phase II drug metabolism and in detoxification of a wide range of molecules, including carcinogens and biologically active steroid hormones. The UDP-1A1 locus (UGT1A1) enzyme is a major UGT involved in estradiol glucuronidation. Genetic variation and breast cancer susceptibility at the UGT1A1 locus was examined in a population-based case–control study of 200 African-American women with breast cancer and 200 controls of African ancestry. The study revealed a 1.8-fold (95% CI, 1.0–3.1; $p = 0.06$) elevated risk in premenopausal women and a 1.0-fold (95% CI, 0.5–1.7; $= 0.9$) risk in postmenopausal women. For premenopausal women, the association was strongest for ER negative (OR, 2.1; 95% CI, 1.0–4.2; $p = 0.04$) than for ER positive (OR, 1.3; 95% CI, 0.6–3.0; $p = 0.5$). These findings suggest a strong association between the UGT1A1 genotype and premenopausal breast cancer and estrogen negativity (51).

4. SUMMARY

There are marked variations in cancer incidence among multiracial and multiethnic population subgroups of the United States. Variations in health measures reflect host, environmental, and genetic attributes of the populations. The dynamics of cultural experiences and differences in risk factor profiles and behaviors modulate how biological disease is expressed among different races and ethnic groups. Alterations in cell growth, biological markers and genetic polymorphisms in racial and ethnic groups provide unique opportunities to examine the relationship of these changes to disease outcomes. Future advancements in knowledge and understanding of cancer biology, gene–environment interactions, and differential rates of disease expression will require adequate data on individuals from multiracial and multiethnic population groups.

REFERENCES

1. Jemal A, Thomas A, Murray T, Thun M. Cancer Statistics, 2002. CA Cancer J Clin 2002; 52:23–47.
2. Edwards BK, Howe HL, Ries LA, Thun MJ, Rosenberg HM, Yancik R, Wingo PA, Jemal A, Feigal EG. Annual report to the Nation on status of cancer, 1973–1999, featuring implications of age and aging on U.S. cancer burden. Cancer 2002; 94:2766–2792.
3. U.S. Bureau of the Census, Department of Commerce, 2002.
4. Greenlee RT, Hill-Harmon MB, Murray T, Thun M. Cancer Statistics, 2001. CA Cancer J Clin 2001; 51:15–36.
5. Ries LAG, Eisner MP, Kosary CL, Hankey BF, Miller BA, Clegg LX, Edwards BK, eds. SEER Cancer Statistics Review, 1973–1997. NIH Publication No. 00-2789. Bethesda, MD: National Cancer Institute, 2000.
6. Howe HL, Wingo PA, Thun MJ, Reis LAG, Rosenberg HM, Fiegal EG, Edwards BK. Annual report to the Nation on the status of cancer (1973–1998), featuring cancers with recent increasing trends. J Nat Cancer Inst 2001; 93:824–842.
7. Miller BA, Kolonel LN, Bernstein L, Young JL, Jr, Swanson GM, West D, Key CR, Liff JM, Glover CS, Alexander GA, et al., eds. Racial/ethnic patterns of cancer in the United States 1992–1998. NIH Publication. No. 96–4104. Bethesda, MD:National Cancer Institute, 1996.
8. Nazario CM, Figueroa-Valles N, Rosario RV. Breast cancer patterns and lifestyle risk of developing breast cancer among Puerto Rican females. P R Health Sci J 2000; 19:7–13.
9. Parkin DM, Khlat M. Studies of cancer in migrants: rationale and methodology. Eur J Cancer 1996; 32A:761–771.
10. Shimizi H, Ross RK, Bernstein L, et al. Cancers of the prostate and breast among Japanese and white immigrants in Los Angeles County. Br J Cancer 1991; 63:963–966.
11. Kelsey JL, Horm-Ross PL. Breast cancer: magnitude of the problem and descriptive epidemiology. Epidemiol Rev 1993; 15:7–16.
12. Velentgas P, Daling J. Risk factors for breast cancer in younger women. J Natl Cancer Inst 1994; 16:15–24.
13. Mayberry RM, Stoddrd-Wright C. Breast cancer risk factors among black women and white women: similarities and differences. Am J Epidemiol 1992; 136:1445–1456.
14. Mayberry RM. Age-specific patterns of association between breast cancer and risk factors in black women, ages 20–39 and 40–54. Ann Epidemiol 1994; 4:205–213.
15. Schatzkin A, Palmer JR, Rosenberg L, Helmrich SP, Miller DR, Kaufman DW, Lesko SM, Shapiro S. Risk factors for breast cancer in black women. J Natl Cancer Inst 1987; 78:213–217.
16. Pathak DR, Osuch JR, He J. Breast carcinoma etiology. Current knowledge and new insights into the effects of reproductive and hormonal risk factors in black and white populations. Cancer 2000; 88:1230–1238.

17. Brinton LA, Benichou J, Gammon MD, Brogan DR, Coates R, Schoenberg JB. Ethnicity and variation in breast cancer incidence. Int J Cancer 1997; 73: 349–355.

18. Newell GR, Borrod LG, McPherson RS, Nichaman MZ, Pillow PC. Prev Med 1998; 5:622–633.

19. Zang EA, Barrett NO, Cohen LA. Differences in nutritional risk factors for breast cancer among New York City white, Hispanic, and black college girls. Ethn Dis 1994; 4:28–40.

20. Wu AH. Diet and breast cancer in multiethnic populations. Cancer 2000; 88:1239–1244.

21. Wu AH, Ziegler RG, Horn-Ross PL, Nomura AM, West DW, Kolonel LN, Rosenthal JF, Hoover RN, Pike MC. Tofu and risk of breast cancer in Asian-Americans. Cancer Epidemiol Biomarkers Prev 1996; 5:901–906.

22. Krieger N, Wolff MS, Hiatt RA, Rivera M, Vogelman, Orentreich N. Breast cancer and serum organochlorines: a prospective study among white, black, and Asian women. J Natl Cancer Inst 1994; 86:589–599.

23. Adami H, Lipworth L, Titus-Ernstoff L, Hsieh C, Hanberg A, Ahlborg U, Baron J, Trichopoulos D. Organochlorine compounds and estrogen-related cancers in women. Cancer Causes Control 1995; 6:551–566.

24. Calle EE, Frumkin H, Henley SJ, Savitz DA, Thun MJ. Organochlorines and breast cancer risk. CA Cancer J Clin 2002; 52:301–309.

25. Chen VW, Correa P, Kurman RJ, Wu X, Eley JW, Austin D, Muss H, Hunter CP, Redmond C, Sobhan M, Coates RC, Reynolds P, Herman AA, Edwards BK. Histological characteristics of breast carcinoma in blacks and whites. Cancer Epidemiol Biomarkers Prev 1994; 3:127–135.

26. Elledge RM, Clark GM, Chamness GC, Osborne CK. Tumor biologic factors and breast cancer prognosis among white, Hispanic, and black women in the United States. J Nat Cancer Inst 1994; 86:705–712.

27. Blaszyk H, Vaughn CB, Hartmann A, McGovern RM, Schroeder JJ, Cunningham J, Schaid D, Sommer SS, Kowach JS. Novel pattern of p53 mutations in an American black cohort with high mortality from breast cancer. Lancet 1994; 343:1195–1197.

28. Thomas PA, Raab SS, Lannin DR, Slagel DD, Silverman JF. Racial differences in breast cancer in a rural population: comparison of cytologic nuclear grade, other prognostic factors, and outcomes for tumors diagnosed by fine-needle aspiration biopsy. Breast J 1998; 4:104–111.

29. Weiss SE, Tartter PI, Ahmed S, Brower ST, Brusco C, Bossolt K, Amberson JB, Bratton J. Ethnic differences in risk and prognostic factors for breast cancer. Cancer 1995; 76:268–274.

30. Rose DP, Royak-Schaler R. Tumor biology and prognosis in black breast cancer patients: a review. Cancer Detect Prev 2001; 25:16–31.

31. Krieger N, van den Eeden SK, Zava D, Okamoto A. Race/ethnicity, social class, and prevalence of breast cancer prognostic biomarkers: a study of white, black, and Asian women in the San Francisco Bay area. Ethnicity 1997; 7:137–149.

32. Shiao Y, Chen VW, Scheer WD, Wu XC, Correa P. Racial disparity in the association of p53 gene alterations with breast cancer survival. Cancer Res 1995; 55:1485–1490.

33. Shiao Y, Chen VW, Wu X, Scheer WD, Lehmann HP, Malcom GT, Boudreau DA, Ruiz B, Correa P. Racial comparison of p53 alterations in breast cancer: difference in prognostic value. In Vivo 1996; 10:169–174.

34. Xie D, ShuXO, Deng Z, Wen WQ, Creek KE, Dai Q, Gao YT, Jin F, Zheng W. Population-based case–control study of HER2 genetic polymorphism and breast cancer risk. J Natl Cancer Inst 2000; 92:412–417.

35. Ameyaw M, Thornton N, McLeod HL. Re: Population-based case–control study of HER2 genetic polymorphisms and breast cancer risk. J Natl Cancer Inst 2000; 92:1947.

36. McKean-Cowdin R, Kolonel LN, Press MF, Pike MC, Henderson BE. Cancer Res 2001; 61:8393–8394.

37. Joe AK, Arber N, Bose S, Heitjan D, Zhang Y, Weinstein IB, Hibshoosh H. Cyclin D1 overexpression is more prevalent in non-Caucasian breast cancer. Anticancer Res 2001; 21:3535–3540.

38. Abeliovic D, Kaduri L, Lerer I, Weinberg N, Amir G, Sagi M, Zlotogora J, Heching N, Peretz T. Am J Hum Genet 1997; 60:505–514.

39. Gao Q, Neuhausen S, Cumming S, Luce M, Olopade O. Recurrent germ-line BRCA1 mutations in extended African-American-families with early-onset breast cancer. Am J Hum Genet 1997; 60:1233–1236.

40. Panguluri RCK, Brody LC, Modali R, Utley K, Adams-Campbell L, Day AA, Whitfield-Broome C, Dunston GM. Hum Genet 1999; 105:28–31.

41. Yawitch TM, van Rensburg EJ. Absence of commonly recurring BRCA1 mutations in black South African women with breast cancer. S Afr Med Assoc 2000; 90:788.

42. Miki Y, Swenson J, Shattuck-Eidens D, Futreal PA, Harshman K, Tavitigian S, Liu Q et al. A strong candidate for breast and ovarian cancer susceptibility genes BRCA1. Science 1994; 266:66–71.

43. Mefford HC, Bambach L, Panguluri RCK, Whitfield-Broome C, Szabo C, Smith S, King M-C, Dunston G, Stoppa-Llyonnet D, Arena F. Evidence for a BRCA 1 founder mutation in families of west African ancestry. Am J Hum Genet 1999.

44. Whittemore AS, Gong G, Itnyre J. Prevalence and contribution of BRCA1 mutations in breast cancer and ovarian cancer: results from three U.S. population-based case–control studies of ovarian cancer. Am J Hum Genet 1997; 60:496–504.

45. Newman B, Mu H, Butler LM, Millikan RG, Moorman PG, King MC. Frequency of breast cancer attributable to BRCA1 in a population-based series of American women. J Am Med Assoc 1998; 279:915–921.

46. Dunning AM, Healey CS, Pharoah PDP, Teare MD, Ponder BAJ, Easton DF. A systematic review of genetic polymorphisms and breast cancer risk. Cancer Epidimiol Biomarkers Prev 1999; 8:843–854.

47. Taioli E, Bradlow HL, Garbers SV, Sepkovic DW, Osborne MP, Trachman J, Ganguly S, Garte SJ. Role of estradiol metabolism and CYP1A1 polymorphisms in breast cancer risk. Cancer Detect Prev 1999; 23:232–237.

48. Taioli E, Trachman J, Cen X, Toniolo P, Garte SJA. Cyp1A1 restriction fragment length polymorphism is associated with breast cancer African-American women. Cancer Res 1995; 55:3757–3758.

49. Bailey LR, Roodi N, Dupont WD, Parl FF. Association of cytochrome P450 1B1 (CYP1B1) polymorphism with steroid receptor status in breast cancer. Cancer Res 1998; 58:5038–5041.
50. Ambrosone CB, Coles BF, Freudenheim JL, Shields PG. Gluththione S-transferase (GSTM1) genetic polymorphisms do not affect human breast cancer risk, regardless of dietary antioxidants. J Nutr 1999; 129:565S–568S.
51. Guillemette C, Millikan RC, Newman B, Housman DE. Genetic polymorphisms in uridine diphospho-glucuronosyltransferase 1A1 and association with breast cancer among African-American. Cancer Res 2000; 60:950–956.

19

Respiratory Tract Cancer

Aage Haugen

Department of Toxicology, National Institute of Occupational Health,
Oslo, Norway

1. OVERVIEW
1.1. Lung Cancer Occurrence

Respiratory tract cancer was a rare disease at the beginning of the twentieth century with only a few hundred cases of lung cancer reported. In 1912, Adler was able to collect data on 374 lung cancer cases from the literature. In the beginning of his paper, he asked the following question, "Is it worthwhile to write a monograph on the subject of primary malignant tumors of the lung?" (1). A century later, lung cancer is a global problem. The cancer is now the most frequent and one of the deadliest in the world and is predicted to remain a major cause of world wide cancer death in the twenty first century (2). The global incidence of lung cancer is increasing 0.5% per year (3).

The World Health Organization (WHO) estimates that there are presently about 1.1 billion smokers in the world and about one-third of the world population older than 15 years are smokers. Tobacco smoking caused about 3 million deaths in 1995 and it is estimated that in 2025 about 10 million deaths annually will be related to tobacco smoking (4). The tobacco industry has suffered some setbacks in more developed countries, but they now focus on developing countries to maintain their profits. China is now the world's biggest producer and consumer of tobacco. Every fourth Chinese now smokes and there are about 750,000 deaths in China every year due to tobacco-related disease. This number will increase to 2 million in year 2025 if the trend continues (5).

Tobacco smoking has been identified not only as a cause of lung cancer but also cancers of oral cavity and pharynx, in addition to cancers at more remote sites. More than 100 years ago oral cancer was the most common cancer in many parts of the world. Oral cancer rates then transiently decreased, but presently oropharyngeal cancers are a significant health problem in various parts of the world; its prevalence ranges from 5% of malignancies in the United States to 50% in India and Southeast Asia (6). The incidence of oral cancers also varies throughout the European countries.

1.2. Lung Cancer Histology

Various respiratory epithelial cell types are exposed chronically to tobacco smoke. This is reflected in the many histological subtypes of lung cancer. There are four main histological subtypes: adenocarcinoma (AC), squamous cell carcinoma (SC), small cell lung carcinoma (SCLC), and large cell carcinoma (LC). Adenocarcinoma (including bronchiolo-alveolar carcinoma) and SC are the most frequent subtypes. These two cancers, plus LC are sometimes referred to as nonsmall cell lung cancer (NSCLC), and represents about 80% of lung cancers. Many lung tumors are heterogeneous and contain malignant cells of more than one subtype complicating pathological characterization.

Cigarette smoking can cause any type of lung cancer, while nonsmokers usually get AC. A dramatic change in the frequency of the various histological subtypes has taken place during the twentieth century. Squamous cell carcinoma was the most frequent histological type but now AC is more frequent (7). It has been suggested that a combination of changing diagnostic criteria and changes in cigarette components and smoking behavior may have caused the rise in the proportion of AC (8). Cigarettes were mainly high tar and nonfilter before the 1960s, resulting in deposition of tar particulates at the branches of central bronchi. The delivery from cigarettes of benzo(a)pyrene (B(a)P) and nicotine decreased in U.S. cigarettes by about 50% between 1965 and 1975 while 4-(methylnitrosamino) -1-(3-pyridyl)-1-butanone (NNK) increased similarly between the late 1970s and the early 1990s (9). Due to the lower nicotine yield, the smokers inhale more deeply, resulting in higher exposure of the peripheral lung to nitrosamines and nitrogen oxides, which are thought to induce AC. Furthermore, the smoke produced by the low tar cigarettes are less irritating for the bronchial epithelium, permitting deeper inhalation bringing the compounds to deposit primarily in the lower respiratory tract epithelium and the alveoli, and to a lesser degree in the upper respiratory tract.

2. LUNG CANCER ETIOLOGY
2.1. Cigarettes

Smoke from cigarettes, both mainstream (inhaled directly by the smoker) and sidestream (smoke emitted from the burning cigarette), are composed of many toxic and carcinogenic compounds. A smoker inhales gas-phase smoke as well as particulates (tar). At least 50 carcinogenic compounds have been identified in the tar and vapor phase thus far, namely polycyclic aromatic hydrocarbons (PAHs), *N*-nitrosamines, aromatic amines, aza-arenes, aldehydes, various organic compounds, inorganic compounds such as hydrazine, metals, and free radical species (Fig. 1) (10). The highly carcinogenic compounds PAHs (mainly B(a)P) and tobacco-specific nitrosamines (mainly NNK) have been postulated to be of major importance in human lung carcinogenesis (see above).

Experimental studies suggest etiological differences between SC and AC. Mutations in the *p53* tumor suppressor gene are frequently altered in human lung cancer, and are found twice as common in SC compared to AC along with a higher frequency of guanine to thymine transversions (11). Benzo(a)pyrene has been shown to form adducts at guanines in codon 157, 248, and 273, which are major hotspots, consistent with a mechanistic link between PAHs in tobacco smoke and guanine to thymine transversions (12). Separately, AC containing mutations in codon 12 in k-*ras* oncogene is induced when rodents are exposed to tobacco-specific nitrosamines. Such mutations are frequent in human lung AC (13).

Cigarette tar contains high concentration of free radicals (14). Alkenes, nitrosamines, aromatic hydrocarbons, amines, catechols and hydroquinone are well-known sources of reactive oxygen species.

Concerning oral cancers, alcohol consumption is an important risk factor in addition to cigarette smoking (15). The effect of these two risk factors may be synergistic. An association between tobacco chewing and oral cancer has also been found (16).

2.2. Air Pollution

Studies have shown that air pollution, such as industrial emissions and traffic exhaust, is a risk factor for lung cancer. These pollutants include PAHs, benzene, ethylene oxide, gasoline vapors, and metals. However, the

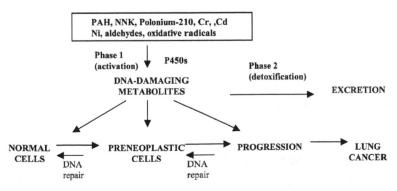

Figure 1 Lung carcinogenesis.

etiological importance of air pollution as a contributory factor is still under debate. An association between lung cancer and air pollution have been reported in studies from cities with a high level of air pollution. Urban residents seem to have an increased risk of lung cancer of 1.5–2.0 times that of rural residents. The effect of air pollution on lung cancer may be identifiable only above a certain threshold level. However, the analysis is complicated due to the fact that air pollution is a complex mixture with numerous air pollutants that also varies over time (17).

2.3. Occupation

There is evidence of human lung cancer associated with industrial exposure. Lung is the major target concerning exposure at work to asbestos, radon, mustard gas, coal tar and soot, chloromethyl ethers, beryllium, chromium, nickel, and inorganic arsenic (18). The contribution of occupational exposure to diesel exhaust is still under debate. There is a strong evidence regarding the synergistic relation between smoking and asbestos exposure. Occupational risk factors for oral cancers are less well established. Nickel, chromium, and mustard gas have been reported as risk factors. In general, occupation appears to have little substantial effect on the development of oral cancers.

2.4. Environmental Tobacco Smoke

Cigarettes generate large amount of environmental tabacco smoke (ETS). ETS is a combination of sidestream smoke and smoke that is exhaled by the smoker. Environmental tabacco smoke contains essentially all the same carcinogens and toxic/irritating agents that have been identified in mainstream smoke inhaled by the smokers. Sidestream smoke is composed of approximately 4000 chemicals and has a higher concentration of many of the possible carcinogenic compounds such as benzene, formaldehyde, hydrazine, nitrosamines, 4-aminobiphenyl, B(a)P, benzo(a)anthracene, and others (19). Several studies have shown an increased risk of lung cancer among nonsmokers who live in the same household as smokers. A recent meta-analysis concluded that marriage to a smoker increased the risk of lung cancer by 26% (20). A recent large European study demonstrated that lung cancer risk after ETS exposure is relatively small (21). Many authors are skeptical to the observed association due to misclassification bias (smoker/nonsmoker nonsmoker and ETS exposure). However, there is evidence that prolonged ETS exposure during childhood can lead to an increased risk of lung cancer.

3. LUNG CARCINOGENESIS
3.1. Genetic Changes in Lung Cancer

The karyotype of lung cancer is very complex and many genetic changes have been identified including specific alterations of proto-oncogens (c-*myc*, K-*ras*, *cyclin D₁*, *erb-B2* and *bcl-2*) and tumor suppressor genes (*p53*, *Rb*, *FHIT*, *RASSF1A*, *SEMA3B*, *p16^{INK4}*) as well as chromosomal losses (22). Epigenetic inactivation, such as aberrant promoter hypermethylation, is a major mode of inactivation of expression of many genes, e.g., *p16^{INK4}*, *DAPK*, *RARβ*, *SEMA3B*, *MGMT*, *P14^{ARF}*, and *GSTP1* (23). Chromosomal regions including 1p, 3p, 4p, 4q, 5q, 8p, 9p, 9q, 10, 11p, 13q, 17p, 18q, 19p, and 22p are frequently deleted in lung cancer (22). NSCLC and SCLC have different regions of frequent loss of heterozygosity (LOH). Allelic losses on 3p have been reported as the most frequent event in lung cancer and many candidate genes have been identified in this region (24). As with lung cancer, multiple genetic alterations have been reported in oral tumors (25).

The evolutionary sequence of genetic alterations that take place during the stepwise progression of lung cancer is not known due to lack of macroscopic premalignant areas in lung epithelium. In SCC, there is a defined sequence of histological events, begining with hyperplasia and advancing to metaplasia, dysplasia, carcinoma in situ (CIS), and then invasive cancer. The whole sequence takes about 20–30 years. In AC, precursor lesions are also possible, but preneoplastic changes have not been established to date (26).

Due to the continuous insult of cigarette smoke, the entire respiratory tract can be damaged. There is a very high incidence of allelic loss, identified though the LOH studies, which can be found in histologically normal and abnormal epithelium of both current and former smokers. These multifocal changes in the mucosa are referred to as field cancerization. In preinvasive lesions, allelic loss (deletions) occurs in chromosomal regions 3p, 9p21, and 17p13. Loss of heterozygosity of 3p is an early change found in dysplastic lesions, 90% of SCLC and about 50% of tumors from NSCLC. Allelic loss at several 3p regions (e.g., 3p12, 3p14 (*FHIT*), 3p21 and 3p24–25) occurs frequently in the tumor. The size of the 3p deletion in the early stages are small, but 3p is lost in CIS (27). *p53* mutations also appear relatively early in lung carcinogenesis (bronchial dysplasia and CIS) (22). About 80% of the SCLC tumors and 50% of NSCLC have *p53* mutations (28). *p53* mutations are also observed in premalignant lesions associated with head and neck carcinomas (29). K-*ras* is frequently activated oncogene in NSCLC (13). Mutations in K-*ras* oncogene, predominantly in codon 12, have been shown to occur in approximately 30% of pulmonary AC. Results suggest that K-*ras* mutations may occur at a relatively early stage in the development of lung cancer and play a role in the conversion of dysplastic cells to preinvasive cancer cells. Apart from *p53* and K-*ras, Rb* gene is frequently inactivated in lung cancer, especially in SCLC where 90% of the tumors have abnormalities in *Rb*. In contrast to *Rb*, loss of *p16*^{INK4} occur more frequently in NSCLC than in SCLC (30). Most of the RB-positive lung tumors are *p16* ^{INK4} inactive indicating that loss of function of both *pRb* and *p16* ^{INK4} does not contribute to increased selective cellular growth potential during the process of tumor development. The literature clearly indicates that the cycline D1/p16/pRb pathway is frequently deregulated in lung cancer. Similarly, in oral cancer deregulated expression in some of these components have been demonstrated.

3.2. Metabolism of Lung Carcinogens

Metabolic activation of procarcinogens, such as PAHs and *N*-nitrosamines, and the covalent binding of the reactive metabolites to DNA forming DNA-adducts are considered key events in tumor initiation. Other forms of genetic damage including chromosomal aberrations also can occur. Lung carcinogens are metabolically activated via complex enzymatic mechanisms and detoxified by combinations of phase I and phase II enzymes. Enzyme families involved in these reactions are the cytochrome P450 (CYP) enzymes, epoxide hydrolases, glutathione *S*-transferases, uridine 5-diphospho-glucorynyltransferases, and *N*-acetyltransferases. Phase I enzymes, which are mainly cytochrome P450s, insert one atom of oxygen into the substrate; and phase II enzymes which act on oxygenated substrates conjugate them with various endogenous moieties producing hydrophilic products which are excreted easily from the cells (31). The extent of DNA-adduct formation depends on the balance between the rates of oxidation of the compound and rates of detoxification of the reactive products via conjugation.

Cytochrome P450 (CYP) enzymes are expressed at significant levels in the lung so that reactive genotoxic metabolites from PAHs and *N*-nitrosamines can be formed directly in the lung epithelium. Reactive metabolites may also migrate to the lung from distal organs (i.e., the liver) through the bloodstream inducing DNA damage. Several forms of P450 have been identified as playing a role in lung carcinogenesis. CYP1A1 and CYP2E1 are of critical importance for the activation of PAH and nitrosamines (and other low molecular weight compounds), respectively (31). The gene product of CYP1A1 catalyzes the first step in the metabolism of PAH. Recent studies indicate that the pulmonary system expresses several CYP enzymes although at low levels (32). Results show that CYP3A4, CYP1B1, and CYP2C9 also catalyze the formation of mutagenic intermediates from PAH. In addition to CYP2E1, the nitrosamines are also metabolically activated by CYP1A2, CYP2A6, and CYP2D6. CYP1A2 is expressed in peripheral lung, CYP2A6 is expressed in both bronchial epithelium and peripheral tissue. There is no detectable CYP2D6 expression in bronchus and lungs.

Although a number of different mechanisms can detoxify PAH-diol epoxides, the most important mechanism in their detoxification is the glutathione *S*-transperase (GST)-catalyzed conjugation with reduced glutathione (GSH). These enzymes have an important role in protecting

DNA against damage and DNA-adduct formation through conjugation to electrophilic substances, particularly those with lipophilic groups. The GSTs comprise a supergene family of phase II enzymes that catalyze GSH-dependent reactions with many electrophiles. The products of the alpha, mu, theta, pi, and zeta gene families have been identified (31). The various enzymes have different but often overlapping substrate specificities. Epoxides are effective substrates for both mu and pi GST. The GSTP1 enzyme is abundantly expressed in the lung and is relatively more active than other classes of GSTs in the GSH conjugation of tobacco-derived B(a)P diol epoxide (33). GSTM1, GSTM2, and GSTM3 also have reactivity towards epoxides. GSTM1 is expressed at low level in the lung, and at high level in the liver (31). Many of the substrates of the GSTs also influence the expression of the GST genes indicating the presence of a adaptive response mechanisms to chemical stress.

Arylamines in tobacco smoke are carcinogenic and metabolized by *N*-acetyltransferases, NAT1 and NAT2 enzymes. These enzymes catalyze *N*- and *O*-acetylation of aromatic and heterocyclic amines. The arylamines have a higher affinity for NAT2 than for NAT1. *N*-acetyltransferases are found in a large number of tissues. Both NAT1 and NAT2 are expressed in the lung but NAT1 is the predominant form. NAT2 is predominantly expressed in the liver (31).

Microsomal epoxide hydrolase (mEPHX) is one of the most important phase II detoxification enzymes. The role of mEPHX is to transform arene, alkene, and aliphatic epoxides to less reactive, less toxic, and more water soluble forms. It also activates some PAHs in tobacco smoke into a more carcinogenic form. Althrough mEPHX is considered a detoxifying enzyme, the dihydrodiols derived from PAHs may be further catalyzed by CYPs into still more reactive forms (32).

4. LUNG CANCER SUSCEPTIBILITY

4.1. Cytochrome P450s Polymorphisms

The interplay between genetic and environmental exposures is thought to be critical factor in lung carcinogenesis despite the fact that tobacco smoke is very deleterious to the lung; only 1 of 10 lifetime smokers contracts lung cancer and some degree of familial aggregation of lung cancer is evident in family studies. Lung cancer susceptibility may be modulated by host-specific factors including differences in xenobiotic metabolism, DNA repair, and alterations in oncogenes and tumor suppressor gene functions. The role of metabolic genes in individual susceptibility to the carcinogenic effects of tobacco smoke have been investigated in several studies in various populations. Polymorphisms exist in the several genes responsible for both activation and inactivation of tobacco carcinogens and may contribute to the observed susceptibility to lung carcinogens.

So far the polymorphic genes most studied in lung cancer include *CYP1A1, CYP2E1, CYP2D6* (Table 1), and the phase II genes *GSTM1, GSTP1, NAT2 and EPHX* (Table 2). At least four polymorphic variants of the *CYP1A1* gene have been identified, two of which are thought to result in increased enzyme activity. Japanese studies have shown that high susceptibility to lung cancer is associated with *CYP1A1* gene polymorphisms (homozygosity for the rare *MspI* allele (m2 variant), and exon 7 substitution (*Val* allele) (34). The association has not been confirmed in European and North American studies. The *CYP1A1* genotype frequencies like many other genes show inter–ethnic differences. The frequency of the m2 and Val variant is much less in Caucasians and it will require about 500–1000 cases to study the association in this ethnic population. This lung cancer susceptibility is dependent on the cigarette dose, showing a high relative risk at low dose level of cigarette smoking for individuals with susceptible genotypes (35,36). However, further studies are required in this area since the *MspI* and the exon 7 polymorphisms are not strictly linked and large differences in catalytic activities for these different alleles have not been shown.

Several studies have examined lung cancer risk and CYP2D6 phenotype but the results have been conflicting. Several mutant *CYP2D6* have been identified (37). Individuals with two defective alleles have been shown to exhibit decreased CYP2D6 activity (poor metabolizers, PM) when compared to those having one or two wildtype alleles (extensive metabolizers, EM). The highest risk of lung cancer was observed among smokers having the highest levels of both tobacco smoking exposure and CYP2D6 activity (38). Since *CYP2D6* is not expressed in the lung, but in the liver, this may reflect that the NNK-metabolites are transported to the lung during high exposures to tobacco carcinogens.

In Japanese studies, individuals homozygous for the rare *Dra I* alleles of *CYP2E1* were reported to have decreased lung cancer risk (39). However,

Table 1 Polymorphic *CYP* Genes Associated with Lung Cancer

Genes	Polymorphism alleles	Carcinogen	Remarks
CYP1A1	*2 MspI mutation *3 Ile-Val mutation	PAHs	Increased risk
CYP2D6	*2 Amplification/ duplication *3 Frameshift *4 Frameshift *5 Deletion	NNK	Poor metabolizers: decreased risk
CYP2EI	Dra I, intron 2 Rsa I/Pst I	NNK, butadiene Benzene, styrene	Decreased risk (DraI) Increased risk (Rsa I)

Table 2 Phase II Polymorphic Genes Associated with Lung Cancer

Genes	Polymorphism alleles	Carcinogen	Remarks
GSTM1	*0 gene deletion	PAH epoxides	Higher risk
	B Ile-Val, exon 5 *C	PAH epoxides	Higher risk
GSTP1	Ile-Val + Ala-Val exon 5		
NAT	*10	Aromatic amines	Lower risk (*10)
	*11		
	*14		
	*15		
EPHX	Tyr113 → His	PAH epoxides and aromatic amines	Higher risk
	His 139 → Arg		(conflicting results)

among Caucasians no association has been found (40,41). Homozygosity for the *Rsa I* variant has been associated with increased risk of lung cancer in some studies, but no association was found in other studies.

4.2. Glutathione *S*-Transferase Polymorphisms

Several studies support the view that GST polymorphism influence the susceptibility to lung cancer. A deletion of both copies of the *GSTM1* gene is present in 40–60% of the general population (with an ethnic variation ranging from 30% to 80%) producing a complete lack of GSTM1 enzyme (null genotype). The *GSTM1* gene product is suggested to be particularly important for detoxifying BP diol epoxide. Individuals lacking GSTM1 activity can potentially be at an enhanced risk for smoking-related lung cancer. A meta-analysis suggests a statistically significant but modest increase in odds ratio for the *GSTM1-null* genotype among lung cancer patients compared to controls (42). It appears that the *GSTM1* genotype is not associated with oral cancer risk (43). When the influence of the *GSTM1* genoptype on the level of PAH–DNA adduct was evaluated, a higher level in the lung was found in patients with the *null* genotype compared to patients with at least one allele intact. Furthermore, the different genotype distribution found in patients with transversion and transition mutations in the *p53* and K-*ras* genes also supports these results (44). G to T transversion mutations at GC base pairs have been particularly associated with certain PAH compounds which are known to be metabolized by the GSTM1 enzyme. Other studies indicate that PAH–DNA adduct levels and *CYP1A1* and/or *GSTM1* genotypes to be independent lung cancer risk factors (45).

A major GST protein in human lung is GSTP1-1. The *GSTP1* gene has been shown to be polymorphic in humans. A polymorphic site at codon

104 (Ile105Val substitution) in the *P1* gene is known to change the enzyme's kinetic properties. A study from our laboratory indicates that individuals with the low activity alleles had a higher lung cancer risk (44). It appeared that the described difference was found in the group of SCC and not among patients with AC. The *GSTP1* polymorphism also influences susceptibility to SCC at the upper aerodigestive tract (46). The impact of the different *GSTP1* genotype on the formation of PAH–DNA adducts in the lung was also investigated and elevated levels were observed among the low activity alleles (44).

4.3. *N*-Acetyltransferase Polymorphisms

The *NAT2* and *NAT1* genes are known to be polymorphic in humans. Several genetic polymorphisms have been shown to be associated with decreased enzyme activity and/or variable stability for the NAT2 gene. Individuals with slow-acetylator *NAT2* alleles have little or no enzyme activity. This slow acetylator genotype occurs at a frequency of about 50% in Caucasians, but the prevalence varies significantly among ethnic populations. Since aromatic amines are abundant in tobacco smoke, the *NAT2* polymorphism is also of interest with respect to lung cancer susceptibility. However, most of the studies on lung cancer show no overall lung cancer risk related to the slow acetylator genotype (47). In a recent Swedish study, an increased odds ratio was associated with the slow acetylator genotype among never-smokers and an increased risk for rapid acetylators among smokers (48). For the slow acetylator genotype, a Japanese study reported a raised odds ratio for AC (49). The *NAT1*10* allele has been linked to increased risk of lung cancer and other cancer types. Several different NAT1 mutations have later been reported but with respect to lung cancer the results are conflicting.

4.4. EPHX Polymorphisms

Two variants of the human mEPHX alleles have been associated with altered enzyme activity; one in exon 3 (His or Tyr substitution at position 113 decreasing mEPHX activity), another in exon 4 (His or Arg substitution at position 139 enhancing enzyme activity). However, inconsistent relationships have been found with respect to lung cancer risk. London et al. found no association between mEPHX and lung cancer risk. The data indicated that genetically reduced EPHX may be prodective (50). A recent study by Zhao et al. indicated that the two polymorphisms modulate lung cancer risk (51).

4.5. Alcohol Dehydrogenase

The association between alcohol and tobacco intake with oral and oropharyngeal carcinoma has been well documented. Ethanol is mainly converted to acetaldehyde by ADH forming adducts with DNA. Acetaldehyde may also inhibit DNA repair processes. *ADH3* is polymorphic (two common alleles, designated 1 and 2), and comparison of the enzymatic properties have shown that individuals homozygous for ADH3 allele 1 (ADH3-1,1) metabolize ethanol to acetaldehyde faster than individuals who carry at least one ADH_3 allele 2 (AEH3-1,2 or ADH3-2,2) (52). Recent data show that the *ADH*3-1,1 genotype appear to increase the risk of ethanol-related oral cancers (53).

4.6. Combinations of Risk Genotypes on Lung Cancer Susceptibility

Individuals with particular combinations of at risk polymorphisms, i.e., in the P450, GST, NAT, EPHX enzyme systems, may have a higher risk of contracting lung cancer. Individual genotypes may have a relatively weak influence on susceptibility, but the effect of genotype combination should be more pronounced.

Hayashi et al. described a 5.8-fold relative risk for all lung cancer type and a 9.1-fold relative risk for SCC in Japanese individuals who were homozygous for both the *CYP1A1* val and *GSTM1 null* risk alleles (54). Nakashi et al. found that among SCC patients individuals with the *CYP1A1 Msp1* genotype combined with deficient *GSTM1* were at remarkable high risk of developing SCC with an odds ratio of 16 (55). These results are consistent with the notion that some procarcinogens in cigarette smoke are activated by CYP1A1 and inactivated by GSTM1 enzymes. Case–control studies have also been combined with genotype analysis and DNA adduct and mutation measurements. In a study where combined *GSTM1* and *GSTP1* genotypes were examined, lung cancer patients with the combined null and AG/GG had significantly higher adduct levels than all other genotype combinations. The distribution of combined genotypes was also significantly different in cases and controls, mainly due to increased frequency of the combination *GSTM1 null* and *GSTP1* AG or GG among patients (44). The *NAT2* slow genotype, in particular when combined with the *GSTM1 null* genotype, may confer increased susceptibility to adduct formation, gene mutation in somatic cells (HPRT) and lung cancer when the smoking dose is low (45). In a recent study, the joint effects of genotype combinations (*GSTP1*, GG, *GSTM1-null* and *GSTP1* GG, *p53* variant) were found to be associated with lung cancer risk and the risk was greatest among individuals ≤55 years of age (46).

5. DNA REPAIR

Susceptibility to lung cancer may also be modulated by DNA repair but whether defects in DNA repair may be a common predisposing factor for lung cancer has not yet been established. There is, however, some evidence indicating that defects in DNA repair may be involved in the development of lung cancer. Recent findings suggest that individuals with reduced DNA repair capacity (DRC) are at an increased risk of lung cancer: in vitro lymphocyte assays has been utilized to measure individual variation in DRC. Sensitivity to mutagen damage, based on the quantification of bleomycin-induced chromatid breaks in vitro, may be a significant determinant of susceptibility. In case–control studies, lung cancer patients, and head and neck cancer patients expressed increased sensitivity to mutagens (56,57). The underlying mechanisms that account for the observed differences in chromosomal sensitivity to bleomycin among individuals are multiple, one mechanism may be alteration in the DNA repair process. Further, studies have shown that this assay can be used to assess the sensitivity also to other carcinogens such as B(a)P. Molecular epidemiological studies have also been conducted in which DNA repair capacity is measured in the host-cell reactivation assay (HCR) where a damaged recombinant plasmid, i.e., by UV or B(a)P, harboring a chloramphenicol acetyltransferase reporter gene is introduced into lymphocytes (58). Since B(a)P-adducts and thymine dimer repair can block reporter gene expression, the measured chloramphenicol transferase activity is the net result of DNA repair in the cell. B(a)P-adducts are repaired by the nucleotide excision repair (NER) pathway and XPD is one of the genetic complementation groups encoding for proteins involved in the NER pathway. One study on DRC and XPD genotypes suggested that the *XPD* variant *Gln751Gln* (exon 23) and *Asp312Asn* (exon 11) genotypes were associated with less DRC and significantly increased risk for lung cancer (59). In a case–control study the *XPD Asp312Asp* genotype was found to have almost twice the risk of lung cancer when the Asp/Asn plus Asn/Asn combined genotype served as reference. In light smokers, the *XPD Asp312Asp* genotype was more frequent among cases than in controls and was associated with increase risk for NSCLC (60). *XPD* variant alleles have also been associated with reduced repair of aromatic DNA adducts (61). In a case–control study, a significant interaction between cumultative cigarette smoking and *XPD* polymorphisms (*Asp312Asn* and *Lys751Gln*) were found (62). *XRCC1* protein is involved in the base excision repair (BER) through the interaction with poly (ADP-ribose) polymerase, DNA polymerase β, and DNA ligase III. Three polymorphisms have been identified (63). Recently, *XRCC1* polymorphisms have been show to modulate lung cancer susceptibility (64,65). The human *OGG1 (hOGG1)* gene encodes a DNA glycosylase/AP-lyase that catalyzes the removal of 8-OH-dG adducts. Several polymorphisms at the hOGG1 locus have been found and recent studies have suggested that the *Ser326Cys hOGG1* polymorphism may be associated with increased lung cancer risk and orolaryngeal cancer risk (66,67).

6. GENDER DIFFERENCES IN LUNG CANCER RISK

Smoking rates among women are increasing, as are the number of smoking-related casualties. However, relatively few women in underdeveloped countries are smokers today. For instance, in China only 20 million women are smokers compared to 280 million men, but the number of women smokers will inevitably increase. Tobacco companies have identified women as a key target group.

Women may be particularly sensitive to certain carcinogenic compounds in tobacco smoke (68). Several recent epidemiological studies indicate that women may have a higher risk of lung cancer than men (69,70). These studies are supported by data showing a higher level of hydrophobic DNA adduct in female lung compared to men (71,72). Moreover, a higher frequency of G to T mutations in the *p53* gene in lung tumors of females than in males was observed (73,74). In human lung, *CYP1A1* mRNA are induced by PAH in tobacco smoke. One study showed that women smokers have significantly higher expression of lung *CYP1A1* (72). In the same study, hydrophobic DNA adducts were found to be significantly associated to the level of *CYP1A1* expression. Together, these data indicate that women may be more susceptible for lung cancer than males. The mechanism(s) is unknown but hormones may be involved, modulating the expression of enzymes involved in the metabolism of PAH. Estrogen receptors (ER-alpha and ER-beta) have been identified in human lung cells (75). There is also recently presented evidence that the observed sex difference in lung cancer risk may be explained by the expression of gastrin-releasing peptide receptor (*GRPR)* at a significant lower exposure to tobacco smoke in females than males (76). Studies have shown that bombesin-like peptides such as GRP induce cell proliferation in several cell types, also human bronchial cells and may thereby stimulate promotion in lung carcinogenesis (77).

7. CONCLUSION

Lung carcinogenesis is mediated through an interaction between several putative carcinogens. The interplay between genetics and environmental exposures is thought to be an important factor in lung carcinogenesis. Several genetically controlled polymorphic enzymes and enzyme systems have been recognized which are linked to tobacco carcinogen activation and deactivation. Genetic differences in DNA repair may also be important determinants of susceptibility. However, their interaction and control as well as their contribution to lung cancer susceptibility and tumor development is presently not well understood. Recent studies may indicates sex difference in lung cancer risk. The mechanisms are still unknown.

REFERENCES

1. Adler I. Primary Malignant Growths of the Lungs and Bronchi. New York: Longmans, Green and Company, 1912.
2. Parkin DM, Pisani P, Ferlay J. Estimates of the worldwide incidence of eighteen major cancers in 1985. Int J Cancer 1993; 54:594–603.
3. Schottenfield D. Epidemiology of lung cancer. In: Pass HI, Mitchell JB, Johnson DH, Turrisi AT, eds. Lung Cancer: Principles and Practice. Philadelphia: Lippincott-Raven, 1996:305–321.
4. Mackay J, Crofton J. Tobacco and the developing world. Br Med Bull 1996; 52:206–221.
5. Liu BQ, Peto R, Chen ZM, Boreham J, Wu YP, Li JY, Campbell TC, Chen JS. Tobacco hazards in China: retrospective proportional mortality study of one million deaths. Br Med J 1998; 317:1411–1422.
6. Brachman DG, Graves D, Vokes E, Beckett M, Haraf D, Montag A, Dunphy E, Mick R, Yandell D, Weichselbaum RR. Occurence of p53 gene deletions and human papilloma virus infections in human head and neck cancer. Cancer Res 1992; 52:4832–4836.
7. Travis WD, Linder J, Mackay B. Classification, histology, cytology and electron microscopy. In: Pass HI, Mitchell JB, Johnson DH, Turrisi AT, eds. Lung Cancer: Principles and Practice. Philadelphia: Lippincott-Raven, 1996:305–321.
8. Thun MJ, Lally CA, Flannery JT, Calle EE, Flanders WD, Health CW Jr. Cigarette smoking and changes in the histopathology of lung cancer. J Natl Cancer Inst 1997; 89:1580–1586.
9. Hoffmann D, Rivenson A, Murphy SE, Chung F-L, Amin S, Hecht SS. Cigarette smoking and adenocarcinoma of the lung: the relevance of nicotine-derived N-nitrosamines. J Smok Relat Disord 1993; 4:165–189.
10. Hoffmann D, Hoffmann I. The changing cigarette, 1950–1995. J Toxicol Environ Health 1997; 50:307–364.
11. Greenblatt MS, Bennett WP, Hollstein M, Harris CC. Mutations in the p53 tumor suppressor gene: clues to cancer etiology and molecular pathogenesis. Cancer Res 1994; 54:4855–4878.
12. Denissenko MF, Pao A, Tang M-S, Pfeifer GP. Preferential formation of benzo(a)pyrene adducts at lung cancer mutational hotspots in p53. Science 1996; 274:430–432.
13. Mills NE, Fishman CL, Rom WN, Dubin N, Jacobson D. Increased prevalence of k-ras oncogene mutations in lung adenocarcinoma. Cancer Res 1995; 55:1444–1447.
14. Pryor WA. Cigarette smoke radicals and the role of free radicals in chemical carcinogenicity. Environ Health Perspect 1997; 105:875–882.
15. Brennan JA, Boyle JO, Koch WM, Goodman SN, Hruban RH, Eby YJ, Couch MJ, Forastiere AA, Sidransky D. Association between cigarette smoking and mutation of the p53 gene in squamous-cell carcinoma of the head and neck. New Engl J Med 1995; 332:712–717.
16. Notani PN, Jayant K. Role of diet in upper digestive cancers. Nutr Cancer 1987; 10:103–113.

17. Engholm G, Palmgren F, Lynge E. Lung cancer, smoking, and environment: a cohort study of the Danish population. Br Med J 1996; 312:1259–1263.
18. Searle CE, Teale OJ. Occupational carcinogens. In: Cooper CS, Grover PL, eds. Chemical Carcinogenesis and Mutagenesis I. Vol. 94/I, Berlin: Springer Verlag, 1990:103–151.
19. Dockery DW, Trichopoulos D. Risk of lung cancer from environmental exposures to tobacco smoke. Cancer Causes Control 1997; 8:333–345.
20. Hackshaw AK, Law M, Wald NJ. The accumulated evidence on lung cancer and environmental tobacco smoke. Br Med J 1997; 315:980–988.
21. Bofetta P, Agudo A, Ahrens W, Benhamou E, Benhamou S, Darby SC, Ferro G, Fortes C, Gonzalez CA, Jöckel KH, Krauss M, Kreienbrock L, Kreuzer M, Mendes A, Merletti F, Nyberg F, Pershagen G, Pohlabeln H, Riboli E, Schmid G, Simonato L, Trédaniel J, Whitley E, Wichmann H-E, Winck C, Zambon P, Saracci R. Multicenter case–control study of exposure to environmental tobacco smoke and lung cancer in Europe. J Natl Cancer Inst 1998; 90: 1440–1450.
22. Fong KM, Sekido Y, Minna JD. Molecular pathogenesis of lung cancer. J Thorac Cardiovasc Surg 1999; 118:1136–1152.
23. Zöchbauer-Müller S, Fong KM, Virmani AK, Geradts J, Gajdar AF, Minna JD. Aberrant promoter methylation of multiple genes in non-small cell lung cancer. Cancer Res 2001; 61:249–255.
24. Maitra A, Wistuba II, Washington C, Virmani AK, Ashfaq R, Milchgrub S, Gazdar AF, Minna JD. High-resolution chromosome 3p allelotyping of breast carcinomas and precursor lesions demonstrates frequent loss of heterozygosity and a discontinuous pattern of allele loss. Am J Pathol 2001; 159:119–130.
25. Wolff E, Girod S, Liehr T, Vorderwulbecke U, Ries J, Steininger H, Gebhart E. Oral squamous cell carcinomas are characterized by a rather uniform pattern of genomic imbalances detected by comparative genomic hybridisation. Oral Oncol 1998; 34:186–190.
26. Gazdar AF, Minna JD. Cigarettes, sex, and lung adenocarcinoma. J Natl Cancer Inst 1997; 89:1563–1565.
27. Thiberville L, Payne P, Vielkinds J, LeRiche J, Horsman D, Nouvet G, Palcic B, Lam S. Evidence of cumultative gene losses with progression of premalignant epithelial lesions to carcinoma of the bronchus. Cancer Res 1995; 55:5133–5139.
28. Hainaut P, Olivier M, Pfeifer GP. TP53 mutation spectrum in lung cancers and mutagenic signature of components of tobacco smoke: lesson form the IARC TP53 mutation database. Mutagenesis 2001; 16:551–553, 555–556.
29. Chung KY, Mukhopadhyay T, Kim J, Casson A, Ro JY, Goepfert H. Discordant p53 gene mutations in primary head and neck cancers and corresponding second primary cancers of the upper aerodigestive tract. Cancer Res 1993; 53:1676–1683.
30. Salgia R, Skarin AT. Molecular abnormalities in lung cancer. J Clin Oncol 1998; 16:1207–1217.
31. Wormhoudt LW, Commandeur JNM, Vermeulen NPE. Genetic polymorphisms of human N-acetyltransferase, cytochrome P450, glutathione S-transferase, and epoxide hydrolase enzymes: relevance to xenobiotic metabolism and toxicity. Crit Rev Toxicol 1999; 29:59–124.

32. Seidegård J, DePierre JW. Microsomal epoxide hydrolase. Properties, regulation and function. Biochim Biophys Acta 1983; 695:251–270.

33. Hayes JD, Pulford DJ. The glutathione S-transferase supergene family: regulation of GST and the contribution of the isoenzymes to cancer chemoprotection and drug resistance. Crit Rev Biochem Mol Biol 1995; 30:445–600.

34. Kawajiri K, Nakachi K, Imai K, Watanabe J, Hayashi S. The CYP1A1 gene and cancer susceptibility. Crit Rev Oncol Hematol 1993; 14:77–87.

35. Tefre T, Ryberg D, Haugen A, Nebert DW, Skaug V, Brøgger A, Børresen A-L. Human CYP1A1 (cytochrome P$_1$450) gene: lack of association between the MspI restriction fragment length polymorphism and incidence of lung cancer in a Norwegian population. Pharmacogenetics 1991; 1:20–25.

36. Shields PG, Caporaso NE, Falk RT, Sugimura H, Trivers GE, Trump BF, Hoover RN, Westin A, Harris CO. Lung cancer, race and a CYP1A1 genetic polymorphism. Cancer Epidemiol Biomarkers Prev 1993; 2:481–485.

37. Daly AK, Brockmoller J, Broly F, Eichelbaum M, Evans WE, Gonzalez FJ, Huang J-D, Idle JR, Ingelman-Sundberg M, Ishizaki T, Jacqz-Aigrain E, Meyer UA, Nebert DW, Steen VM, Wolf CR, Zanger UM. Nomenclature for human CYP2D6 alleles. Pharmacogenetics 1996; 6:193–201.

38. Bouchardy C, Benhamou S, Dayer P. The effect of tobacco on lung cancer risk depends on CYP2D6 activity. Cancer Res 1996; 56:251–253.

39. Uematsu F, Kikuchi H, Motomiya M, Abe T, Sagami I, Ohmachi T, Wakui A, Kanamaru R, Watanabe M. Association between restriction fragment length polymorphism of the human cytochrome P450IIE1 gene and susceptibility to lung cancer. Jpn J Cancer Res 1991; 82:254–256.

40. Hirvonen A, Husgafvel-Pursiainen K, Karjalainen A, Vainio H. The human CYP2E1 gene and lung cancer: DraI and RsaI restriction fragment length polymorphisms in a Finnish study population. Carcinogenesis 1993; 14:85–88.

41. Persson I, Johansson I, Berling H, Dahl M-L, Seidegård J, Rylander R, Rannug A, Hogberg J, Ingelman-Sundberg M. Genetic polymorphism of cytochrome P4502E1 in a Swedish population. Relationship to incidence of lung cancer. FEBS Lett 1993; 319:207–211.

42. Rebbeck TR. Molecular epidemiology of human glutathione S-transferase genotypes GSTM1 and GSTT1 in cancer susceptibility. Cancer Epidemiol Biomarkers Prev 1997; 6:733–743.

43. Park JY, Muscat JE, Ren Q, Schantz SP, Harwick RD, Stern JC, Pike V, Richie JP Jr, Lazarus P. CYP1A1 and GSTM1 polymorphisms and oral cancer risk. Cancer Epidemiol Biomarkers Prev 1997; 6:791–797.

44. Ryberg D, Skaug V, Hewer A, Phillips DH, Harries LW, Wolf CR, Øgreid D, Ulvik A, Vu P, Haugen A. Genotypes of glutathione transferase M1 and P1 and their significance for lung DNA adduct levels and cancer risk. Carcinogenesis 1997; 18:1285–1289.

45. Hou S-M, Fält S, Yang K, Nyberg F, Pershagen G, Hemminki K, Lambert B. Diffrential interactions between GSTM1 and NAT2 genotypes on aromatic DNA adduct level and HPRT mutant frequency in lung cancer patients and population controls. Cancer Epidemiol Biomarkers Prev 2001; 10:133–140.

46. Miller DP, Liu G, Vivo ID, Lynch TJ, Wain JC, Su L, Christiani DC. Combinations of the variant genotypes of GSTP1, GSTM1 and p53 are associated with an increased lung cancer risk. Cancer Res 2002; 62:2819–2823.

47. Cascorbi I, Brockmöller J, Mrozikiewicz PM, Bauer S, Loddenkemper R, Roots I. Homozygous rapid arylamine N-acetyltransferase (NAT2) genotype as a susceptibility factor for lung cancer. Cancer Res 1996; 56:3961–3966.

48. Nyberg F, Hou S-M, Hemminki K, Lambert B, Pershagen G. Glutathione S-transferase μ1 and N-acetyltransferase 2 genetic polymorphisms and exposure to tobacco smoke in nonsmoking and smoking lung cancer patients and population controls. Cancer Epidemiol Biomarkers Prev 1998; 7: 875–883.

49. Oyama T, Kawamoto T, Mizoue T, Yasumoto K, Kodama Y, Mitsudomi T. N-acetylation polymorphism in patients with lung cancer and its association with p53 gene mutation. Anticancer Res 1997; 17:577–581.

50. London SJ, Smart J, Daly AK. Lung cancer risk in relation to genetic polymorphisms of microsomal epoxide hydrolase among African–American and Caucasian in Los Angeles Country. Lung Cancer 2000; 2:147–155.

51. Zhao H, Spitz MR, Gwyn KM, Wu X. Microsomal epoxide hydrolase polymorphisms and lung cancer risk in non-hispanic whites. Mol Carcinog 2002; 33:99–104.

52. Bosron WF, Li TK. Genetic polymorphism of human liver alcohol and aldehyde dehydrogenases, and their relationship to alcohol metabolism and alcoholism. Hepatology 1986; 6:502–510.

53. Harty LC, Caporaso NE, Hayes RB, Winn DM, Bravo-Otero E, Blot WJ, Kleinman DW, Brown LM, Armenian HK, Fraumeni JF Jr, Shields PG. Alcohol dehydrogenase 3 genotype and risk of oral cavity and pharyngeal cancers. J Natl Cancer Inst 1997; 89:1698–1705.

54. Hayashi S, Watanabe J, Kawajiri K. High susceptibility to lung cancer analyzed in terms of combined genotypes of P4501A1 and mu-class glutathione S-transferase genes. Jpn J Cancer Res 1992; 83:866–870.

55. Nakachi K, Imai K, Hayashi S, Kawajiri K. Polymorphism of the CYP1A1 and glutathione S-transferase genes associated with susceptibility to lung cancer in relation to cigarette dose in a Japanese population. Cancer Res 1993; 53:2994–2999.

56. Wei Q, Cheng L, Hong WK, Spitz MR. Reduced DNA repair capacity in lung cancer patients. Cancer Res 1996; 56:4103–4107.

57. Cheng L, Eicher SA, Guo Z, Hong WK, Spitz MR, Wei Q. Reduced DNA repair capacity in head and neck cancer patients. Cancer Epidemiol Biomarkers Prev 1998; 7:465–468.

58. Wei Q, Spitz MR. The role of DNA repair capacity in susceptibility to lung cancer: a review. Cancer Metast Rev 1997; 16:295–307.

59. Spitz MR, Wu X, Wang Y, Wang LE, Shete S, Amos CI, Guo Z, Lei L, Mohrenweiser H, Wei Q. Modulation of nucleotide excision repair capacity by XPD polymorphisms in lung cancer patients. Cancer Res 2001; 61:1354–1357.

60. Butkiewicz D, Rusin M, Enewold L, Shields PG, Chorazy M, Harris CC. Genetic polymorphisms in DNA repair genes and risk of lung cancer. Carcinogenesis 2001; 22:593–597.

61. Hou SM, Fält S, Angelini S, Yang K, Nyberg F, Lambert B, Hemminki K. The XPD variant alleles are associated with increased aromatic DNA adduct level and lung cancer risk. Carcinogenesis 2002; 23:599–603.

62. Zhou W, Liu G, Miller DP, Thurston SW, Xu LL, Wain JC, Lynch TJ, Su L, Christiani DC. Gene–environment interaction for the ERCC2 polymorphisms and cumulative cigarette smoking exposure in lung cancer. Cancer Res 2002; 62:1377–1381.

63. Shen MR, Jones IM, Mohrenweiser H. Nonconservative amino acid substitution variants exist at polymorphic frequency in DNA repair genes in healthy humans. Cancer Res 1998; 58:604–608.

64. Park JY, Lee SY, Jeon HS, Bae NC, Chae SC, Joo S, Kim CH, Park JH, Kam S, Kim IS, Jung TH. Polymorphism of the DNA repair gene XRCC1 and risk of primary lung cancer. Cancer Epidemiol Biomarkers Prev 2002; 11:23–27.

65. David-Beabes GL, London SJ. Genetic polymorphism of XRCC1 and lung cancer among African–Americans and Caucasians. Lung Cancer 2001; 34:333–339.

66. Sugimura H, Kohno T, Wakai K, et al. hOGG1 Ser326Cys polymorphism and lung cancer susceptibility. Cancer Epidemiol Biomarkers Prev 1999; 8:669–674.

67. Elahi A, Zheng Z, Park J, Eyring K, McCaffrey T, Lazarus P. The human OGG1 DNA repair enzyme and its association with orolaryngeal cancer risk. Carcinogenesis 2002; 23:1229–1234.

68. Haugen A. Women who smoke: are women more susceptible to tobacco induced lung cancer? Carcinogenesis 2002; 23:227–229.

69. Zang E, Wynder EL. Differences in lung cancer risk between men and women: examination of the evidence. J Natl Cancer Inst 1996; 88:183–192.

70. Prescott E, Osler M, Hein HO, Borch-Jonsen K, Lange P, Schnohr P, Vestbo J. Gender and smoking-related risk of lung cancer: the Copenhagen center for prospective population studies. Epidemiology 1998; 9:79–83.

71. Ryberg D, Hewer A, Phillips DH, Haugen A. Different susceptibility to smoking-induced DNA damage among male and female lung cancer patients. Cancer Res 1994; 54:5801–5803.

72. Mollerup S, Ryberg D, Hewer A, Phillips DH, Haugen A. Sex differences in lung CYP1A1 expression and DNA adduct levels among lung cancer patients. Cancer Res 1999; 59:3317–3320.

73. Kure EH, Ryberg D, Hewer A, Phillips DH, Skaug V, Bæra R, Haugen A. p53 mutations in lung tumors: relationship to gender lung DNA adduct levels. Carcinogenesis 1996; 17:2201–2205.

74. Guinee DG, Travis WD Jr, Trivers GE, De Bendetti VMG, Cawley H, Welsh JA, Bennett WP, Jett J, Colby TV, Tazelaar H, Abbondanzo SL, Pairolero P, Trastek V, Caparaso NE, Liotta LA, Harris CC. Gender comparisons in human lung cancer: analysis of p53 mutations, anti-p53 antibodies and c-erbB-2 expression. Carcinogenesis 1995; 16:993–1002.

75. Mollerup S, Jørgenen K, Berge G, Haugen A. Expression of estrogen receptors α and β in human lung tissue and cell lines. Lung Cancer 2002; 37:153–159.

76. Shiver SP, Bourdeau HA, Gubish CT, Tirpark DL, Davis LG, Luketich JD, Siegfried JM. Sex-specific expresson of gastrin-releasing peptide receptor:

relationship to smoking history and risk of lung cancer. J Natl Cancer Inst 2000; 92:24–33.
77. Willey J, Lechner J, Harris CC. Bombesin and C-terminal tetradecapeptide of gastrin-releasing peptide are growth factors for normal bronchial epithelial cells. Exp Cell Res 1984; 153:245–248.

20

Head and Neck Cancers

**Qingyi Wei, Hongbing Shen, and
Margaret R. Spitz**

*Department of Epidemiology, M. D. Anderson Cancer Center, University of
Texas, Houston, Texas, U.S.A.*

Erich M. Sturgis

*Department of Head and Neck Surgery, M. D. Anderson Cancer Center,
University of Texas, Houston, Texas, U.S.A.*

Peter G. Shields

*Cancer Genetics and Epidemiology Program, Department of Medicine and
Oncology, Lombardi Cancer Center, Georgetown University Medical
Center, Washington, D.C., U.S.A.*

1. INTRODUCTION

Head and neck cancers, also known as cancers of the upper aerodigestive
tract, are chiefly squamous cell carcinomas arising in the oral cavity,
pharynx, or larynx. About 40,000 persons are diagnosed with squamous cell
carcinoma of the head and neck (SCCHN) in the United States each year,
and about 12,000 die of the disease (1). The male:female ratio of patients
is about 2:1 for oral and pharyngeal cancer but 4:1 for laryngeal
cancer. Only a fraction of individuals exposed to tobacco smoke and/or
alcohol develop SCCHN, suggesting that there are differences in individual
susceptibility to carcinogenesis and that the impact of gene–environment
interactions should be considered. Tobacco carcinogens undergo a series
of metabolic activation and detoxification steps that determine the internal
dose of exposure and ultimately impact the level of DNA damage incurred.

Both endogenous and exogenous exposure to carcinogens or genotoxic agents cause cell-cycle delays (2) that allow cells to repair such DNA damage. Therefore, the cellular DNA repair capacity (DRC) is central to maintaining genomic integrity and normal cellular functions (3). Recently, molecular epidemiological studies of tobacco-induced carcinogenesis were comprehensively reviewed (4–6). Also, studies have shown that polymorphisms of genes that control drug metabolism (7–9) and DNA repair (10–13) may contribute to the variation in tobacco-induced carcinogenesis in the general population. This chapter focuses on recent molecular epidemiological studies with an emphasis on the role of DNA repair in susceptibility to SCCHN.

2. RISK FACTORS FOR SCCHN
2.1. Tobacco and Alcohol Exposure

Tobacco initiates a linear dose–response carcinogenic effect in which the duration of exposure is more important than the intensity of exposure. The major carcinogenic activity of cigarette smoke resides in the particulate (tar) fraction, which contains a complex mixture of interacting cancer initiators, promoters, and co-carcinogens. In the late 1950s, a landmark case–control study by Dr. Ernst Wynder established the link between tobacco use and oral cavity cancer (14). This was followed a year later by a cohort study of more than 180,000 men that demonstrated an increased risk of death due to SCCHN in cigarette smokers when compared with men who never smoked (15). These studies also demonstrated an elevated risk of death due to SCCHN in cigar and pipe smokers. Due to limitations because of the sample size and follow-up time, Hill's classic cohort study of more than 40,000 British physicians showed only a borderline risk of SCCHN related to smoking (16). In 1964, the Advisory Committee to the Surgeon General on Smoking and Health published a report linking smoking with cancer based on many of Doll & Hill's classic criteria of disease causality, and these criteria have been clearly demonstrated linking SCCHN and tobacco smoking over the past 40 years in multiple independent studies (17–20). Most importantly, the strength and consistency of the association between smoking and SCCHN have been demonstrated in numerous case–control and cohort studies with significant relative risks or odds ratios (ORs) in the 3–12-fold range. Furthermore, these studies consistently showed a dose–response effect of the duration and dose of smoking on increasing risk of SCCHN and of the time since quitting on decreasing risk of SCCHN (17,18,21). The specificity of the link between tobacco exposure and SCCHN (not identifying nonmucosal/unexposed head and neck malignancies), coherence and analogy of the explanation of tobacco-induced SCCHN to lung carcinogenesis, and biological plausibility of the well-established tobacco-induced carcinogenesis model have all helped establish tobacco as the chief etiological agent in SCCHN.

Although the risk of bronchogenic carcinoma appears to be less significant for cigar and pipe smokers than for cigarette smokers, these forms of tobacco use are clearly associated with an increased risk of SCCHN (21–23). The pooling of saliva containing carcinogens in gravity-dependent regions may account for the frequent occurrence of oral carcinomas along the lateral and ventral surfaces of the tongue and in the floor of the mouth (24). Smokeless tobacco use has also been demonstrated to be associated with cancer of the oral cavity (25). Smokeless tobacco users and pipe smokers who habitually use the same position for their quid and pipe stem, respectively, often develop carcinomas and dysplasias at the specific site of use, which suggests that physical and thermal trauma may be contributing factors.

While the smoking rate is declining by approximately 1.5% annually in the developed world, it is rising by 2% annually in developing countries, home to four-fifths of the world's population. In the United States, the smoking rate has declined since the Surgeon General's warning in 1964 (26). Specifically, in 1965, 42.4% of the U.S. adult population were current smokers, while in 1999, only 23.5% were current smokers. While the reduction in cigarette smoking has been much greater in men than in women over the past three decades, the rate of current cigarette use remains higher in men (25.7%) than in women (21.5%). Furthermore, 40.8% of Native Americans continue to smoke (27). Other concerns include the increasing rate of cigarette smoking among high school seniors and dramatic increase in the number of new cigar smokers over the past decade (26). A dramatic increase in smokeless tobacco use among younger people has been implicated by some in the rise of oral cancer mortality rates in this group (28,29). Striking variations in head and neck cancer sites and incidence seen among different regions, cultures, and demographic groups are due in large part to differing patterns of abuse of tobacco and other substances (30). For example, smokeless tobacco and similar products are used greatly in parts of Asia and Africa (30–32). In south central Asia in particular, "pano" (betel leaf, lime, catechu, and areca nut) is commonly chewed and is a strong risk factor independent of tobacco use for carcinoma of the oral cavity, one of the most common cancers in men and women in this region (32).

However, tobacco is not the only factor in the complex causality equation for these cancers. Alcohol is an important promoter of carcinogenesis and a contributing factor in at least 75% of SCCHNs (17,18). Furthermore, alcohol consumption appears to have an effect on the risk of SCCHN independent of tobacco smoking, but this effect is consistently significant only at the highest level of alcohol consumption (14,17,21). While studies attempting to correlate the different types of alcoholic beverages with specific cancer risks have been conflicting, most investigators believe that ethanol itself is the main causative factor (14,21,33). Nevertheless, it appears

that the major clinical significance of alcohol consumption is that it potenti-
ates the carcinogenic effect of tobacco at every level of tobacco exposure.
However, this effect is most striking at the highest levels of exposure, and
its magnitude is at least additive but may be multiplicative dependent on
the subsite of SCCHN and level of exposure (17,18).

2.2. Genetic Susceptibility

The predominant risk factor for SCCHN is a history of tobacco and alcohol
use. However, because only a fraction of smokers ever develop cancer,
variations in genetic susceptibility may be equally important in the disease
etiology. A genetic component of this disease is supported by large family
studies demonstrating a three- to eight-fold increased risk of SCCHN in
first-degree relatives of patients with SCCHN (34). Furthermore, there
is molecular epidemiological evidence supporting the concept of genetic
susceptibility in head and neck cancer patients (35). Emerging data from
case–control studies of several phenotyping and genotyping assays support
the hypothesis that genetic susceptibility plays an important role in the
etiology of SCCHN. According to this hypothesis, inherited differences in
the efficiency of carcinogen-metabolizing, DNA repair, and/or cell cycle
control/apoptosis systems influence one's risk of tobacco-induced cancers.
Identifying such at-risk individuals in the general population using these
biomarker assays would have a profound impact on primary prevention,
early detection, and secondary prevention strategies.

2.3. Infectious Agents

While it has been suggested that various infectious agents play a role in
head and neck carcinogenesis, only Epstein–Barr virus (EBV) and human
papilloma virus (HPV) can be implicated as etiological agents in head and
neck carcinogenesis based on current scientific evidence. Epstein–Barr virus
appears to be associated with most nasopharyngeal carcinomas, while
HPV (most commonly, type 16) is associated with approximately 50% of
oropharyngeal carcinomas. Although herpes simplex viruses have been
suggested as risk factors for oral cavity cancer (36) and *Helicobacter pylori*
has been suggested as a risk factor for laryngeal cancer (37), confirmation of
these findings is lacking (38).

   While laboratory evidence supporting the role of HPV as a risk
factor for SCCHN is largely circumstantial, HPV has been established as
an etiological agent in cervical cancer (39). More recently, several investigators suggested that infection with HPV, especially the high-risk HPV-16, is a
risk factor for SCCHN (40). The chief oncoproteins of HPV-16 are encoded
by the E6 and E7 genes. The E6 oncoprotein targets the tumor suppressor
gene *p53* for ubiquitination and degradation; in fact, degradation of *p53*

in HPV-positive cells is fully dependent on the presence of E6 (41). The E7 oncoprotein is involved in suppression of pRb function; reduced pRb expression is common in HPV-positive tonsillar cancers (42). In vitro experiments support the tumorigenicity of HPV-16 in human epithelial cells. Furthermore, numerous studies using methods such as polymerase chain reaction (PCR), Southern blotting, and in situ hybridization detected HPV DNA in the tumor tissue and sera of SCCHN patients (40). In those studies, oropharyngeal tumors and tumors in nonsmokers were the most frequently positive for HPV DNA. However, because they did not include cancer-free controls, most of these studies were unable to estimate the risk of SCCHN attributable to HPV-16. Molecular epidemiological evidence with a case–control design supporting the role of HPV-16 in SCCHN has emerged, however (36,43). In a recent nested case–control study of 292 cases and 1568 controls from a Scandinavian cohort of almost 900,000 subjects, Mork et al. (44) reported that HPV-16 seropositivity was associated with a 2.2-fold increased risk of SCCHN after multivariate adjustment. However, 25% of the cases in that study were not classic SCCHN: 3% were nasopharyngeal cancers, 20% were lip cancers, and 2% were sinus cancers. Because subjects with cancers at these sites were less frequently seropositive for HPV-16, Mork and colleagues may have underestimated the risk of SCCHN associated with HPV-16 exposure. In their subgroup analysis of oropharyngeal cancer, Mork et al. reported an estimated risk of 14.4 [95% confidence interval (CI), 3.6–58.1]. An additional serological study using a population-based case–control study design of 284 subjects with newly diagnosed oral or oropharyngeal carcinoma and 477 cancer-free controls demonstrated a significantly elevated risk associated with HPV-16 seropositivity (adjusted OR, 2.3; 95% CI, 1.6–3.3) (45). While the researchers did not perform a subgroup risk analysis for oropharyngeal cancer, the chief effect again appeared to be in the oropharyngeal cancer subgroup, approximately 35% of whom had cancer positive for HPV-16 DNA. The circumstantial, mechanistic, and molecular epidemiological evidence strongly supports the role of HPV-16 infection in oropharyngeal carcinogenesis.

2.4. Environmental Tobacco Smoke

A recent high-profile legal case in Australia has brought significant interest to the risk of SCCHN secondary to exposure to environmental tobacco smoke. In May 2001, the New South Wales Supreme Court found that SCCHN in a 62-year-old nonsmoker was associated with long-term exposure to environmental tobacco smoke in her job as a bar attendant significant enough to impose liability on her employer (46). Two case–control studies supported the court's finding. In the first study of 173 SCCHN patients and 176 cancer-free controls, environmental tobacco smoke exposure was associated with a greater than two fold increased risk of SCCHN, and a dose–response relationship was observed (47). In the second study of 44 nonsmokers with SCCHN and 132 cancer-free nonsmoking controls, environmental tobacco smoke exposure was associated with a significantly increased risk of SCCHN (OR, 5.34), particularly in female subjects (OR, 8.00) and those reporting exposure at their workplace (OR, 10.16) (48).

2.5. Laryngopharyngeal Reflux

Observational and anecdotal studies have long suggested that gastroesophageal reflux is associated with laryngeal cancer (49,50). Furthermore, multiple studies have objectively documented a high prevalence of gastric reflux into the laryngopharynx using 24-h pH probe monitoring (50,51). Recently, a retrospective case–control study of 10,140 inpatients and 12,061 outpatients with laryngeal or pharyngeal cancer and 40,560 inpatients and 48,244 outpatient controls was performed using computerized hospital and outpatient databases of the U.S. Department of Veterans Affairs (52). A diagnosis of gastroesophageal reflux disease was associated with a significantly elevated risk of laryngeal cancer (OR, 2.40; 95% CI, 2.15–2.69; and OR, 2.31; 95% CI , 2.10–2.53 for inpatients and outpatient groups, respectively) and of pharyngeal cancer (OR, 2.38; 95% CI, 1.87–3.02 and OR, 1.92; 96% CI, 1.72–2.15 for inpatients and outpatient groups, respectively). These risk estimates were adjusted for age, gender, ethnicity, smoking, and alcohol consumption.

2.6. Marijuana

Compared with tobacco smoke, marijuana smoke has a four times greater tar burden and 50% higher concentration of benzo[a]pyrene and aromatic hydrocarbons. While anecdotal evidence has long suggested that marijuana smoking is a risk factor for SCCHN, few reports have found direct evidence of marijuana as an etiological factor for SCCHN because most users of marijuana are also exposed to tobacco and alcohol (53). A recent case–control study that included 173 SCCHN patients and 176 cancer-free controls demonstrated a cigarette smoking-adjusted risk of SCCHN of 2.6 (95% CI, 1.1–6.6) associated with marijuana use with evidence of a dose–response relationship (54). However, a large retrospective cohort of 64,855 health maintenance organization members found no association with tobacco-related cancers (55).

2.7. Diet

Epidemiological evidence from studies using traditional case–control study designs suggests that a diet high in animal fats and low in fruits and vegetables may be a risk factor for SCCHN (56–59). Specifically, Winn and colleagues found that the risk of oral and pharyngeal cancer in women was inversely related to consumption of fresh fruits and vegetables (56). Similarly, in a study of 871 individuals with oral or pharyngeal cancer and 979 cancer-free controls, McLaughlin et al. (57) demonstrated an inverse relationship between fruit intake and oral and pharyngeal cancer risk. In a Chinese population-based case–control study, intake of citrus fruits and dark green/yellow vegetables was associated with a decreased risk of laryngeal cancer, while intake of salted fish and meat as well as deep-fried foods was associated with an increased risk of laryngeal cancer (58). More recently, both European and U.S. studies have confirmed the protective effects of eating fruits and vegetables and the risk of animal fat consumption after adjustment for smoking and alcohol use (59,60). Some evidence suggests that vitamin A and beta-carotene are responsible for the protective effect of a diet high in fruits and vegetables and that a deficiency of carotenoids appears to be a risk factor for SCCHN and lung cancers (58). It is not known, however, which of the more than 500 carotenoids are protective, which chemical interactions may occur, and which protective roles other micronutrients in carotenoid-rich foods may play. Others have found that total intake of vitamins C and E is also protective (56,60). Moreover, diets are complex and difficult to assess and validate; in particular, there are often inaccuracies in translating foods into constituent nutrients. Further studies are needed to more precisely define the relationship between dietary intake and serum levels of the various carotenoid components. It may be impossible to determine which of the vast array of compounds is most beneficial, and controlling for other dietary variables and confounding risk factors has remained a difficult problem. Further confounding this situation is that smoking has been associated with reduced dietary intake and serum levels of carotenoids. Despite these many problems, prospective and retrospective nutritional (serum and dietary) epidemiological studies have provided important clues about the development and prevention of these cancers.

3. MOLECULAR EPIDEMIOLOGY OF SCCHN

The study of genetic susceptibility can improve the accuracy of estimates of association with carcinogen exposure (61). Tobacco toxicants affect people to variable degrees. There is considerable interindividual variation in cellular responses, for example, in metabolism and detoxification of toxicants, and DRC. As other cellular responses to DNA damage are identified (e.g., cell cycle delays, heat shock, etc.), interindividual variation in risk is likely to be attributed to these responses as well. Interindividual effects of cellular responses may be due to genetically determined differences in enzyme expression, kinetics, or stability. Induction of enzymes from previous exposure or comorbidity also may contribute to cancer risk, and induction has a genetic component.

Disease risk due to genetic variations ranges from small to large depending on the genetic penetrance. Highly penetrant cancer susceptibility genes cause familial cancers but account for less than 1% of all cancers (62). Lowly penetrant genes cause common sporadic cancers and have greater public health consequences (4) because they are highly prevalent.

Genetic susceptibility can be assessed either phenotypically (measuring the resultant enzymatic function) or genotypically (determining the genetic code). Phenotypic assays may include determination of enzymatic activity by administering probe drugs and measuring blood levels or urinary metabolites, assessing the carcinogen metabolic capacity in cultured lymphocytes, or establishing the ratios of endogenously produced substances, such as estrogen metabolites. One of the most extensively studied phenotypes in relation to smoking risk is aryl hydrocarbon hydroxylase activity (63). In general, using a genotypic assay is preferable to using a phenotypic assay to assess cancer risk because DNA is easier to obtain and the assays are technically simpler. However, phenotypes represent a multigenic trait and may not be adequately characterized with one genetic assay. Therefore, there is a role for both genotype- and phenotype-based assays in research studies of cancer risk.

3.1. Xenobiotic Metabolisms of Carcinogens in SCCHN

Mucosa of the upper aerodigestive tract can metabolically activate tobacco-smoke carcinogens, resulting in DNA damage (64). The highest levels of *CYP1A1* expression have been reported in these tissues compared with that in other sites (65). Also, *NAT1* but not *NAT2* activity has been demonstrated in the mucosa of the head and neck, and there is evidence that *CYP2C* plays an important role in these tissues. Furthermore, aromatic DNA and 4-ABP adducts have been detected in laryngeal tissues at higher levels in smokers than in nonsmokers (66,67).

N-nitroso compounds in smokeless tobacco have been demonstrated to cause cancers of the mouth and lip, nasal cavity, esophagus, stomach, and lungs in laboratory animals. Urinary metabolites of tobacco-specific nitrosamines have been measured in persons using smokeless tobacco products, with higher levels associated with oral leukoplakia, indicating greater use of such products. Hemoglobin adducts to these carcinogens are measurable in the blood of smokeless tobacco users (68) and thus may be useful biomarkers for measuring exposure levels in them. For instance, hemoglobin adduct levels have been found to be higher in snuff users than in nonusers. Other exposures that occur with the use of smokeless tobacco products include those to compounds that cause oxidative DNA damage (69). Several studies have indicated that there is an increased risk of SCCHN among individuals who have a heritable trait, such as genetic polymorphisms of these genes, although which marker plays the greatest role is not known (70–73), and there is evidence of a greater effect in persons at lower levels of smoking (73). In one study, heritable traits in carcinogen metabolism increased the frequency of *p53* mutations (74).

The *p53* gene is commonly mutated in cancers associated with the use of smokeless tobacco products. While some differences in the spectrum have been reported in different regions of the world, there are no consistent hotspots or patterns when compared with oral cavity cancers related to smoking. The mutational spectrum of *p53* in SCCHN is similar to that in lung cancer (75), although some disagree (76). Additionally, mutations occur more often in smokers than in nonsmokers (75,77,78). In a study by Brennan et al. (77), the frequency of *p53* mutations was higher in tobacco and alcohol users than in those who did not use tobacco or alcohol.

3.2. DNA Repair Phenotype and Risk of SCCHN

Through the process of evolution, species of all living organisms have developed sophisticated DNA repair pathways and mechanisms to battle genomic insults from environmental hazards to survive and maintain genomic integrity. The DRC appears to meet the challenge from the natural environment. For instance, the human skin repair capacity just meets the repair demand from sunlight exposure at midday (79). Overloaded DNA damage leads to either cell death or mutant cancerous cells that have escaped from repair systems. It has been reported that more than 150 human genes are involved in various repair pathways, a number that is likely to increase when the Human Genome Project refines its published draft of the human genome (80). These repair genes are grossly categorized into the four most important and well-characterized repair pathways: base excision repair (BER), nucleotide excision repair (NER), mismatch repair (MMR), and homologous recombinational repair (HRR).

Assays that measure cellular DNA repair are now being applied in population studies to investigate the association between DNA repair and susceptibility to cancer. Generally, cellular responses to DNA damage fall into three major categories: direct reversal of damage, e.g., enzymatic photore activation; excision of damage by BER or NER; and postreplication repair, namely, MMR and HRR (3). While the presence of only one unrepaired DNA lesion can block the transcription of an essential gene (81,82), there is a wide range of repair ability in the general population (83,84), with xeroderma pigmentosum (XP) patients representing the lowest end of the repair spectrum (85). Because there is a shortage of target tissues for laboratory experiments, peripheral blood lymphocytes have been used extensively as surrogate tissues (83,86).

3.2.1. Host-Cell Reactivation Assay for Nucleotide Excision Repair

While there are many assays that measure the efficiency of multiple steps of excision repair individually, the ability to test the whole pathway is needed for population studies, in which time, cost, and repeatability of the measurements are major concerns. Therefore, the host-cell reactivation (HCR) assay, which measures the level of expression of a damaged reporter gene as a marker of the repair proficiency in the host cell is the assay of choice (87,88). The HCR assay uses undamaged cells, is relatively fast, and is an objective method of measuring DRC. In this assay, a damaged nonreplicating recombinant plasmid (pCMV*cat* or pCVM*luv*) harboring a chloramphenicol acetyltransferase (or luciferase) reporter gene is introduced into cultured cells such as primary lymphocytes via transfection (88). For instance, reactivated chloramphenicol acetyltransferase enzyme activity is measured as a function of NER of the damaged reporter gene (87). Both lymphocytes (83) and skin fibroblasts (89) from patients who have basal cell carcinoma but not XP have lower excision-repair rates of a UV-damaged reporter gene than individuals without cancer. This finding suggests that the repair capacity of lymphocytes can be considered a reflection of an individual's overall repair capacity.

To investigate whether differences in DRC for repairing tobacco carcinogen-induced DNA damage are associated with differential susceptibility to tobacco-related cancer, the HCR assay with benzo[a]pyrene diol epoxide (BPDE) -damaged plasmids was used in both an initial pilot study (51 lung cancer patients and 56 frequency-matched controls) (90), and a subsequent large hospital-based case–control study of lung cancer (316 lung cancer patients and 316 cancer-free controls) (84). Statistically significantly lower DRC was observed in the patients when compared with the controls, which was associated with a greater than two-fold increase in risk of lung cancer (84). Compared with the highest DRC quartile in the controls, suboptimal DRC was associated with an increased risk of lung cancer in a dose–response fashion. Patients who were younger at diagnosis (< 60 years), female, lighter smokers, or reported to have a family history of cancer exhibited the lowest DRC and therefore were associated with the highest lung cancer risk, suggesting that these subgroups may be especially susceptible to lung cancer (84). The low DRC found in women in this study is consistent with epidemiological findings showing that women are at higher risk for tobacco-induced cancer than men are at the same exposure level (91–93). Using the same assay, Cheng et al. (94) investigated the role of DRC in head and neck cancers. Again, DRC was significantly lower in the patients than in the controls with a similar dose–response trend, that is, those in the middle and lowest DRC tertiles had a greater than two-fold and four-fold increased risk, respectively. These results suggest that suboptimal DRC may contribute to susceptibility to tobacco carcinogenesis, such as in the lung and head and neck.

3.2.2. Mutagen Sensitivity Assay

The mutagen sensitivity assay is another functional assay that measures chromatid breaks in response to in vitro exposure to carcinogens in short-term cultures of peripheral blood lymphocytes. Several case–control (95–97) and cohort studies (98,99) have suggested that induced and spontaneous lymphocytic chromosome aberrations can be used as markers of susceptibility to cancer. The implications of chromosomal aberrations and genomic instability in carcinogenesis of the head and neck have been comprehensively reviewed elsewhere (100,101).

In the general population, the frequency of spontaneous chromosome aberrations is low (102), and classic cytogenetic assays that assess these types of aberrations may not be applicable to epidemiological studies requiring a large number of samples. Therefore, Hsu et al. developed an assay of mutagen sensitivity to measure genetic susceptibility to cancer by estimating the frequency of in vitro bleomycin-induced breaks in short-term lymphocyte cultures (103,104). Bleomycin is considered radiomimetic (i.e., it causes the generation of free oxygen radicals), which is relevant to tobacco-induced carcinogenesis because numerous compounds in tobacco condensate may generate free oxygen radicals that can induce single- and double-strand breaks. Mutagen sensitivity has consistently been shown to be a significant independent predictor of the risk of upper aerodigestive tract cancers in case–control studies (96,97,103,105,106). For instance, lighter and former smokers appear to be more sensitive than heavier smokers do as measured by this bleomycin assay, as do younger patients compared with older ones. In upper aerodigestive tract cancer patients, bleomycin sensitivity has been found to be highest in those under the age of 30 years among the age groups investigated (107). These results suggest that the mutagen sensitivity assay may serve as a biomarker for susceptibility to tobacco-related cancers.

The bleomycin assay was later modified by using BPDE as the test mutagen (108), and this BPDE sensitivity was found to be associated with a significantly elevated risk for head and neck cancer (109). In this pilot case–control study of 60 SCCHN patients and 112 healthy controls, a high frequency of BPDE-induced chromatid breaks was associated with a greater than two-fold increase in the risk of head and neck cancer, and there was a dose–response relationship between the frequency of BPDE-induced chromatid breaks and risk of SCCHN, suggesting that the number of BPDE-induced breaks per cell is a significant risk factor for head and neck cancer (109). The findings that cancer is more likely to develop in younger people who have the BPDE sensitive phenotype support the hypothesis that the presence of BPDE-induced chromatid breaks is a marker for genetic susceptibility to tobacco-induced carcinogenesis.

It has been suggested that the mutagen sensitivity assay indirectly measures the effectiveness of one or more DNA repair mechanisms (110). A correlation between the cellular DRC measured using the HCR assay and frequency of mutagen-induced in vitro chromatid breaks has been reported (11,90,111). Mutagen sensitivity may also be involved in an inherent chromatin alteration that permits more efficient translation of DNA damage into chromosome damage after exposure to a mutagen (112). Although the mechanism underlying the association between induced chromosomal aberrations and susceptibility to cancer remains to be unraveled, tobacco smoke causes both oxidative damage and bulky adducts. Defects in both BER and NER mechanisms may therefore dramatically increase the risk of smoking-related cancer.

3.2.3. ^{32}P-Postlabeling Assay of DNA Adducts

A relatively large variation has been observed in the level of persistent DNA adducts in vivo believed to be related to smoking (113,114). Although this variation may be partly due to the experimental methodology used, it may also be a true biological variation that is a valid phenotypic marker for the joint effect of host metabolic activities and DNA repair in response to carcinogen exposure (115). Using the ^{32}P-postlabeling assay developed by Reddy and Randerath (116), Phillips et al. (117) noted a linear relationship between the levels of aromatic DNA adducts in the human lung and number of cigarettes smoked per day. While some studies have failed to find a correlation between lymphocyte adduct levels and smoking habits (118,119), one study did report a significant difference between the aromatic DNA adduct levels in smokers and nonsmokers (86).

A large variation in adduct levels in vivo may be driven by a variation in the activities of enzymes involved in carcinogen bioactivation (120,121) such as CYP1A2 (122), which can be induced by smoking in the target tissues (123). To tackle this problem, Li et al. (115) developed a new assay of in vitro induction of carcinogen–DNA adducts by an ultimate carcinogen. In this assay, stimulated lymphocytes were treated with BPDE (the ultimate carcinogen of benzo[a]pyrene, which does not need bioactivation). Therefore, variation in the level of BPDE-induced DNA adducts should reflect only genetic variation in phase II enzymes and DRC. However, phase II enzymes have little, if any, effect on the in vitro formation of adducts in this assay because of the relatively high concentration of BPDE used (4 µM) and the rapid binding of BPDE to DNA, which peaks within 15 min (124). This ultimate carcinogen generates in vitro adduct levels that are 100-fold higher than in vivo adduct levels. Furthermore, the variation in such induced adduct levels is within 100-fold rather than 1000-fold as often seen in vivo.

In a pilot study of 91 patients with SCCHN and 115 cancer-free controls, Li et al. (125) found that the levels of BPDE-induced DNA adducts were significantly higher in patients than in the controls. Using the median level of control values $(35/10^7)$ as the cutoff point, they also found that about 66% of the patients were distributed above this level. High levels of BPDE-induced DNA adducts were associated with a greater than two-fold increased risk. There was a statistically significant dose–response relationship between the quartile levels of BPDE-induced DNA adducts and risk of head and neck cancer, suggesting that this biomarker may compliment others in identifying individuals at increased risk for developing tobacco-related cancers. Indeed, similar findings were observed in lung cancer studies (115,126).

3.2.4. Assays of DNA Repair Gene Transcript (mRNA) Levels

While the DRC phenotype can be affected by polymorphisms of genes that participate in the repair pathway, epigenetic factors may also influence the repair outcome. For instance, the level of expression of repair genes may be affected epigenetically. To investigate the variation in expression, a multiplex RT-PCR assay has been used to measure the levels of several DNA repair gene transcripts relative to those of a ubiquitous housekeeping gene (127). In this technique, transcripts from several repair genes and the β-actin gene are simultaneously amplified, and the transcript levels are quantified in relation to the β-actin level using computerized densitometry analysis of gel electrophoresis of the multiplex RT-PCR products. This assay is also flexible in that it groups the genes involved in the same repair pathway such as MMR (128) or NER (129) into one experiment.

Using this multiplex RT-PCR assay, Wei et al. (130) simultaneously evaluated the relative levels of expression of five MMR genes (*hMSH2*, *hMLH*1, *hPMS*1, *hPMS*2, and *hGTBP/hMSH6*) in the peripheral blood lymphocytes of 78 patients with head and neck cancer and 86 cancer-free controls. The relative MMR gene expression was not correlated with the disease stage or tumor site in the patients or with smoking and alcohol use in the controls, but it did increase with age in both patients and controls. The mean level of expression of *hMLH1*, *hPMS1*, and *hGTBP/hMSH6* was significantly lower in the patients than in the controls. Low expression of *hMLH1* was associated with a greater than four-fold increase in risk, while low expression of *hGTBP/hMSH6* was associated with a greater than two-fold increase in risk. Cheng et al. (131) used this assay to measure the relative level of expression of five NER genes *ERCC1* (ERCC, excision repair cross-complementing), *XPB/ERCC3*, *XPG/ERCC5*, *CSB/ERCC6* (CSB, Cockayne's syndrome complementary group B), and *XPC* and in phytohemagglutinin-stimulated peripheral blood lymphocytes obtained from 57 SCCHN patients and 105 cancer-free controls. They found that the levels of *ERCC1*, *XPB/ERCC3*, *XPG/ERCC5*, and *CSB/ERCC6* transcripts were lower in the patients than in the controls. In a multivariate logistic regression analysis (adjusting for age, gender, race, smoking status, and alcohol use), low expression of *ERCC1, XPB/ERCC3, XPG/ERCC5,* and *CSB/ERCC6* was associated with a statistically significantly increased risk of SCCHN (adjusted OR (95% CI), 6.42 (2.63–15.69), 2.86 (1.39–5.90), 3.69 (1.73–7.90), and 2.46 (1.19–5.09), respectively). These results suggest that individuals with low expression of DNA repair genes may be at higher risk for SCCHN.

3.3. DNA Repair Genotypes and Risk of SCCHN

Polymorphisms of DNA repair genes may also contribute to variations in DRC. Clearly, functional (phenotypic) studies of DNA repair in individuals with various DNA repair genotypes are needed. However, it will be difficult to detect subtle differences in DRC in such studies due to a single polymorphism of a single gene in a very complex pathway. Recently, the entire coding regions of the following DNA repair genes on chromosome 19 were resequenced in 12 normal individuals (132): three NER genes (*ERCC1, XPD/ERCC2,* and *XPF/ERCC4*), one HRR gene (*XRCC3*), and one BER gene (*XRCC1*). Among these, 7 variants of *ERCC1,* 17 variants of *XPD/ERCC2,* 6 variants of *XPF/ERCC4,* 4 variants of *XRCC3,* and 12 variants of *XRCC1* were identified. Of these variants, 4 of *XPD/ERCC2,* 3 of *XRCC1,* 1 of *XRCC3* and 1 of *XPF/ERCC4* result in an amino acid sequence change. Later, another 6 variants of *XPF/ERCC4* were identified in 38 individuals (133), 2 variants of *XPA* (chromosome 9), and 2 variants of *XPB/ERCC3* (chromosome 2) were identified in 35 individuals, and 2 variants of *XPC* (chromosome 3) (134) and 3 variants of *XPG/ERCC5* (chromosome 13) (135) were also identified. Although the significance of these variants is largely unknown, the implication is those that cause amino acid substitutions may have an impact on the function of the proteins and therefore on the efficiency of DNA repair. Variants that do not cause an amino acid change may also have an impact on the DNA repair function through altered splicing, mRNA instability, or linkage with other genetic changes. Therefore, knowing the impact of these polymorphisms on disease risk is important to ultimately understanding their functional relevance.

The XPD protein is an evolutionarily conserved helicase, a subunit of transcription factor IIH (TFIIH) that is essential for transcription and NER (136). Mutations in *XPD* prevent its protein from interacting with *p44,* another subunit of TFIIH (137), and decrease helicase activity, resulting in a defect in NER. Furthermore, mutations at different sites result in distinct clinical phenotypes (138). *XPD* is also thought to be involved in the repair of genetic damage induced by tobacco carcinogens (111).

Several *XPD* polymorphisms were recently identified in the coding regions of different exons at a relatively high frequency (132,139). These common polymorphisms (allele frequencies > 0.20) included C22541A (156Arg) of exon 6, C35326T (711Asp) without amino acid changes and G23592A (Asp312Asn) of exon 10, and A35931C (Lys751Gln) with amino acid changes of exon 23. The Lys751Gln polymorphism is located about 50 bp upstream from the poly(A) signal and therefore may alter XPD protein function (139). In a study of 31 women, those with the 751Gln/Gln genotype were found to have a higher number of chromatid aberrations induced by X-rays (140). However, this finding was not confirmed in another study that measured the frequency of smoking-induced sister chromatid exchanges and polyphenol DNA adducts ($n = 61$) (141).

In a case–control study of 189 SCCHN patients and 496 cancer-free controls, Sturgis et al. (111) found that the frequency of the XPD 22541 AA homozygous genotype was lower in the patients (15.9%) than in the controls (20.4%), but that the difference was not statistically significant. However, the frequency of the 751Gln/Gln homozygous genotype was higher in the patients (16.4%) than in the controls (11.5%) and was associated with a borderline increased risk (OR, 1.55). The risk was higher in older subjects (OR, 2.22), current smokers (OR, 1.83), and current drinkers (OR, 2.59). Although no studies reported the role of the Asp312Asn variant in the etiology of SCCHN, the Asp312Asn variant was found to be associated with a nearly two fold increase in the risk of lung cancer in two independent studies (142,143). The *XPD* C22541A and C35326T polymorphisms are silent, resulting in no amino acid substitutions (132), and they were not found to be associated with an increased risk of cancer (11,144). However, it is possible that such a sequence variation could affect RNA stability or otherwise disturb protein synthesis (139).

Several polymorphisms of *XRCC1* have also been identified (132). They include those that result in a nonconservative amino acid substitution at C26304T of codon 194 (Arg194Trp) in exon 6, G27466A of codon 280 (Arg280His) in exon 9, and G28152A of codon 399 (Arg399Gln) in exon 10. Although the functional relevance of these variants is unknown, codon 399 is within the *XRCC1* BRCT (breast cancer susceptibility protein-1) domain (codons 314–402) (145), which is highly homologous to *BRCA1* (a gene also involved in DNA repair) and contains a binding site for poly(ADP-ribose) polymerase (PARP) (146). Because the role of *XRCC1* in BER involves bringing together DNA polymerase β (β-pol), DNA ligase III, and PARP at the site of DNA damage (147–149), the codon 399 variant may have an impact on repair activity. The codon 194 polymorphism resides in the linker regions of the *XRCC1* N-terminal domain separating the helix 3 and β-pol involved in the binding of a single-nucleotide gap DNA substrate (150). Lunn et al. (151) reported that the codon 399 variant was associated with higher levels of both aflatoxin B1-DNA adducts and glycophorin A variants in a normal population, suggesting that this variant is an adverse genotype. However, few studies have examined the associations between polymorphisms of the DNA repair gene *XRCC1* and risk of cancer.

In another case–control study, Sturgis et al. (10) reported that 89% of 203 SCCHN patients and 86% of 424 cancer-free controls lacked the XRCC1 codon 194 Trp variant, resulting in a significant risk of oral cavity and pharyngeal cancers (OR, 2.46). Thirty-two patients (16%) and 46 controls (11%) were homozygous for the codon 399 Gln variant (adjusted OR, 1.59 for all cases). Furthermore, when the two genotypes were combined, the adjusted OR was 1.51 for either risk genotype and 2.02 for both risk genotypes. In addition, the codon 399 Arg/Gln and Gln/Gln genotypes were associated with increased risk of breast cancer in African Americans (152) and gastric cancer in a Chinese population (153), the codon 280 Arg/His and His/His genotypes were associated with increased risk of lung cancer in a Chinese population (154), and the 194Trp and 399Gln variant alleles were associated with increased risk of colon cancer in an Egyptian population (155). However, not all of these polymorphisms were found to be associated with increased risk of cancer in other studies (143,144,156). Despite some conflicting reports, the variants of *XRCC1* and their impact on cancer risk have generated much interest recently (157).

The *hOGG*1 gene is localized on chromosome 3p25 and encodes two proteins that result from alternative splicing of a single messenger RNA (158,159). The alpha-hOGG1 protein undergoes nuclear localization, whereas the beta-hOGG1 protein is targeted to a mitochondrion. A polymorphism at codon 326 (Ser326Cys) produces the hOGG1-Ser326 and hOGG1-Cys326 proteins (160). Also, the mutant forms hOGG1-Gln46 and hOGG1-His154 are defective in their catalytic capacity, especially for 8-OH-Gua (161). The activity in the repair of 8-hydroxyguanine appears to be greater with the Ser326 protein than with the Cys326 protein. Because tobacco carcinogens produce 8-hydroxyguanine residues, the capacity to repair these lesions can be involved in cancer susceptibility. This polymorphism was identified in European patients with head and neck or kidney cancer but not associated with increased risk (162).

In a study using buccal cell DNA isolated from 169 white orolaryngeal cancer patients and 338 race-, sex-, and age-matched controls, Elahi et al. (162) screened normal orolaryngeal tissue specimens for hOGG1 expression and assessed the role of the hOGG1 Ser326Cys polymorphism in the risk of orolaryngeal cancer. They detected hOGG1 mRNA in all aerodigestive tract tissues tested, including the tonsil, tongue, floor of the mouth, larynx, and esophagus. They also found significantly increased risk of orolaryngeal cancer with the hOGG1 326(Ser)/326(Cys)(OR, 1.6; 95% CI, 1.04–2.60) and hOGG1 326(Cys)/326(Cys) genotypes (OR, 4.1; 95% CI, 1.3–13). However, no significant differences in risk of orolaryngeal cancer were observed with hOGG1 genotypes in never smokers and never drinkers of alcohol, suggesting that the hOGG1 Ser326Cys polymorphism plays an important role in the risk of tobacco- and alcohol-related orolaryngeal cancer.

In conclusion, studies of the correlation between the DNA repair genotype and phenotype are needed, and large well-designed, confirmatory case–control or cohort studies will be required to verify the impact of the DNA repair phenotype and its genetic variants on cancer risk.

ACKNOWLEDGMENTS

The authors thank Mrs Joanne Sider for assistance in preparing the manuscript. This investigation was supported in part by National Institutes of Health grants CA86390 and CA97007 and National Institute of Environmental Health Sciences grants ES11740 and ES07784.

REFERENCES

1. Jemal A, Thomas A, Murray T, Thun M. Cancer statistics, 2002. CA Cancer J Clin 2002; 52:23–47.
2. Hartwell LH, Weinert TA. Checkpoints: controls that assure the order of cell cycle events. Science 1989; 246:629–633.
3. Sancer A. DNA repair in humans. Annu Rev Genet 1995; 29:69–105.
4. Shields PG, Harris CC. Cancer risk and low-penetrance susceptibility genes in gene–environment interactions. J Clin Oncol 2000; 18:2309–2315.
5. Perera FP. Molecular epidemiology: on the path to prevention? J Natl Cancer Inst 2000; 92:602–612.
6. Christiani DC. Smoking and the molecular epidemiology of lung cancer. Clin Chest Med 2000; 21:87–93.
7. Autrup H. Genetic polymorphisms in human xenobiotic metabolizing enzymes as susceptibility factors in toxic response. Mutat Res 2000; 464: 65–76.
8. Bartsch H, Nair U, Risch A, Rojas M, Wikman H, Alexandrov K. Genetic polymorphism of CYP genes, alone or in combination, as a risk modifier of tobacco-related cancers. Cancer Epidemiol Biomarkers Prev 2000; 9:3–28.
9. Nair U, Bartsch H. Metabolic polymorphisms as susceptibility markers for lung and oral cavity cancer. IARC Sci Publ 2001; 154:271–290.
10. Sturgis EM, Castillo EJ, Li L, Zheng R, Eicher SA, Clayman GL, et al. Polymorphisms of DNA repair gene XRCC1 in squamous cell carcinoma of the head and neck. Carcinogenesis 1999; 20:2125–2129.
11. Sturgis EM, Clayman GL, Guan Y, Guo Z, Wei Q. DNA repair in lymphoblastoid cell lines from patients with head and neck cancer. Arch Otolaryngol Head Neck Surg 1999; 125:185–190.
12. Sturgis EM, Zheng R, Li L, Castillo EJ, Eicher SA, Chen M, et al. XPD/ERCC2 polymorphisms and risk of head and neck cancer: a case–control analysis. Carcinogenesis 2000; 21:2219–2223.

13. Berwick M, Vineis P. Markers of DNA repair and susceptibility to cancer in humans: an epidemiologic review. J Natl Cancer Inst 2000; 92:874–897.
14. Wynder EL, Bross IJ, Feldman RM. A study of the etiological factors in cancer of the mouth. Cancer 1957; 10:1300–1323.
15. Hammond EC, Horn D. Smoking and death rates—Report on forty-four months of follow-up of 187,783 men. J Am Med Assoc 1958; 166: 1294–1308.
16. Doll R, Hill AB. Lung cancer and other causes of death in relation to smoking: a second report on the mortality of British doctors. Br Med J 1956; 2: 1071–1081.
17. Franceschi S, Levi F, La Vecchia C, Conti E, Dal Maso L, Barzan L, et al. Comparison of the effect of smoking and alcohol drinking between oral and pharyngeal cancer. Int J Cancer 1999; 83:1–4.
18. Schlecht NF, Franco EL, Pintos J, Negassa A, Kowalski LP, Oliveira BV, et al. Interaction between tobacco and alcohol consumption and the risk of cancers of the upper aero-digestive tract in Brazil. Am J Epidemiol 1999; 150: 1129–1137.
19. Cattaruzza MS, Maisonneuve P, Boyle P. Epidemiology of laryngeal cancer. Eur J Cancer B Oral Oncol 1996; 32B:293–305.
20. LaVecchia C, Tavani A, Franceschi S, Levi F, Corrao G, Negri E. Epidemiology and prevention of oral cancer. Oral Oncol 1997; 33:302–312.
21. Schlecht NF, Franco EL, Pintos J, Kowalski LP. Effect of smoking cessation and tobacco type on the risk of cancers of the upper aero-digestive tract in Brazil. Epidemiology 1999; 10:412–418.
22. Iribarren C, Tekawa IS, Sidney S, Friedman GD. Effect of cigar smoking on the risk of cardiovascular disease, chronic obstructive pulmonary disease, and cancer in men. N Engl J Med 1999; 340:1773–1780.
23. Baker F, Ainsworth SR, Dye JT, Crammer C, Thunn MJ, Hoffmann D, et al. Health risks associated with cigar smoking. J Am Med Assoc 2000; 284: 735–740.
24. Moore C, Catlin D. Anatomic origins and locations of oral cancer. Am J Surg 1967; 114:510–513.
25. Winn DM. Smokeless tobacco and cancer: the epidemiologic evidence. CA Cancer J Clin 1988; 38:236–243.
26. CDC. Tobacco use—United States, 1900–1999. MMWR Morb Mortal Wkly Rep 1999; 48:986–993.
27. CDC. Cigarette smoking among adults—United States, 1999. MMWR Morb Mortal Wkly Rep 2001; 50:869–873.
28. Marwick C. Increasing use of chewing tobacco, especially among younger persons, alarms Surgeon General. J Am Med Assoc 1993; 269:195.
29. Schantz SP, Yu GP. Head and neck cancer incidence trends in young Americans, 1973–1997, with a special analysis for tongue cancer. Arch Otolaryngol Head Neck Surg 2002; 128:268–274.
30. Scully C, Bedi R. Ethnicity and oral cancer. Lancet 2000; 1:37–42.
31. Idris AM, Ahmed HM, Malik MOA. Toombak dipping and cancer of the oral cavity in the Sudan: a case–control study. Int J Cancer 1995; 63: 477–480.

32. Merchant A, Husain SSM, Hosain M, Fikree FF, Pitiphat W, Siddiqui AR, et al. Paan without tobacco: an independent risk factor for oral cancer. Int J Cancer 2000; 86:128–131.

33. Kabat GC, Wynder EL. Type of alcoholic beverage and oral cancer. Int J Cancer 1989; 43:190–194.

34. Foulkes WD, Brunet JS, Sieh W, Black MJ, Shenouda G, Narod SA. Familial risks of squamous cell carcinoma of the head and neck: retrospective case–control study. Br Med J 1996; 313:716–721.

35. Sturgis EM, Wei Q. Genetic susceptibility–molecular epidemiology of head and neck cancer. Curr Opin Oncol 2002; 14:310–317.

36. Maden C, Beckmann AM, Thomas DB, McKnight B, Sherman KJ, Ashley RL, et al. Human papillomaviruses, herpes simplex viruses, and the risk of oral cancer in men. Am J Epidemiol 1992; 135:1093–1102.

37. Aygenc E, Selcuk A, Celikkanat S, Ozbek C, Ozdem C. The role of *Helicobacter pylori* infection in the cause of squamous cell carcinoma of the larynx. Otolaryngol Head Neck Surg 2001; 125:520–521.

38. Grandis JR, Perez-Perez GI, Yu VL, Johnson JT, Blaser MJ. Lack of serologic evidence for *Helicobacter pylori* infection in head and neck cancer. Head Neck 1997; 19:216–218.

39. ZurHausen H. Papillomaviruses causing cancer: evasion for host-cell control in early events in carcinogenesis. J Natl Cancer Inst 2000; 92:690–698.

40. Gillison ML, Shah KV. Human papillomavirus-associated head and neck squamous cell carcinoma: mounting evidence for an etiologic role for human papillomavirus in a subset of head and neck cancers. Curr Opin Oncol 2001; 13:183–188.

41. Hengstermann A, Linares LK, Ciechanover A, Whitaker NJ, Scheffner M. Complete switch from Mdm2 to human papillomavirus E6-mediated degradation of p53 in cervical cancer cells. Proc Natl Acad Sci USA 2001; 98: 1218–1223.

42. Andl T, Kahn T, Pfuhl A, Nicola T, Erber R, Conradt C, et al. Etiological involvement of oncogenic human papillomavirus in tonsillar squamous cell carcinomas lacking retinoblastoma cell cycle control. Cancer Res 1998; 58: 5–13.

43. Strome SE, Savva A, Brissett AE, Gostout BS, Lewis J, Clayton AC, et al. Squamous cell carcinoma of the tonsils: a molecular analysis of HPV associations. Clin Cancer Res 2002; 8:1093–1100.

44. Mork J, Lie AK, Glattre E, Hallmans G, Jellum E, Koskela P, et al. Human papilloma virus infection as a risk factor for squamous-cell carcinoma of the head and neck. N Engl J Med 2001; 344:1125–1131.

45. Schwartz SM, Daling JR, Doody DR, Wipf GC, Carter JJ, Madeleine MM, et al. Oral cancer risk in relation to sexual history and evidence of human papillomavirus infection. J Natl Cancer Inst 1998; 90:1626–1636.

46. Loff B, Cordner S. Passive smoking test case wins in Australia. Lancet 2001; 357:1511.

47. Zhang ZF, Morgenstern H, Spitz MR, Tashkin DP, Yu GP, Hsu TC, et al. Environmental tobacco smoking, mutagen sensitivity, and head and neck squamous cell carcinoma. Cancer Epidemiol Biomark Prev 2000; 9:1043–1049.

48. Tan EH, Adelstein DJ, Droughton MLT, Van Kirk MA, Lavertu P. Squamous cell head and neck cancer in nonsmokers. Am J Clin Oncol 1997; 20:146–150.

49. Morrison MD. Is chronic gastroesophageal reflux a causative factor in glottic carcinoma? Otolaryngol Head Neck Surg 1988; 99:370–373.

50. Biacabe B, Gleich LL, Laccourreye O, Hartl DM, Bouchoucha M, Brasnu D. Silent gastroesophageal reflux disease in patients with pharyngolaryngeal cancer: further results. Head Neck 1998; 20:510–514.

51. Copper MP, Smit CF, Stanojcic LD, Devriese PP, Schouwenburg PF, Mathus-Vliegen LM. High incidence of laryngopharyngeal reflux in patients with head and neck cancer. Laryngoscope 2000; 110:1007–1011.

52. El-Serag HB, Hepworth EJ, Lee P, Sonnenberg A. Gastroesophageal reflux disease is a risk factor for laryngeal and pharyngeal cancer. Am J Gastroenterol 2001; 96:2013–2018.

53. Caplan GA, Brigham BA. Marijuana smoking and carcinoma of the tongue: is there an association? Cancer 1990; 66:1005–1006.

54. Zhang ZF, Morgenstern H, Spitz MR, Tashkin DP, Yu GP, Marshall JR, et al. Marijuana use and increased risk of squamous cell carcinoma of the head and neck. Cancer Epidemiol Biomark Prev 1999; 8:1071–1078.

55. Sidney S, Quesenberry CP, Friedman GD, Tekawa IS. Marijuana use and cancer incidence (California, United States). Cancer Causes Control 1997; 8:722–728.

56. Winn DM, Ziegler RG, Pickle LW, Gridley G, Blot WJ, Hoover RN. Diet in the etiology of oral and pharyngeal cancer among women from the southern United States. Cancer Res 1984; 44:1216–1222.

57. McLaughlin JK, Gridley G, Block G, Winn DM, Preston-Martin S, Schoenberg JB, et al. Dietary factors in oral and pharyngeal cancer. J Natl Cancer Inst 1988; 80:1237–1243.

58. Zheng W, Blot WJ, Shu XO, Gao YT, Ji BT, Ziegler RG, et al. Diet and other risk factors for laryngeal cancer in Shanghai, China. Am J Epidemiol 1992; 136:178–191.

59. Levi F, Pasche C, LaVecchia C, Lucchini F, Franceschi S, Monnier P. Food groups and risk of oral and pharyngeal cancer. Int J Cancer 1998; 77:705–709.

60. Schantz SP, Zhang ZF, Spitz MS, Sun M, Hsu T. Genetic susceptibility to head and neck cancer: interaction between nutrition and mutagen sensitivity. Laryngoscope 1997; 107:765–781.

61. Khoury MJ, Wagener DK. Epidemiological evaluation of the use of genetics to improve the predictive value of disease risk factors. Am J Hum Genet 1995; 56:835–844.

62. Fearon ER. Human cancer syndromes: clues to the origin and nature of cancer. Science 1997; 278:1043–1050.

63. Kellermann G, Shaw CR, Luyten-Kellerman M. Aryl hydrocarbon hydroxylase inducibility and bronchogenic carcinoma. N Engl J Med 1973; 289:934–937.

64. Nath RG, Ocando JE, Guttenplan JB, Chung FL. 1,N2-propanodeoxyguanosine adducts: potential new biomarkers of smoking-induced DNA damage in human oral tissue. Cancer Res 1998; 58:581–584.

65. Ullrich D, Munzel PA, Beck-Gschaidmeier S, Schroder M, Bock KW. Drug-metabolizing enzymes in pharyngeal mucosa and in oropharyngeal cancer tissue. Biochem Pharmacol 1997; 54:1159–1162.
66. Flamini G, Romano G, Curigliano G, Chiominto A, Capelli G, Boninsegna A, et al. 4-Aminobiphenyl–DNA adducts in laryngeal tissue and smoking habits: an immunohistochemical study. Carcinogenesis 1998; 19:353–357.
67. Szyfter K, Hemminki K, Szyfter W, Szmeja Z, Banaszewski J, Yang K. Aromatic DNA adducts in larynx biopsies and leukocytes. Carcinogenesis 1994; 15:2195–2199.
68. Carmella SG, Kagan SS, Kagan M, Foiles PG, Palladino G, Quart AM, et al. Mass spectrometric analysis of tobacco- specific nitrosamine hemoglobin adducts in snuff dippers, smokers, and nonsmokers. Cancer Res 1990; 50: 5438–5445.
69. Nair J, Ohshima H, Nair UJ, Bartsch H. Endogenous formation of nitrosamines and oxidative DNA-damaging agents in tobacco users. Crit Rev Toxicol 1996; 26:149–161.
70. Geisler SA, Olshan AF. GSTM1, GSTT1, and the risk of squamous cell carcinoma of the head and neck: a mini-HuGE review. Am J Epidemiol 2001; 154:95–105.
71. Olshan AF, Weissler MC, Watson MA, Bell DA. GSTM1, GSTT1, GSTP1, CYP1A1, and NAT1 polymorphisms, tobacco use, and the risk of head and neck cancer. Cancer Epidemiol Biomarkers Prev 2000; 9:185–191.
72. Rebbeck TR. Molecular epidemiology of the human glutathione S-transferase genotypes GSTM1 and GSTT1 in cancer susceptibility. Cancer Epidemiol Biomarkers Prev 1997; 6:733–743.
73. Jourenkova N, Reinikainen M, Bouchardy C, Dayer P, Benhamou S, Hirvonen A. Larynx cancer risk in relation to glutathione S-transferase M1 and T1 genotypes and tobacco smoking. Cancer Epidemiol Biomarkers Prev 1998; 7:19–23.
74. Lazarus P, Sheikh SN, Ren Q, Schantz SP, Stern JC, Richie JP Jr, et al. p53, but not p16 mutations in oral squamous cell carcinomas are associated with specific CYP1A1 and GSTM1 polymorphic genotypes and patient tobacco use. Carcinogenesis 1998; 19:509–514.
75. Liloglou T, Scholes AG, Spandidos DA, Vaughan ED, Jones AS, Field JK. p53 mutations in squamous cell carcinoma of the head and neck predominate in a subgroup of former and present smokers with a low frequency of genetic instability. Cancer Res 1997; 57:4070–4074.
76. Olshan AF, Weissler MC, Pei H, Conway K. p53 mutations in head and neck cancer: new data and evaluation of mutational spectra. Cancer Epidemiol Biomarkers Prev 1997; 6:499–504.
77. Brennan JA, Boyle JO, Koch WM, Goodman SN, Hruban RH, Eby YJ, et al. Association between cigarette smoking and mutation of the p53 gene in squamous-cell carcinoma of the head and neck. N Engl J Med 1995; 332:712–717.
78. Field JK, Zoumpourlis V, Spandidos DA, Jones AS. p53 expression and mutations in squamous cell carcinoma of the head and neck: expression correlates with the patients' use of tobacco and alcohol. Cancer Detect Prev 1994; 18:197–208.

79. Setlow RB. DNA repair, aging, and cancer. Natl Cancer Inst Monogr 1982; 60:249–255.
80. Wood RD, Mitchell M, Sgouros J, Lindahl T. Human DNA repair genes. Science 2001; 291:1284–1289.
81. Protic-Sabljic M, Kraemer KH. One pyrimidine dimer inactivates expression of a transfected gene in xeroderma pigmentosum cells. Proc Natl Acad Sci USA 1985; 82:6622–6626.
82. Koch KS, Fletcher RG, Grond MP, Inyang AI, Lu XP, Brenner DA, et al. Inactivation of plasmid reporter gene expression by one benzo(a)pyrene diol-epoxide DNA adduct in adult rat hepatocytes. Cancer Res 1993; 53: 2279–2286.
83. Wei Q, Matanoski GM, Farmer ER, Hedayati MA, Grossman L. DNA repair and aging in basal cell carcinoma: a molecular epidemiology study. Proc Natl Acad Sci USA 1993; 90:1614–1618.
84. Wei Q, Cheng L, Amos CI, Wang LE, Guo Z, Hong WK, et al. Repair of tobacco carcinogen-induced DNA adducts and lung cancer risk: a molecular epidemiological study. J Natl Cancer Inst 2000; 92:1764–1772.
85. Hoeijmakers JHJ. Human nucleotide excision repair syndromes: molecular clues to unexpected intricacies. Eur J Cancer 1994; 30:1912–1921.
86. Gupta RC, Earley K, Sharma S. Use of human peripheral blood lymphocytes to measure DNA binding capacity of chemical carcinogens. Proc Natl Acad Sci USA 1988; 85:3513.
87. Athas WF, Hedayati M, Matanoski GM, Farmer ER, Grossman L. Development and field-test validation of an assay for DNA repair in circulating lymphocytes. Cancer Res 1991; 51:5786–5793.
88. Qiao Y, Spitz MR, Guo Z, Hadeyati M, Grossman L, Kraemer KH, Wei Q. Rapid assessment of repair of ultraviolet DNA damage with a modified host-cell reactivation assay using a luciferase reporter gene and correlation with polymorphisms of DNA repair genes in normal human lymphocytes. Mutat Res 2002; 509:165–174.
89. Alcalay J, Freeman SE, Goldberg LH, Wolf JE. Excision repair of pyrimidine dimers induced by simulated solar radiation in the skin of patients with basal cell carcinoma. J Invest Dermatol 1990; 95:506–509.
90. Wei Q, Cheng L, Hong WK, Spitz MR. Reduced DNA repair capacity in lung cancer patients. Cancer Res 1996; 56:4103–4107.
91. Brownson RC, Chang JC, Davis JR. Gender and histologic type variations in smoking-related risk of lung cancer. Epidemiology 1992; 3:61–64.
92. Risch HA, Howe GR, Jain M, Burch JD, Holowaty EJ, Miller AB. Are female smokers at higher risk for lung cancer than male smokers? A case–control analysis by histologic type. Am J Epidemiol 1993; 138:281–293.
93. Zang EA, Wynder EL. Differences in lung cancer risk between men and women: examination of the evidence. J Natl Cancer Inst 1996; 88: 183–192.
94. Cheng L, Eicher SA, Guo Z, Hong WK, Spitz MR, Wei Q. Reduced DNA repair capacity in head and neck cancer patients. Cancer Epidemiol Biomarkers Prev 1998; 7:465–468.

95. Spitz MR, Hoque A, Trizna Z, Schantz SP, Amos CI, King TM. Mutagen sensitivity as a risk factor for second malignant tumors following upper aerodigestive tract malignancies. J Natl Cancer Inst 1994; 86:1681–1684.

96. Strom SS, Wu X, Sigurdson AJ, Hsu TC, Fueger JJ, Lopez J, et al. Lung cancer, smoking patterns, and mutagen sensitivity in Mexican-Americans. Monogr Natl Cancer Inst 1995; 18:29–33.

97. Wu X, Delclos GL, Annegers FJ, Bondy ML, Honn SE, Henry B, et al. A case–control study of wood-dust exposure, mutagen sensitivity, and lung-cancer risk. Cancer Epidemiol Biomarkers Prev 1995; 4:583–588.

98. Hagmar L, Brogger A, Hansteen I, Heim S, Hogstedt B, Knudsen L, et al. Cancer risk in humans predicted by increased levels of chromosome aberrations in lymphocytes: Nordic study group on the health risk of chromosome damage. Cancer Res 1994; 54:2919–2922.

99. Bonassi S, Abbondandolo A, Camurri L, Dal Pra L, De Ferrari M, Degrassi F, et al. Are chromosome aberrations in circulating lymphocytes predictive of future cancer onset in humans? Preliminary results of an Italian cohort study. Cancer Genet Cytogenet 1995; 79:133–135.

100. Field JK. Genomic instability in squamous cell carcinoma of the head and neck. Anticancer Res 1996; 16:2421–2431.

101. Scully C, Field JK, Tanzawa H. Genetic aberrations in oral or head and neck squamous cell carcinoma 2: chromosomal aberrations. Oral Oncol 2000; 36:311–327.

102. Dutrillaux, B. Pathways of chromosome alteration in human epithelial cancers. Adv Cancer Res 1995; 67:59–82.

103. Hsu TC, Johnston DA, Cherry LM, Ramkissoon D, Schantz SP, Jessup JM, et al. Sensitivity to genotoxic effects of bleomycin in humans: possible relationship to environmental carcinogenesis. Int J Cancer 1989; 43:403–409.

104. Hsu TC, Spitz MR, Schantz SP. Mutagen sensitivity: a biologic marker of cancer susceptibility. Cancer Epidemiol Biomarkers Prev 1991; 1:83–89.

105. Spitz MR, Fueger JJ, Beddingfield NA, Annegers JF, Hsu TC, Newell GR, et al. Chromosome sensitivity to bleomycin-induced mutagenesis, an independent risk factor for upper aerodigestive tract cancers. Cancer Res 1989; 49:4626–4628.

106. Spitz MR, Hsu TC, Wu XF, Fueger JJ, Amos CI, Roth JA. Mutagen sensitivity as a biologic marker of lung cancer risk in African Americans. Cancer Epidemiol Biomarkers Prev 1995; 4:99–103.

107. Schantz SP, Hsu TC, Ainslie N, Moser RP. Young adults with head and neck cancer express increased susceptibility to mutagen-induced chromosome damage. J Am Med Assoc 1989; 262:3313–3315.

108. Wei Q, Gu J, Cheng L, Bondy ML, Jiang H, Hong WK, Spitz MR. Benzo(a)pyrene diol epoxide-induced chromosomal aberrations and risk of lung cancer. Cancer Res 1996; 56:3975–3979.

109. Wang LE, Sturgis EM, Eicher SA, Spitz MR, Hong WK, Wei Q. Mutagen sensitivity to benzo(a)pyrene diol epoxide and the risk of squamous cell carcinoma of the head and neck. Clin Cancer Res 1998; 4:1773–1778.

110. Hsu TC. Genetic instability in the human population: a working hypothesis. Hereditas 1983; 98:1–9.

111. Sturgis EM, Spitz MR, Wei Q. DNA repair and genomic instability in tobacco induced malignancies of the lung and upper aerodigestive tract. Environ Carcinogen Ecol 1998; C16:1–30.

112. Pandita TK, Hittelman WN. Evidence of a chromatin basis for increased mutagen sensitivity associated with multiple primary malignancies of the head and neck. Int J Cancer 1995; 61:738–743.

113. Everson RB, Randerath E, Santella RM, Cefalo RC, Avitts TA, Randerath K. Detection of smoking-related covalent DNA adducts in human placenta. Science 1986; 231:54–57.

114. Geneste O, Camus AM, Castegaro M, Petruzzelli S, Macchiarini P, Angeletti CA, et al. Comparison of pulmonary DNA adduct levels, measured by 32P-postlabelling and aryl hydrocarbon hydroxylase activity in lung parenchyma of smokers and ex-smokers. Carcinogenesis 1991; 12:1301–1305.

115. Li D, Wang M, Cheng L, Spitz MR, Hittelman WN, Wei Q. In vitro induction of benzo(a)pyrene diol epoxide–DNA adducts in peripheral lymphocytes as a susceptibility marker for human lung cancer. Cancer Res 1996; 56:3638–3641.

116. Reddy MV, Randerath K. Nuclease P1-mediated enhancement of sensitivity of 32P-postlabeling test for structurally diverse DNA adducts. Carcinogenesis 1986; 7:1543–1551.

117. Phillips DH, Hewer A, Grover PL. Aromatic DNA adducts in human bone marrow and peripheral blood leukocytes. Carcinogenesis 1986; 7:2071–2075.

118. Savela K, Hemminki K. DNA adducts in lymphocytes and granulocytes of smokers and nonsmokers detected by the 32P-postlabelling assay. Carcinogenesis 1991; 12:503–508.

119. van Schooten FJ, Hillebrand MJ, van Leeuwen FE, van Zandwijk N, Jansen HM, den Engelse L, et al. Polycyclic aromatic hydrocarbon-DNA adducts in white blood cells from lung cancer patients: no correlation with adduct levels in lung. Carcinogenesis 1992; 13:987–993.

120. Gelboin HV. Benzo(a)pyrene metabolism, activation, and carcinogenesis: role and regulation of mixed function oxidases and related enzymes. Physiol Rev 1980; 60:1107–1166.

121. Gonzalez MV, Alvarez V, Pello MF, Menendez MJ, Suarez C, Coto E. Genetic polymorphism of N-acetyltransferase-2, glutathione S-transferase-M1, and cytochromes P450IIE1 and P450IID6 in the susceptibility to head and neck cancer. J Clin Pathol 1998; 51:294–298.

122. Eaton DL, Gallagher EP, Bammler TK, Kunze KL. Role of cytochrome P4501A2 in chemical carcinogenesis: implications for human variability in expression and enzyme activity. Pharmacogenetics 1995; 5:259–274.

123. Bartsch H, Rojas M, Alexandrov K, Camus AM, Castegnaro M, Malaveille C, et al. Metabolic polymorphism affecting DNA binding and excretion of carcinogens in humans. Pharmacogenetics 1995; 5:S84–S90.

124. Krolewski B, Little JB, Reynolds RJ. Effect of duration of exposure to benzo(a)pyrene diol-epoxide on neoplastic transformation, mutagenesis, cytotoxicity, and total covalent binding to DNA of rodent cells. Teratog Carcinog Mutagen 1988; 8:127–136.

125. Li D, Firozi PF, Chang P, Wang LE, Xiong P, Sturgis EM, et al. In vitro BPDE-induced DNA adducts in peripheral lymphocytes as a risk factor for squamous cell carcinoma of the head and neck. Int J Cancer 2001; 93:436–440.

126. Li D, Firozi PF, Wang LE, Bosken CH, Spitz MR, Hong WK, et al. Sensitivity to DNA damage induced by benzo(a)pyrene diol epoxide and risk of lung cancer: a case–control analysis. Cancer Res 2001; 61:1445–1450.

127. Wei Q, Xu X, Cheng L, Legerski RJ, Ali-Osman F. Simultaneous amplification of four DNA repair genes and beta-actin in human lymphocytes by multiplex reverse transcriptase-PCR. Cancer Res 1995; 55:5025–5029.

128. Wei Q, Guan Y, Cheng L, Radinsky R, Bar-Eli M, Tsan R, et al. Expression of five selected human mismatch repair genes simultaneously detected in normal and cancer cell lines by a nonradioactive multiplex reverse transcription-polymerase chain reaction. Pathobiology 1997; 65:293–300.

129. Cheng L, Guan Y, Li L, Legerski RJ, Einspahr J, Bangert J, et al. Expression in normal human tissues of five nucleotide excision repair genes measured simultaneously by multiplex reverse transcription-polymerase chain reaction. Cancer Epidemiol Biomarkers Prev 1999; 8:801–807.

130. Wei Q, Eicher SA, Guan Y, Cheng L, Xu J, Young LN, et al. Reduced expression of hMLH1 and hGTBP/hMSH6: a risk factor for head and neck cancer. Cancer Epidemiol Biomarkers Prev 1998; 7:309–314.

131. Cheng L, Sturgis EM, Eicher SA, Spitz MR, Wei Q. Expression of nucleotide excision repair genes and the risk for squamous cell carcinoma of the head and neck. Cancer 2002; 94:393–397.

132. Shen MR, Jones IM, Mohrenweiser H. Nonconservative amino acid substitution variants exist at polymorphic frequency in DNA repair genes in healthy humans. Cancer Res 1998; 58:604–608.

133. Fan F, Liu C, Tavare S, Arnheim N. Polymorphisms in the human DNA repair gene XPF. Mutat Res 1999; 406:115–120.

134. Khan SG, Metter EJ, Tarone RE, Bohr VA, Grossman L, Hedayati M, et al. A new xeroderma pigmentosum group C poly(AT) insertion/deletion polymorphism. Carcinogenesis 2000; 21:1821–1825.

135. Emmert S, Schneider TD, Khan SG, Kraemer KH. The human XPG gene: gene architecture, alternative splicing and single nucleotide polymorphisms. Nucleic Acids Res 2001; 29:1443–1452.

136. Coin F, Marinoni JC, Rodolfo C, Fribourg S, Pedrini AM, Egly JM. Mutations in the XPD helicase gene result in XP and TTD phenotypes, preventing interaction between XPD and the p44 subunit of TFIIH. Nat Genet 1998; 20:184–188.

137. Reardon JT, Ge H, Gibbs E, Sancar A, Hurwitz J, Pan ZQ. Isolation and characterization of two human transcription factor IIH (TFIIH)-related complexes: ERCC2/CAK and TFIIH. Proc Natl Acad Sci USA 1996; 93: 6482–6487.

138. Taylor EM, Broughton BC, Botta E, Stefanini M, Sarasin A, Jaspers NG, et al. Xeroderma pigmentosum and trichothiodystrophy are associated with different mutations in the XPD (ERCC2) repair/transcription gene. Proc Natl Acad Sci USA 1997; 94:8658–8663.

139. Broughton BC, Steingrimsdottir H, Lehmann AR. Five polymorphisms in the coding sequence of the xeroderma pigmentosum group D gene. Mutat Res 1996; 362:209–211.

140. Lunn RM, Helzlsouer KJ, Parshad R, Umbach DM, Harris EL, Sanford KK, et al. XPD polymorphisms: effects on DNA repair proficiency. Carcinogenesis 2000; 21:551–555.

141. Duell EJ, Wiencke JK, Cheng TJ, Varkonyi A, Zuo ZF, Ashok TD, et al. Polymorphisms in the DNA repair genes XRCC1 and ERCC2 and biomarkers of DNA damage in human blood mononuclear cells. Carcinogenesis 2000; 21:965–971.

142. Spitz MR, Duphorne CM, Detry MA, Pillow PC, Amos CI, Lei L, et al. Dietary intake of isothiocyanates: evidence of a joint effect with glutathione S-transferase polymorphisms in lung cancer risk. Cancer Epidemiol Biomarkers Prev 2000; 9:1017–1020.

143. Butkiewicz D, Rusin M, Enewold L, Shields PG, Chorazy M, Harris CC. Genetic polymorphisms in DNA repair genes and risk of lung cancer. Carcinogenesis 2001; 22:593–597.

144. Matullo G, Guarrera S, Carturan S, Peluso M, Malaveille C, Davico L, et al. DNA repair gene polymorphisms, bulky DNA adducts in white blood cells and bladder cancer in a case– control study. Int J Cancer 2001; 92:562–567.

145. Zhang X, Morera S, Bates PA, Whitehead PC, Coffer AI, Hainbucher K, et al. Structure of an XRCC1 BRCT domain: a new protein–protein interaction module. EMBO J. 1998; 17:6404–6411.

146. Masson M, Niedergang C, Schreiber V, Muller S, Demarcia JM, Demurcia G. XRCC1 is specifically associated with PARP polymerase and negatively regulates its activity following DNA damage. Mol Cell Biol 1998; 18:3563–3571.

147. Caldecott KW, McKeown CK, Tucker JD, Ljungquist S, Thompson LH. An interaction between the mammalian DNA repair protein XRCC1 and DNA ligase III. Mol Cell Biol 1994; 14:68–76.

148. Kubota Y, Nash RA, Klungland A, Schar P, Barnes DE, Lindahl T. Reconstitution of DNA base excision-repair with purified human proteins: interaction between DNA polymerase beta and the XRCC1 protein. EMBO J 1996; 15:6662–6670.

149. Cappelli E, Taylor R, Cevasco M, Abbondandolo A, Caldecott K, Forsina G. Involvement of XRCC1 and DNA ligase gene products in DNA base excision repair. J Biol Chem 1997; 272:23970–23975.

150. Marintchev A, Mullen MA, Maciejewski MW, Pan B, Gryk MR, Mullen GP. Solution structure of the single-strand break repair protein XRCC1 N-terminal domain. Nat Struct Biol 1999; 6:884–893.

151. Lunn RM, Langlois RG, Hsieh LL, Thompson CL, Bell DA. XRCC1 polymorphisms: effects on aflatoxin B1-DNA adducts and glycophorin A variant frequency. Cancer Res 1999; 59:2557–2561.

152. Duell EJ, Millikan RC, Pittman GS, Winkel S, Lunn RM, Tse CK, et al. Polymorphisms in the DNA repair gene XRCC1 and breast cancer. Cancer Epidemiol Biomarkers Prev 2001; 10:217–222.

153. Shen H, Xu Y, Qian Y, Yu R, Qin Y, Zhou L, et al. Polymorphisms of the DNA repair gene XRCC1 and risk of gastric cancer in a Chinese population. Int J Cancer 2000; 88:601–606.
154. Ratnasinghe D, Yao SX, Tangrea JA, Qiao YL, Andersen MR, Barrett MJ, et al. Polymorphisms of the DNA repair gene XRCC1 and lung cancer risk. Cancer Epidemiol Biomarkers Prev 2001; 10:119–123.
155. Abdel-Rahman SZ, Soliman AS, Bondy ML, Omar S, El-Badawy SA, Khaled HM, et al. Inheritance of the 194Trp and the 399Gln variant alleles of the DNA repair gene XRCC1 are associated with increased risk of early-onset colorectal carcinoma in Egypt. Cancer Lett 2000; 9:79–86.
156. Stern MC, Umbach DM, van Gils CH, Lunn RM, Taylor JA. DNA repair gene XRCC1 polymorphisms, smoking, and bladder cancer risk. Cancer Epidemiol Biomarkers Prev 2001; 10:125–131.
157. Kaiser J. Diversity in mending DNA damage. Science 2001; 292:837–838.
158. Boiteux S, Radicella JP. The human OGG1 gene: structure, functions, and its implication in the process of carcinogenesis. Arch Biochem Biophys 2000; 377:1–8.
159. Audebert M, Radicella JP, Dizdaroglu M. Effect of single mutations in the OGG1 gene found in human tumors on the substrate specificity of the OGG1 protein. Nucleic Acids Res 2000; 28:2672–2678.
160. Kohno T, Shinmura K, Tosaka M, Tani M, Kim SR, Sugimura H, et al. Genetic polymorphisms and alternative splicing of the hOGG1 gene, that is involved in the repair of 8-hydroxyguanine in damaged DNA. Oncogene 1998; 16:3219–3225.
161. Blons H, Radicella JP, Laccoureye O, Brasnu D, Beaune P, Boiteux S, et al. Frequent allelic loss at chromosome 3p distinct from genetic alterations of the 8-oxoguanine DNA glycosylase 1 gene in head and neck cancer. Mol Carcinog 1999; 26:254–260.
162. Elahi A, Zheng Z, Park J, Eyring K, McCaffrey T, Lazarus P. The human OGG1 DNA repair enzyme and its association with orolaryngeal cancer risk. Carcinogenesis 2002; 23:1229–1234.

21

Breast Cancer

Christine B. Ambrosone and Kirsten B. Moysich

*Department of Epidemiology, Roswell Park Cancer Institute,
Buffalo, New York, U.S.A.*

Helena Furberg

*Department of Genetics, University of North Carolina at Chapel Hill,
Chapel Hill, North Carolina, U.S.A.*

1. INTRODUCTION

Despite focused efforts over the last two decades to further understand the causes of breast cancer, little new information has been gained regarding breast cancer etiology. Risk factors that are "known" explain approximately 40% of the variability in incidence (1); the remaining risks for breast cancer are yet to be determined. Breast cancer appears to be extremely heterogeneous, with multiple factors contributing to the etiology of the disease. It is plausible that a number of lifetime events and exposures, in combination with variability in key genes that metabolize steroid hormones, dietary factors, and chemical carcinogens, as well as those involved in DNA repair, signal transduction, and cell cycle control, are likely to be responsible for carcinogenesis in the breast. The focus of this chapter will be to review known and suspected risk factors for breast cancer, and the possible modification of risk relationships by genetic variability in mechanistic pathways.

2. KNOWN BREAST CANCER RISK FACTORS AND PARADIGMS OF CARCINOGENESIS

Perhaps the most consistent risk factor for breast cancer is diagnosis of the disease in a first-degree relative. A positive family history of breast cancer may or may not imply genetic susceptibility, however. It may also be due to similar environments or lifestyle habits, i.e., risk factors that are common to the mother are also common to the daughter(s). It is also possible that familial occurrence due to an inherited susceptibility is heterogeneous in mechanism and strength. Genetic susceptibility may reside in more than one gene locus, i.e., in proto-oncogenes related to signal transduction and cell cycle control, in hormone metabolism or responsiveness, in allelic loss in tumor suppressor genes, or polymorphisms in genes involved in carcinogen metabolism and detoxification, DNA repair, and immune response.

There is considerable clinical and epidemiological evidence to suggest that breast cancer is influenced by hormones, and to a lesser extent environmental exposures. Well-established risk factors for breast cancer include early age at menarche, late age at menopause, late age at first full-term pregnancy, and nulliparity. Body size also appears to influence breast cancer risk, but appears to differ according to menopausal status. High body mass index (BMI) is associated with increased risk of breast cancer among postmenopausal women, but not premenopausal women. Other putative risk factors for breast cancers originate in the environment. The presumed relationship between dietary fat and breast cancer risk has not been supported in most epidemiologic studies. There are somewhat consistent data to suggest that consumption of fruits and vegetables decreases risk, however. There are also consistent data indicating that alcohol consumption, even moderate use, increases risk of breast cancer. Cigarette smoking, despite being a biologically plausible risk factor, has been associated with increased risk of breast cancer only among certain subgroups of women.

There are primarily two paradigms proposed to link the above risk factors to breast carcinogenesis. The historically older model, which has predominated until recently, is that of two-stage carcinogenesis. Based on rodent experiments, this is a model of initiation and promotion; cells that develop mutations through DNA damage replicate and immortalize that damage. In the case of breast cancer, replication would be driven by the mitotic stimulation of circulating steroid hormones. While we now know that there are likely multiple 'hits' that damage DNA, and multiple genetic events occurring over a number of years, this model of DNA damage and cell replication is still plausible. There are a number of factors that could initiate DNA damage, including chemical carcinogens, hormone metabolites, spontaneous errors in replication, and reactive oxygen species (ROS) that could be generated through a number of processes.

The second paradigm of carcinogenesis in hormonally responsive tissue asserts that steroid hormones are complete carcinogens. Biosynthesis and metabolism of estrogens is mediated by a number of enzymes, many which are polymorphic. Some estrogen metabolites, namely the 4-hydroxy catechol estrogen, have been shown to bind to DNA and cause mutations. In this scenario, estrogens would act as both the DNA damaging agent and the mitotic stimulator.

The ability to link breast cancer risk factors to mechanisms of carcinogenesis can be enhanced by exploring the role of genetic polymorphisms in the various pathways related to exposure and response in affecting ultimate agents that can damage DNA. Polymorphisms in genes involved in the metabolism of steroid hormones or chemical carcinogens can be related to levels of ultimate reactive intermediates. The identification of genetic variants that might modify associations between exposure and disease has the potential to elucidate risk relationships more clearly, as well as to identify subsets of the population that are most susceptible to certain exposures.

3. MODIFICATION OF EXPOSURES BY NONGENETIC FACTORS

The primary focus of this chapter will be the effects of genetic variability on associations between risk factors and breast cancer. However, in addition to genetic factors, demographic or lifestyle variables may impact the effects of exposures on ultimate breast cancer risk. The age at which exposures occur may influence breast cancer risk and the impact of risk factors may vary depending on the age at which breast cancer is diagnosed.

3.1. Timing of Exposures

The timing of carcinogenic exposures may be critical to risk of breast cancer. In rats, carcinogens administered before a first pregnancy result in twice the tumor load than in rats exposed after mammary cell differentiation (2). As reviewed by Colditz and Frazier (3) and confirmed by Marcus et al. (4,5), studies of the effects of irradiation, alcohol consumption, and cigarette smoking have shown that breast cancer risk is increased by exposure at an early age. Colditz suggests that genetic damage resulting from exposures before a first pregnancy may be immortalized by cell proliferation during breast development and pregnancy, and that the decrease in cell turnover following pregnancy may prevent further genetic damage, thus reducing risk. An understanding of the importance of the age at which exposures occur may be of key importance for strategies in cancer prevention.

3.2. Age at Diagnosis of Breast Cancer

It is possible that etiologic pathways may differ for pre- and postmenopausal breast cancer, with the effects of specific risk factors having differential effects by menopausal status. For example, research indicates that there is a crossover effect of BMI by menopausal status (6–9). As reviewed by Hunter and Willett (10), the majority of breast cancer studies have found that higher BMI increases risk for postmenopausal women, but leaner women are at increased risk for premenopausal breast cancer. Relationships between exposures and breast cancer risk may also vary between subsets of individuals depending upon numerous other modifying factors, a few of which include dietary intakes of macro- and micronutrients, smoking, and reproductive histories. Another extensively studied putative effect modifier of breast cancer risk is a history of breast cancer in a first-degree relative.

4. MODIFICATION OF EXPOSURE/DISEASE RELATIONSHIPS BY GENETIC FACTORS

4.1. Family History of Breast Cancer

In most epidemiological studies, the presence of breast cancer in a first-degree relative is associated with an approximate twofold elevation in breast cancer. Among women with a family history of breast cancer, a proportion of them may carry mutant alleles in BRCA1 or BRCA2, which confer a high lifetime risk of breast cancer. However, while only a small proportion of the population of women with breast cancer carry BRCA mutations (<3%), most studies indicate that approximately 15% of the cases report breast cancer in a first-degree relative. Some studies have indicated that a family history of breast cancer may alter risks associated with other factors. Sellers and colleagues reported that risks associated with hormone replacement therapy, body fat distribution, and a number of reproductive factors varied by family history of breast cancer (11–14). Other investigators have noted similar modification of risk by reported family history of a number of reproductive and dietary factors (15–22).

4.2. BRCA1 and BRCA2 Genes

The identification of breast cancer susceptibility genes, BRCA1 and BRCA2, has enabled researchers to more clearly evaluate the effects of genetic predisposition on breast cancer risk, particularly among younger women (23,24). The two genes are believed to be responsible for most hereditary breast cancers, particularly early-onset breast cancer. Breast cancer associated with BRCA1 and BRCA2 has high penetrance, and predisposition is inherited as a dominant genetic trait. While this mutation is present in families with hereditary breast cancer, it was also found in 10% of a population-based cohort of women diagnosed with breast cancer before the age of 35 (25). Even for women with hereditary breast cancer, however, it appears that risk and age at onset may be modified by a number of other exogenous and endogenous factors.

There is considerable interest in the effect endogenous hormones have on risk of breast cancer among BRCA1 and BRCA2 mutation carriers. In an investigation of reproductive factors, Narod and colleagues found that low parity, but not age at first or last pregnancy, was associated with risk of developing breast cancer among women who carried the BRCA1 mutation (26). More recent evidence indicates that risk of breast cancer may be significantly reduced among BRCA1 carriers with a history of bilateral prophylactic oophorectomy (27). The proposed mechanism for this protective effect relates to the reduced exposure to endogenous ovarian hormones associated with such a procedure.

Polymorphic genes involved in endocrine processes may also influence risk of breast cancer among BRCA1 carriers. Rebbeck et al. reported that among women with a BRCA1 mutation, those with the CAG repeat-length polymorphism in the androgen receptor (AR) gene (28) and the variant AlB1 genotype (29) were at greater risk of developing breast cancer than those without these alterations. Four subsequent studies did not confirm these findings (30–33), however, Haiman et al. using data from the Nurses' Health Study, found that longer AR repeat alleles were overrepresented among women with a family history of breast cancer (34).

There is little existing research on the effects of exogenous exposures on BRCA1/BRCA2-associated breast cancer risk. Brunet and colleagues (35) evaluated the effect of smoking on risk of breast cancer among BRCA1 or BRCA2 mutation carriers. Results from this investigation showed that smokers were at significantly reduced risk of BRCA1/BRCA2-associated breast cancer, possibly the result of the suspected antiestrogenic effect associated with cigarette smoking. Johansson et al. and Jernstrom et al. both reported that BRCA1/BRCA2 mutation status modified the effects of pregnancy-related factors on breast cancer risk (36,37).

5. TRADITIONAL AND SUSPECTED RISK FACTORS FOR BREAST CANCER

5.1. Diet

While ecological and animal studies indicate that dietary fat intake may increase risk, cohort and case–control studies generally do not supported this hypothesis (38). Investigators have also studied possible associations with other related variables, such as total calories, animal fat and meat consumption (10,39,40), with mixed findings. There have been somewhat consistent data to indicate that a diet high in fruits and vegetables decrease risk of breast cancer, and the data strongly suggest moderate alcohol intake is associated with increased risk (41,42). Whether or not associations between these factors and risk are of the same magnitude for all women, however, has not been established. It is likely that for some women, the deleterious or protective effects of diet are more pronounced than for other women, based on metabolic variability.

5.2. Animal Products, Dietary Fat, and Heterocyclic Amines

Studies of the consumption of animal products, particularly meat, have yielded inconsistent results, although a meta-analysis of 5 cohort and 12 case–control studies by Boyd and colleagues revealed a summary relative risk of 1.54 [95% Confidence interval (CI) 1.31–1.82] associated with consumption of red meat (43). A more recent investigation, however, involving a pooled analysis of cohort studies found no association between meat consumption and breast cancer (40). The assessment of meat as a risk factor for breast cancer has focused primarily on its role as a source of dietary fat or animal protein. Dietary fat intake has long been hypothesized to be associated with breast cancer risk (44) based on animal studies (45), ecologic studies (46,47), and studies of migrants from areas with low fat intake to those with high fat intake (48). However, many analytic epidemiological studies have not shown an effect of fat, including the results of a pooled analysis of seven cohort studies (38). Recently, it has been suggested that diet in childhood and at the time of puberty may be of importance (49). Evidence from animal studies suggests that only fat intake before the first pregnancy affects risk (50). It is possible that the failure to identify an association of fat intake with breast cancer in epidemiological studies may be because intake early in life, rather than recent consumption, is most important. Failure to detect an association may also be due to fact that there is not enough variability in fat consumption within populations (i.e., there are too few individuals with low intakes) (51,52), or because of measurement error inherent in dietary questionnaires (52). It may also be that specific types of dietary fat are more important than total fat, and investigators have not been evaluating the proper variables.

Blood levels of lipoproteins have been investigated in relation to breast cancer etiology as a potential mediating factor on the relationship between dietary fat and risk and as an independent risk factor. The associations between serum and plasma total cholesterol, high-density lipoprotein (HDL) cholesterol, low-density lipoprotein (LDL) cholesterol, and triglycerides have been widely studied, but results from these investigations are inconsistent.

The apoE protein plays an important role in lipid metabolism (53) and has three common isoforms (E2, E3, and E) coded by the alleles e2, e3, and e4. In general, compared to individuals with the e3 allele, levels of total and LDL cholesterol tend to be lower for those with the e2 allele and higher for those with the e4. The e4 allele has been associated with increased risk for coronary heart disease (54,55) and Alzheimer's disease (56) and has been found to be underrepresented in elderly populations

(57), including elderly coronary heart disease patients (55) and elderly smokers (58). With respect to breast cancer, Moysich et. al. (59) reported that women with the highest serum triglyceride levels had an increase in risk compared to women with the lowest levels. This effect was not apparent among women with the e2 or e3 alleles, but much stronger among women with at least one e4 allele, suggesting that the apoE 4 genotype may modify the association between serum triglycerides and breast cancer risk.

If meat consumption does increase breast cancer risk, it may not be due to its fat content, but rather to other components. Three recent studies found that breast cancer risk was significantly increased by consumption of meat, after controlling for total fat or protein (39,60,61). It is possible that meat consumption may impact breast cancer risk as a result of mutagens and carcinogens, such as heterocyclic amines, which are formed in the cooking of meats and are potent mammary mutagens and carcinogens in rodent models (62,63). One of the most abundant heterocyclic amines, PhIP, has been detected in breast milk indicating direct exposure of ductal epithelial cells to this potent mutagen (64–66). Ultimate levels of heterocyclic amines depend on cooking method, cooking time, cooking temperature, and protein source (63).

In addition, metabolism of heterocyclic and aromatic amines varies among individuals and depends, in part, on polymorphisms in genes involved in their metabolism, such as N-acetyltransferases NAT1 and NAT2 and cytochrome P4501A2 (CYP1A2) (67). Several polymorphic sites have been identified at the NAT2 locus, and result in decreased N-acetyltransferase activity (68). Slow NAT2 acetylation of aromatic amines is associated with increased risk for bladder cancer (69) and may increase postmenopausal breast cancer risk associated with cigarette smoking (70). Heterocyclic amines appear to be poor substrates for N-acetylation at the liver, however, and rapid O-acetylation of the activated metabolites by NAT2 in the target tissue appears to be associated with increased risk of colon cancer related to consumption of red meat (71).

In a pilot study of colon cancer, Lang et al. found that individuals with rapid activation by CYP1A2 and rapid O-acetylation by NAT2 had almost three times the risk of colon cancer as those with slow phenotypes (72). More recently, LeMarchand et al. confirmed this finding in a population-based, case–control study in Hawaii (73). They found that well-done meat intake increases risk of colorectal cancer, particularly in people who inherited the rapid phenotype for both NAT2 and CYP1A2. This association was only observed among smokers, however, presumably since CYP1A2 is induced by cigarette smoking. Because heterocyclic amines appear to be mammary carcinogens, it is possible that rapid hepatic activation by CYP1A2 and further activation by NAT1 or NAT2, may be related to breast cancer risk (74–76). Thus, heterocyclic amines may be associated with increased breast cancer risk among women with rapid CYP1A2 and rapid NAT2 status. Findings from epidemiological studies, however, have been inconsistent.

We found no associations between meat consumption, NAT2, and breast cancer in a study of Caucasian women in western New York (77). However, the questionnaire used was not designed to evaluate heterocyclic amines per se, thus substantial misclassification was possible. Using Sinha's questionnaire specifically designed for heterocyclic amine exposure, Zheng et al. (78) recently reported that consumption of well-done meats increased breast cancer risk in a dose-dependent manner. Deitz et al. also reported an elevated association between well-done meats and breast cancer risk among rapid/intermediate NAT2 acetylators (79). In a subsequent paper (80), Zheng et al. examined the role of NAT1 genetic polymorphisms and risk related to smoking and meat consumption. They reported that the NAT1*11 allele, thought to result in rapid activation, resulted in a significant sixfold increase in breast cancer risk among women who were high consumers of red meat. Among women with low intake, there was a nonsignificant risk of less than three associated with that putative allele. Contrary to these findings, Gertig and colleagues (81) and Delfino et al. (79) did not report an increased risk with read meat consumption, and risk was not modified by NAT2 status.

5.3. Fruit and Vegetable Consumption

There are fairly consistent data indicating that higher consumption of fruits and vegetables is associated with decreased breast cancer risk (82,83), although not all studies support such an association (84,85). Fruits and vegetables are sources of a number of nutrients, including antioxidant vitamins such as carotenoids, the tocopherols, and vitamin C. Several nutritional epidemiological studies have noted inverse associations between dietary antioxidants and breast cancer risk (86–88). The mechanistic relationship of these putative risk factors, however, has not been elucidated. One hypothesis is that dietary antioxidants affect oxidative stress and the production of reactive oxygen species (ROS) by altering the balance between prooxidant cellular activity and antioxidant defenses (89). Reactive oxygen species are produced by normal cellular respiration and as a result of inflammation and cellular stress (90). When ROS are the result of normal metabolism, and there is sufficient antioxidant power and repair capacity, there are presumably few harmful effects. Excessive production of ROS resulting from toxic agents, such as tobacco smoke, or from insufficient in vivo defense mechanisms, can result in oxidative stress, leading to damage to DNA and cell membranes, mitochondrion, and protein (91–96). It is also possible that a diet low in fruits and vegetables could contribute to excessive ROS and oxidative stress. Oxidative damage has been reported to be higher in women with breast cancer, compared to controls, although studies to date remain small (97–99), and these levels vary with the consumption of meats, vegetables, and fruits (100–102).

Endogenous defenses against ROS include glutathione peroxidase, catalase, and superoxide dismutase (SOD) (90). There are three known forms of SOD: the cytosolic and extracellular copper/zinc SODs and the mitochondrial manganese SOD (MnSOD). MnSOD is synthesized in the cytosol and post-transcriptionally modified for transport into the mitochondrion (103,104). In the mitochondrion, it catalyzes the dismutation of two superoxide radicals, producing H_2O_2 and oxygen. MnSOD is induced with free radical challenge (105) and cigarette smoke (106). Recently, two genetic variants of MnSOD were identified. A nucleotide T to C substitution in the mitochondrial targeting sequence was found that changes an amino acid. The investigators who identified the polymorphism predicted that the resulting amino acid change would alter the secondary structure of the protein (104), and Rosenblum and colleagues (107) suggested that the alteration might affect the cellular allocation of the enzyme and mitochondrial transport of MnSOD into the mitochondrion. They further suggested that inefficient targeting of MnSOD could leave mitochondria without their full defense against superoxide radicals, which could lead to protein oxidation, as well as mitchondrial DNA mutations.

We hypothesized that the polymorphism in MnSOD would result in higher levels of ROS, and that in women whose diets were low in fruits and vegetables, this polymorphism would increase risk of breast cancer (108). Interestingly, we found this to be the case, particularly for premenopausal women (108). Those who were homozygous for the variant allele had a fourfold increase in breast cancer risk in comparison to those with who were homozygous or heterozygous for the common allele [odds ratio (OR) = 4.3, 95% CI, 1.7–10.8]. Risk was most pronounced among women below the median consumption of fruits and vegetables, and of dietary ascorbic acid and a-tocopherol, with little increased risk for those with diets rich in these foods. These findings were supported by Mitrunen et al. in their study of pre- and postmenopausal Finnish women (109).

These data support the hypothesis that MnSOD and oxidative stress play a significant role in breast cancer risk, particularly in premenopausal women. The finding that risk was greatest among women who consumed lower amounts of dietary antioxidants, and was minimal among high consumers, suggests that a diet rich in sources of antioxidants may compensate for the effects of the MnSOD polymorphism, thereby supporting public health recommendations for consumption of diets rich in fruits and vegetables as a preventive measure against cancer.

5.4. Alcohol

The potential effect of alcohol consumption on breast cancer risk has been widely studied in the past decades. The importance of determining such an association has been emphasized due to the major public health problem associated with breast cancer as well as the notion that alcohol consumption is fairly common, yet modifiable (110). Based on findings from two meta-analyses, there appears to be a modest increase in breast cancer risk associated with daily consumption of alcoholic beverages (42,111). Several mechanisms for a role of alcohol consumption in breast carcinogenesis have been proposed, including increases of bioavailable estrogen and direct toxic effects associated with ethanol exposure (112,113).

Recently, efforts have been made to evaluate the role of alcohol metabolizing genes as a potential susceptibility marker for the adverse effect of alcohol consumption on breast cancer risk. The polymorphic alcohol dehydrogenase 3 (ADH3) gene is involved in the oxidation of ethanol to carcinogenic acetaldehyde and plays a rate-limiting role in the metabolic pathway for most human ethanol oxidation (114). The presence of the ADH3[1] allele, coding for the more rapid form of the ADH3 enzyme, has previously been associated with increased risk of cancer of the oral cavity and pharynx (115,116) and of hepatic cirrhosis and chronic pancreatitis (117).

In a population–based case–control study, Freudenheim et al. (118) observed an increased risk of premenopausal breast cancer among women with the highest self-reported alcohol consumption and at least one ADH3[1] allele. These findings are supported by a preliminary report (119) indicating that among women with at least one ADH3[1] allele, those who drank alcohol were at greater risk of breast cancer compared to those who abstained. Furthermore, there was also evidence for a risk elevation for women who drank and who carried the GSTM1 null genotype and at least ADH3[1] allele. Hines et al. conducted a prospective study on the effect of alcohol consumption, ADH3 genotype on plasma steroid hormone levels and breast cancer risk (120). While a modest association was seen for plasma hormones and alcohol consumption, no association was found between ADH3 genotype and breast cancer risk, regardless of alcohol consumption or menopausal status.

The genetic polymorphism in cytochrome P4502E1 (CYP2E1) may also modify the association between alcohol consumption and breast cancer risk. Ethanol-inducible CYP2E1 is an enzyme of major toxicological interest because it metabolizes a wide range of environmental compounds to reactive metabolites (121). Shields et al. (122) found a smoking-associated risk elevation to be restricted to women with the CYP2E1 variant genotype, but did not investigate associations with alcohol consumption due to small numbers in groups with varying alcohol intake and variant alleles. In fact, molecular epidemiological studies on the CYP2E1 genetic polymorphism may pose substantial methodological challenges, due to the low prevalence of the CYP2E1 variant genotype in the general population.

5.5. Reproductive Factors and Hormones

Because epidemiological studies indicate that key breast cancer risk factors are related to endogenous exposure to steroid hormones, intensive epidemiological research has been targeted at serum and urinary measurement of parent hormones and their metabolites in both case–control and cohort studies, yielding inconsistent results (123,124). However, measurement of serum levels of estrogens may reflect levels quite different from those hormone metabolites to which the target tissue is exposed. Many of the genes involved in the biosynthesis and metabolism of estrogen are polymorphic, and research attention has begun to focus on the impact of these variants on breast cancer risk. Investigating the distribution of functionally relevant genetic polymorphisms that alter the bioavailability of steroid hormones among persons with disease and persons without may provide more direct evidence for estrogen and estrogen metabolites as modifiers of human diseases, including breast cancer. A number of studies, to date, have evaluated relationships between breast cancer risk and genetic polymorphisms in CYP1A1, CYP17, CYP19, and COMT.

5.5.1. CYP1A1

Early studies of genetic polymorphisms in cytochrome P450 (CYP) 1A1 focused primarily on its role in lung cancer risk, since it activates polycyclic aromatic hydrocarbons, which are potent tobacco smoke carcinogens. However, CYP1A1 is also involved in the metabolism of estradiol. To date, four polymorphisms have been identified within this gene, one of which is specific to African-Americans (125). A number of studies have been conducted to evaluate associations between CYP1A1 and breast cancer risk, with mixed results (126–129). In a study with African-American and Caucasian women, Taioli and colleagues (128) noted that among African-American women, the m1 polymorphism significantly increased breast cancer risk (OR = 9.7, 95% CI: 2.0–47.9). Numbers in these stratified analyses, however, were quite small. In both the western New York study (129) and the Harvard study (129) it was found that while there were no main effects of CYP1A1 on breast cancer risk, the effects of CYP1A1 polymorphisms were modified by cigarette smoking. Women who were light smokers with variant alleles were at increased risk of breast cancer in the Ambrosone study (127), and those with variant alleles who began smoking before age 16 in the Ishibe study (129). Recently, Bailey et al. evaluated all four known CYP1A1 polymorphisms in relation to breast cancer risk, in a case–control study. None of these polymorphisms, including that specific to African-Americans, was associated with increased risk; smoking status "ever/never" did not modify risk. Furthermore, Basham et al. who combined data from their own study with those of four previously published, failed to observe an association between CYP1A1 genotype and breast cancer (130). No interactions were noted between genotype and alcohol or smoking habits.

5.5.2. CYP17

Another cytochrome P450 enzyme that has received much attention of late is the P45017a encoded by the CYP17 gene. This enzyme functions at key branch points in human steroidogenesis. The CYP17 polymorphism has also been evaluated by a number of groups; again, studies have had conflicting results. Feigelson and colleagues initially found that the variant allele conferred more than a twofold increase in risk among women with advanced disease (131). They also noted that late age at menarche was protective only among women who were homozygous for common allele. Several subsequent studies have not corroborated these findings (132–137), although analyses in the Nurses' Health study (135) demonstrated that the protective effect of later age at menarche (>13 years) was only observed among women with the common allele and not among women carrying variant alleles. The recent meta-analysis involving data from 15 case–control studies (138) also showed that the variant allele in CYP17 acts as a weak modifier of breast cancer risk but is not an independent risk factor.

5.5.3. CYP19

Aromatase or estrogen synthetase, encoded by the CYP19 gene, converts androgens to estrogens, and completes the pathway for estrogen biosynthesis from cholesterol (139). The conversion of testosterone to estradiol in adipose tissue is the main source of estrogens in postmenopausal women. A polymorphic tetranucleotide repeat (TTTA)n has been identified and although relatively rare, Kristensen et al. (140) noted a significant association with breast cancer risk in carriers of the longest repeat variant (TTTA)12, designated the A1 allele, in a case–control study with 366 cases and 252 controls. The A1 allele was present in less than 2% of the control population, but in almost 4% of cases. Siegelmann-Danieli (141) also evaluated this association and found increased risk with the variant A1 allele. Baxter et al. confirmed this association in a study of breast cancer in England (142). These findings were not confirmed, however, by Haiman et al. who evaluated CYP19 polymorphisms in relation to breast cancer and estrogen levels in the Nurses' Health study (143).

5.5.4. Catechol-O-Methyltransferase

Catechol-O-methyltransferase (COMT) is one of several phase II enzymes involved in the conjugation and inactivation of catechol estrogens (144). Because there is evidence that catechol estrogens, particularly the 4-hydroxy catechol estrogen, may bind to DNA and result in DNA damage (145), the possible role of lower activity in the enzyme in relation to breast cancer risk is important. Several groups to date, all with conflicting results, have evaluated the role of the COMT genetic polymorphism in relation to breast cancer risk. Lavigne et al. (146) found that women who were postmenopausal had a greater than twofold increase in risk with the low activity alleles, but inverse associations were noted for premenopausal women with the same genotype. Thompson et al. (147) performed similar analyses and observed that, among premenopausal women with breast cancer, those with at least one low activity allele showed significantly increased risk (OR = 2.4, CI, 1.4–4.3). In contrast to premenopausal women, there was an inverse association between low activity alleles and postmenopausal breast cancer. Mitrunen et al. (148) noted inverse associations for women with low activity COMT alleles in relation to premenopausal breast cancer risk, and elevated associations for postmenopausal women, particularly those using exogenous estrogens or early age at menarche. The authors hypothesized that there may be an opposing role of catechol estrogen metabolism in breast cancer etiology depending on the hormonal environment. Yim et al. (149) also reported that the low activity COMT allele was associated with increased risk of breast cancer among Asian women. Millikan (150) and Bergman-Jungestrom (151), however, found no associations with COMT genotypes and increased breast cancer risk for pre- or postmenopausal women. These discrepancies may be due to small sample sizes in the previous studies, or there may be biological factors that differentially impact risk associations.

5.6. Chemical Exposures

Environmental factors have been implicated in breast cancer etiology, due to the steady increase in incidence over the last decades (152), regional and international differences in incidence, and observed changes in incidence rates in migrant populations (153).

5.6.1. Organochlorines

One group of environmental exposures that has been examined in relation to breast cancer includes organochlorine compounds, such as 2,2-bis(4-chlorophenyl)-1,1-dichloroethane (DDE), the major metabolite of 2,2-bis(p-chlorophenyl)-1,1,1-trichloroethane (DDT), and polychlorinated biphenyls (PCBs). Evidence from laboratory studies has demonstrated a complex diversity of biological effects associated with these compounds. DDE and some PCB congeners have been associated with induction of cytochrome P450 enzymes (154,155), which may or may not be associated with estrogenic (156–158) and antiestrogenic effects (158) shown in some investigations. Studies have also noted changes in immune responses (159) and tumor promoting effects (154,160,161).

Several recent epidemiologic studies have investigated the role of DDE and PCBs in breast cancer etiology (162–175), but results from these studies are inconsistent. While results from an earlier investigation pointed to a potential role of organochlorine exposure in breast carcinogenesis, most subsequent studies did not observe significant risk elevations among women with the highest blood or adipose levels of these compounds.

Some efforts have been made to examine the effect of environmental organochlorine exposure among susceptible subgroups, defined by reproductive or genetic factors. Moysich et al. (163) observed a significant increase in risk of breast cancer among parous postmenopausal women who never lactated with the highest serum PCB levels compared to those with the lowest levels. Organochlorine levels were also associated with age and serum lipids, but not fruit intake (176). It is possible that women who had lactated were less susceptible to the adverse effect of organochlorine exposure due to the fact that they had eliminated a substantial amount of organochlorine body burden at a biologically relevant period of time. Alternatively, lactation in itself may contribute to the terminal differentiation of the mammary epithelium, resulting in larger compartments of nonproliferating cells (2). It has also been suggested that organochlorine body burden may have been measured more accurately among women who had never breastfed an infant. Serum levels in this group may represent a more valid measure of chronic exposure, uninterrupted by elimination of these compounds through lactation. Based on the same study population, these investigators also attempted to determine whether or not the genetic polymorphism in the CYP1A1 gene affected the association between PCB exposure and risk (177).

In laboratory studies, PCBs are potent inducers of CYP1A1, a drug-metabolizing gene, involved in the activation of potentially genotoxic endogenous and exogenous substances (178,179). Their results indicated that postmenopausal women with the highly inducible CYP1A1 variant genotype and high PCB levels were at significantly increased risk for breast cancer compared to women with the CYP1A1 wild genotype and lower PCB levels. A potential mechanism for this finding relates to the PCB mediated enhanced induction of polymorphic CYP1A1, leading to increased activation of environmental carcinogens and subsequently resulting in the production of reactive intermediates and DNA damage. Thus, by inducing CYP1A1, PCBs, and other inducers can trigger the activation of xenobiotics, such as those found in tobacco, into mutagenic compounds.

5.6.2. Cigarette Smoking and Breast Cancer

Environmental contaminants other than organochlorines could also be associated with breast cancer risk, including aryl and heterocyclic aromatic amines, nitro- and polycyclic aromatic hydrocarbons, and *N*-nitroso compounds, all of which are known mammary mutagens and carcinogens. In addition to their presence in an industrialized environment, these carcinogens are present in cigarette smoke. Aromatic amines form DNA adducts in cultured human epithelial cells (180), and cause unscheduled DNA synthesis (180). In vivo activated aromatic amine metabolites have been shown to cause DNA damage in rodents (181,182) to transform mouse mammary glands (183), and to induce rodent mammary tumors (184,185). Polycyclic aromatic hydrocarbons are also likely human breast carcinogens. The PAHs benzo(a)pyrene and 7,12-dimethylbenz(a)anthracene induce mammary tumors in rodents (186,187) and cause transformation in human breast epithelial cell lines in vitro (188).

The mutational spectrum of the p53 tumor suppressor gene also supports a role for chemical carcinogens in breast cancer risk. While the pattern of p53 mutations in breast cancer differs from the fingerprint mutations associated with smoking in lung cancer, they occur on sites that are suggestive of an unknown, environmental exposure (189,190). Furthermore, it is clear that chemical carcinogens reach the breast in laboratory animals and humans, and because they are lipophilic, they are stored in breast adipose tissue (191,192). Ductal epithelial cells are directly exposed to nicotine (193) and mutagenic compounds (194). Heterocyclic amines administered to nursing rat dams were found at high levels in the breast tissue, and were excreted in the milk (195). Three studies have identified DNA adducts in normal breast tissue from women with and without breast cancer (66, 196–199), some of which were putatively related to tobacco smoking. Therefore, the breast is certainly exposed to chemical carcinogens, and can be susceptible to the carcinogenic process.

If these compounds are human mammary carcinogens, one would expect to see an association between smoking and breast cancer risk. However, in the majority of epidemiological studies, an association between smoking and breast cancer risk has not been found (200–202). However, most previous studies combined passive smokers with non-smokers in the reference category. Sidestream smoke contains higher levels of aromatic amines than mainstream smoke, as much as 10 mg of aniline per cigarette, as well as many other aromatic amines [e.g., multiple isomers of toluidine, naphthylamine and aminobiphenyl (ABP)]. Thus, passive smoke exposure may result in different circulating levels of carcinogens than active smoking. The presence of passive smokers in the referent 'non-smoking' category would certainly dilute risk estimates. Studies that confined the referent group to those never exposed to passive smoke all found increased breast cancer risk for active and passive smokers (203–208). Using data from the Nurses' Health study, however, Egan et al. did not find a positive association between passive smoking and breast cancer risk, but a small increase in risk was noted for smoking initiated at young ages (<17 years old) (201).

It has been suggested that some components of tobacco smoke may have antiestrogenic effects (209,210). For example, cigarette smoking induces CYP1A2, which decreases the level of circulating estradiol. It is possible that genetic variability in metabolism of chemical carcinogens may make some women more susceptible to their carcinogenic effects from ubiquitous exposure, dietary intake, and exposure through active and passive cigarette smoke. Other women may be more affected by the putative antiestrogenic effect of tobacco smoke. When these subgroups are grouped together, however, as in population-based studies, the effects of a particular exposure may not be observable above the background of other exposures and susceptibilities. In this case, the effects may be diluted and thus, not statistically significant. Several molecular epidemiological studies have been conducted to ascertain possible associations between smoking and breast cancer risk among women likely to be susceptible to their carcinogenic effects. By evaluating genetic polymorphisms for enzymes involved in the metabolism of classes of chemical carcinogens, subgroups of the population who may be susceptible to tobacco smoke carcinogens may be identified.

Aromatic Amine Metabolism: Aromatic amines are likely to be first metabolized in the liver via two competing pathways. They may be either activated by CYP1A2, or detoxified through *N*-acetylation by NAT2. We hypothesized that among women who had inherited mutations NAT2 encoding a less efficient form of the enzyme and were thus, 'slow acetylators'; aromatic amines would be more likely to be activated by CYP1A2. In this scenario, activated hydroxylamines could be further activated either in the liver or in the breast, DNA adducts could form, and breast cancer could result. In a study of several hundred pre- and postmenopausal women in western New York (70), we found that neither smoking nor the slow NAT2 genotype impacted breast cancer risk. However, postmenopausal women who had slow NAT2 and smoked were at dose-dependent, increased risk. This hypothesis was subsequently explored by other groups, with mixed results (207,211,212).

Polycyclic Aromatic Hydrocarbon Metabolism: PAHs are metabolized by a complex of phase I and phase II enzymes. Those studied in relation to smoking and breast cancer include CYP1A1 and glutathione *S*-transferase M1 (GSTM1). CYP1A1 activates PAHs, and as mentioned previously, Ambrosone et al. found that the exon 7 polymorphism (m2) increased risk among postmenopausal women who were light smokers. This finding was supported by data from the Nurses' Health study (m1 and m2) (129), but Bailey and colleagues found no associations with any of the polymorphisms (m1–m4) (125). Earlier, Taioli et al. (128) evaluated CYP1A1 polymorphisms (m1–m3) among Caucasians and African-Americans, and found that the m1 allele increased risk among African-American women. These data were not presented in relation to smoking, however.

Phase II metabolism includes detoxification of reactive metabolites by conjugation with glutathione, which is catalyzed by glutathione *S*-transferases. GSTM1 has a deletion that is present in approximately 50% of Caucasian populations, resulting in loss of the enzyme. A number of groups have evaluated the possible association of the GSTM1 polymorphism with breast cancer risk. For the most part, studies have found no association between the null allele and breast cancer regardless of smoking status (125,127,213–217). Helzlsouer et al., however, reported an increased risk of postmenopausal breast cancer associated with GSTM1 deletion (218). This association was not modified by exposure to tobacco smoke.

6. FUTURE DIRECTIONS

While molecular epidemiology studies hold the promise of elucidating mechanisms behind breast cancer risk factors, it is still subject to limitations of traditional epidemiological studies. Much of the molecular epidemiology literature is rife with inconsistencies, as described in this chapter. This is likely due to the small sample sizes of the studies, which result in low power to detect associations. A recent article described the sobering numbers of participants required to detect stable estimates from epidemiological studies of gene–environment interactions (219).

Additionally, examining one gene at a time in relation to breast cancer risk is likely too simplistic. Future studies should consider the roles of other genes involved in metabolic pathways and examine several genes at a time in relation to cancer risk (220). Multigenic studies have been conducted recently with suggestive findings. Feigelson et al. examined CYP17 and 17β-HSD in combination, in relation to breast cancer risk in a large, multi-ethnic population. They demonstrated an increased risk from high-risk alleles limited to advanced stage breast cancer and postulated that these tumors may be more aggressive as a result of increased estrogenic exposure (221). Huang et al. also considered the effect of several estrogen-metabolizing genes involved at different points within the pathway, including CYP17, CYP1A1, and COMT (222). A trend in increasing risk was observed with increasing number of at risk genotypes. This effect was especially pronounced in women with prolonged estrogen exposure, providing further support of the possibility that breast cancer can be initiated by estrogen exposure and is influenced by genotypes. Eventually, techniques that provide simultaneous assessment of tens-to-hundreds-to-thousands of genes at a time will be useful in studies of cancer. However, it is unrealistic to anticipate the incorporation of a large number of genes into current molecular epidemiological practice, since proper statistical methods are not in place.

7. CONCLUSION

It is becoming quite clear that the etiology of human breast cancer is exceedingly complex, with probable multiple factors involved in its etiology. Molecular epidemiology and the use of markers of susceptibility, internal dose, and early effects may elucidate not only mechanisms, but also clarify relationships between risk factors and disease among subsets of the population who are specifically at risk. For the public, however, lifestyle modification to maintain normal weight, eat a diet high in fruits and vegetables, and refraining from tobacco use and alcohol consumption, should be advised for all women, regardless of genetic makeup.

REFERENCES

1. Madigan MP, Ziegler RG, Benichou J, Byrne C, Hoover RN. Proportion of breast cancer cases in the United States explained by well-established risk factors. J Natl Cancer Inst 1995; 87:1681–1685.
2. Russo J, Russo IH. Biological and molecular bases of mammary carcinogenesis. Lab Invest 1987; 57:112–37.
3. Colditz GA, Frazier AL. Models of breast cancer show that risk is set by events of early life: prevention efforts must shift focus. Cancer Epidemiol Biomarkers Prev 1995; 4:567–571.
4. Marcus PM, Newman B, Moorman PG, Millikan RC, Baird DD, Qaqish B, et al. Physical activity at age 12 and adult breast cancer risk (United States). Cancer Causes Control 1999; 10:293–302.
5. Marcus PM, Newman B, Millikan RC, Moorman PG, Baird DD, Qaqish B. The associations of adolescent cigarette smoking, alcoholic beverage consumption, environmental tobacco smoke, and ionizing radiation with subsequent breast cancer risk (United States). Cancer Causes Control 2000; 11:271–278.
6. Janerich DT, Hoff MB. Evidence for a crossover in breast cancer risk factors. Am J Epidemiol 1982; 116:737–742.
7. Lubin F, Ruder AM, Wax Y, Modan B. Overweight and changes in weight throughout adult life in breast cancer etiology. A case–control study. Am J Epidemiol 1985; 122:579–588.
8. Velentgas P, Daling JR. Risk factors for breast cancer in younger women. J Natl Cancer Inst Monogr 1994; 15–24.
9. Hislop TG, Coldman AJ, Elwood JM, Brauer G, Kan L. Childhood and recent eating patterns and risk of breast cancer. Cancer Detect Prev 1986; 9:47–58.
10. Hunter DJ, Willett WC. Diet, body size, and breast cancer. [Review]. Epidemiol Rev 1993; 15:110–132.
11. Sellers TA, Kushi LH, Potter JD, Kaye SA, Nelson CL, McGovern PG, et al. Effect of family history, body-fat distribution, and reproductive factors on the risk of postmenopausal breast cancer. N Engl J Med 1992; 326:1323–1329.
12. Sellers TA, Potter JD, Severson RK, Bostick RM, Nelson CL, Kushi LH, et al. Difficulty becoming pregnant and family history as interactive risk factors for postmenopausal breast cancer: the Iowa Women's Health Study. Cancer Causes Control 1993; 4:21–28.
13. Tutera AM, Sellers TA, Potter JD, Drinkard CR, Wiesner GL, Folsom AR. Association between family history of cancer and breast cancer defined by estrogen and progesterone receptor status. Genet Epidemiol 1996; 13:207–221.

14. Sellers TA, Minks T, Cerhan JR, Zheng W, Anderson KE, Kushi LH, et al. The role of hormone replacement therapy in the risk for breast cancer and total mortality in women with a family history of breast cancer. Ann Intern Med 1997; 127:973–980.

15. Andrieu N, Duffy SW, Rohan TE, Le MG, Luporsi E, Renaud R, et al. Familial risk, abortion and their interactive effect on the risk of breast cancer—a combined analysis of six case–control studies. Br J Cancer 1995; 72:744–751.

16. Ambrosone CB, Marshall JR, Vena JE, Laughlin R, Graham S, Nemoto T, et al. Interaction of family history of breast cancer and dietary antioxidants with breast cancer risk (New York, United States). Cancer Causes Control 1995; 6:407–415.

17. Brinton LA, Hoover R, Fraumeni JF Jr. Interaction of familial and hormonal risk factors for breast cancer. J Natl Cancer Inst 1982; 69:817–822.

18. Byrne C, Brinton LA, Haile RW, Schairer C. Heterogeneity of the effect of family history on breast cancer risk. Epidemiology 1991; 2:276–284.

19. Dupont WD, Page DL. Breast cancer risk associated with proliferative disease, age at first birth, and a family history of breast cancer. Am J Epidemiol 1987; 125:769–779.

20. Parazzini F, La Vecchia C, Negri E, Franceschi S, Bocciolone L. Menstrual and reproductive factors and breast cancer in women with family history of the disease. Int J Cancer 1992; 51:677–681.

21. Colditz GA, Rosner BA, Speizer FE. Risk factors for breast cancer according to family history of breast cancer. J Natl Cancer Inst 1996; 88:365–371.

22. Egan KM, Stampfer MJ, Rosner BA, Trichopoulos D, Newcomb PA, Mittendorf R, et al. Risk factors for breast cancer in women with a breast cancer family history. Cancer Epidemiol Biomarkers Prev 1998; 7:359–364.

23. Miki Y, Swensen J, Shattuck-Eidens D, Futreal PA, Harshman K, Tavtigian S, et al. A strong candidate for the breast and ovarian cancer susceptibility gene BRCA1. Science 1994; 266:66–71.

24. Wooster R, Neuhausen SL, Mangion J, Quirk Y, Ford D, Collins N, et al. Localization of a breast cancer susceptibility gene, BRCA2, to chromosome 13q12-13. Science 1994; 265:2088–2091.

25. Langston AA, Malone KE, Thompson JD, Daling JR, Ostrander EA. BRCA1 mutations in a population-based sample of young women with breast cancer. N Engl J Med 1996; 334:137–142.

26. Narod SA, Goldgar D, Cannon-Albright L, Weber BL, Moslehi R, Ives E, et al. Risk modifiers in carriers of BRCA1 mutations. Int J Cancer 1995; 64:394–398.

27. Rebbeck TR, Levin AM, Eisen A, Snyder C, Watson P, Cannon-Albright L, et al. Breast cancer risk after bilateral prophylactic oophorectomy in BRCA1 mutation carriers. J Natl Cancer Inst 1999; 91:1475–1479.

28. Rebbeck TR, Kantoff PW, Krithivas K, Neuhausen S, Blackwood MA, Godwin AK, et al. Modification of BRCA1-associated breast cancer risk by the polymorphic androgen-receptor CAG repeat. Am J Hum Genet 1999; 64:1371–1377.

29. Rebbeck TR, Kantoff PW, Krithivas K, Neuhausen S, Blackwood MA, Godwin AK, et al. Modification of breast cancer risk in BRCA1 mutation carriers by the A1B1 gene. Proc Amer Assoc Cancer Res 1999; 40:194.

30. Menin C, Banna GL, De Salvo G, Lazzarotto V, De Nicolo A, Agata S, et al. Lack of association between androgen receptor CAG polymorphism and familial breast/ovarian cancer. Cancer Lett 2001; 168:31–36.

31. Given HF, Radbourne R, Oag H, Merritt S, Barclay E, Hanby AM, et al. The androgen receptor exon 1 trinucleotide repeat does not act as a modifier of the age of presentation in breast cancer. Eur J Cancer 2000; 36:533–534.

32. Kadouri L, Easton DF, Edwards S, Hubert A, Kote-Jarai Z, Glaser B, et al. CAG and GGC repeat polymorphisms in the androgen receptor gene and breast cancer susceptibility in BRCA1/2 carriers and non-carriers. Br J Cancer 2001; 85:36–40.

33. Spurdle AB, Dite GS, Chen X, Mayne CJ, Southey MC, Batten LE, et al. Androgen receptor exon 1 CAG repeat length and breast cancer in women before age forty years. J Natl Cancer Inst 1999; 91:961–966.

34. Haiman CA, Brown M, Hankinson SE, Spiegelman D, Colditz GA, Willett WC, et al. The androgen receptor CAG repeat polymorphism and risk of breast cancer in the Nurses' Health Study. Cancer Res 2002; 62:1045–1049.

35. Brunet JS, Ghadirian P, Rebbeck TR, Lerman C, Garber JE, Tonin PN, et al. Effect of smoking on breast cancer in carriers of mutant BRCA1 or BRCA2 genes. J Natl Cancer Inst 1998; 90:761–766.

36. Jernstrom H, Lerman C, Ghadirian P, Lynch HT, Weber B, Garber J, et al. Pregnancy and risk of early breast cancer in carriers of BRCA1 and BRCA2. Lancet 1999; 354:1846–1850.

37. Johannsson O, Loman N, Borg A, Olsson H. Pregnancy-associated breast cancer in BRCA1 and BRCA2 germline mutation carriers. Lancet 1998; 352:1359–1360.

38. Hunter DJ, Spiegelman D, Adami HO, Beeson L, van den Brandt PA, Folsom AR, et al. Cohort studies of fat intake and the risk of breast cancer—a pooled analysis. N Engl J Med 1996; 334:356–361.

39. Toniolo P, Riboli E, Shore RE, Pasternack BS. Consumption of meat, animal products, protein, and fat and risk of breast cancer: a prospective cohort study in New York [see comments]. Epidemiology 1994; 5:391–397.

40. Missmer SA, Smith-Warner SA, Spiegelman D, Yaun SS, Adami HO, Beeson WL, et al. Meat and dairy food consumption and breast cancer: a pooled analysis of cohort studies. Int J Epidemiol 2002; 31:78–85.

41. Hunter DJ, Willett WC. Nutrition and breast cancer. Cancer Causes Control 1996; 7:56–68.

42. Singletary KW, Gapstur SM. Alcohol and breast cancer: review of epidemiologic and experimental evidence and potential mechanisms. J Am Med Assoc 2001; 286:2143–2151.

43. Boyd NF, Martin LJ, Noffel M, Lockwood GA, Tritchler DL. A meta-analysis of studies of dietary fat and breast cancer risk. Br J Cancer 1993; 68: 627–636.

44. Willett WC. The search for the causes of breast and colon cancer. Nature 1989; 338:389–394.

45. Cave WT. Dietary fat effects on animal models of breast cancer. In: Weisburger EK, ed. Diet and Breast Cancer. New York: Plenum Press, 1994.

46. Armstrong B, Doll R. Environmental factors and cancer incidence and mortality in different countries, with special reference to dietary practices. Int J Cancer 1975; 15:617–631.
47. Caroll KK, Braden LM, Bell JM, Kalamegham R. Fat and cancer. Cancer 1986; 58:1818–1825.
48. Dunn JE. Breast cancer among American Japanese in the San Francisco bay area. J Natl Cancer Inst Monogr 1975; 47:157–160.
49. Potischman N, Weiss HA, Swanson CA, Coates RJ, Gammon MD, Malone KE, et al. Diet during adolescence and risk of breast cancer among young women. J Natl Cancer Inst 1998; 90:226–233.
50. Ip C. Controversial issues of dietary fat and experimental mammary carcinogenesis. Prev Med 1993; 22:728–737.
51. Goodwin PJ, Boyd NF. Critical appraisal of the evidence that dietary fat intake is related to breast cancer risk in humans. J Natl Cancer Inst 1987; 79: 473–485.
52. Bingham SA, Gill C, Welch A, Day K, Cassidy A, Khaw KT, et al. Comparison of dietary assessment methods in nutritional epidemiology: weighted records v. 24h recalls, food frequency questionnaires and estimated diet records. Br J Nutr 1994; 72:643.
53. Beisiegel U, Weber W, Ihrke G. The LDL-receptor related protein, LPR, is an apolipoprotein E binding protein. Nature 1989; 341:162–170.
54. Uterman G. Apoliproprotein E polymorphism in health and disease. Am Heart J 1987; 113:433–440.
55. Davignon J, Gregg RE, Sing CF. Apolipoprotein E polymorphism and atherosclerosis. Arteriosclerosis 1988; 8:1–21.
56. Kuusisto J, Koivisto K, Kervinen K, Mykkanen L, Helkala EL, Vanhanen M, et al. Association of apolipoprotein E phenotypes with late onset Alzheimer's disease: population based study. Br Med J 1994; 309:636–638.
57. Kervinen K, Savolainen MJ, Salokannel J, Hynninen A, Heikkinen J, Ehnholm C, et al. Apolipoprotein E and B polymorphisms—longevity factors assessed in nonagenarians. Atherosclerosis 1994; 105:89–95.
58. Bowman ED, Broemke B, Lensing W, Shields PG. Apolipoprotein E allelic frequency in elderly smokers. Am J Med Genet 1998; 76:32–36.
59. Moysich KB, Freudenheim JL, Baker JA, Ambrosone CB, Schisterman EF, Vena JE, Shields PG. Apolipoprotein E polymorphism, cholesterol, and breast cancer risk. Mol Carcinog 2000; 27:2–9.
60. Ronco A, Destefani E, Mendilaharsu M, Deneopellegrini H. Meat, fat and risk of breast cancer—a case–control study from Uruguay. Int J Cancer 1996; 65:328–331.
61. Destefani E, Ronco A, Mendilaharsu M, Guidobono M, Deneo-Pellegrini H. Meat intake, heterocyclic amines, and risk of breast cancer: a case–control study in Uruguay. Cancer Epidemiol Biomarkers Prev 2001; 6:573–581.
62. Snyderwine EG. Some perspectives on the nutritional aspects of breast cancer research. Food-derived heterocyclic amines as etiologic agents in human mammary cancer. [Review]. Cancer 1994; 74:1070–1077.

63. Felton JS, Knize MG, Salmon CP, Malfatti MA, Kulp KS. Human exposure to heterocyclic amine food mutagens/carcinogens: relevance to breast cancer. Environ Mol Mutagen 2002; 39:112–118.
64. DeBruin LS, Martos PA, Josephy PD. Detection of PhIP (2-amino-1-methyl-6-phenylimidazo[4,5-b]pyridine) in the milk of healthy women. Chem Res Toxicol 2001; 14:1523–1528.
65. Gorlewska-Roberts K, Green B, Fares M, Ambrosone CB, Kadlubar FF. Carcinogen–DNA adducts in human breast epithelial cells. Environ Mol Mutagen 2002; 39:184–192.
66. Thompson PA, DeMarini DM, Kadlubar FF, McClure GY, Brooks LR, Green BL, et al. Evidence for the presence of mutagenic arylamines in human breast milk and DNA adducts in exfoliated breast ductal epithelial cells. Environ Mol Mutagen 2002; 39:134–142.
67. Lang NP, Butler MA, Massengill J, Lawson M, Stotts C, Kadlubar FF. Aromatic amine metabolism and diet in colorectal cancer polyp and cancer patients. International Conference on Environment Mutations, Satellite Meeting, Auckland, New Zealand, 1993.
68. Bell DA, Taylor JA, Butler MA, Stephens EA, Wiest J, Brubaker LH, et al. Genotype/phenotype discordance for human arylamine N-acetyltransferase (NAT2) reveals a new slow-acetylator allele common in African-Americans. Carcinogenesis 1993; 14:1689–1692.
69. Cartwright RA. Epidemiological studies on N-acetylation and C-center ring oxidation in neoplasia. In: Omenn GS, Gelboin HV, eds. Genetic variability in Responses to Chemical Exposure. Cold Spring Harbor, NY: : Cold Spring Harbor Press, 1984:359–368.
70. Ambrosone CB, Freudenheim JL, Graham S, Marshall JR, Vena JE, Brasure JR, et al. Cigarette smoking, N-acetyltransferase 2 genetic polymorphisms, and breast cancer risk. J Am Med Assoc 1996; 276:1494–1501.
71. Welfare MR, Cooper J, Bassendine MF, Daly AK. Relationship between acetylator status, smoking, diet and colorectal cancer risk in the north-east of England. Carcinogenesis 1997; 18:1351–1354.
72. Lang NP, Butler MA, Massengill J, Lawson M, Stotts RC, Hauer-Jensen M, et al. Rapid metabolic phenotypes for acetyltransferase and cytochrome P4501A2 and putative exposure to food-borne heterocyclic amines increase the risk for colorectal cancer or polyps. Cancer Epidemiol Biomarkers Prev 1994; 3:675–682.
73. Le Marchand L, Hankin JH, Wilkens LR, Pierce LM, Franke A, Kolonel LN, et al. Combined effects of well-done red meat, smoking, and rapid N-acetyltransferase 2 and CYP1A2 phenotypes in increasing colorectal cancer risk. Cancer Epidemiol Biomarkers Prev 2001; 10:1259–1266.
74. Debiec-Rychter M, Land SJ, King CM. Tissue-specific expression of human acetyltransferase 1 and 2 detected by non-isotopic in situ hybridization (Abstract). Proc Am Assoc Cancer Res 1996; 37:133.
75. Sadrieh N, Davis CD, Snyderwine EG. N-Acetyltransferase expression and metabolic activation of their food-derived heterocyclic amines in the human mammary gland. Cancer Res 1996; 56:2683–2687.

76. Dubuisson JG, Gaubatz JW. Bioactivation of the proximal food mutagen 2-hydroxyamino-1-methyl-6-phenylimidazo [4,5-b]pyridine (N-OH-PhIP) to DNA-binding species by human mammary gland enzymes. Nutrition 1998; 14:683–686.
77. Ambrosone CB, Freudenheim JL, Sinha R, Graham S, Marshall JR, Vena JE, et al. Breast cancer risk, meat consumption and N-acetyltransferase (NAT2) genetic polymorphisms. Int J Cancer 1998; 75:825–830.
78. Zheng W, Gustafson DR, Sinha R, Cerhan JR, Moore D, Hong C-P, et al. Well-done meat intake and the risk of breast cancer. J Natl Cancer Inst 1998; 90:1724–1729.
79. Delfino RJ, Sinha R, Smith C, West J, White E, Lin HJ, et al. Breast cancer, heterocyclic aromatic amines from meat and N-acetyltransferase 2 genotype. Carcinogenesis 2000; 21:607–615.
80. Deitz AC, Zheng W, Leff MA, Gross M, Wen WQ, Doll MA, et al. N-Acetyltransferase-2 genetic polymorphism, well-done meat intake, and breast cancer risk among postmenopausal women. Cancer Epidemiol Biomarkers Prev 2000; 9:905–910.
81. Gertig DM, Hankinson SE, Hough H, Spiegelman D, Colditz GA, Willett WC, et al. *N*-Acetyltransferase 2 genotypes, meat intake and breast cancer risk. Int J Cancer 1999; 80:13–17.
82. Steinmetz KA, Potter JD. Vegetables, fruit, and cancer prevention: a review. J Am Diet Assoc 1996; 96:1027–1039.
83. Zhang S, Hunter DJ, Forman MR, Rosner BA, Speizer FE, Colditz GA, et al. Dietary carotenoids and vitamins A, C, and E and risk of breast cancer. J Natl Cancer Inst 1999; 91:547–556.
84. Byers T. Nutritional risk factors for breast cancer. Cancer 1994; 74:288–295.
85. Smith-Warner SA, Spiegelman D, Yaun SS, Adami HO, Beeson WL, van den Brandt PA, et al. Intake of fruits and vegetables and risk of breast cancer: a pooled analysis of cohort studies. J Am Med Assoc 2001; 285:769–776.
86. Graham S, Zielezny M, Marshall J, Priore R, Freudenheim J, Brasure J, et al. Diet in the epidemiology of postmenopausal breast cancer in the New York State Cohort [see comments]. Am J Epidemiol 1992; 136:1327–1337.
87. Graham S, Hellmann R, Marshall J, Freudenheim J, Vena J, Swanson M, et al. Nutritional epidemiology of postmenopausal breast cancer in western New York [see comments]. Am J Epidemiol 1991; 134:552–566.
88. Freudenheim JL, Marshall JR, Vena JE, Laughlin R, Brasure JR, Swanson M, et al. Premenopausal breast cancer risk and intake of vegetables, fruits, and related nutrients. J Natl Cancer Inst 1996; 88:340–348.
89. Ambrosone CB. Oxidants and antioxidants in breast cancer. Antioxid Redox Signal 2000; 2:903–917.
90. Oberly TD, Oberly LW. Antioxidant enzyme levels in cancer. Histol Histopathol 1997; 12:525–535.
91. Schwartz JL, Antoniades DZ, Zhao S. Molecular and biochemical reprogramming of oncogenesis through the activity of prooxidants and antioxidants. Ann N Y Acad Sci 1993; 686:262–278.
92. Halliwell B, Gutteridge JMC. Free Radicals in Biology and Medicine. Oxford: Oxford University Press, 1989.

93. Cerutti PA. Oxy-radicals and cancer. Lancet 1994; 344:862–863.
94. Emerit I. Reactive oxygen species, chromosome mutation and cancer: possible role of clastogenic factors in carcinogenesis. Free Radic Biol Med 1994; 16: 99–109.
95. Esterbauer H, Jurgens G. Mechanistic and genetic aspects of susceptibility of LDL to oxidation. Curr Opin Lipidol 1993; 4:114–124.
96. Halliwell B. Why and how should we measure oxidative DNA damage in nutritional studies? How far have we come? Am J Clin Nutr 2000; 72: 1082–1087.
97. Musarrat J, Arezina-Wilson J, Wani AA. Prognostic and aetiological relevance of 8-hydroxyguanosine in human breast carcinogenesis. Eur J Cancer 1996; 32A:1209–1214.
98. Djuric Z, Heilbrun L, Simon MS, Smith D, Luongo DA, LoRusso PM, et al. Levels of 5-hydroxymethyl-2'-deoxyuridine in DNA from blood as a marker of breast cancer. Cancer 1996; 77:696.
99. Li D, Zhang W, Zhu J, Chang P, Sahin A, Singletary E, et al. Oxidative DNA damage and 8-hydroxy-2-deoxyguanosine DNA glycosylase/apurinic lyase in human breast cancer. Mol Carcinog 2001; 31:214–223.
100. Djuric Z, Depper JB, Uhley V, Smith D, Lababidi S, Martino S, et al. Oxidative DNA damage levels in blood from women at high risk for breast cancer are associated with dietary intakes of meats, vegetables, and fruits. J Am Diet Assoc 1998; 98:524–528.
101. Rehman A, Bourne LC, Halliwell B, Rice-Evans CA. Tomato consumption modulates oxidative DNA damage in humans. Biochem Biophys Res Commun 1999; 262:828–831.
102. Verhagen H, Poulsen HE, Loft S, van Poppel G, Willems MI, van Bladeren PJ. Reduction of oxidative DNA-damage in humans by brussels sprouts. Carcinogenesis 1995; 16:969–970.
103. Wispe JR, Clark JC, Burhans MS, Dropp KE, Korfhagen TR, Whitsett JA. Synthesis and processing of the precursor for human mangano-superoxide dismutase. Biochim Biophys Acta 1989; 994:30–36.
104. Shimoda-Matsubayashi S, Matsumine H, Kobayashi T, Nakagawa-Hattori Y, Shimizu Y, Mizuno Y. Structural dimorphism in the mitochondrial targeting sequence in the human manganese superoxide dismutase gene. A predictive evidence for conformational change to influence mitochondrial transport and a study of allelic association in Parkinson's disease. Biochem Biophys Res Commun 1996; 226:561–565.
105. Rohrdanz E, Kahl R. Alterations of antioxidant enzyme expression in response to hydrogen peroxide. Free Rad Biol Med 1998; 24:27–38.
106. Gilks CB, Price K, Wright JL, Churg A. Antioxidant gene expression in rat lung after exposure to cigarette smoke. Am J Pathol 1998; 152:269–278.
107. Rosenblum JS, Gilula NB, Lerner RA. On signal sequence polymorphisms and diseases of distribution. Proc Natl Acad Sci 1996; 93:4471–4473.
108. Ambrosone CB, Freudenheim JL, Thompson PA, Bowman ED, Vena JE, Marshall JR, et al. Manganese superoxide dismutase (MnSOD) genetic polymorphisms, dietary antioxidants and risk of breast cancer. Cancer Res 1999; 59:602–606.

109. Mitrunen K, Sillanpaa P, Kataja V, Eskelinen M, Kosma V-M, Benhamou S, et al. Association between manganese superoxide dismutase (MnSOD) gene polymorphism and breast cancer risk. Carcinogenesis 2001; 22:827–829.

110. Schatzkin A, Longnecker MP. Alcohol and breast cancer. Cancer 1994; 74:1101–1110.

111. Longnecker MP. Alcoholic beverage consumption in relation to breast cancer risk: meta-analysis and review. Cancer Causes Control 1994; 5:73–82.

112. Ginsburg ES, Mello NK, Mendelson JH, Barbieri RL, Teoh SK, Rothman M, et al. Effects of alcohol ingestion on estrogens in postmenopausal women. J Am Med Assoc 1996; 276:1747–1751.

113. Dorgan JF, Reichman ME, Judd JT, Brown C, Longcope C, Schatzkin A, et al. The relation of reported alcohol ingestion to plasma levels of estrogens and androgens in premenopausal women. Cancer Causes Control 1994; 5:53–60.

114. Bosron WF, Li TK. Genetic polymorphisms of human liver alcohol and aldehyde dehydrogenases, and their relationship to alcohol metabolism and alcoholism. Hepatology 1986; 6:502–510.

115. Harty LC, Caporaso NE, Hayes RB, Winn DM, Bravo-Otero E, Blot WJ, et al. Alcohol dehydrogenase 3 genotype and risk of oral cavity and pharyngeal cancers. J Natl Cancer Inst 1997; 89:1698–1705.

116. Coutelle C, Ward PJ, Fleury B, Quattrocchi P, Chambrin H, Iron A, et al. Laryngeal and oropharyngeal cancer, and alcohol dehydrogenase 3 and glutathione S-transferase M1 polymorphisms. Hum Genet 1997; 99:319–325.

117. Bashir R, James OFW, Bassendine MF, Crabb DW, Thomasson HR, Li TK, et al. Investigation of the role of polymorphisms at the alcohol and aldehyde dehydrogenase loci in genetic predisposition to alcohol-related end-organ damage. Hepatology 1991; 6:502–510.

118. Freudenheim JL, Ambrosone CB, Moysich KB, Vena JE, Graham S, Marshall JR, et al. Alcohol dehydrogenase 3 genotype and risk of breast cancer associated with alcohol consumption. Cancer Causes Control 1999; 10:369–377.

119. Visvanathan K, Bell DA, Strickland PT, Alberg AJ, Hoffman S, Helzlsouer KJ. Association of ADH3, GSTM1 and alcohol and the risk of breast cancer. Proc Amer Assoc Cancer Res 1999; 40:194.

120. Hines LM, Hankinson SE, Smith-Warner SA, Spiegelman D, Kelsey KT, Colditz GA, et al. A prospective study of the effect of alcohol consumption and ADH3 genotype on plasma steroid hormone levels and breast cancer risk. Cancer Epidemiol Biomarkers Prev 2000; 9:1099–1105.

121. Hu Y, Oscarson M, Johansson I, Yue Q-Y, Dahl M-L, Tabone M, et al. Genetic polymorphism of human *CYP2E1*: characterization of two variant alleles. Mol Pharmacol 1997; 51:370–376.

122. Shields PG, Ambrosone CB, Graham S, Bowman ED, Harrington A, Gillenwater K, et al. A cytochrome P4502E1 genetic polymorphism and tobacco smoking in breast cancer. Molec Carc 1996; 17:144–150.

123. Pike MC, Spicer DV, Dahmoush L, Press MF. Estrogens, progestogens, normal breast cell proliferation, and breast cancer risk. [Review]. Epidemiol Rev 1993; 15:17–35.

124. Dorgan JF, Longcope C, Stephenson HE, Falk RT, Miller R, Franz C, et al. Serum sex hormone levels are related to breast cancer risk in postmenopausal women. Environ Health Perspect 1997; 105:583–585.

125. Bailey LR, Roodi N, Verrier CS, Yee CJ, Dupont WD, Parl FF. Breast cancer and *CYP1A1, GSTM1*, and *GSTT1* polymorphisms: evidence of a lack of association in Caucasians and African Americans. Cancer Res 1998; 58:65–70.

126. Rebbeck TR, Rosvold EA, Duggan DJ, Zhang J, Buetow KH. Genetics of CYP1A1: coamplification of specific alleles by polymerase chain reaction and association with breast cancer. Cancer Epidemiol Biomarkers Prev 1994; 3:511–514.

127. Ambrosone CB, Freudenheim JL, Graham S, Marshall JR, Vena JE, Brasure, et al. Cytochrome P4501A1 and glutathione S-transferase (M1) genetic polymorphisms and postmenopausal breast cancer risk. Cancer Res 1995; 55:3483–3485.

128. Taioli E, Trachman J, Chen X, Toniolo P, Garte SJ. A CYP1A1 restriction fragment length polymorphism is associated with breast cancer in African-American women. Cancer Res 1995; 55:3757–3758.

129. Ishibe N, Hankinson SE, Colditz GA, Spiegelman DL, Willett WC, Speizer FE, et al. Cigarette smoking, cytochrome P4501A1 polymorphisms, and breast cancer risk in the Nurses' Health Study. Cancer Res 1998; 58:667–671.

130. Basham VM, Pharoah PD, Healey CS, Luben RN, Day NE, Easton DF, et al. Polymorphisms in CYP1A1 and smoking: no association with breast cancer risk. Carcinogenesis 2001; 22:1797–1800.

131. Feigelson HS, Coetzee GA, Kolonel LN, Ross RK, Henderson BE. A polymorphism in the CYP17 gene increases the risk of breast cancer. Cancer Res 1997; 57:1063–1065.

132. Dunning AM, Healey CS, Pharoah PDP, foster NA, Lipscombe JM, Redman KL, et al. No association between a polymorphism in the steroid metabolism gene CYP17 and risk of breast cancer. Br J Cancer 1998; 77:2045–2047.

133. Helzlsouer KJ, Huang H-Y, Strickland PT, Hoffman S, Alberg AJ, Comstock GW, et al. Association between CYP17 polymorphisms and the development of breast cancer. Cancer Epidemiol Biomarkers Prev 1998; 7:945–949.

134. Weston A, Pan C-F, Bleiweiss IJ, Ksieski HB, Roy N, Maloney N, et al. CYP17 genotype and breast cancer risk. Cancer Epidemiol Biomarkers Prev 1998; 7:941–944.

135. Haiman CA, Hankinson SE, Spiegelman D, Colditz GA, Willett WC, Speizer FE, et al. Relationship between a polymorphism in CYP17 with plasma hormone levels and breast cancer. Cancer Res 1999; 59:1015–1020.

136. Mitrunen K, Jourenkova N, Kataja V, Eskelinen M, Kosma V-M, Benhamou S, et al. Steroid metabolism gene *CYP17* polymorphism and the development of breast cancer. Cancer Epidemiol Biomarkers Prev 2000; 9:1343–1348.

137. Lai J, Vesprini D, Chu W, Jernstrom H, Narod SA. CYP gene polymorphisms and early menarche. Mol Genet Metab 2001; 74:449–457.

138. Ye Z, Parry JM. The CYP17 MspA1 polymorphism and breast cancer risk: a meta-analysis. Mutagenesis 2002; 17:119–126.

139. Sasano H, Nagura H, Harada N, Goukon Y, Kimura M. Immunolocalization of aromatase and other steroidogenic enzymes in human breast disorders. Hum Pathol 1994; 25:535.

140. Kristensen VN, Andersen TI, Lindblom A, Erikstein B, Magnus P, Borresen-Dale AL. A rare CYP19 (aromatase) variant may increase the risk of breast cancer. Pharmacogenetics 1998; 8:43–48.

141. Siegelmann-Danieli N, McGlynn KA, Buetow KH. Human aromatase as a candidate for breast cancer susceptibility. Am J Hum Genetics 1996; 59:A82.

142. Baxter SW, Choong DY, Eccles DM, Campbell IG. Polymorphic variation in CYP19 and the risk of breast cancer. Carcinogenesis 2001; 22:347–349.

143. Haiman CA, Hankinson SE, Spiegelman D, Brown M, Hunter DJ. No association between a single nucleotide polymorphism in CYP19 and breast cancer risk. Cancer Epidemiol Biomarkers Prev 2002; 11:215–216.

144. Guldberg HC, Marsden CA. Catechol-O-methyltransferase: pharmacological aspects and physiological role. Pharmacol Rev 1975; 27:135–206.

145. Cavalieri EL, Stack DE, Devanesan PD, Todorovic R, Dwivedy I, Higginbotham S, et al. Molecular origin of cancer: catechol estrogen-3-4-quinones as endogenous tumor initiators. Proc Natl Acad Sci USA 1997; 94: 10937–10942.

146. Lavigne JA, Helzlsouer KJ, Huang H-Y, Strickland PT, Bell DA, Selmin O, et al. An association between the allele coding for a low activity variant of catechol-O-methyltransferase and the risk for breast cancer. Cancer Res 1997; 57:5493–5497.

147. Thompson PA, Shields PG, Freudenheim JL, Stone AA, Vena JE, Marshall JR, et al. Genetic polymorphisms in catechol-O-methyltransferase (COMT), menopausal status and breast cancer risk. Cancer Res 1998; 58:2107–2110.

148. Mitrunen K, Jourenkova N, Kataja V, Eskelinen M, Kosma VM, Benhamou S, et al. Polymorphic catechol-O-methyltransferase gene and breast cancer risk. Cancer Epidemiol Biomarkers Prev 2001; 10:635–640.

149. Yim DS, Parkb SK, Yoo KY, Yoon KS, Chung HH, Kang HL, et al. Relationship between the Val158Met polymorphism of catechol O-methyl transferase and breast cancer. Pharmacogenetics 2001; 11:279–286.

150. Millikan RC, Pittman GS, Tse CK, Duell E, Newman B, Savitz D, et al. Catechol-O-methyltransferase and breast cancer risk. Carcinogenesis 1998; 19: 1943–1947.

151. Bergman-Jungestrom M, Wingren S. Catechol-O-methyltransferase (COMT) gene polymorphism and breast cancer risk in young women. Br J Cancer 2001; 85:859–862.

152. American Cancer Society. Cancer Facts and Figures—1999. Atlanta, GA: American Cancer Society, Inc., 1999.

153. Kelsey JL, Horn-Ross PL. Breast cancer: magnitude of the problem and descriptive epidemiology. [Review]. Epidemiol Rev 1993; 15:7–16.

154. International Agency for Research on Cancer. DDT and associated compounds. IARC Monogr 1992; 53:179–249.

155. Safe S, Bandiera SM, Sawyer T, Robertson L, Safe L, Parkinson A, et al. PCBs: structure–function relationships and mechanism of action. Environ Health Perspect 1985; 60:47–56.

156. Bulger WH, Kupfer D. Polychlorinated biphenyls as hormonally active structural analogues. Environ Health Perspect 1994; 102:290–294.
157. McKinney JD, Waller CD. Polychlorinated biphenyls as hormonally active structural analogues. Environ Health Perspect 1994; 102:290–297.
158. Jansen HT, Cooke PS, Poecelli J, Liu TC, Hansen LG. Estrogenic and antiestrogenic actions of PCBs in the female rat: in vitro and in vivo studies. Reprod Toxicol 1993; 7:237–241.
159. Banerjee BD. Effects of sub-chronic DDT exposure on humoral and cell-mediated immune responses in albino rats. Bull Environ Contam Toxicol 1987; 39:827–834.
160. Kimbrough RD. Laboratory and human studies on polychlorinated biphenyls (PCBs) and related compounds. Environ Health Perspect 1985; 59:99–106.
161. Norback DH, Weltman RH. Polychlorinated biphenyl induction of hepatoellular carcinoma in the Sprague–Dawley rat. Environ Health Perspect 1985; 60:97–105.
162. Wolff MS, Toniolo PG, Lee EW, Rivera M, Dubin N. Blood levels of organochlorine residues and risk of breast cancer. J Natl Cancer Inst 1993; 85: 648–652.
163. Moysich KB, Ambrosone CB, Vena J, Mendola P, Marshall JR, Graham S, et al. Environmental organochlorine exposure and postmenopausal breast cancer risk. Cancer Epidemiol Biomarkers Prev 1998; 7:181–188.
164. Hunter DJ, Hankinson SE, Laden F, Colditz GA, Manson JE, Willett WC, et al. Plasma organochlorine levels and the risk of breast cancer. N Engl J Med 1997; 337:1253–1258.
165. Helzlsouer KJ, Alberg AJ, Huang H-Y, Hoffman SC, Strickland PT, Brock JW, et al. Serum concentrations of organochlorine compounds and the subsequent development of breast cancer. Cancer Epidemiol Biomarkers Prev 1999; 8:525–532.
166. Krieger N, Wolff MS, Hiatt RA, Rivera M, Vogelman JH, Orentreich N. Breast cancer and serum organochlorines: a prospective study among white, black, and Asian women. J Natl Cancer Inst 1994; 86:589–599.
167. Olaya-Contreras P, Rodriguez-Villamil J, Posso-Valencia HJ, Cortez JE. Organochlorine exposure and breast cancer risk in Colombian women. Cadernos de Saude Publica 1998; 14S:125–132.
168. Lopez-Carrillo L, Blair A, Lopez-Cervantes M, Cebrian M, Rueda C, Reyes R, et al. Dichlorodiphenyltrichloroethane serum levels and breast cancer risk: a case–control study from Mexico. Cancer Res 1997; 57:3728–3732.
169. Schecter A, Toniolo P, Dai LC, Thuy LT, Wolff MS. Blood levels of DDT and breast cancer risk among women living in the North of Vietnam. Arch Environ Contam Toxicol 1997; 33:453–456.
170. Hoyer AP, Grandjean P, Jorgensen T, Brock JW, Hartvig HB. Organochlorine exposure and risk of breast cancer. Lancet 1998; 352:1816–1820.
171. Guttes S, Failing K, Neumann K, Kleinstein J, Georgii S, Brunn H. Chlororganic pesticides and polychlorinated biphenyls in breast tissue of women with benign and malignant breast disease. Arch Environ Contam Toxicol 1998; 35:140–147.

172. Van't Veer P, Lobbezoo IE, Martin-Moreno JM, Guallar E, Gomez-Aracena J, et al. DDT (dicophane) and postmenopausal breast cancer in Europe: case–control study. Br Med J 1997; 315:81–85.

173. Wolff M, Berkowitz G, Brower S, Senie R, Bleiweiss I, Tartter P, et al. Organochlorine exposures and breast cancer risk in New York City Women. Environ Res 2000; 84:151–161.

174. Millikan R, DeVoto E, Duell EJ, Tse CK, Savitz DA, Beach J, et al. Dichlorodiphenyldichloroethene, polychlorinated biphenyls, and breast cancer among African-American and white women in North Carolina. Cancer Epidemiol Biomarkers Prev 2000; 9:1233–1240.

175. Laden F, Collman G, Iwamoto K, Alberg AJ, Berkowitz GS, Freudenheim JL, et al. 1,1-Dichloro-2,2-bis(p-chlorophenyl)ethylene and polychlorinated biphenyls and breast cancer: combined analysis of five U.S. studies. J Natl Cancer Inst 2001; 93:768–776.

176. Moysich KB, Ambrosone CB, Mendola P, Kostyniak PJ, Greizerstein HB, Vena JE, et al. Exposures associated with serum organochlorine levels among postmenopausal women from western New York State. Am J Ind Med 2002; 41:102–110.

177. Moysich KB, Shields PG, Freudenheim J, Vena JE, Kotake T, Grenberg-Funes RA, et al. Polychlorinated biphenyls, cytochrome P4501A1 polymorphism, and postmenopausal breast cancer risk. Cancer Epidemiol Biomarkers Prev 1999; 8:41–44.

178. Drahushuk AT, Choy CO, Kumar S, McReynolds JH, Olson JR. Modulation of cytochrome P450 by 5,5'-bis-triflouromethyl-2,2'-dicholrobiphenyl, a unique environmental comtaminant. Toxicology 1997; 120:197–205.

179. Bandiera SM, Torok SM, Letcher RJ, Norstrom RJ. Immunoquantification of cytochromes P450 1A and P450 2B and comparison with chlorinated hydrocarbon levels in archived polar bear liver samples. Chemosphere 1997; 34:1469–1479.

180. Swaminathan S, Frederickson SM, Hatcher JF. Metabolic activation of N-hydroxy-4-acetylaminobiphenyl by cultured human breast epithelial cell line MCF 10A. Carcinogenesis 1994; 15:611–617.

181. Wang CY, Yamada H, Morton KC, Zukowski K, Lee MS, King CM. Induction of repair synthesis of DNA in mammary and urinary bladder epithelial cells by N-hydroxy derivatives of carcinogenic arylamines. Cancer Res 1988; 48:4227–4232.

182. Allaben WT, Weis CC, Fullerton NF, Beland FA. Formation and persistence of DNA adducts from the carcinogen N-hydroxy-2-acetylaminofluorene in rat mammary gland in vivo. Carcinogenesis 1983; 4:1067–1070.

183. Tonelli QJ, Custer RP, Sorof S. Transformation of cultured mouse mammary glands by aromatic amines and amides and their derivatives. Cancer Res 1979; 39:1784–1792.

184. Shirai T, Fysh JM, Lee MS, Vaught JB, King CM. Relationship of metabolic activation of N-hydroxy-N-acylarylamines to biological response in the liver and mammary gland of the female CD rat. Cancer Res 1981; 41:4346–4353.

185. International Agency for Research on Cancer. Monographs on the evaluation of the Carcinogenic Risk of Chemicals to Humans. 1972; 1:74–79.

186. Cavalieri E, Rogan E, Sinha D. Carcinogenicity of aromatic hydrocarbons directly applied to rat mammary gland. J Cancer Res Clin Oncol 1988; 114:3–9.

187. Chatterjee M, Banerjee MR. Selenium mediated dose-inhibition of 7,12-dimethylbenz[a] anthracene-induced transformation of mammary cells in organ culture. Cancer Lett 1982; 17:187–195.

188. Calaf G, Russo J. Transformation of human breast epithelial cells by chemical carcinogens. Carcinogenesis 1993; 14:483–492.

189. Olivier M, Hainaut P. TP53 mutation patterns in breast cancers: searching for clues of environmental carcinogenesis. Semin Cancer Biol 2001; 11:353–360.

190. Biggs PJ, Warren W, Venitt S, Stratton MR. Does a genotoxic carcinogen contribute to human breast cancer? The value of mutational spectra in unravelling the aetiology of cancer. [Review]. Mutagenesis 1993; 8:275–283.

191. Obana H, Hori S, Kashimoto T, Kunita N. Polycyclic aromatic hydrocarbons in human fat and liver. Bull Environ Contam Toxicol 1981; 27:23–27.

192. Martin FL, Carmichael PL, Crofton-Sleigh C, Venitt S, Phillips DH, Grover PL. Genotoxicity of human mammary lipid. Cancer Res 1996; 56:5342–5346.

193. Petrakis NL, Gruenke LD, Beelen TC, Castagnoli N Jr, Craig JC. Nicotine in breast fluid of nonlactating women. Science 1978; 199:303–305.

194. Martin FL, Venitt S, Carmichael PL, Crofton-Sleigh C, Stone EM, Cole KJ, Gusterson BA, Grover PL, Phillips DH. DNA damage in breast epithelial cells: detection by the single-cell gel (comet) assay and induction by human mammary lipid extracts. Carcinogenesis 1997; 18:2299–2305.

195. Ghoshal A, Snyderwine EG. Excretion of food-derived heterocyclic amine carcinogens into breast milk of lactating rats and formation of DNA adducts in the newborn. Carcinogenesis 1993; 14:2199–2203.

196. Perera FP, Estabrook A, Hewer A, Channing K, Rundle A, Mooney LA, et al. Carcinogen-DNA adducts in human breast tissue. Cancer Epidemiol Biomarkers Prev 1995; 4:233–238.

197. Li D, Wang M, Dhingra K, Hittelman WN. Aromatic DNA adducts in adjacent tissues of breast cancer patients: clues to breast cancer etiology. Cancer Res 1996; 56:287–293.

198. Seidman LA, Moore CJ, Gould MN. 32P-postlabeling analysis of DNA adducts in human and rat mammary epithelial cells. Carcinogenesis 1988; 9:1071–1077.

199. Li D, Wang M, Firozi PF, Chang P, Zhang W, Baer-Dubowska W, et al. Characterization of a major aromatic DNA adduct detected in human breast tissues. Environ Mol Mutagen 2002; 39:193–200.

200. Morabia A. Smoking (active and passive) and breast cancer: epidemiologic evidence up to June 2001. Environ Mol Mutagen 2002; 39:89–95.

201. Egan KM, Stampfer MJ, Hunter D, Hankinson S, Rosner BA, Holmes M, et al. Active and passive smoking in breast cancer: prospective results from the Nurses' Health Study. Epidemiology 2002; 13:138–145.

202. Palmer JR, Rosenberg L. Cigarette smoking and the risk of breast cancer. [Review]. Epidemiol Rev 1993; 15:145–156.

203. Wells AJ. Breast cancer, cigarette smoking, and passive smoking [letter]. Am J Epidemiol 1991; 133:208–210.

204. Wells AJ. Breast cancer, cigarette smoking, and passive smoking. The author replies (letter). Am J Epidemiol 1992; 135:710–712.
205. Smith SJ, Deacon JM, Chilvers CE. Alcohol, smoking, passive smoking and caffeine in relation to breast cancer risk in young women. UK National Case Study Group. Br J Cancer 1994; 70:112–119.
206. Lash TL, Aschengrau A. Active and passive cigarette smoking and the occurrence of breast cancer. Am J Epidemiol 1999; 149:5–12.
207. Delfino RJ, Smith C, West JG, Lin HJ, White E, Liao SY, et al. Breast cancer, passive and active cigarette smoking and N-acetyltransferase 2 genotype. Pharmacogenetics 2000; 10:461–469.
208. Morabia A, Bernstein M, Heritier S, Khatchatrian N. Relation of breast cancer with passive and active exposure to tobacco smoke. Am J Epidemiol 1996; 143:918–928.
209. MacMahon B, Trichopoulos D, Cole P, Brown J. Cigarette smoking and urinary estrogens. N Engl J Med 1982; 307:1062–1065.
210. Baron JA. Smoking and estrogen-related disease. [Review]. Am J Epidemiol 1984; 119:9–22.
211. Millikan R, Pittman G, Newman B, Tse C-K, Selmin O, Rockhill B, et al. Cigarette smoking, N-acetyltransferases 1 and 2, and breast cancer risk. Cancer Epidemiol Biomarkers Prev 1998; 7:371–378.
212. Hunter DJ, Hankinson SE, Hough H, Gertig DM, Garcia-Closas M, Spiegelman D, et al. A prospective study of NAT2 acetylation genotype, cigarette smoking, and risk of breast cancer. Carcinogenesis 1997; 18:2127–2132.
213. Ambrosone CB, Coles BF, Freudenheim JL, Shields PG. Glutathione S-transferase (GSTM1) genetic polymorphisms do not affect human breast cancer risk, regardless of dietary antioxidants. J Nutr 1999; 129:565S–568S.
214. Garcia-Closas M, Kelsey KT, Hankinson SE, Spigelman D, Springer K, Willett WC, et al. Glutathione S-transferase mu and theta polymorphisms and breast cancer susceptibility. J Natl Cancer Inst 1999; 91:1960–1964.
215. Kelsey KT, Hankinson SE, Colditz GA, Springer K, Garcia-Closas M, Spiegelman D, et al. Glutathione S-transferase μ deletion polymorphism and breast cancer: results from prevalent *versus* incident cases. Cancer Epidemiol Biomarkers Prev 1997; 6:511–5.
216. Zhong S, Wyllie AH, Barnes D, Wolf CR, Spurr NK. Relationship between the GSTM1 genetic polymorphism and susceptibility to bladder, breast and colon cancer. Carcinogenesis 1993; 14:1821–1824.
217. Garcia-Closas M, Kelsey KT, Wiencke JK, Xu X, Wain JC, Christiani DC. A case–control study of cytochrome P450 1A1, glutathione S-transferase M1, cigarette smoking and lung cancer susceptibility (Massachusetts, United States). Cancer Causes Control 1997; 8:544–553.
218. Helzlsouer KJ, Selmin O, Huang H-Y, Strickland PT, Hoffman S, Alberg AJ, et al. Association between glutathione S-transferase M1, P1, and T1 genetic polymorphisms and development of breast cancer. J Natl Cancer Inst 1998; 90:512–518.
219. Garcia-Closas M, Lubin JH. Power and sample size calculations in case–control studies of gene–environment interactions: comments on different approaches. Am J Epidemiol 1999; 149:689–692.

220. Pharoah PD, Antoniou A, Bobrow M, Zimmern RL, Easton DF, Ponder BA. Polygenic susceptibility to breast cancer and implications for prevention. Nat Genet 2002; 31:33–36.

221. Feigelson HS, McKean-Cowdin R, Coetzee GA, Stram DO, Kolonel LN, Henderson BE. Building a multigenic model of breast cancer susceptibility: CYP17 and HSD17B1 are two important candidates. Cancer Res 2001; 61:785–789.

222. Huang CS, Chern HD, Chang KJ, Cheng CW, Hsu SM, Shen CY. Breast cancer risk associated with genotype polymorphism of the estrogen-metabolizing genes CYP17, CYP1A1, and COMT: a multigenic study on cancer susceptibility. Cancer Res 1999; 59:4870–4875.

22

Gynecological Cancer—Ovarian, Endometrial, Cervical

Kala Visvanathan

*Bloomberg School of Public Health, Johns Hopkins University,
Baltimore, Maryland, U.S.A.*

Kathy J. Helzlsouer

*Bloomberg School of Public Health, Johns Hopkins University,
Baltimore, Maryland, U.S.A. and Prevention and Research Center,
Mercy Medical Center, Baltimore, Maryland, U.S.A.*

1. INTRODUCTION

Gynecological malignancies can result in significant morbidity and mortality. In the United States alone, it is estimated that about 24,000 women will die from cancers of the ovary, endometrium, and cervix annually (1). Women diagnosed with ovarian cancer have the highest mortality, when compared to those with endometrial or cervical cancer. This difference in mortality for ovarian cancer has been attributed to the delay in the diagnoses due to a lack of symptoms in early stage disease, and the fact that we do not have a curative treatment for advanced stage disease (2). The 5-year survival rate for localized disease is 95% (3). Therefore, we could potentially decrease the overall mortality if we are able to detect ovarian cancer at an earlier stage. This has been the focus of current research, along with the search for effective treatment and prevention strategies. In the case of endometrial cancer the issues are different. Despite being detected at an early stage, due to symptoms such as vaginal bleeding, the 5-year survival rates for local-regional disease are still lower than that for breast cancer suggesting a need for better treatments. In comparison with ovarian and endometrial cancer, major advances have been made in cervical cancer. High-risk human papilloma viruses (HPVs) have been identified as the primary etiologic factor and early detection testing with regular pap smears is available the possibility of primary prevention with vaccines exist (4). In addition, a current challenge is identifying women infected with HPV who will go on refer sheet attached to develop cervical cancer. At any one time, up to 6 million women in the United States alone are thought to have contracted HPV (5). Additional challenges include developing effective treatments for HPV, behavioral programs, and effective vaccines to decrease the rates of high-risk HPV infection.

The focus of this chapter is to review the risk and susceptibility factors associated with ovarian, endometrial, and cervical cancer. Knowledge of these factors, help us gain a better understanding of the various carcinogenesis pathways and may help us identify susceptible individuals in whom preventive measures can potentially be implemented (Fig. 1).

2. OVARIAN CANCER
2.1. Overview

During the last three decades, there has been little change in the incidence of ovarian cancer in North America and Europe (the high-risk countries). However, a steady increase in the incidence has been observed in developing countries. This may reflect a true increase in incidence or an increase in reporting or both. Japan has always been classified along developing countries as a low-risk country. Up to a fourfold difference in the risk of ovarian cancer has been reported between the high- and low-risk countries (6).

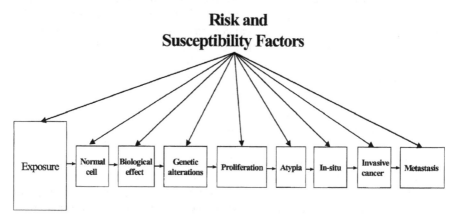

Figure 1   The influence of risk and susceptibility factors on the carcinogenesis pathway. *Source*: Adapted from Schulte and Perera 1993.

In the United States, the incidence rate of ovarian cancer in the general population is 14 per 100,000 persons and the mortality rate is 9 per 100,000 persons (3). Incidence rates and mortality rates have decreased over time primarily among women less than 65 years of age. The decrease in mortality varies according to race and ethnicity; the largest decline was seen among American Indians (3.3%), Blacks (1.7%), and Asians (1.6%) and the smallest decrease among the White non-Hispanics (0.6%). A recent study demonstrated that migrants take on the risk of their adoptive country after successive generations suggesting environmental and lifestyle factors, such as use of the oral contraceptive pill (7).

Survival varies by age and stage of disease at diagnosis. The 5-year survival for ovarian cancer, irrespective of stage is 50% (3). It is 95% for localized disease, 79% for regional disease, and 28% for distant disease (3). The 5-year survival of women under 65 was 64% and for 65 years and over 30% (3).

2.2. Histological Types

Epithelial ovarian tumors are the most common type accounting for between 80% and 90% of neoplasms, and the remaining are either sex-cord stromal or germ cell tumors (8). Approximately 10–20% of epithelial carcinomas that are primarily serous can be classified as borderline tumors, which implies that they are of low malignant potential (2). Ovarian cancer is primarily a disease of peri- and postmenopausal women, with 80–90% occurring after the age of 40 (3). The peak incidence of epithelial ovarian cancer is 63 years of age, whereas germ cell tumors commonly occur in younger patients (2).

2.3. Etiology

The etiology of ovarian cancer is poorly understood. From epidemiological studies it is evident that multiple pathways are involved, incorporating genetic, hormonal, and environmental factors. Three major theories or models of carcinogenesis have been suggested. The first was Fathalla's theory of "incessant ovulation" (9). This theory suggests that repeated ovulation traumatizes the ovarian epithelium, increasing the likelihood of errors occurring during DNA repair and the exposure of the epithelial cells to the estrogen-rich follicular fluid that is present during ovulation, thereby making the cells within the ovary more susceptible to malignant change.

Cramer and Welch proposed a second theory related to persistent elevation of gonadotropins (10). From their observations that the ovarian epithelium repeatedly invaginates throughout life to form clefts and inclusion cysts, they proposed a theory that under excessive stimulation by gonadotropins (FSH and LH), estrogen and its precursors, the ovarian epithelium may undergo malignant transformation.

Risch suggested that ovarian cancer may be increased by factors associated with excess androgenic stimulation of ovarian epithelial cells, and may be decreased by factors related to greater progesterone stimulation (11).

2.4. Risk and Susceptibility Factors

2.4.1. Inherited Factors

Family History: Approximately 5–10% of women diagnosed with ovarian cancer report a positive family history (12). Depending on the number of affected relatives on either the maternal and paternal side, and a family history of breast cancer below the age of 50, the relative risk of developing ovarian cancer can range anywhere between 2 and 18 times the average population risk (13). A case–control study by Tavani et al. found that women with both a positive family history and other known risk factors had three and a half times the risk of developing ovarian cancer compared to women without a family history or any other risk factors (14).

In 1990, Lynch et al. reported three separate hereditary ovarian cancer syndromes; site-specific ovarian cancer; hereditary ovarian and breast cancer; and Lynch type II or hereditary nonpolyposis colorectal cancer (HNPCC), (in which case there is an increased risk of ovarian, colorectal, endometrial, and/or genitourinary cancers) (15–18). All three syndromes are associated with an autosommal dominant pattern of inheritance with variable penetrance and early onset cancer (17,19,20). This means that each first-degree relative of an individual with a mutation has a 50% chance of inheriting it. Clues in a family history to suggest such a strong hereditary predisposition include; multiple cancers occurring in close relatives over multiple generations, early age of onset of cancer (i.e., before 40 or 50 years), multiple cancers occurring in a single individual and a pattern consistent with an autosommal dominant inheritance or a familial association with tumors of other organs, particularly the breast, colon, and uterus.

Germline Mutations: Specific mutations in two known cancer susceptibility genes, BRCA1 and BRCA2 can explain some of the "cancer families" with breast and ovarian cancer. They are both tumor suppressor genes and may also be involved in DNA repair (21–23). The BRCA1 gene was cloned in 1994 and codes for a protein of 1863 amino acids (24,25) whereas the BRCA2 gene was identified in 1995, is located on the 13q12–13, and codes for a protein twice its size (26). Both these proteins are expressed in large quantities in the breast and ovaries (24,25). Eighty percent of the known mutations are due to the insertion or deletion of bases in the coding sequence (frame shifts) or nonsense mutations that convert the to a stop codon and results in the truncation of the protein (27). All of the breast-ovarian cancer families cannot be explained by these two mutations, it is estimated that between 10% and 20% of cancer families do not have a

BRCA1 or 2 mutations suggesting the possibility of further mutations in these genes or unidentified genes (28).

The probability that a woman with ovarian cancer is a mutation carrier has been shown to vary by the stringency of family history criteria. Prevalence rises with increasing number of ovarian cancer families and the early onset of breast cancer. The frequency of BRCA1 mutations in breast/ovarian cancer families range from 30% to 81%, and the frequency of a BRCA2 mutation ranges from 7% to 14% (19,29–34). When BRCA1 mutation testing was done in women with ovarian cancer for whom there was no information on family history, only 5% of women were found to be mutation carriers (35–38). In the general population between 0.04% and 0.20% of individuals have been estimated to be BRCA1 mutation carriers (39).

The estimated lifetime risk for women with a BRCA1 mutation of ovarian cancer varies from 16–63% by the age of 70, to 20–30% for BRCA2 mutation carriers (19,40–43). The range of estimates reflects variation in penetrance, due to the selection of families into the studies, the analysis of specific mutations or other unknown genetic or environmental modifying factors.

BRCA1 and BRCA2 mutations also are associated with an increased risk of other malignancies. Individuals from high-risk families with BRCA1 mutations have up to 85% cumulative risk for breast cancer by age 70, while the specific risk varies by mutation and other modifying factors, there is a 6% risk for colon and prostate cancer (39,44). The estimated risk of breast cancer in BRCA2 mutation carriers is 85% (44). The risk of other cancers associated with BRCA2 include a 6–14% risk in prostate cancer and gall bladder and bile duct cancer as well as a threefold increase in pancreatic cancer and an increase in stomach cancer and malignant melanoma (44).

Certain ethnic populations, for example, the Ashkenazi Jews and the Icelandic population, have specific founder mutations that account for most of the mutations identified on the BRCA1 and BRCA2 genes. These mutations occur at a higher than average frequency than in a population of unrelated families within a certain ethnic or racial group. Specifically, three mutations, two in the BRCA1 gene (185delAG and 5382 insC) and one in the BRCA2 gene (6174delT) 185 have been found in the Ashkenazi Jewish population (43,45–47). The combined frequency of these three mutations among 5318 Ashkenazi Jewish volunteers from the Washington, DC area, (both male and female) was 2.3% (95% CI 1.9–2.7). The individual prevalences were 0.8% (185delAG), 0.4% (5382insC), and 1.2% (6174delT). The probability of an Ashekanzi Jewish women in the study of having one of the three specific mutations was higher if they were less than 50 years of age, at the time of breast cancer diagnosis (14%) or had at least one first-degree relative with ovarian or breast cancer (5.1%). In Iceland, the 999del5 BRCA1 mutation has been described and the 5382insC in the Eastern European population (48–50).

HNPCC contributes to approximately 1–2% of all hereditary ovarian cancers. An individual with HNPCC has a 9–12% lifetime risk of developing ovarian cancer (51,52). Cancer susceptibility genes in the form of DNA repair genes (hMSH2, hMLH1, PMS1, PMS2, hMSH6) have also been identified with the respect to the HNPCC syndrome (53–55). The HNPCC genes will be discussed further in the section on endometrial cancer.

Genetic Polymorphisms: The role of other inherited factors such as low penetrant mutations that commonly occur in the population are unclear. Polymorphisms are genetic mutations occurring with a frequency of >1% in the general population. These genetic polymorphisms may code for enzymes involved in the metabolism or detoxification of carcinogens or in DNA repair. In conjunction with particular exposures they may be associated with either an increase or decrease an individual's risk of particular cancers. Given that the both polymorphisms and exposures are prevalent in the population, the attributable risk of such a gene environment association with respect to the development of ovarian cancer could be high. However, because ovarian cancer is rare, studies of these associations are challenging due to the need for large sample sizes. Examples of such genetic polymorphisms relevant to ovarian cancer include microsomal epoxide hyrolase and galactose-1-phosphate uridyl transferase (GALT).

Epoxide hydrolases (EPHX) play an important role in both the activation and detoxification of exogenous chemicals such as polycyclic aromatic hydrocarbons, a carcinogen found in cigarette smoke. Microsomal epoxide hydrolase is one of many enzymes that are part of the epoxide hydrolase family and is strongly expressed in the human ovary (56). A number of genetic polymorphisms coding for the EPHX gene have been described. In 1994, Hassett et al. identified the Tyr113His polymorphism on the EPHX gene that is the result of a substitution of Histidine for Tyrosine at codon 113. Further, a 40% decrease in EPHX activity has been demonstrated in vitro DNA expression studies for the His113His allelic variant compared to the Tyr113His variant (57). Consistent with these laboratory findings, a greater than twofold increase in the risk of ovarian cancer was observed in a case–control study among women who were homozygous for this polymorphism (Tyr113Tyr) compared to those who were homozygous or heterozygous (56). A limitation of the study was the lack of information on other risk factors. In order to confirm these results further replication is required.

A number of other polymorphisms in genes involved in hormone biosynthesis and detoxification pathways have also been examined. CYP17 and COMT are examples of two that code for enzymes that are part of the hormone biosynthesis pathway (59, 59a, Goodman et al., 2001,). Polymorphisms of the androgen receptor (AR) gene and progesterone receptor (PR) gene have also been studied (59b). Results from these studies have been inconsistent so far. No association has been observed between polymorphisms of the glutathione S-transferases (GSTM1 and GSTT1), which encode for enzymes that are responsible for the detoxification of a large number of carcinogens in the liver (Coughlin SS et al., 2002).

2.4.2. Hormonal Factors

Hormones, both endogenous and exogenous have been thought to play an important role in the etiology of ovarian cancer.

Endogenous: *Menstrual factors*: Early age at menarche and late age of menopause have not been consistently associated with an increased risk of ovarian cancer, as one might have expected based on Fathalla's theory of incessant ovulation. Some studies have suggested a modest increase in risk of 10–20% in women who began to menstruate at less than or equal to 12 years of age compared to women greater than 15 years old (61,62). Similarly late age of menopause has been associated with anywhere between 1.4 and 4.6 times the risk of ovarian cancer (62–68) while others have reported no association (69,70).

Serum levels: Consistent with Risch's androgen hypothesis theory, serum androgen levels have been shown to be potential predictors of increased ovarian cancer risk (71). In a nested case–control study after an average follow up time of 8 years mean levels of androstenedione and dehydroepiandrosterone (DHEAS) were significantly higher among cases than controls (p trend $= 0.008$, and 0.11, respectively). Increasing levels of androstenedione were associated with increasing risk. Whereas decreasing levels of gonadotropin, in particular FSH was lower among cases than controls (p for trend $= 0.02$). A similar increase in risk was not reported when urinary androgen levels were measured (72). Along with hormones, growth factors, such as insulin are believed to be important in cancer by regulating cell proliferation, differentiation, and apoptosis. In a pooled case control analysis of 3 prospective studies there was no overall association between insulin growth factor (IGF) binding proteins 1 and 2 (Lukanova et al., 2003). However, a protective effect was observed in women diagnosed before the age of 55 for both binding proteins. However, the odds ratios were not statistically significant.

Exogenous: *Oral contraceptive pill (OCP)*: The complex numerical instructions that may predispose to ovarian cancer require further investigation. Numerous cohort and case–control studies have demonstrated a 40–50% reduction in the risk of ovarian cancer in women taking the combined oral contraceptive pill for at least 5 years (62,69,73–78). Biologically, it has been hypothesized that by inducing ovarian suppression the oral contraceptives decreases the degree of trauma to the ovary and thereby an individual's risk of ovarian cancer (9,79,80). In some studies the protective association increased further with longer duration of use for up to 10 years (77,78,81–83) and continued for up to 15 years after cessation of use (69,82,84,85). A 40% reduction in mortality from ovarian cancer was also observed by Beral et al. among women who had ever used the OCP compared to those who had not (relative risk, 0.6; 95% CI, 0.3, 1.0) (77). A protective association was also observed in women with epithelial borderline tumors but the sample size was small (75,79,86).

The results have been mixed in BRCA1 and BRCA2 mutation carriers (87,88). Narod et al. in a family study, reported a similar risk reduction of ovarian cancer among mutation carriers compared to non mutation carriers in a population-based case–control study conducted in Israel (88). However, Modan et al. did not observe a risk reduction associated with OCP use among mutation carriers. Risk was reduced with increasing parity similar to what has been observed in the general population of women similar risk (87).

Hormone replacement therapy (HRT): Several studies have observed a small increase in the risk of ovarian cancer associated with HRT. The American Cancer Society's Cancer Prevention Study II, a prospective cohort study of 211,581 postmenopausal women observed a 20% increase in mortality from ovarian cancer among women who gave a history of HRT use compared to those who did not (89). This risk was higher among current users (relative risk = 1.51; 95% CI 1.16, 1.96) and those who used estrogen replacement therapy (ERT) for 10 or more years (relative risk = 2.20; 95% CI 1.53, 3.17). After 15 years of cessation of use women were no longer at risk. Similar results were observed in a large case control study (Riman et al., 2002). They observed that the risk of invasive epithelial ovarian cancer was increased among women who use regimens that sequentially added progestins and not regimens in which progestins were continually added. In a prospective cohort study only women who used estrogen only replacements were at significantly increased risk of ovarian cancer (R.R. 1.6, 95% CI 1.2, 2.0). The risk increase with increasing duration of use. An increase in risk was not observed in women who used short term estrogen and progestin replacement therapy (89a). Other studies have reported no association (60,90) or a modest association between estrogen replacement therapy use and the risk of ovarian cancer (62,75,91–93).

2.4.3. Reproductive Factors

Pregnancy: A large number of studies have focused on the association between reproductive factors and the risk of ovarian cancer. Women who develop ovarian cancer are significantly more likely to be nulliparous or to have fewer pregnancies. Pregnancy has been consistently shown to be associated with a decreased the risk of ovarian cancer by between 10% and 50% (61,62,65,74,83,94–97). The risk reduction increases with increasing number of births. In a combined analysis of 12 U.S. case–control studies, a 40% reduction in risk was found for the first full term pregnancy, and a 14% reduction for each subsequent birth when compared to nulliparous women (69). The number of years since last pregnancy has also been associated with an increased risk of ovarian cancer (98). A twofold increase in risk was observed among women who had been pregnant greater than or equal to 25 years ago (99). A similar risk reduction has also been reported in BRCA1 and BRCA2 mutation carriers (87). This protective association was not seen for mucinous tumors (93). The decreased risk of ovarian cancer associated with multiparity, pregnancy, and lactation is consistent with Fathalla's theory of incessant ovulation.

Tubal ligation has been associated with a decreased risk of ovarian cancer by between 10% and 40% and persists up to 25 years after surgery (73,100–102). It has been hypothesized that tubal ligation interrupts utero-ovarian blood flow decreasing the number of ovulations (10,69,100). Intrauterine devices (IUD) and the barrier method have all been shown to decrease the risk of ovarian cancer by 10–20% (73). It has been suggested that these methods of contraception may protect the ovaries from toxins reaching the ovaries (103,104).

Lactation has also been shown to be protective resulting in a 10–30% reduction in the risk of ovarian cancer (10,61,62,80,83,105,106). Whittemore et al. reported that ovarian cancer risk decreases almost 1% for each month of lactation (69). The protective association was strongest the months immediately following the birth.

Infertility: It is unclear whether infertility or medications used to treat infertility are risk factors for ovarian cancer. One of the difficulties in assessing the impact of infertility is separating the effect of infertility or its treatment from that of nulliparity by choice. Whittemore et al. in a collaborative analysis of 12 case–control studies used information on length of longest pregnancy attempt and total duration of unprotected intercourse as surrogate measurements for infertility along with information on parity, seperating women who never had children, women who conceived but did not carry to term and those who had children. A 60% increase in the risk of ovarian cancer was reported among women who had greater than or equal to 15 years of unprotected intercourse compared to less than 2 years. Among studies having information on physician diagnosis of infertility and type of infertility, women that had an ovulatory abnormality had a twofold increase in risk compared to women with no physician diagnosed infertility (69). A 60% increase in the risk of ovarian cancer among a cohort of 2496 infertile Israeli women was observed compared to the general population rates (107). However, this increase could be partially explained by the increase in positive family history of ovarian cancer among the cohort compared to the general population.

Controversy has been raised regarding the impact of fertility drugs. Whittemore et al. reported almost a threefold increase in the risk of invasive epithelial ovarian cancer in women taking fertility drugs (OR = 2.8, 95% CI 1.3, 6.1) (69). This risk was significantly greater among nulliparous women and in women with borderline tumors. Parity was protective, in that infertile women who used fertility drugs and subsequently became pregnant did not have a significantly increased risk of ovarian cancer. This finding is consistent with other studies (69,75,108). A large case–cohort study that found infertile women had an increased risk of developing both invasive epithelial carcinoma significant (relative risk = 1.5; 95% CI 0.4, 3.7) and borderline tumors (relative risk = 3.3; 95% CI 1.1, 7.8) compared to the general population. Though, in the case of invasive epithelial tumors this association was not statistically significant. This study had good detail with regard to type of infertility and drugs used to treat it, with the majority of women using Clomiphene as the ovulation induction agent (109). These results are consistent with other studies that have shown an association between fertility drug use and the risk of borderline ovarian cancers (108). In a cohort of of women from in vitro fertilisation (IVF) clinics in Australia, Venn et al. found no increase in the risk of ovarian cancer among women who had undergone treatment (110).

Hysterectomy without oophorectomy has been associated with a 10–60% decrease in the risk of ovarian cancer (69,101). This risk attenuates with time since hysterectomy. The risk reduction may be greater in women who have hysterectomies before the age of 40 (69). Proposed mechanisms for this risk reduction include a decrease in androstendione which has been observed in women who have had hysterectomy and would be consistent with Risch's hypothesis of androgen excess and a decreased exposure of the ovaries to external toxins (111,112).

2.4.4. Lifestyle Factors

Diet: The majority of dietary studies have been case–control studies and the results have been inconsistent. Despite an observed association between milk consumption and the risk of ovarian cancer and biological evidence that galactose is toxic to the oocytes, a positive association was not found between the consumption of lactose or free galactose and the risk of ovarian cancer (83,113–115). Associations between enzymes involved in the metabolism of galactose and the risk of ovarian cancer have also been inconsistent. Cramer et al. found the mean activity of erythrocyte galactose-1-phosphate uridyl transferase, a key enzyme in galactose metabolism, to be lower among cases who had a family history of ovarian cancer compared to controls, however, these findings were not replicated by Herrington et al. (115,116). A number of studies have reported an increased risk of ovarian cancer due to the intake of saturated fats (68,83) and a protective association between the intake of green leafy vegetables, total dietary fiber, fiber from vegetables, crude fiber, carotenoids, and carrots (83,117–122). Low serum levels of vitamin A and selenium among cases compared to controls has been observed but no differences in the levels of total carotenoids and vitamin E were reported (123–125).

A few prospective studies have also examined the association between dietary intake or serum micronutrients and the risk of ovarian cancer. Kushi et al. using information from a dietary questionnaire demonstrated an increasing risk of ovarian cancer with increasing intake of lactose (p trend $= 0.12$) and cholesterol (p trend $= 0.06$). Total vegetable intake was inversely associated with risk of ovarian cancer (p trend $= 0.21$) in particular green leafy vegetables (P trend $= 0.010$) (117). Knekt et al. found no association between prediagnostic alpha-tocopherol levels and the risk of gynecological cancers (126). These results were similar to those seen in case–control studies. In another prospective study, Helzlsouer et al. examined the association between serum micronutrients and the risk of ovarian cancer. A protective association was only observed between serum selenium and the risk of ovarian cancer (p trend $= 0.02$) (127). The findings on selenium were not replicated in a prospective study by Garland et al. (128). An incidental finding of the study by Helzlsouer et al. (127) was an increase in the risk of ovarian cancer in women with cholesterol levels greater than 200 mg/dL that has also been reported by Kushi et al. (117) but not by Hiatt and Fireman (129).

Weight: The available studies suggest that distribution of body fat may be a more important risk factor than absolute weight. Further studies are needed to confirm this. Mink et al., in a prospective study, observed almost a two fold increase in the incidence of ovarian cancer among women who had the greatest waist to hip ratio (>0.89) (130). A similar association was not seen between BMI and ovarian cancer. The results of other studies with respect to BMI have been mixed (70,131,132). In a nested case–control study in England, women with ovarian cancer were found to have gained significantly more weight during their first year of life than controls (133). In a prospective study of more than 900,000 U.S. adults, women with a BMI of 35.0 were at a greater risk of dying from ovarian cancer (R.R. 1.51, 95% CI 1.12, 2.02) (Calle et al., 2003).

Physical Activity: Only a few studies have specifically examined the association between physical activity and the risk of ovarian cancer and their results have been conflicting. In a prospective study of 31,396 women, Mink et al. reported a twofold increase in the risk of ovarian cancer in postmenopausal women who currently were undertaking vigorous physical activity compared to those who took part in low or no physical activity. This risk was greatest among women who took part in vigorous physical activity more than four times per week (relative risk $= 2.52$, 95% CI 1.01, 6.8) (130). Whereas Couttreau et al. in a case–control study, found high levels of lifetime leisure-time physical activity to be protective. A 27% reduction in risk was observed among women in the highest category of lifetime leisure physical activity compared with those in the lowest level (134). The degree of reduction correlated with the number of hours of leisure physical activity. It is difficult to explain the conflicting results of these two studies even after taking into consideration the limitations of their respective study designs. Possible explanations include the potential difference in risk between pre and post-menopausal women and current and lifetime physical activity. In the study by Mink et al. all women were between 55 and 69, whereas in Couttreau's study the mean age in the high physical activity group was 47 years (130,134). Two other studies, one retrospectively comparing the incidence of reproductive cancers among former college nonathletes compared to athletes, and the other comparing physical education teachers and language teachers with respect to physical activity, reported opposite results (135,136). In terms of etiology, it is easier to explain why physical activity may be protective rather than associated with an increased risk of ovarian cancer, as continuous vigorous activity can delay menarche and cause ammenorrhea, and anovulatory cycles in young women, as well alterations in hormonal and metabolic pathways (137–144).

Medications: A number of case–control studies have examined the association between over-the-counter analgesics and the risk of ovarian cancer, initially based on the protective association seen with colorectal cancer. Cramer et al. looked at aspirin, ibuprofen, paracetamol, and prescribed analgesics in a case–control study (145). A 48% decrease in the risk of ovarian cancer was observed among those women who took paracetamol compared to those who did not. Paracetamol is the same medication as acetaminophen. This risk decreased further with frequency and duration of use. Whereas Rosenberg et al. reported a 20% decrease in the risk of ovarian cancer among women who took nonsteroidal anti-inflammatory drugs (NSAIDS) 1 day per week for at least 6 months that began a year before hospital admission compared with those who did not take NSAIDS (146). A further reduction up to 50% was found with increasing frequency of use. They did not observe a decrease in risk in those women taking acetaminophen. In another case–control study by Moysich et al. aspirin users were not at a reduced risk but women who took acetaminophen were (43%) (147). A decrease in risk was seen with increasing frequency and duration of use. In a prospective study looking at mortality, a 45% decrease in the death rate from ovarian cancer was observed among current paracetamol users compared to nonusers. The risk was not lowered with increased frequency of use (148). The biological mechanism under lying this decrease in risk seen with acetaminophen is unknown, however, Cramer et al. did demonstrate lower gonadotropin and estradiol levels in women taking acetaminophen compared to women taking no drugs or other analgesics (149).

The use of psychotropic medications was found to increase the risk of ovarian cancer in three case–control studies done in the North Eastern part of the United States. It is hypothesized that these medications may increase the risk of ovarian cancer by inducing gonadotropin secretion (150). Self-reported use of psychotropic medications, including amphetamines, sedatives, antidepressants, and antipsychotics for 6 months or longer was associated with between a 1.6 and twofold increase in the risk of invasive ovarian cancer compared to nonusers (150,151). The risk was greater with longer duration of use.

Other Exposures: Talc powder, has been studied as a potential risk factor for ovarian cancer for almost 20 years. It was originally examined because of its chemical similarity to the rod like asbestoses that has been shown to be associated with ovarian cancer in the occupational setting (152–155). Talc is thought to cause damage to the ovary by retrograde entry through fallopian tubes. When 14 case–control studies were combined that included eight studies with more than 200 cases, women who used talc in the genital area had a small excess risk compared to those who did not use talc (OR = 1.36; 95% CI 1.24, 1.49) (156). No dose response was seen. However, in a prospective study of 78,630 women no association was seen for talc (relative risk = 1.09; 95% CI = 0.86, 1.37) (152). A modest association was observed among women who used talc and had invasive serous carcinoma (relative risk = 1.40; 95% CI 1.02, 1.91). However, there were certain limitations to the study including no information on duration of use and a short follow-up of 9 years. A case–control study by Cramer et al. also suggested that women might be at an increased risk of ovarian cancer if the male partner used talc on their genital area (156). In the same study, genital talc use that began after a first pregnancy appeared to be associated with lower risk compared to use, which began before the first pregnancy. In summary, further prospective studies are needed to address possible recall or selection bias and to help decide whether perineal talc is in fact a risk factor for ovarian cancer.

Weak associations have been reported between tobacco smoke, radiation exposure, mumps virus, caffeine, hair dye and the development of ovarian cancer (86,158–160).

2.4.5. Diseases Associated with Ovarian Cancer

Polycystic Ovarian Disease and Endometriosis: The data relating polycystic ovarian disease (PCOD) to ovarian cancer are conflicting. Based on Fathalla's hypothesis one may expect women with polycystic ovarian disease to have a lower risk of ovarian cancer due to decrease ovulation whereas based on Risch's or Cramer and Welch's theories women may have a higher risk due to endogenous hormone profiles. The increased use of fertility drugs among women with PCOD may also affect risk further. From a population-based case–control study a diagnosis of PCOD was associated with greater than a twofold increase in the risk of ovarian cancer (OR = 2.5, 95% CI 1.1, 5.9) (161). Data from a Mayo Clinic cohort study did not demonstrated a similar association (162). Further studies are required.

An increased risk of ovarian cancer has also been observed in women with a history of endometriosis. Brinton et al. examined the records of 20,686 women who were hospitalized for endometriosis and found almost a twofold increase in the risk of ovarian cancer compared to the general population (SIR = 1.9, 95% CI 1.3, 2.8) (163).

2.5. Biomarkers of Early Detection

The search for effective screening marker(s) for ovarian cancer is ongoing. An ideal screening test should have a high sensitivity, that is the ability to detect true positives, and a high specificity, that is a low number of false positives, to avoid unnecessary testing and anxiety, particularly when the prevalence of the disease is low. The positive predictive value (the probability that a positive test indicates the presence of disease) is influenced by the specificity of the test and the prevalence of the disease in the screened population. One method of increasing the positive predictive value of the test is to target high-risk groups, who have higher prevalence rather than the general population. For this to be effective at a population level, the factors used to select the high-risk groups should capture most of the women who have disease. Qualities of a good marker of early detection include the ease at which it can be done, cost effectiveness, and ultimately, the demonstration that early detection translates into a reduction in mortality.

2.5.1. CA125

CA125 is a serum marker associated with ovarian cancer first described by Bast et al. (164). CA125 is a glycoprotein (molecular weight = 200,000) detected by the murine monoclonal antibody OC 125 (164). This antibody is produced by the somatic hybridization of spleen cells from mice immunized with ovarian cell lines (164). Its use as a prognostic marker and in the follow-up and therapy of ovarian cancer has been established, but not its use as a marker for early detection (165).

The idea that serum CA125 may be a potential biomarker for early detection came from a report published by Bast et al. in 1985 and was confirmed by Zurawski et al. in 1988 (166,167). Both these studies demonstrated the CA125 levels increase between 1 year and 18 months preceeding diagnosis. Subsequently, a number of studies have attempted to assess the sensitivity and specificity of CA125 as an early detection marker. In a case–control study, Zurawski et al. reported that only 38% of patients with stage 1 disease and 75% of women with stage II disease had CA125 levels in excess of 65 U/mL suggesting that the sensitivity of the test was not optimal. Further, Bast et al. measured the serum CA125 level in 888 healthy women, 143 women with nonmalignant disease, and 101 women with ovarian cancer and found that the specificity was also low (167). One percent of healthy women, 6% of women with nonmalignant disease, and 82% of patients had a CA125 level greater than 35 U/mL (168). In a nested case–control study Zurawaski et al. reported a sensitivity of 20% for a CA125 level over 35 U/mL for a 3-year period prior to the diagnosis (167). They also noticed an increase in specificity with increasing age and in postmenopausal women. In a prospective study of 5500 women, Einhorn et al. reported a specificity of 98.5% for a CA125 level >35 U/mL for women aged 50 years or older for a 3-year period (169). For the same time period similar results were reported by Helzlsouer et al. in a nested case–control study of 37 women who developed ovarian cancer and 73 controls. A maximum sensitivity of 57% for a serum level CA125 greater 35 U/ml within the first 3 years of follow-up and a specificity of 100% was observed. However, the specificity and sensitivity decreased over time (170). The new second generation assays, combining monoclonal antibodies recognize epitopes on two distinct regions and are potentially more sensitive.

The next phase of studies with regard to CA125 involve looking at serial levels or CA125 in combination with other tests. The sensitivity of the screening program can be increased by the use of two parallel tests, to screen for a disease. Zurawski et al. in 1990, demonstrated the increase of serial CA125s compared to a single value in a nested case–control study (171). Among women who had an elevated CA125 level at baseline, they reported a specificity of 99.9% if a woman's CA125 level had doubled over a 6-month period. In a retrospective study of 5550 women from the Stockholm study, a sensitivity of 83%, and a specificity of 99.7% to detect ovarian cancer was reported using serial CA125s (172). Both these studies were limited by sample size.

Another approach has been to increase the specificity of the test by using a two-stage screening procedure, where women who test positive for the first test are then screened using a second test. The drawback is this will lower over-all program sensitivity. Jacobs et al. designed a two-stage screening procedure: 22,000 volunteers had a serum CA125 level and if that was abnormal (defined as greater than 30 U/mL), they were called back for an abdominal ultrasound (173). Those women with an abnormal ultrasound were then referred to their gynecologist. Transvaginal ultrasongraphy has an estimated sensitivity between 80% and 100% and a specificity of around 99.6% (174,175). Eleven ovarian cancers were detected as a result of the two-stage screening. Only 4 of the 11 had early stage disease. As expected within the short follow-up period of 2 years, the screening program achieved an increase in specificity (99.9%), but a sensitivity of only 58% (173). This study was followed by a pilot randomized trial comparing a two-stage screening program (annual CA125 followed by ultrasound screening in those with an abnormal CA125 result) with follow-up without screening. Postmenopausal women aged 45 years and older were randomized to either the screened group ($n = 10,977$) or the control group ($n = 10,958$). The follow-up period was 7 years. The primary aims of the study were to assess feasibility and compliance. Seventy-one percent of women were screened annually over the 3-year period (176). Parallel screening programs also have been instigated in ovarian cancer with the hope to increase the sensitivity of the program. The National Cancer Institute is currently conducting the prostate, lung, colorectal, and ovarian (PLCO) cancer screening trial, in which 148,000 men and women between the ages of 55 and 74 have been enrolled from nine geographic areas in the United States. The women are randomized to a screening or control group. Those women who are being screened are receiving an annual physical examination, CA125 and transvaginal ultrasound.

2.5.2. Other Biomarkers

A number of studies have begun to assess the feasibility of other biomarkers that could be potentially used in conjunction with CA125 or independently. So far no biological marker has been proven to be effective in early detection. Some of the markers that have been investigated include; CEA, CA 19-9, CA 15-3, CA 54-61, CA 72-4, TAG 72, HMFG2, IL-6, IL-10, M-CSF, placental alkaline phosphatase, tissue peptide antigen, lipid associated sialic acid, NB70K, OVX1, D Dimer, prostasin, urinary gonadotropin fragment, and plasma lysophosphatidic acid (177–181).

Proteomics, which examines protein patterns in association with disease states, has offered hope for developing an effective test for the detection of ovarian cancer. Preliminary studies identified a pattern of proteins that could distinguish women with ovarian cancer from healthy women nearly 100% of the time. Clinical research using patterns of proteins as a means for identifying those with disease are underway. The technology is also used to identify specific proteins that could then be developed into clinical tests for early detection. Studies of these has been limited.

3. ENDOMETRIAL CANCER
3.1. Overview

Endometrial cancer, like ovarian cancer, is a disease of the elderly. Most women diagnosed are over the age of 60 and it rarely occurs below the age of 40. The overall age-adjusted incidence of endometrial cancer in the United States is 25 per 100,000 women and the mortality is about 4 per 100,000 women. Stratified by race, the incidence is higher among white females but the mortality is greater among black women. Incidence and mortality increase markedly with age (3). For women 65 and older, the incidence and mortality rates are 94 and 23 per 100,000 women, respectively (3).

Historically, the increased use of estrogen replacement therapy in the late 1960s and early 1970s led to a transient increase in the incidence of endometrial cancer between 1974 and 1976. Once it became clear that unopposed estrogen therapy increased a women's risk of endometrial cancer, a warning was issued by the Food and Drug Administration in 1976 and there was a subsequent decline in the use of unopposed estrogen and less endometrial cancer.

Stage and age also affects mortality rates. Women less than 65 years old have a 5-year survival rate of 88% compared to 80% in those who are 65 years or older (3). The 5-year survival rate for local-regional disease was 64% compared to 25% for distant disease (3).

3.2. Histological Types

The most common histological type of endometrial cancer is endometriod, accounting for 75–80% of cases, (squamous differentiation occurs in one-third of those); 10% are papillary serous carcinomas and 4–5% are clear cell adenocarcinomas.

There is evidence that atypical hyperplasia in endometrial tissue may be a precursor or intermediate marker in the development of endometrial cancer, raising the possibility that early screening or preventive measures could be implemented. A retrospective study of 170 women with endometrial carcinoma who were followed for 13.4 years, only 2% of women with endometrial hyperplasia without atypia developed carcinoma compared to 23% of those with atypical hyperplasia (182). Ho et al. in a retrospective study, reported a 27.6% incidence in emdometrial cancer among patients with atypia compared to a 3.4% incidence among women without atypia (183).

3.3. Etiology

Both epidemiological and laboratory studies strongly implicate hormonal exposure, in particular estrogen, in the etiology of endometrial cancer. The exact mechanism by which estrogen exerts its effect, as well as the contribution of other factors to the carcinogenesis pathway, is still unclear.

The "unopposed estrogen" hypothesis was first coined in the late 1970s and subsequently modified to explain the various associations observed between many of the known risk factors and the development of endometrial cancer (184–186). It is based on the premise that prolonged and uncontrolled mitosis of endometrial cells, as a result of unopposed estrogen exposure, increases the susceptibility of these cells to developing endometrial cancer. During a normal menstrual cycle, the mitotic rate of endometrial cells rises rapidly during menstruation to reach maximum levels early in the cycle and then stays constant until around day 19, where it falls due to an increase in progesterone. The maximum endometrial mitotic rate is induced in the early follicular phase. Progesterone reduces mitotic activity by decreasing the number of available estrogen receptors, increasing the metabolism of estradiol to the less active estrone and promoting the proliferating endometrial cells to move to a secretory state. In postmenopausal women, plasma estrogen is mainly derived from extraglandular conversion of androstenedione to estrone. Obese women have higher estrogen levels. There is a limit to the extent to which estrogen can increase the mitotic rate. Above a threshold, the mitotic rate remains constant. Because leaner postmenopausal women have a lower amount of endogenous estrogen than obese women, exogenous estrogen has greater potential to increase the mitotic rate before the threshold is reached.

3.4. Risk and Susceptibility Factors

The main risk factors can be divided into: inherited factors, hormonal factors, reproductive factors, lifestyle factors, diseases associated with endometrial cancer, and biomarkers of early detection.

3.4.1. Inherited Factors

Germline Mutation: A small percentage of women with endometrial cancer may have inherited genetic susceptibility to colon cancer. Hereditary nonpolyposis colorectal cancer (HNPCC) syndrome is associated with increased risk of colon, endometrial and ovarian cancer. In 1990, the International Collaborative Group on HNPCC proposed the Amsterdam criteria (Table 1) to identify high-risk groups predominantly in the research setting (186a,b). The criteria were revised in 1998 to take into consideration extracolonic malignancies (186c) (Table 1). A second set of criteria that is used, is called the revised Bethesda Guidelines. Clinically (186d) in table. HNPCC is an autosomal dominant disorder that is associated with mutations in DNA mismatch repair genes (53–55,187–191). In particular, germline mutations in hMSH2, hMLH1, PMS1, PMS2, and hMSH6 have been observed in up to 70% of HNPCC families (192). Microsatellite instability was also demonstrated in 75% of endometrial tumors associated with HNPCC (193). It is estimated that between 30% and 60% of women with

Table 1   Amsterdam Criteria for Hereditary Nonpolyposis Colorectal Cancer

---

1. Histologically confirmed colorectal cancer in at least three relatives, one of whom is a first-degree relative of the other two
2. Occurrence of disease in at least two successive generations
3. Age at diagnosis below 50 years in at least one colorectal cancer case
4. Exclusion of familial adenomatous polyposis (FAP)

International Collaborative Group on Hereditary Nonpolyposis Colorectal Cancer (ICG-HNPCC), 1991.
Source: Adapted from Vasen HFA, Mecklin J-P, Meera Khan P, Lynch HT. Dis Colon Rec 1991; 34:424–425.

this syndrome may develop endometrial cancer by the age of 70 (52,194,195). Little is known about the natural history of women with HNPCC. On average, women with the HNPCC syndrome were diagnosed with endometrial cancer 15 years earlier than the general population (52,196). Vassen et al. collected data on 125 endometrial cancer cases that were known to have HNPCC (196). Of the 125 women, 61% had a second primary cancer of which 72% had colorectal cancer, and 9% had both ovary and stomach cancer. There were also a few reports of synchronous cancers. In this group the mortality from endometrial cancer was 7% higher than the expected population rate.

Genetic Polymorphisms: As in ovarian cancer, the role of other inherited factors in endometrial cancer causation such as low penetrant mutations that commonly occur in the population are unclear. The focus has been on polymorphisms in genes encoding for enzymes involved in hormone biosynthesis in particular CYP17, and the androgen receptor CAG repeat length (197,198). Few studies have been done. Himan et al. examined the association between a single nucleotide change (T to C) in the 5' region of CYP17, which encodes a cytochrome P450 enzyme involved in androgen biosynthesis and the risk of endometrial cancer (197). This polymorphism was found to be protective in women who were homozygous for the allelic variant (OR = 0.43, 95% CI 0.23, 0.80). In another study, Yaron et al. examined the CAG length of the androgen receptor gene and the association with endometrial cancer (198). The mean number of CAG repeats was 19.8 in cases and 17.9 in controls ($p < 0.01$).

3.4.2. Hormonal Factors

Endogenous: *Menstrual factors*: consistent with the estrogen hypothesis both early menarche and late menopause are associated with an increased risk of endometrial cancer. An early menarche, defined as less than or equal to 12 years of age, increases a women's risk of endometrial cancer anywhere between 1.6 and 3.9 times the risk of women who undergo menarche at a later age (159,199–204). Similarly, an increased risk, between 1.7 and 2.4, was observed in women who became postmenopausal at the age of 52 or greater compared to those who were less than 49 years old (159,199,201–207). Increasing years of ovulation and longer duration of flow during each menstrual cycle were also observed to be risk factors (199,200,208).

Serum levels: in line with the "unopposed estrogen" hypothesis and other risk factors that have been discussed above, several studies have demonstrated an increased risk of endometrial cancer in women who have higher endogenous plasma levels of estrogen and androgens and a decreased risk in women with high levels of sex hormone binding globulin that tightly bind estrogen (209–213). In a study by Potischman et al. these hormonal differences were only seen among postmenopausal women and they observed a relative progesterone deficiency among premenopausal women with endometrial cancer compared to controls, suggesting that progesterone exposure may be a more important factor in premenopausal women (213).

Exogenous: *Oral contraceptive pill*: the majority of epidemiological studies have reported a risk reduction in endometrial cancer of approximately 50% in women who have used an OCP that contains both progesterone and estrogen for at least a year (78,82,84,201,203,210,214–222). This risk continues to decrease with increasing duration of use. Studies also suggest that the protective effect continues for 15 years or more even after cessation of the OCP (82,214,217). In some studies, OCPs that contained higher levels of progesterone correlated with a greater reduction in risk of endometrial cancer (216,223). It is unclear whether this is due to the dose of progestogen or their duration of use (224).

In the mid-1970s, case reports indicated an association between sequential oral contraceptive use (in particular a brand called Oracon that used a strong estrogen and weak progesterone dose) and a range of endometrial lesions including proliferative lesions, severe atypical hyperplasia, and endometrial cancer and as a result it was withdrawn from the market (215,225–228).

Hormone replacement therapy: HRT is used to treat many of the symptoms and prevent further health risks such as osteporosis and cardiovascular disease in postmenopausal women. It can be administered in two forms, as estrogen replacement alone or a combination of both estrogen and progesterone. Estrogen alone carries an increased risk of endometrial cancer. In observational studies, the relative risk of endometrial cancer has been estimated between 1.3 and 12 for women who used estrogen replacement compared to nonusers (159,203,229–245). In some studies, the risk increased with duration of use (242–247), and although the risk gradually decreased after cessation of use, it did not return to that of nonusers (240,247–249). Most of these cancers occurring among users of estrogen replacement therapy have been detected at an early stage and are well differentiated (232,234,241,242). In some studies, an increased risk was not seen in women who took estrogen replacement therapy for less than 6 months (232,233,235,238). In the meta-analysis by Grady et al. in 1995 a twofold increase in risk for estrogen users when compared to nonusers was found and the risk for less than 1 year of use was 1.4, and for greater than 10 years was 9.5 (250). Irrespective of estrogen dose or the manner it was administered (continuously or cyclically), an elevated risk in endometrial cancer was observed (250). Combining progesterone therapy with estrogen for women with a uterus attenuates the risk of endometrial cancer (220,243,245,246,251–253). In a randomized double blind placebo controlled trial continuous combines estrogen plus progestin therapy does not increase a women's risk of endometrial cancer (H.R. 0.81, 95% CI 0.48, 1.36) (253a).

In some studies, the association between estrogen therapy and endometrial cancer has been modified by weight and smoking. In women taking estrogen therapy alone, those who did not smoke had a higher risk of developing endometrial cancer than nonsmokers. It appears that smoking negates the risk associated with estrogen therapy and may be due to the anti-estrogen effects of smoking (201,260,261). Leaner women on estrogen therapy demonstrated a higher risk for endometrial cancer compared to women with a higher BMI (262).

3.4.3. Reproductive Factors

Pregnancy: Compared with nulliparous women, parous women have a 10–50% reduction in the risk of endometrial cancer (79,199,200,203, 263–265). Increasing number of pregnancies and increasing age of first and last pregnancy were also found to be protective in some studies (82,199,200,203,204,217,264,266). These findings are also consistent with the estrogen hypothesis since pregnancy reduces the time of exposure to unopposed estrogens. The increased exposure to progesterone may also lower the risk.

An ongoing question is whether the increased risk associated with nulliparity may be related to infertility. Brinton et al. reported a twofold increase in risk among nulliparous women who had difficulty conceiving compared to nulliparous women with no difficulty, and a sevenfold increase in risk among nulliparous women who had sought medical advice regarding infertility (200). Infertility is one of the factors attributed to the increased risk of endometrial cancer observed among nulliparous women who have married and never had children (264,267).

Studies on the role of induced and spontaneous abortions/miscarriages as risk factors for endometrial cancer have mixed results (199,200,264,265,267). McPherson et al. observed 2.5 times the risk of endometrial cancer in women who had an induced abortion compared to those who did not but the sample size was small (199). In contrast, Parazzini et al. had reported a protective association in women who had either an induced or spontaneous abortion, with a greater effect in premenopausal women (267). An increased risk was observed among women whose last pregnancy ended in a miscarriage compared with women who had a miscarriage during their first or middle pregnancy suggesting that the timing of the unopposed estrogen surge that occurs when in the case of a miscarriage may be an important risk factor (199).

3.4.4. Lifestyle Factors

Diet: Evaluating the association of various dietary factors and the risk of endometrial cancer is complicated by the variations in study design, dietary assessment tools, and information on potential confounding factors. However, most of these studies suggest that diets low in fat, high in fiber, and rich in fruits and vegetables may reduce the risk of endometrial cancer.

Dietary fat has been consistently associated with an increased risk of endometrial cancer. Reported odds ratios range between 1.5 and 5.6 (268–272). Both, animal fat (269,270), and saturated fat such as oleic acid and linoleic acid (269) have been associated with increased risk, whereas, mono-unsaturated fats may be protective (272). There are some data linking low fat diets to a reduction in serum estrogen levels or a shift in estrogen metabolism towards less active metabolites which may explain the association (273–275). In a clinical study, premenopausal women given a low-fat diet were observed to have decreased plasma levels of free estradiol and free testosterone (276).

Some studies suggest that the consumption of fruit and vegetables are protective. A 30–60% reduction in endometrial cancer was observed among women who consumed the highest fourth of fruit consumption compared to the lowest fourth (248,270,277). A risk reduction of 50–70% was also seen with the consumption of green vegetables (271), carotene, which is found in green and yellow vegetables (248,270,271,278,279), and lycopene (279). Decreased plasma estradiol levels have been observed in women whose diet contains large amounts of plant food. Lower plasma estradiol and urinary estrogen levels have also been measured among postmenopausal women who are vegetarian compared to those who are nonvegetarians (280,281). Carotene may alter estrogen metabolism by producing less active metabolites (278).

Increased soy and dietary fiber intakes from cereal, vegetable and fruit, have also been associated with a decreased risk of endometrial cancer (279,282). A risk reduction between 29% and 50% for women in the highest fourth of consumption of cereal, vegetable and fruit fiber compared to the lowest fourth has been reported (279,282). High consumption of soy products was associated with a 54% decrease in the risk of endometrial cancer compared to the lowest soy intake. Potentially, both soy and fiber could alter estrogen levels in the following ways; (1) altering the metabolism of estrogen at the receptor site (283,284), (2) decreased enterohepatic circulation and increased elimination of estrogen (281,285), or (3) increasing levels of sex hormone binding globulin resulting in lower levels of free estrogen (286,287).

Other dietary factors such as alcohol (248,271,288–292), protein intake (268–270,278,279), and total energy (248,268–270,278,293) have not been consistently associated with an increased or decreased risk of endometrial cancer (269,278).

Weight: In postmenopausal women, increasing BMI and increasing body weight has been consistently associated with an increased risk of endometrial cancer. Odds ratios ranging between 1.5 and 4.0 have been reported in postmenopausal women with BMI of greater than 28 kg/m^2 or body weight of greater than 165 lb when compared to women with a BMI of less than 22.5 kg/m^2 or less than 130 lb (199,202–204,232,233,235,236,282,294–301). A few studies have observed an even greater risk among obese premenopausal women with odds ratio between 17 and 20 (159,184). In postmenopausal women, the increased conversion of androstenedione to estrogens in adipose tissue and the decreased levels of sex hormone binding globulins results in an increased availability of free estrogen (302,303), which could explain these findings. DeWaard et al. demonstrated a positive correlation between changes in body weight and the excretion of estrone, estriol, and total estrogen (304). In premenopausal women, increased BMI has been associated with anovulatory cycles and diminished production of progesterone suggesting a different mechanism of action (305,306). Although current weight seems to be the strongest predictor of risk, an increased risk was also seen in women with a past history of obesity. The risk appears to persist regardless of age (295,296). It is unclear whether rate of change in weight is an independent risk factor (295). In a large prospective study increasing BMI was associated with and increased risk of dying from endometrial cancer (Calle et al., 2003). The increase in risk was 6-fold in women with a BMI of 40 (Calle et al., 2003).

Physical Activity: Low levels of physical activity have been associated with a modest increase in the risk of endometrial cancer (odds ratios of 1.3–2.5) independent of age and after adjusting for BMI and caloric intake (248,282,294,307–310). A greater risk was observed among women who reported lower levels of occupational activity compared to those who reported lower levels of recreational activities (282,309–312). Sturgeon et al. reported an increased risk only in inactive women who had a BMI greater than 28 suggesting that decreased physical activity is a surrogate marker for high BMI (294). Higher levels of physical activity have been associated with lower estrogen levels (313,314) and a reduction in the length of the luteal phase and/or frequency of ovulatory cycles (139,315–317). Based on existing studies, it is unclear whether physical activity is an independent risk factor for endometrial cancer.

Smoking: In observational studies a risk reduction of up to 40% has been consistently observed in postmenopausal women who currently smoke (203,242,243,260,261,298–321). However, in most studies a clear dose–response has not been observed (243,260,261,321), and studies have not consistently shown decreasing risk with increasing duration of use (201,243,299,320). The protective association with smoking may be due to a decrease in estrogen levels. Women who smoke are known to have an earlier menopause and decreased urinary estrogen secretion (214,322–324).

The antiestrogenic effects of smoking may also be mediated by induction of microsomal mixed function oxidase systems that metabolize sex hormones (298).

Medications: *Tamoxifen*: tamoxifen is a nonsteroidal hormone that has both estrogen antagonist and agonist properties. In some tissues, like the breast, it exhibits antiestrogenic properties, whereas, in other tissues such as the endometrium, bone, and liver, it acts as an estrogen agonist. In 1978, tamoxifen was approved for the treatment of metastatic breast cancer and then subsequently for the adjuvant treatment of breast cancer and to reduce risk of the onset of breast cancer.

The risk of endometrial cancer is increased among tamoxifen users. The initial report of an association between endometrial cancer and tamoxifen appeared in the literature in 1985 (325). Subsequently, at least 14 randomized trials and a number of observational studies have confirmed this association (326–331). Tamoxifen has been classified as a human carcinogen by IARC based on these studies (332).

Women on tamoxifen as part of the adjuvant treatment for breast cancer were observed to have between 1.5 and 6 times the risk of endometrial cancer when compared with those who were not taking it (328–331,333). This risk increased with longer duration of use (328,331), a history of prior use of hormone replacement therapy (331) and BMI greater than 24.5 kg/m^2 (331). A twofold increase in risk of endometrial cancer was also observed in women participating in the Breast Cancer Prevention Trial (BCPT). The risk of endometrial cancer occurred primarily in women over 50 years, RR $= 4.01$ (95% CI $= 1.70$–10.90) (334).

3.4.5.   Diseases Associated with Endometrial Cancer

Diabetes: A number of studies have reported a significant association between diabetes mellitus and cancer of the endometrium with odds ratios ranging from 1.2 to 3.3 even after adjusting for body weight suggesting that diabetes may also be an independent risk factor (204,207,335–338). Consistent with the unopposed estrogen hypothesis, increased levels of estrogen and decreased levels of luteinizing hormones and follicular stimulating hormone have been reported in postmenopausal diabetic women (339,340). In most studies, an increased risk has been observed in diabetic women over the age of 40 suggesting an association between noninsulin dependent diabetes and endometrial cancer. Abnormalities in glucose tolerance have also been associated with an increased risk of endometrial cancer (341–343).

Polycystic Ovarian Syndrome: It is unclear whether polycystic ovarian syndrome (PCOS) increases a women's risk of endometrial cancer because factors such as obesity, infertility, and nulliparity are commonly associated with PCOS (69,344). Chamlian et al. also reported a 25% increase in the incidence of PCOS among women with endometrial hyperplasia (345).

4. CERVICAL CANCER
4.1. Overview

Cervical cancer is the third most common cancer in women in the world today, accounting for approximately 9.8% of all new cancer cases. In the United States alone, in the year 2005, an estimated 10,370 new cervical cancers will be diagnosed and 3710 deaths from cervical cancer will occur (1). During the period 1973–1999 there was a 44% decrease in the incidence and a 47% decrease in the mortality of cervical cancer in the United States (3). A similar trend has been observed in other developed countries. The decline in mortality rates predated the implementation of widespread screening programs therefore it is felt that factors other than screening may have been responsible for the initial decline (346–348). These factors include; increasing affluence, improvements in standard of living, nutrition, increasing use of barrier contraceptives, and decline in sexually transmitted diseases (349).

Unfortunately, racial, ethnic, and socioeconomic disparities exist. The incidence of cervical cancer is at least three times higher in women living in developing countries, in areas where there are no screening programs, and in lower socioeconomic groups (346–348). The incidence and mortality rates in the United States are higher for Black women, (11.2 per 100,000 and 2.8 per 100,000, respectively), compared to White women (7.9 per 100,000 and 5.9 per 100,000), respectively. White Hispanics, Hispanics, American Indians, and Asian Pacific Islanders also have higher incidence and mortality rates compared to White women (3).

The incidence of cervical cancer is two times higher among women 65 and over compared to those under 65 (3). This difference could be due to poor access to screening as well as to decreased participation in screening programs (349). The 5-year survival rate for women 65 and over is 52% compared to 74% for women under 65 years of age (3). With respect to staging, the 5-year survival rate for localized disease is 91% compared to 13% for distant disease (3).

4.2. Histological Types

Invasive carcinoma of the cervix can be divided into three types; squamous, adenocarcinoma, and adeno squamous. Squamous carcinoma accounts for approximately 80% of cervical cancers while adenocarcinoma and adenosquamous carcinomas account for 10%. The other 10% are usually classified as undefined (350). The peak incidence of squamous carcinoma occurs between the ages of 48 and 55 years, whereas adenocarcinoma of the cervix is seen more often among younger women (267,351).

The majority of invasive squamous cell carcinomas are thought to arise from premalignant intraepithelial or dysplastic lesions (352). Dysplastic changes in the cervical epithelium were first described in the 1940s by Papanicolau (353). These lesions were classified into histological grades based on the degree of dysplasia (CIN I–III) (354). In 1988, the histological and cytological changes were combined to form a new classification known as the Bethesda System (355). Using this system, cervical lesions were classified into low-grade squamous intraepithelial lesions (LSIL) and high-grade squamous intraepithelial lesions (HSIL). The CIN and Bethesda system are often interchanged. LSIL contains CIN I and HSIL includes CIN II and CIN III. In 1998, a separate category for atypical squamous cells of uncertain significance (ASCUS) was added followed by categories for atypical glandular cells of uncertain significance (AGUS) and adenocarcinoma in situ (AIS) (356). These squamous intraepithelial lesions can spontaneously regress, persist or progress to invasive cancer (357). CIN I lesions are more likely to regress, whereas CIN II lesions are more likely to progress on to CIN III or invasive cancer (358–360). Spontaneous regression has been reported in up to 56% of women with CIN I, and 43% with CIN II. Whereas up to 11% of women with CIN I, and 22% of women with CIN II progress to CIN III, and 1% of women with CIN I and 5% of women with CIN III progress to invasive cancer (361,362).

4.3. Etiology

Human papilloma virus (HPV) infection is necessary for the development of cervical cancer (363). HPV is a member of the papovaviridae family of double-strand DNA viruses (364). It measures about 50–55 nm in diameter. The papilloma virus genome is about 7900 base pairs and can be divided into three regions: the long control region, required for DNA expression and replication, the early region that codes for proteins involved in the regulation of viral transcription (E2), DNA replication (E1 and E2) and cell proliferation (E5, E6, and E7), and the late region that contains two genes which code for the capsid proteins, (L1 and L2) (332). There are over 100 genotypes that have been identified, of which 35 are known to infect the anogenital tract (365). In order to be classified as a specific type of HPV there must be less than 90% homology between base pairs (366). HPVs have been categorized into low-risk (6,11,39,41–44,51), intermediate, and high-risk types (16,18,45,31,33,35,52–59) based on their oncogenic potential (367).

From an international prevalence study of 1035 frozen biopsies, HPV DNA was detected in 93% of invasive squamous cervical tumors (368). Twenty different strains were detected. Fiftyone percent of the 881 cases of invasive squamous carcinoma were positive for HPV 16, and 12% were positive for HPV 18. Human papilloma virus 16 was the predominant type seen in all countries, except Indonesia where HPV 18 was found to be more prevalent. Among the HPV 16 positive specimens, just over half were well differentiated as opposed to moderately or poorly differentiated and no difference in prevalence was found according to clinical stage. HPV 45 was also common in western Africa and HPV 39 and 59 in Central and South America. In contrast, among 25 specimens of adenocarcinoma, 28% were positive for HPV 16 and 56% were positive for HPV 18 (368). A similar pattern was also seen in the adenosquamous specimens. HPV type 40, 42, 53, 54, 66 and PAP155 were not detected in any of the specimens. When the negative cases from this study were reanalyzed in 1999 with a more sensitive HPV DNA test, the prevalence of HPV in those specimens increased even further to 99.7% (363). HPV infections, have also been closely linked to CIN I–III and carcinoma in situ (369).

Genital HPV is acquired primarily through sexual intercourse. Once a cell is infected it undergoes cellular differentiation, followed by replication and transcription of the HPV DNA virus (364). In two prospective studies involving young women in Western countries aged between 15 and 23, the incidence of HPV infection over 36 months ranged from 26% to 43% (370,371). Whereas in a population-based prospective study of 1425 low income women between the ages of 18 and 80, the cumulative incidence was 38% at 18 months (372). In all these studies, incident cases were defined as women who were HPV negative at baseline and became positive on subsequent testing. Thus, the incidence rate may represent recurrent infections as well as new infections. In all three studies, HPV 16 was one of the most common types detected (370–372). The medium duration of infection by type 16 ranged from between 8.1 and 11 months (370–372). The average incubation period for all types of HPV infection was between 3 and 7 months (370,372). However, for those women with type 16 the medium duration varied from 8.1 to 11 months (370–372).

A number of prospective and nested case–control studies have examined the association between positive HPV antibodies and the risk of cervical cancer reporting odds ratios ranging from 2.0 to 7.5 (373–376). The association between HPV DNA typing, a more sensitive test, and the risk of high-grade squamous epithelial lesions have also been examined in a number of prospective studies (371,372,377,378). Women who were HPV DNA 16 positive had between 8.5 and 13 times the risk of developing CIN II &III compared to CIN I (371,372,377,378). Given that only a small number of women who are infected with the HPV develop cervical cancer, other inherited and environmental factors must play an important role in the carcinogenesis pathway.

4.4. Risk and Susceptibility Factors
4.4.1. Risk Factors for Oncogenic HPV Infections

Exposures increasing the incidence of oncogenic HPV infections are also important risk factors for the development of cervical cancer (379,380).

These factors include young age, duration of oral contraceptive use, number of lifetime sexual partners, sexual practices, and HIV infection (379,380). Rousseau et al. reported a 70% reduction in the incidence of high-risk HPV infection in women greater than 45 years of age compared to women 24 years or less (379,380). A threefold increase in the incidence of high-risk HPV infection was observed in women who used the oral contraceptive pill (OCP) for greater than or equal to 6 years compared to women who used the OCP for less than 6 years (OR 3.36, 95% CI 1.30, 8.68). Silins et al. observed that women with a history of greater than six lifetime sexual partners were at a tenfold increase in the risk of oncogenic HPV infections compared to women who had one lifetime sexual partner (OR 10.2, 95% CI 3.5, 29.6) (380). Increased rates of HPV infection have also been reported among HIV-positive women who took part in high-risk sexual practices compared to HIV-negative women (381–385). Among HIV positive women, higher viral load and lower CD4 count was also associated with an increased risk of HPV infection (381–385).

4.4.2. Persistence of HPV Infection and Viral Load

Persistence of high-risk HPV infection is thought to be related to the development of CIN III and invasive cervical cancer (372,386,387). Nobbenhius found that 95% of women with CIN III had persistent HPV infection (386). Factors such as viral load may directly affect persistence of infection. In a nested case–control study, the risk of developing cervical cancer in women with a high viral load increased steadily up to 23% (95% CI 12.4, 31.8) after 15 years of surveillance (388). Josefsson et al. demonstrated a 60-fold increase in the risk of cervical cancer in women with a high HPV 16 viral load compared to women who were HPV 16 negative. Viral load was measured 7.8 years prior to the diagnosis of cervical cancer (389). Studies suggest that an individual's HIV status may also affect viral persistence (385,390). In a longitudinal study, 20% of HIV positive women were positive for HPV types 16 and 18 infection on repeated measurements compared to 3% in HIV negative women ($p < 0.001$) (385).

4.4.3. Inherited Factors

Genetic Polymorphisms: *Human leukocyte antigen polymorphisms*: An individual's level of immunity is one factor that may be associated with a woman's risk of CIN III or invasive cervical cancer. Human leukocyte antigen (HLA) classes I and II genes, are known to be involved in the immune response (364). There are 20 class I genes in the HLA region, three of these, HLA-A, B, and C, are mainly involved in the immune response. Class I genes are expressed in most somatic cells and class II are expressed by a subgroup of immune cells including B cells, activated T cells, macrophages, dendritic cells and thymic epithelial cells. The function of both class I and II molecules is to present short peptides to T cells thereby initiate an immune response (391). A number of studies have shown an association between particular HLA polymorphisms and cervical neoplasia. Hildeshem et al. reported a ninefold increased risk of HSIL if a woman was homozygous for DQB1*302 or a carrier of both B7 and DQB1*(302,392,393). Neuman et al. reported a positive association, between HLA DQB1*0303 and the risk of invasive cancer, only among HPV positive patients ($p = 0.005$) (394). Cuzick et al. reported similar findings of increased risk but with different variants of HLADQB1 (395).

MTHFR polymorphisms: Given that folate may be protective for cervical cancer, Piyathilake et al. investigated the association between a polymorphism of MTHFR and the risk of cervical cancer using cervical tissue from 64 women with CIN lesions and 31 controls (396). MTHFR is a critical enzyme regulating the metabolism of folate and methionine that are important in DNA methylation and repair. A common base change from C to T at the nucleotide position 677 of the MTHFR gene results in substitution of valine for alanine (397). Both heterozygous (Ala/Val) and homozygous (Val/Val) variants have been shown to have reduced MTHFR enzyme activity and significantly higher circulating homocysteine levels compared to those homozygous for (Ala/Ala) (398,399). Therefore, it is postulated that women who had at least one valine allele would be at an increased risk of cervical cancer. Piyathilake et al. found a threefold increase in the risk of cervical cancer among women who were homozygous or heterozygous for the valine allele (396). The greatest risk was seen among parous women who had the mutant polymorphism. This may be explained by the fact that pregnancy stresses folate status, making the folate deficiency even greater.

Glutathione S-transferase polymorphisms: The glutathione *S*-transferases (GSTs) are enzymes that detoxify a large number of carcinogens by catalyzing the conjugation of reactive chemical intermediates to soluble glutathione in the liver. The GSTM1 and GSTT1 polymorphisms result in a reduction in enzyme activity due to the inheritance of two null alleles. Both GSTM1 and GSTT1 polymorphisms occur in slightly less than 50% of Caucasians (400).

Two studies have examined the association between the GSTM1 and GSTT1 genotypes and the risk of cervical cancer in Caucasians (401,402). Neither study reported a positive association. However, a study in Japan where GSTT1 null is more prevalent, a twofold increase in the risk in women who had the GSTT1 null genotype compared to those with the GSTT1 was observed present. This risk increased when GSTT1 and GSTM1 were analyzed in combination. No information on other risk factors, such as smoking, was available (403).

P53 Arg72Pro polymorphisms: HPV 16 and HPV 18 encode two major oncoproteins E6 and E7. The E6 protein binds to the tumor suppressor protein P53 and directs its degradation (404,405). The tumor suppressor gene P53 inhibits cell growth through the activation of cell-cycle arrest and apoptosis. Alteration or inactivation of p53 by mutation or the interaction of p53 with DNA tumor viruses can lead to cancer (404). In early cervical tumors, the P53 protein is usually not mutated. Inactivation of p53 by E6 oncoprotein may be analogous to being inactivated by a mutation (404,406). In 1987, a polymorphism of wild type p53 was identified from human cells amino acid residue 72 resulting in the substitution of arginine for proline (407). There have been at least 37 studies examining this association. A meta-analysis of these studies demonstrated a 20% increased risk of cervical cancer in women who were homozygous for the *Arg* variant compared to those who were heterozygous for the *Arg* variant (Jee SH et al., 2004). When stratified by cancer type, the risk of adenocarcinoma of the cervix was increased but not squamous cell carcinoma.

4.4.4. Hormonal Factors

Oral Contraceptives: Results from studies that have examined the association between OCP use and the risk of carcinoma of the cervix, taking into consideration HPV status have been mixed. Ylitalo et al. reported almost a fourfold increase among current users compared with nonusers (OR = 3.78, 95% CI 2.09, 6.85) and an increasing risk with increasing duration of use (p trend < 0.001) (417). Kruger-Kjaer et al. reported an increased risk only among women who had HSIL (OR = 1.6, 95% CI 0.8, 3.2) (418). Five other studies that also tested for HPV DNA did not observe an association between OCP and cervical cancer (420–424). The mixed picture may reflect the difficulty in fully assessing other factors that might confound the association between OCP use and the risk of cervical cancer, both positively and negatively. For example, OCP use is highly correlated with sexual behaviors that increase exposure to HPVs. On the other hand, women who use OCPs also tend to have more regular Pap smears, which is associated with a decreased risk of cervical cancer (425,426). In a meta-analysis of 28 studies, the relative risk of cervical cancer increased with increasing duration of use (Smith JS., 2003). The relative risk of cervical cancer in women who had used oral contraceptives for 10 years or more was 2.2 (95 % CI 1.9, 2.4) irrespective of HPV status. In HPV positive women the relative risk was similar, as would be expected (RR 2.5, 95% CI 1.6, 3.9). A direct association between OCP use and cervical cancer is biologically plausible, through a mechanism involving folic acid. Studies have detected megaloblastic changes in the cervical epithelium of women associated with the OCP that were reversed by folic acid (427,428). Folate deficiency can lead to impaired DNA methylation and repair. These changes were then reversed by folic acid.

4.4.5. Reproductive Factors

Parity has been consistently found to be a risk factor for cervical cancer even after taking HPV DNA into account (429,430). The biological mechanism behind this association is obscure but is thought to be due to either hormonal effects, low folic acid, or trauma to the cervix (429).

4.4.6. Lifestyle Factors

Diet: In a number of case–control studies, high dietary carotene, vitamins C and E, folate, and low levels of carotenoids have been associated with a reduced risk of cervical cancer (277,431–439). Unfortunately, the majority of studies were completed before sensitive HPV DNA tests were available and few studies took into consideration the effect of both smoking and oral contraceptive use on these associations (440). Oral contraceptive use appears to reduce both plasma levels of vitamin C and red blood cell folate even in women whose dietary intake is adequate (427,428). Smoking decreases plasma β-carotene, folate, and Vitamin C levels (441).

A number of dietary and serological studies have shown that the low intake of carotenoids are associated with an increased risk of cervical dysplasia and invasive carcinoma (436,439,442–448). The risk of cervical cancer was increased threefold in women with serum levels of β-carotene and α-carotene in the lower third compared to the highest tertile in a prospective study (439). Similar results have been reported in case–control studies (442,449,450). An increased risk in cervical cancer was also been observed in women with low serum levels of cryptoxanthin and lycopene (439,441,446,449).

Vitamin C, or ascorbic acid, has been consistently associated with decreased risk of both dysplasia and invasive cancer (437,444,445,451–454). Few studies have been able to assess serological levels of ascorbic acid, as it is necessary to use fresh blood samples for valid assays or samples specifically preserved (387,446). Two studies found that vitamin C was protective only among smokers (432,433). A study of in situ disease noted a protective association of vitamin C supplements (455). A sixfold risk was observed among women with the lowest intake of dietary vitamin C supplements compared to the highest group (456). In a clinic-based case–control study, HPV seropositive women with plasma levels of reduced ascorbic acid greater than 0.803 mg/dL were found to have a 60% reduction in the risk of developing intraepithelial neoplasia compared to women with less than 0.803 mg/dL (95% CI 0.19, 0.89) (457).

Low serum levels of retinol have also been associated with an increased risk of cervical cancer (449). An increased rate of progression (4.5 times) to carcinoma in situ or invasive cancer was observed among women with cervical dysplasia who had low serum retinol levels compared to those with high serum levels (449). In a prospective study, the association between HPV 16, 18, and 33 and the risk of cervical cancer was greater in women with lower serum level of retinol compared to higher levels (relative risk = 2.6, 95% CI 0.7, 8.8) (458).

The association between vitamin E and the risk of cervical cancer is unclear. Verreault et al. in a case–control study, reported a 60% decreased risk of cervical cancer among women with highest intake of vitamin E (≥ 5.9 mg/day) compared to the lowest intake (444). Two case–control studies reported lower α-tocopherol levels in women with CIN and cervical cancer (387,442) but these results were not observed in two nested case–control studies and one case–control study controlling for HPV infection (439,443,458).

Folate has been postulated to have a protective role in the etiology of cervical dysplasia and cancer. The majority of studies have been case–control and demonstrated either a mild protective association with increasing amounts folate intake or serum concentration (428,432,444,445,452,455, 459,460). A nonstatistically significant trend in the protective direction was reported in a prospective study for increasing serum concentration of folate and vitamin B12 (431). Human papilloma virus status was known for all study participants. In the same study, the serum levels of homocysteine, a marker of low vitamin B12 levels was increased twofold in women with cervical cancer (431). Folate intake may be associated with HPV and cervical cancer. In case–control studies, low levels of folic acid was associated with HPV infection (428). Women with HPV and lower level of folic acid had a sevenfold risk of CIN (OR 7.5, 95% CI 1.2, 9.7) (461).

Smoking: Like so many other factors, smoking was initially thought to be a surrogate for HPV infection because women who were heavy smokers also had many of the other high-risk behaviors that were associated with cervical cancer (Trimble et.al.). However, subsequent studies suggest that smoking may be an independent cofactor, where there is a modest increase in the risk of cervical cancer associated with cigarette smoking (OR between 1.5 and 2.6) after taking into consideration HPV status (417,418,422–424,430,457,462,463). A dose response was seen in some studies (417,457,464,465). An increased risk of cervical cancer was also observed with longer duration of smoking (417,465). A strong association between smoking and cervical cancer was observed among women infected with HPV 16 or 18 high-risk genotypes (418,423,424,457,463,466,467). A positive association has also been reported between smoking and adenocarcinoma of the cervix, although the sample sizes were much smaller (422).

Biological plausibility for this positive association stems from a number of findings among smokers including the detection of mutagenic cervical fluids (468), high concentrations of nicotine and tobacco-specific *N*-nitrosamines in cervical mucus of smokers (469), increased levels of DNA adducts of benzo(a)pyrene and its metabolites in cervical mucus (470) and evidence of decreased cervical epithelial immunity which may increase persistence of the HPV infection (471). In support of a causal link between smoking and cervical cancer, Szarewski, et al. demonstrated a significant correlation between the extent of smoking reduction and the change in cervical lesion size in a randomized intervention trial (472).

4.4.7. Diseases Associated with Cervical Cancer

Chlamydia Trachomatis: Although there is often a correlation in sexual behavior between HPV and other sexually transmitted diseases, studies suggest that *Chylamydia trachomatis* may be an independent risk factor for cervical cancer.

In a nested case–control study of 182 cases and matched controls, serum samples were analyzed for IgG antibodies to *C. trachomatis* (a test for past infection) and HPV types 16, 18, and 33 (473). Positive IgG antibodies were associated with a twofold increase in the risk of cervical cancer after adjusting for smoking and HPV status (OR = 2.2, 95% CI 1.3, 3.5). There was no difference according to type of HPV infection. An increased risk was not seen for adenocarcinoma of the cervix. These results are consistent with prior case–control studies (474,475). A longitudinal study by Anttila et al. demonstrated a sixfold increase in the risk of cervical squamous carcinoma among women who had been exposed to a specific *C. trachomatis* serotype, G (OR = 6.6, 95% CI 1.6, 27.0) (476).

4.4.8. Biomarkers of Early Detection

Human Papilloma Virus DNA Testing as a Screening Tool: Despite the advent of HPV DNA testing its exact role in cervical cancer screening is yet to elucidated. Initial studies suggest that HPV DNA testing may be more sensitive but less specific compared to conventional cytological screening and therefore is unlikely to replace pap smears (477–479). However, a modest improvement in screening efficacy has been observed when the two tests are used in combination (477).

A greater focus is being placed on the use of HPV DNA testing as a second screening test in women who have equivocal pap smears (ASCUS). To avoid missing women with high-risk lesions, many physicians currently refer all women with atypical smears for colposcopy, which is an expensive and invasive procedure (480–485). In a group of women diagnosed with atypical smears repeat pap smears had a sensitivity of 60% and a specificity of 77% compared to a sensitivity of 86% and a specificity of 71% for HPV DNA using hybrid capture which identifies 14 HPV viruses as the second line test. When the two tests were used concurrently the sensitivity increased to 90% but the specificity decreased to 58%. Manos et al. reported similar results (479). There is a multicenter randomized clinical trial study organized by the National Cancer Institute in progress to evaluate three alternative methods of managing low grade and atypical cervical cytologic diagnoses. Women who have either of these two diagnoses are referred to immediate referral for colposcopy, follow up with cytology alone, or use of HPVDNA to triage to colposcopy. All women are being followed every 6 months for 2 years (486).

5. FUTURE RESEARCH NEEDS

Significant advances have been made in understanding the etiology of ovarian, endometrial, and cervical cancers. This chapter highlights the importance of both inherited and environmental factors as risk and susceptibility factors. With the sequencing of the human genome research there has been a greater focus on understanding the role of inherited factors in the different cancers and how they interact with particular environmental factors. With advancements in the laboratory a greater understanding of the biological mechanisms underlying these environmental exposures is also ongoing. These developments should be able to yield new approaches for the prevention of these cancers and biomarkers to assist in early detection.

ACKNOWLEDGMENTS

We would like to thank Gomathi Visvanathan, Ram Tenkasi, Megan McSorley, Patti Gravitt, and Gloria Zepp for their help.

REFERENCES

1. American Cancer Society. Cancer Facts and Figures—2005. Atlanta, GA: American Cancer Society, 2005.
2. Ozols F, Schwartz PE, Eifel PJ. Ovarian cancer, fallopian tube carcinoma, and peritoneal carcinoma In: Devita VT, Heilman S, Rosenberg SA, eds. Cancer: Principles and Practices of Oncology. 4th ed. Philadelphia: The Lippincott Company, 1993:1597–1628.
3. Ries LAG, Eisner MP, Kosary CL, Hankey BF, Miller BA, Clegg L, Mariotlo A, Feuer EJ, Edwards BK (eds). SEER Cancer Statistics Review 1975–2001, National Cancer Institute, Bethesda, MD http://seer.cancer.sov/esr/1975_2001/2004.
4. Munoz. Human papillomavirus and cervical cancer: epidemiological evidence. In: Franco E, Monsonego J, eds. New Development in Cervical Cancer Screening and Prevention. Oxford: Blackwell Science Ltd, 1997:3–13.
5. Schiffman M, Adrianza ME. ASCUS-LSIL Triage Study. Design, methods and characteristics of trial participants. Acta Cytol 2000; 44(5):726–742.
6. Coleman MP, Esteve J, Damiecki P, Arslan A, Renard H. Trends in cancer incidence and mortality. IARC Scientific publication No. 121. Lyon: International Agency for Research on Cancer, 1993.
7. Kliewer V, Smith KR. Ovarian cancer mortality among immigrants in Australia and Canada. Cancer Epidemiol Biomarkers Prev 1995; 4(5):453–458.

8. Thigpen T. Ovaries and fallopian tubes. In: Abeloff MD, Armitage JO, Lichter AS, Niederhuber JE, eds. Clinical Oncology. Philadelphia: Churchill Livingstone 2000:2016–2040.
9. Fathalla F. Incessant ovulation—a factor in ovarian neoplasia? Lancet 1971; 2(7716):163.
10. Cramer DW, Welch WR. Determinants of ovarian cancer risk. II. Inferences regarding pathogenesis. J Natl Cancer Inst 1983; 71:717–721.
11. Risch A. Hormonal etiology of epithelial ovarian cancer, with a hypothesis concerning the role of androgens and progesterone. J Natl Cancer Inst 1998; 90(23):1774–1786.
12. Easton DF, Peto J. The contribution of inherited predisposition to cancer incidence. Cancer Survey 1990; 9:395415.
13. Parazzini F, Franceschi S, La Vecchia C, Fasoli M. The epidemiology of ovarian cancer. Gynecol Oncol 1991; 43:9–23.
14. Tavani, Ricci E, La Vecchia C, Surace M, Benzi G, Parazzini F, Franceschi S. Influence of menstrual and reproductive factors on ovarian cancer risk in women with and without family history of breast or ovarian cancer. Int J Epidemiol 2000; 29:799–802.
15. Lynch HT, Guirgis HA, Albert S, Brennan M, Lynch J, Kraft C, Pocekay D, Vaughns C, Kaplan A. Familial association of carcinoma of the breast and ovary. Surg Gynecol Obstet 1974; 138(5):717–724.
16. Lynch HT, Albano W, Black L, Lynch JF, Recabaren J, Pierson R. Familial excess of cancer of the ovary and other anatomic sites. J Am Med Assoc 1981; 245(3):261–264.
17. Lynch HT, Fitzsimmons ML, Conway TA, Bewtra C, Lynch J. Hereditary carcinoma of the ovary and associated cancers: a study of two families. Gynecol Oncol 1990; 36(1):48–55.
18. Watson P, Lynch HT. Extracolonic cancer in hereditary nonpolyposis colorectal cancer. Cancer 1993; 71:677–685.
19. Laplace-Marieze V, Presneau N, Sylvain V, Kwiatkowski F, Lortholary A, Hardouin A, Bignon YJ. Systematic sequencing of the BRCA-1 coding region for germ-line mutation detection in 70 French high-risk families. Int J Oncol 1999; 14(5):971–977.
20. Shattuck-Eidens D, Oliphant A, McClure M, McBride C, Gupte J, Rubano T, Pruss D, Tavtigian SV, Teng DH, Adey N, Staebell M, Gumpper K, Lundstrom R, Hulick M, Kelly M, Holmen J, Lingenfelter B, Manley S, Fujimura F, Luce M, Ward B, Cannon-Albright L, Steele L, Offit K, Thomas A, et al. BRCA1 sequence analysis in women at high risk for susceptibility mutations. Risk factor analysis and implications for genetic testing. J Am Med Assoc 1997; 278(15):1242–1250.
21. Scully R, Ganesan S, Vlasakova K, Chen J, Socolovsky M, Livingston DM. Genetic analysis of BRCA1 function in a defined tumor cell line. Mol Cell 1999; 4(6):1093–1099.
22. Chen Y, Lee WH, Chew HK. Emerging roles of BRCA1 in transcriptional regulation and DNA repair. J Cell Physiol 1999; 181(3):385–392.

23. Holt JT, Thompson ME, Szabo C, Robinson-Benion C, Arteaga CL, King M-C, Jenson RA. Growth retardation and tumour inhibition. Nat Genet 1996; 12: 298–302.

24. Hall JM, Lee MK, Newman B, Morrow JE, Anderson LA, Huey B, King M-C. Linkage of early-onset familial breast cancer to chromosome 17q21. Science 1990; 250:1684–1689.

25. Miki Y, Swensen J, Shattuck-Eidens D, Futreal PA, Harshman K, Tavtigian S, Liu Q, Cochran C, Bennett LM, Ding W, et al. A strong candidate for the breast and ovarian cancer susceptibility gene BRCA1. Science 1994; 266(5182):66–71.

26. Wooster R, Neuhausen SL, Mangion J, Quirk Y, Ford D, Collins N, Nguyen K, Seal S, Tran T, Averill D, et al. Localization of a breast cancer susceptibility gene, BRCA2, to chromosome 13q12–13. Science 1994; 265(5181):2088–2090.

27. Merajver SD, Pham TM, Caduff RF, Chen M, Poy EL, Cooney KA, Weber BL, Collins FS, Johnston C, Frank TS. Somatic mutations in the BRCA1 gene in sporadic ovarian tumours. Nat Genet 1995; 9(4):439–443.

28. Eeles R, Kodouri. BRCA1/2 carriers and endocrine risk modifiers. Endocr Relat Cancer 1999; 6:521–528.

29. Hakansson S, Johannsson O, Johansson U, Sellberg G, Loman N, Gerdes AM, Holmberg E, Dahl N, Pandis N, Kristoffersson U, Olsson H, Borg A. Moderate frequency of BRCA1 and BRCA2 germ-line mutations in Scandinavian familial breast cancer. Am J Hum Genet 1997; 60(5):1068–1078.

30. Stoppa-Lyonnet D, Laurent-Puig P, Essioux L, Pages S, Ithier G, Ligot L, Fourquet A, Salmon RJ, Clough KB, Pouillart P, Bonaiti-Pellie C, Thomas G. BRCA1 sequence variations in 160 individuals referred to a breast/ovarian ovarian family cancer clinic. Institut Curie Breast Cancer Group. Am J Hum Genet 1997; 60(5):1021–1030.

31. Wagner TM, Moslinger RA, Muhr D, Langbauer G, Hirtenlehner K, Concin H, Doeller W, Haid A, Lang AH, Mayer P, Ropp E, Kubista E, Amirimani B, Helbich T, Becherer A, Scheiner O, Breiteneder H, Borg A, Devilee P, Oefner P, Zielinski C. BRCA1-related breast cancer in Austrian breast and ovarian cancer families: Specific BRCA1 mutations and pathological characteristics. Int J Cancer 1998; 77(3):354–360.

32. Pharoah PD, Stratton JF, Mackay J. Screening for breast and ovarian cancer: the relevance of family history. Br Med Bull 1998; 54(4):823–838.

33. Frank F, Manley SA, Olopade OI, Cummings S, Garber JE, Bernhardt B, Antman K, Russo D, Wood ME, Mullineau L, Isaacs C, Peshkin B, Buys S, Venne V, Rowley T, Loader S, Offit K, Robson M, Hampel H, Brener D, Winer EP, Clark S, Weber B, Strong LC, Thomas A, et al. Sequence analysis of BRCA1 and BRCA2: correlation of mutations with family history and ovarian cancer risk. J Clin Oncol 1998; 16(7):2417–2425.

34. Gayther SA, Russell P, Harrington P, Antoniou AC, Easton DF, Ponder BA. The contribution of germline BRCA1 and BRCA2 mutations to familial ovarian cancer: no evidence for other ovarian cancer-susceptibility genes. Am J Hum Genet 1999; 65(4):1021–1029.

35. Berchuck A, Heron KA, Carney ME, Lancaster JM, Fraser EG, Vinson VL, Deffenbaugh AM, Miron A, Marks JR, Futreal PA, Frank TS. Frequency of

germline and somatic BRCA1 mutations in ovarian cancer. Clin Cancer Res 1998; 4(10):2433–2437.

36. Stratton JF, Gayther SA, Russell P, Dearden J, Gore M, Blake P, Easton D, Ponder BA. Contribution of BRCA1 mutations to ovarian cancer. N Engl J Med 1997; 336(16):1125–1130.

37. Whittemore AS, Gong G, Itnyre J. Prevalence and contribution of BRCA1 mutations in breast cancer and ovarian cancer: results from three U.S. population-based case–control studies of ovarian cancer. Am J Hum Genet 1997; 60(3):496–504.

38. Takahashi H, Behbakht K, McGovern PE, Chiu HC, Couch FJ, Weber BL, Friedman LS, King MC, Furusato M, LiVolsi VA, et al. Mutation analysis of the BRCA1 gene in ovarian cancers. Cancer Res 1995; 55(14):2998–3002.

39. Ford D, Easton DF, Peto J. Estimates of the gene frequency of BRCA2 and its contribution to breast and ovarian cancer incidence. Am J Hum Genet 1995; 57(6):1457–1462.

40. Ford D, Easton DF. The genetics of breast and ovarian cancer. Br J Cancer 1995; 72(4):805–812.

41. Easton DF, Ford D, Bishop DT. Breast and ovarian cancer incidence in BRCA1-mutation carriers. The Breast Cancer Linkage Consortium. Am J Hum Genet 1995; 56(1):265–271.

42. Ford D, Easton DF, Stratton M, Narod S, Goldgar D, Devilee P, Bishop DT, Weber B, Lenoir G, Chang-Claude J, Sobol H, Teare MD, Struewing J, Arason A, Scherneck S, Peto J, Rebbeck TR, Tonin P, Neuhausen S, Barkardottir R, Eyfjord J, Lynch H, Ponder BA, Gayther SA, Zelada-Hedman M, et al. Genetic heterogeneity and penetrance analysis of the BRCA1 and BRCA2 genes in breast cancer families. The Breast Cancer Linkage Consortium. Am J Hum Genet 1998; 62(3):676–689.

43. Struewing JP, Hartge P, Wacholder S, Baker SM, Berlin M, McAdams M, Timmerman MM, Brody LC, Tucker MA. The risk of cancer associated with specific mutations of BRCA1 and BRCA2 among Ashkenazi Jews. N Engl J Med 1997; 336(20):1401–1408.

44. The Breast Cancer Linkage Consortium. Cancer risks in BRCA2 mutation carriers. J Natl Cancer Inst 1999; 91(15):1310–1316.

45. Struewing JP, Abeliovich D, Peretz T, Avishai N, Kaback MM, Collins FS, Brody LC. The carrier frequency of the BRCA1 185delAG mutation is approximately 1 percent in Ashkenazi Jewish individuals. Nat Genet 1995; 11(2):198–200.

46. Roa BB, Boyd AA, Volcik K, Richards CS. Ashkenazi Jewish population frequencies for common mutations in BRCA1 and BRCA2. Nat Genet 1996; 14(2):185–187.

47. Oddoux C, Struewing JP, Clayton CM, Neuhausen S, Brody LC, Kaback M, Haas B, Norton L, Borgen P, Jhanwar S, Goldgar D, Ostrer H, Offit K. The carrier frequency of the BRCA2 6174delT mutation among Ashkenazi Jewish individuals is approximately 1%. Nat Genet 1996; 14(2):188–190.

48. Thorlacius S, Olafsdottir G, Tryggvadottir L, Neuhausen S, Jonasson JG, Tavtigian SV, Tulinius H, Ogmundsdottir HM, Eyfjord JE. A single BRCA2

mutation in male and female breast cancer families from Iceland with varied cancer phenotypes. Nat Genet 1996; 13(1):117–119.

49. Gayther SA, Harrington P, Russell P, Kharkevich G, Garkavtseva RF, Ponder BA. Frequently occurring germ-line mutations of the BRCA1 gene in ovarian cancer families from Russia. Am Hum J Genet 1997; 60(5): 1239–1242.

50. Ramus SJ, Kote-Jarai Z, Friedman LS, van der Looij M, Gayther SA, Csokay B, Ponder BA, Olah E. Analysis of BRCA1 and BRCA2 mutations in Hungarian families with breast or breast-ovarian cancer. Am J Hum Genet 1997; 60(5):1242–1246.

51. Aarnio M, Mecklin JP, Aaltonen LA, Nystrom-Lahti M, Jarvinen HJ. Lifetime risk of different cancers in hereditary non-polyposis colorectal cancer (HNPCC) syndrome. Int J Cancer 1995; 64(6):430–433.

52. Aarnio M, Sankila R, Pukkala E, Salovaara R, Aaltonen LA, de la Chapelle A, Peltomaki P, Mecklin JP, Jarvinen HJ. Cancer risk in mutation carriers of DNA-mismatch-repair genes. Int J Cancer 1999; 81(2):214–218.

53. Peltomaki P, Vasen HFA. Mutations predisposing to hereditary nonpolyposis colorectal cancer: database and results of a collaborative study. The International Collaborative Group on HNPCC. Gastroenterology 1997; 113: 1146–1158.

54. Miyaki M, Konishi M, Tanaka K, Kikuchi-Yanoshita R, Muraoka M, Yanuso M, Igari T, Kolkechiba M, Mori T. Germline mutation of MSH6 as the cause of hereditary nonpolyposis colorectal cancer. Nat Genet 1997; 17:271–272.

55. Akiyama Y, Sato H, Yamada T, Nagasaki H, Tsuchiya A, Abe R, Yuasa Y. Germline mutation of the hMSH6/GTBP in an atypical hereditary nonpolyposis colorectal cancer kindred. Cancer Res 1997; 57:3920–3923.

56. Lancaster JM, Brownlee HA, Bell DA, Futreal PA, Marks JR, Berchuck A, Wiseman RW, Taylor JA. Microsomal epoxide hydrolase polymorphism as a risk factor for ovarian cancer. Mol Carcinog 1996; 17(3):160–162.

57. Hassett C, Robinson KB, Beck NB, Omiecinski CJ. The human microsomal epoxide hydrolase gene (EPHX1): complete nucleotide sequence and structural characterization. Genomics 1994; 23(2):433–442.

58. Goodman A. Role of routine human papillomavirus subtyping in cervical screening. Curr Opin Obstet Gynecol 2000; 12:11–14.

59. Spurdle AB, Chen X, Abbazadegan M, Martin N, Khoo SK, Hurst T, Ward B, Webb PM, Chenevix G-Trench G. CYP17 promotor polymorphism and ovarian cancer risk. Int J Cancer 2000; 86(3):436–439.

59a. Garner EI, Stokes EE, Berkowitz RS, Mok SC, Cramer DW. Polymorphisms of the estrogen-metabolizing genes CYP17 and catechol-O-methyltransferase and risk of epithelial ovarian cancer. Cancer Res 2002; 62(11):3058–3062.

59b. Modugno F. Ovarian cancer and polymorphisms in the androgen and progesterone receptor genes: a HuGE review. Am J Epidemiol 2004; 159(4):319–335.

60. Hengstler JG, Kett A, Arand M, Oesch-Bartlomowicz B, Oesch F, Pilch H, Tanner B. Glutathione S-transferase T1 and M1 gene defects in ovarian carcinoma. Cancer Lett 1998; 130(1–2):43–48.

61. Titus-Ernstoff L, Perez K, Cramer DW, Harlow BL, Baron JA, Greenberg ER. Menstrual and reproductive factors in relation to ovarian cancer risk. Br J Cancer 2001; 84(5):714–721.
62. Chiaffarino F, Pelucchi C, Parazzini F, Negri E, Franceschi S, Talamini R, Conti E, Montella M, La Vecchia C. Reproductive and hormonal factors and ovarian cancer. Ann Oncol 2001; 12:337–341.
63. Franceschi S, La Vecchia C, Helmrich SP, Mangioni C, Tognoni G. Risk factors for epithelial ovarian cancer in Italy. Am J Epidemiol 1982; 115(5): 714–719.
64. Tzonou A, Day NE, Trichopoulos D, Walker A, Saliaraki M, Papapostolou M, Polychronopoulou A. The epidemiology of ovarian cancer in Greece: a case–control study. Eur J Cancer Clin Oncol 1984; 20(8):1045–1052.
65. Wu ML, Whittemore AS, Paffenbarger RS Jr, Sarles DL, Kampert JB, Grosser S, Jung DL, Ballon S, Hendrickson M, Mohle Boetani J. Personal and environmental characteristics related to epithelial ovarian cancer. I. Reproductive and menstrual events and oral contraceptive use. Am J Epidemiol 1988; 128(6):1216–1227.
66. Booth M, Beral V, Smith P. Risk factors for ovarian cancer: a case–control study. J Cancer 1989; 60(4):592–598.
67. Parazzini F, La Vecchia C, Negri E, Gentile A. Menstrual factors and the risk of epithelial ovarian cancer. J Clin Epidemiol 1989; 42(5):443–448.
68. Shu XO, Brinton LA, Gao YT, Yuan JM. Population-based case–control study of ovarian cancer in Shanghai. Cancer Res 1989; 49(13):3670–3674.
69. Whittemore AS, Harris R, Itnyre J. Characteristics relating to ovarian cancer risk: collaborative analysis of 12 US case–control studies. IV. The pathogenesis of epithelial ovarian cancer. Collaborative Ovarian Cancer Group. Am J Epidemiol 1992; 136(10):1212–1220.
70. Purdie D, Green A, Bain C, Siskind V, Ward B, Hacker N, Quinn M, Wright G, Russell P, Susil B. For the Survey of Women's Health Study Group. Reproductive and other factors and risk of epithelial ovarian cancer: An Australian case–control study. Int J Cancer 1995; 62:678–684.
71. Helzlsouer KJ, Alberg AJ, Gordon GB, Longcope C, Bush TL, Hoffman SC, Comstock GW. Serum gonadotropins and steroid hormones and the development of ovarian cancer. J Am Med Assoc 1995; 274(24):1926–1930.
72. Cuzick J, Bulstrode JC, Stratton I, Thomas BS, Bulbrook RD, Hayward JL. A prospective study of urinary androgen levels and ovarian cancer. Int J Cancer 1983; 32(6):723–726.
73. Ness RB, Grisso JA, Vergona R, Klapper J, Morgan M, Wheeler JE. For the study of Health Reproduction (SHARE) study group. Oral contraceptives, other methods of contraception and risk reduction for ovarian cancer. Epidemiology 2001; 12:307–312.
74. Hankinson SE, Colditz GA, Hunter DJ, Willett WC, Stampfer MJ, Rosner B, Hennekens CH, Speizer FE. A prospective study of reproductive factors and risk of epithelial ovarian cancer. Cancer 1995; 76(2):284–290.
75. Harris R, Whittemore AS, Itnyre J. Characteristics relating to ovarian cancer risk: collaborative analysis of 12 US case–control studies. III. Epithelial

tumors of low malignant potential in white women. Collaborative Ovarian Cancer Group. Am J Epidemiol 1992; 136(10):1204–1211.

76. John M, Whittemore AS, Harris R, Itnyre J. Characteristics relating to ovarian cancer risk: collaborative analysis of seven U.S. case–control studies. Epithelial ovarian cancer in black women. Collaborative Ovarian Cancer Group. J Natl Cancer Inst 1993; 85(2):142–147.

77. Beral V, Hannaford P, Kay C. Oral contraceptive use and malignancies of the genital tract. Results from the Royal College of General Practitioners' Oral Contraception Study. Lancet 1988; 2(8624):1331–1335.

78. Vessey MP, Painter R. Endometrial and ovarian cancer and oral contraceptives—findings in a large cohort study. Br J Cancer 1995; 71:1340–1342.

79. Parazzini F, La Vecchia C, Negri E, Fedele L, Balotta F. Reproductive factors and risk of endometrial cancer. Am J Obstet Gynecol 1991; 164(2):522–527.

80. Casagrande JT, Louie EW, Pike MC, Roy S, Ross RK, Henderson BE. "Incessant ovulation" and ovarian cancer. Lancet 1979; 2(8135):170–173.

81. Weiss NS, Lyon JL, Liff JM, Vollmer WM, Daling JR. Incidence of ovarian cancer in relation to the use of oral contraceptives. Int J Cancer 1981; 28: 669–671.

82. Combination oral contraceptive use and the risk of endometrial cancer. The cancer and Steroid Hormone Study of the Centers for Disease Control and the National Institute of Child Health and Human Development. J Am Med Assoc 1987; 257:796–800.

83. Risch HA, Marrett LD, Howe GR. Parity, contraception, infertility, and the risk of epithelial ovarian cancer. Am J Epidemiol 1994; 140(7):585–597.

84. WHO Collaborative Study of Neoplasia and Steroid Contraceptives. Endometrial cancer and combined oral contraceptives. Int J Epidemiol 1988; 17: 263–269.

85. Rosenberg L, Palmer JR, Zauber AG, Warshauer ME, Lewis JL Jr, Strom BL, Harlap S, Shapiro S. A case–control study of oral contraceptive use and invasive epithelial ovarian cancer. Am J Epidemiol 1994; 139(7):654–661.

86. Harlow BL, Weiss NS, Roth GJ, Chu J, Daling JR. Case–control study of borderline ovarian tumors: reproductive history and exposure to exogenous female hormones. Cancer Res 1988; 48:5849–5852.

87. Modan B, Hartge P, Hirsh-Yechezkel G, Chetrit A, Lubin F, Beller U, Ben-Baruch G, Fishman A, Menczer J, Struewing JP, Tucker MA, Wacholder S. For the National Israel Ovarian Cancer Study Group Parity, oral contraceptives, and the risk of ovarian cancer among carriers and noncarriers of a BRCA1 or BRCA2 mutation. N Engl J Med 2001; 345:235–240.

88. Narod S, Risch H, Moslehi R, Dorum A, Neuhasen S, Olsson H, Provencher D, Radice P, Evans G, Bishop S, Brunet J-S, Ponder B, et al. Oral contraceptives and the risk of hereditary ovarian cancer. N Engl J Med 1998; 339: 424–428.

89. Rodriguez C, Patel AV, Calle EE, Jacob EJ, Thun MJ. Estrogen replacement therapy and ovarian cancer mortality in a large prospective study of US women. J Am Med Assoc 2001; 285:1460–1465.

89a. Lancy JV, Brinton LA, Abbas FM, Barnes WA, Gravitt PE, Greenbery MD, Greene SM, Hadjimichael OC, McGowan L, Mortel R, Schwartz PE,

Silverberg SG, Hildesheim A. Oral contraceptiues as risk factors for Cervical Adenocarcinomas and squamous Cell Carcinomas. Can Epid Bio Pre 1999; 8:1079–1085.

90. Adami HO, Hsieh CC, Lambe M, Trichopoulos D, Leon D, Persson I, Ekbom A, Janson PO. Parity, age at first childbirth, and risk of ovarian cancer. Lancet 1994; 344(8932):1250–1254.

91. Kaufman DW, Kelly JP, Welch WR, Rosenberg L, Stolley PD, Warshauer ME, Lewis J, Woodruff J, Shapiro S. Noncontraceptive estrogen use and epithelial ovarian cancer. Am J Epidemiol 1989; 130(6):1142–1151.

92. Parazzini F, La Vecchia C, Negri E, Villa A. Estrogen replacement therapy and ovarian cancer risk. Int J Cancer 1994; 57(1):135–136.

93. Risch HA, Marrett LD, Jain M, Howe GR. Differences in risk factors for epithelial ovarian cancer by histologic type. Results of a case–control study. Am J Epidemiol 1996; 144(4):363–372.

94. Mori M, Harabuchi I, Miyake H, Casagrande JT, Henderson BE, Ross RK. Reproductive, genetic, and dietary risk factors for ovarian cancer. Am J Epidemiol 1988; 128(4):771–777.

95. McGowan L, Norris HJ, Hartge P, Hoover R, Lesher L. Risk factors in ovarian cancer. Eur J Gynaecol Oncol 1988; 9(3):195–199.

96. Annegers JF, Strom H, Decker DG, Dockerty MB, O'Fallon WM. Ovarian cancer: Incidence and case–control study. Cancer 1979; 43(2):723–729.

97. Joly DJ, Lilienfeld AM, Diamond EL, Bross ID. An epidemiologic study of the relationship of reproductive experience to cancer of the ovary. Am Epidemiol J 1974; 99(3):190–209.

98. Albrektsen G, Heuch I, Kvale G. Reproductive factors and incidence of epithelial ovarian cancer: a Norwegian prospective study. Cancer Causes Control 1996; 7(4):421–427.

99. Cooper GS, Schildkraut JM, Whittemore AS, Marchbanks PA. Pregnancy recency and risk of ovarian cancer. Cancer Causes Control 1999; 10(5): 397–402.

100. Hankinson SE, Hunter DJ, Colditz GA, Willett WC, Stampfer MJ, Rosner B, Hennekens CH, Speizer FE. Tubal libation, hysterectomy, and risk of ovarian cancer: a prospective study. J Am Med Assoc 1993; 270:2813–2818.

101. Green A, Purdie D, Bain C, Siskind V, Russell P, Quinn M, Ward B. Tubal sterilisation, hysterectomy and decreased risk of ovarian cancer. Survey of Women's Health Study Group. Int J Cancer 1997; 71(6):948–951.

102. Miracle-McMahill HL, Calle EE, Kosinski AS, Rodriguez C, Wingo PA, Thun M, Heath Cw. Tubal ligation and fatal ovarian cancer in a large prospective cohort study. Am J Epidemiol 1997; 145:349–357.

103. Ness RB, Cottreau C. Possible role of ovarian epithelial inflammation in ovarian cancer. J Natl Cancer Inst 1999; 91:1459–1467.

104. Ness RB, Grisso JA, Cottreau C, Klapper J, Vergona R, Wheeler JE, Morgan M, Schlesselman JJ. Factors related to inflammation of the ovarian epithelium and risk of ovarian cancer. Epidemiology 2000; 11:111–117.

105. Rosenblatt KA, Thomas DB. Lactation and the risk of epithelial ovarian cancer. The WHO Collaborative Study of Neoplasia and Steroid Contraceptives. Int J Epidemiol 1993; 22(2):192–197.

106. Demopoulos RI, Seltzer V, Dubin N, Gutman E. The association of parity and marital status with the development of ovarian carcinoma: clinical implications. Obstet Gynecol 1979; 54(2):150–155.

107. Modan B, Ron E, Lerner-Geva L, Blumstein T, Menczer J, Rabinovici J, Oelsner G, Freedman L, Mashiach S, Lunenfeld B. Cancer incidence in a cohort of infertile women. Am J Epidemiol 1998; 147:1038–1042.

108. Bristow RE, Karlan BY. Ovulation induction, infertility, and ovarian cancer risk. Fertil Steril 1996; 66(4):499–507.

109. Rossing MA, Daling JR, Weiss NS, Moore DE, Self SG. Ovarian tumors in a cohort of infertile women. N Engl J Med 1994; 331(12):771–776.

110. Venn A, Watson L, Bruinsma F, Giles G, Healy D. Risk of cancer after use of fertility drugs with in-vitro fertilisation. Lancet 1999; 354:1586–1590.

111. Laughlin GA, Barrett-Connor E, Kritz-Silverstein D, von Muhlen D. Hysterectomy, oophorectomy, and endogenous sex hormone levels in older women: the Rancho Bernardo Study. J Clin Endocrinol Metab 2000; 85(2): 645–651.

112. Cramer DW, Xu H. Epidemiologic evidence for uterine growth factors in the pathogenesis of ovarian cancer. Ann Epidemiol 1995; 5(4):310–314.

113. Mettlin CJ, Piver MS. A case–control study of milk-drinking and ovarian cancer risk. Am J Epidemiol 1990; 132(5):871–876.

114. Cramer DW. Lactase persistence and milk consumption as determinants of ovarian cancer risk. Am J Epidemiol 1989; 130(5):904–910.

115. Cramer DW, Harlow BL, Willett WC, Welch WR, Bell DA, Scully RE, Ng WG, Knapp RC. Galactose consumption and metabolism in relation to the risk of ovarian cancer. Lancet 1989; 2(8654):66–71.

116. Herrinton LJ, Weiss NS, Beresford SA, Stanford JL, Wolfla DM, Feng Z, Scott CR. Lactose and galactose intake and metabolism in relation to the risk of epithelial ovarian cancer. Am J Epidemiol 1995; 141(5):407–416.

117. Kushi LH, Mink PJ, Folsom AR, Anderson KE, Zheng W, Lazovich D, Sellers TA. Prospective study of diet and ovarian cancer. Am J Epidemiol 1999; 149(1):21–31.

118. Steinmetz KA, Potter JD. Vegetables, fruit, and cancer. II. Mechanisms. Cancer Causes Control 1991; 2(6):427–442.

119. Byers T, Marshall J, Graham S, Mettlin C, Swanson M. A case–control study of dietary and nondietary factors in ovarian cancer. J Natl Cancer Inst 1983; 71(4):681–686.

120. Slattery ML, Schuman KL, West DW, French TK, Robison LM. Nutrient intake and ovarian cancer. Am J Epidemiol 1989; 130(3):497–502.

121. Engle A, Muscat JE, Harris RE. Nutritional risk factors and ovarian cancer. Nutr cancer 1991; 15(3–4):239–247.

122. La Vecchia C, Decarli A, Negri E, Parazzini F, Gentile A, Cecchetti G, Fasoli M, Franceschi S. Dietary factors and the risk of epithelial ovarian cancer. J Natl Cancer Inst 1987; 79(4):663–669.

123. Sundstrom H, Ylikorkala O, Kauppila A. Serum selenium and thromboxane in patients with gynaecological cancer. Carcinogenesis 1986; 7(7):1051–1052.

124. Drozdz M, Tomala J, Jendryczko A, Banas K. Concentration of selenium and vitamin E in the serum of women with malignant genital neoplasms and their family members. Ginekol Pol 1989; 60(6):301–305.

125. Heinonen PK, Kuoppala T, Koskinen T, Punnonen R. Serum vitamins A and E and carotene in patients with gynecologic cancer. Arch Gynecol Obstet 1987; 241(3):151–156.
126. Knekt P, Aromaa A, Alfthan G, Maatela J, Hakama M, Hakulinen T, Teppo L. Re: Prospective study of serum micronutrients and ovarian cancer. J Natl Cancer Inst 1996; 88(19):1408.
127. Helzlsouer KJ, Alberg AJ, Norkus EP, Morris JS, Hoffman SC, Comstock GW. Prospective study of serum micronutrients and ovarian cancer. J Natl Cancer Inst 1996; 88(1): 32–37.
128. Garland M, Morris JS, Stampfer MJ, Colditz GA, Spate VL, Baskett CK, Rosner B, Speizer FE, Willett WC, Hunter DJ. Prospective study of toenail selenium levels and cancer among women. J Natl Cancer Inst 1995; 87(7):497–505.
129. Hiatt RA, Fireman BH. Serum cholesterol and the incidence of cancer in a large cohort. J Chronic Dis 1986; 39(11):861–870.
130. Mink PJ, Folsom AR, Sellers TA, Kushi LH. Physical activity, waist-to-hip ratio, and other risk factors for ovarian cancer: a follow-up study of older women. Epidemiology 1996; 7(1):38–45.
131. Farrow DC, Weiss NS, Lyon JL, Daling JR. Association of obesity and ovarian cancer in a case-control study. Am J Epidemiol 1989; 129:1300–1304.
132. Shu XO, Gao YT, Yuan JM, Ziegler RG, Brinton LA. Dietary factors and epithelial ovarian cancer. Br J Cancer 1989; 59(1):92–96.
133. Barker DJ, Winter PD, Osmond C, Phillips DI, Sultan HY. Weight gain in infancy and cancer of the ovary. Lancet 1995; 345(8957):1087–1088.
134. Cottreau CM, Ness RB, Kriska AM. Physical activity and reduced risk of ovarian cancer. Obstet Gynecol 2000; 96(4):609–614.
135. Frisch RE, Wyshak G, Albright NL, Albright TE, Schiff L, Jones JP, et al. Lower prevalence of breast cancer and cancers of the reproductive system among former college athletes compared to non-athletes. Br J Cancer 1985; 52:885–891.
136. Pukkala E, Poskiparta M, Apter D, Vihko V. Life-long physical activity and cancer risk among Finnish female teachers. Eur J Cancer Prev 1993; 2: 369–376.
137. Frisch RE, Wyshak G, Vincent L. Delayed menarche and amenorrhea in ballet dancers. N Engl J Med 1980; 303(1):17–19.
138. Frisch RE, Gotz-Welbergen AV, McArthur JW, Albright T, Witschi J, Bullen B, Birnholz J, Reed RB, Hermann H. Delayed menarche and amenorrhea of college athletes in relation to age of onset of training. J Am Med Assoc 1981; 246(14):1559–1563.
139. Bernstein L, Ross RK, Lobo RA, Hanisch R, Krailo MD, Henderson BE. The effects of moderate physical activity on menstrual cycle pattern in adolescence: implications for breast cancer prevention. Br J Cancer 1987; 55: 681–685.
140. Russell JB, Mitchell D, Musey PI, Collins DC. The relationship of exercise to anovulatory cycles in female athletes: hormonal and physical characteristics. Obstet Gynecol 1984; 63(4):452–456.

141. Moisan J, Meyer F, Gingras S. Leisure physical activity and age at menarche. Med Sci Sports Exerc 1991; 23(10):1170–1175.

142. Peiris AN, Mueller RA, Smith GA, Struve MF, Kissebah AH. Splanchnic insulin metabolism in obesity. Influence of body fat distribution. J Clin Invest 1986; 78(6):1648–1657.

143. Kissebah AH, Vydelingum N, Murray E, Evans DJ, Hartz AJ, Kalkhoff RK, et al. Relation of body fat distribution to metabolic complications of obesity. J Clin Endocrinol Metab 1982; 54:254–260.

144. Kaye SA, Folsom AR. Is serum cortisol associated with body fat distribution in postmenopausal women? Int J Obes 1991; 15(7):437–439.

145. Cramer DW, Harlow BL, Titus-Ernstoff L, Bohlke K, Welch WR, Greenberg ER. Over-the-counter analgesics and risk of ovarian cancer. Lancet 1998; 351:104–107.

146. Rosenberg L, Palmer JR, Rao RS, Coogan PF, Strom BI, Zauber AG, Stolley PD, Shapiro S. A case–control study of analgesic use and ovarian cancer. Cancer Epidemiol Biomarkers Prev 2000; 9(9):933–937.

147. Moysich KB, Mettlin C, Piver MS, Natarajan N, Menezes RJ, Swede H. Regular use of analgesic drugs and ovarian cancer risk. Cancer Epidemiol Biomarkers Prev 2001; 10(8):903–906.

148. Rodriguez C, Henley SJ, Calle EE, Thun MJ. Paracetamol and risk of ovarian cancer mortality in a prospective study of women in the USA. Lancet 1998; 352:1354–1355.

149. Cramer DW, Liberman RF, Hornstein MD, McShane P, Powers D, Li EY, Barbieri R. Basal hormone levels in women who use acetaminophen for menstrual pain. Fertil Steril 1998; 70:371–373.

150. Harlow BL, Cramer DW, Baron JA, Titus-Ernstoff L, Greenberg ER. Psychotropic medication use and risk of epithelial ovarian cancer. Cancer Epidemiol Biomarkers Prev 1998; 7(8):697–702.

151. Harlow BL, Cramer DW. Self-reported use of antidepressants or benzodiazepine tranquilizers and risk of epithelial ovarian cancer: evidence from two combined case–control studies. (Massachusetts, United States). Cancer Causes Control 1995; 6(2):130–134.

152. Gertig DM, Hunter DJ, Cramer DW, Colditz GA, Speizer FE, Willett WC, Hankinson SE. Prospective study of talc use and ovarian cancer. J Natl Cancer Inst 2000; 92:249–252.

153. Keal EE. Asbestosis and abdominal neoplasms. Lancet 1960; 2:1211–1216.

154. Acheson ED, Gardner MJ, Pippard EC, Grime LP. Mortality of two groups of women who manufactured gas masks from chrysotile and crocidolite asbestos: a 40-year follow-up. Br J Ind Med 1982; 39(4):344–348.

155. Heller DS, Gordon RE, Katz N. Correlation of asbestos fiber burdens in fallopian tubes and ovarian tissue. Am J Obstet Gynecol 1999; 181(2):346–347.

156. Cramer DW, Liberman RF, Titus-Ernstoff L, Welch WR, Greenberg ER, Baron JA, Harlow BL. Genital talc exposure and risk of ovarian cancer. Int J Cancer 1999; 81(3):351–356.

157. Doll R. The epidemiology of cancer. Cancer 1980; 45(10):2475–2485.

158. Cramer DW, Hutchison GB, Welch WR, Scully RE, Ryan KJ. Determinants of ovarian cancer risk. I. Reproductive experiences and family history. J Natl Cancer Inst 1983; 71(4):711–716.

159. La Vecchia C, Franceschi S, Decarli A, Gallus G, Tognomi G. Risk factors for endometrial cancer at different ages. J Natl Cancer Inst 1984; 73:667–671.

160. Tzonou A, Polychronopoulou A, Hsieh CC, Rebelakos A, Karakatsami A, Trichopoulos D. Hair dyes, analgesics, tranquilizers and perineal talc application as risk factors for ovarian cancer. Int J Cancer 1993; 55(3):408–410.

161. Schildkraut JM, Schwingl PJ, Bastos E, Evanoff A, Hughes C. Epithelial ovarian cancer risk among women with polycystic ovary syndrome. Obstet Gynecol 1996; 88(4 pt 1):554–559.

162. Coulam CB, Annegers JF, Kranz JS. Chronic anovulation syndrome and associated neoplasia. Obstet Gynecol 1983; 61(4):403–407.

163. Brinton LA, Gridley G, Persson I, Baron J, Bergqvist A. Cancer risk after a hospital discharge diagnosis of endometriosis. Am J Obstet Gynecol 1997; 176(3):572–579.

164. Bast C, Feeney M, Lazarus H, et al. Reactivity of a monoclonal antibody with human ovarian carcinoma. J Clin Invest 1981; 68:1331–1337.

165. Bast RC, Klug TL, Schaetzl E, Lavin P, Niloff JM, Greber TF, Zurawski VR, Knapp RC. Monitoring human ovarian carcinoma with a combination of CA 125, CA 19.9 and carcinoembryonic antigen. Am J Obstet Gynecol 1994; 149:553–559.

166. Bast RC Jr, Siegal FP, Runowicz C, Klug TL, Zurawski VR Jr, Schonholz D, Cohen CJ, Knapp RC. Elevation of serum CA 125 prior to diagnosis of an epithelial ovarian carcinoma. Gynecol Oncol 1985; 22(1):115–120.

167. Zurawski VR Jr, Orjaseter H, Andersen A, Jellum E. Elevated serum CA 125 levels prior to diagnosis of ovarian neoplasia: relevance for early detection of ovarian cancer. Int J Cancer 1988; 42(5):677–680.

168. Bast RC Jr, Klug TL, St John E, Jenison E, Niloff JM, Lazarus H, Berkowitz RS, Leavitt T, Griffiths CT, Parker L, Zurawski VR Jr, Knapp RC. A radioimmunoassay using a monoclonal antibody to monitor the course of epithelial ovarian cancer. N Engl J Med 1983; 309(15):883–887.

169. Einhorn N, Sjovall K, Knapp RC, Hall P, Scully RE, Bast RC Jr, Zurawski VR Jr. Prospective evaluation of serum CA 125 levels for early detection of ovarian cancer. Obstet Gynecol 1992; 80(1):14–18.

170. Helzlsouer KJ, Bush TL, Alberg AJ, Bass KM, Zacur H, Comstock GW. Prospective study of serum CA-125 levels as markers of ovarian cancer. J Am Med Assoc 1992; 269(9): 1123–1126.

171. Zurawski VR Jr, Sjovall K, Schoenfeld DA, et al. Prospective evaluation of serum CA 125 levels in a normal population, phase I. The specificities of single and serial determinations in testing for ovarian cancer. Gynecol Oncol 1990; 36(3):299–305.

172. Skates SJ, Xu FJ, Yu YH, Sjovall K, Einhorn N, Chang Y, Bast RC Jr, Knapp RC. Toward an optimal algorithm for ovarian cancer screening with longitudinal tumor markers. Cancer 1995; 76(10 suppl):2004–2010.

173. Jacobs I, Davies AP, Bridges J, Stabile I, Fay T, Lower A, Grudzinskas JG, Oram D. Prevalence screening for ovarian cancer in postmenopausal women by CA 125 measurement and ultrasonography. Br Med J 1993; 306(6884):1030–1034.

174. Karlan BY. The status of ultrasound and color Doppler imaging for early detection of ovarian carcinoma. Cancer Invest 1997; 15:265–269.

175. De Priest PD. Transvaginal sonography as a screening method for the detection of early ovarian cancer. Gynecol Oncol 1997; 65:408–414.

176. Jacobs I, Skates SJ, MacDonald N, Menon U, Rosenthal AN, Davies AP, Woolas R, Jeyarajah AR, Sibley K, Lowe DG, Oram DH. Screening for ovarian cancer: a pilot randomised controlled trial. Lancet 1999; 353(9160): 1207–1210.

177. Berek JS, Bast RC Jr. Ovarian cancer screening. The use of serial complementary tumor markers to improve sensitivity and specificity for early detection. Cancer 1995; 76(10 suppl):2092–2096.

178. Mok SC, Chao J, Skates S, Wong K-K, Yiu GK, Muto MG, Berkowitz RS, Cramer DW. Prostasin, a potential serum marker for ovarian cancer: identification through microarray technology. J Natl Cancer Inst 2001; 93(19): 1458–1464.

179. Woolas RP, Conaway MR, Xu F, Jacobs IJ, Yu Y, Daly L, Davies AP, O'Briant K, Erchuck A, Soper JT. Combinations of multiple serum markers are superior to individual assays for discriminating malignant from benign pelvic masses. Gynecol Oncol 1995; 59:111–116.

180. Gadducci A, Baichhi U, Marrai R, Ferdegini M, Bianchi R, Facchini V. Preoperative evaluation of D-dimer and CA 125 levels in differentiating benign from ovarian malignant masses. Gynecol Oncol 1996; 60:197–202.

181. Xu Y, Shen Z, Wiper D, Wu M, Morton R, Elson P, Kennedy A, Belinson J, Markman M, Casey G. Lysophosphatidic acid as a potential biomarker for ovarian cancer and other gynecologic cancers. J Am Med Assoc 1998; 280(8):719–723.

182. Kurman RJ, Kaminski PF, Norris HJ. The behavior of endometrial hyperplasia: a long-term study of "untreated" hyperplasia in 170 patients. Cancer 1985; 56(2):403–412.

183. Ho SP, Tan KT, Pang MW, Ho TH. Endometrial hyperplasia and the risk of endometrial carcinoma. Singapore Med J 1997; 38:11–15.

184. Henderson BE, Ronald KR, Malcolm CP, Casagrande JT. Endogenous hormones as a major factor in human cancer. Cancer Res 1982; 42:3232–3239.

185. Siiteri PK. Adipose tissue as a source of hormones. Am J Clin Nutr 1987; 45:277–282.

186. Key TJ, Pike MC. The dose-effect relationship between 'unopposed' estrogens and endometrial mitotic rate: its centgral role in explaining and predicting endometrial cancer risk. Br J Cancer 1988; 57:205–212.

186a. Pettomäki P, Vasen HF. Mutations predisposing to hereditary nonploypopsis colorectal cancer: database and results of a collaborative study. The International Collaboration Group on Hereditary Nonpolyposis colorectal Cancer. Gastroenterology 1997; 113(4): 1146–1158.

186b. Beck NE, Tomlilnson IP, Homfray T, et al. Genetic testing is important in families with a history suggestive of hereditary non-polyposis colorectal cancer if the Amsterdam criteria are not fulfilled. Br J Surg 84 1997; (2): 233–237.

186c. Vasen HF, Watson P, Mecklin JP, et al. New clinical criteria for hereditary nonpolyposis colorectial cancer (HNPCC, Lynch syndrome) proposed by the International Collaborative group on HNPCC. Gastroenterology 1999; 116 (6):1453–1456.

186d. Umar A, Boland CR, Terdiman JP, et al. Revised Bethesda Guidelines for hereditary nonpolyposis colorectal cancer (Lynch syndrome) and microsatellite. J Nati Cancer Inst 2004; 96(4):261–268.

187. Lynch HT, Smyrk TC, Watson P, Lanspa SJ, Lynch JF, Lynch PM, Cavalieri RJ, Boland CR. Genetics, natural history, tumor spectrum, and pathology of hereditary onpolyposis colorectal cancer: an updated review. Gastroenterology 1993; 104:1535–1549.

188. Marra G, Boland CR. Hereditary nonpolyposis colorectal cancer: the syndrome, the genes, and historical perspectives. J Natl Cancer Inst 1995; 87:1114–1125.

189. Lynch HT, Lemon SJ, Karr B, Franklin B, Lynch JF, Watson P, Tinley S, Lerman C, Carter C. Etiology, natural history, management and molecular genetics of hereditary nonpolyposis colorectal cancer (Lynch syndrome): genetic counseling implications. Cancer Epidemiol Biomarkers Prev 1997; 6:987–991.

190. Utsunomiya J, Miyaki M. Studies of hereditary nonpolyposis colorectal cancer in Japan. Int J Clin Oncol 1998; 353–374.

191. Jass JR. Diagnosis of hereditary non-polyposis colorectal cancer. Histopathology 1998; 32:491–497.

192. Liu B, Parsons R, Papadopoulos N, Nicolaides NC, Lynch HT, Watson P, et al. Analysis of mismatch repair genes in hereditary non-polyposis colorectal cancer patients. Nat Med 1996; 2:169–174.

193. Risinger JI, Berchuck A, Kohler MF, Watson P, Lynch HT, Boyd J. Genetic instability of microsatellites in endometrial carcinoma. Cancer Res 1993; 53:5100–5103.

194. Watson P, Vasen FAH, Mecklin JP, Jarvinen H, Lynch HT. The risk of endometrial cancer in hereditary nonpolyposis colorectal cancer. Am J Med 1994; 96:516–520.

195. Vasen HF, Wijnen JT, Menko FH, Kleibeuker JH, Taal BG, Griffioen G, Nagengast FM, Meijers-Heijboer EH, Bertario L, Varesco L, Bisgaard ML, Mohr J, Fodde R, Khan PM. Cancer risk in families with hereditary nonpolyposis colorectal cancer diagnosed by mutation analysis. Gastroenterology 1996; 110(4):1020–1027.

196. Vasen HF, Watson P, Mecklin JP, Lynch HT. New clinical criteria for hereditary nonpolyposis colorectal cancer (HNPCC, Lynch syndrome) proposed by the International Collaborative Group on HNPCC. Gastroenterology 1999; 116:1453–1456.

197. Haiman CA, Hankinson SE, Colditz GA, Hunter DJ, De Vivo I. A polymorphism in CYP17 and endometrial cancer risk. Cancer Res 2001; 61: 3955–3960.

198. Yaron M, Levy T, Chetrit A, Levavi H, Sabah G, Schneider D, Halperin R, Ben-Rafael Z, Friedman E. The polymorphic CAG repeat in the androgen receptor gene in Jewish Israeli women with endometrial carcinoma. Cancer 2001; 92:1190–1194.

199. McPherson CP, Sellers TA, Potter JD, Bostick RM, Folsom AR. Reproductive factors and risk of endometrial cancer. The Iowa Women's Health Study. Am J Epidemiol 1996; 143:1195–1202.
200. Brinton LA, Berman ML, Mortel R, Twiggs LB, Barrett RJ, Wilbanks GD, Lannom L, Hoover RN. Reproductive, menstrual, and medical risk factors for endometrial cancer: results from a case–control study. Am J Obstet Gynecol 1992; 167:1317–1325.
201. Koumantaki Y, Tzonou A, Koumantakis E, Kaklamani E, Aravantinos D, Trichopoulos D. A case–control study of cancer of endometrium in Athens. Int J Cancer 1989; 43: 795–799.
202. Ewertz M, Schou G, Boice JD Jr. The joint effect of risk factors on endometrial cancer. Eur J Cancer Clin Oncol 1988; 24:189–194.
203. Kelsey JL, LiVolsi VA, Holford TR, Fischer DB, Mostow ED, Schwartz PE, O'Connor T, White C. A case–control study of cancer of the endometrium. Am J Epidemiol 1982; 116:333–342.
204. Elwood JM, Cole P, Rothman JK, Kaplan SD. Epidemiology of endometrial cancer. J Natl Cancer Inst 1977; 59:1055–1060.
205. Fox H, Sen DK. A controlled study of the constitutional stigmata of endometrial adenocarcinoma. Br J Cancer 1970; 24:30–36.
206. Wynder EL, Escher GC, Mantel N. An epidemiological investigation of cancer of the endometrium. Cancer 1966; 19:489–520.
207. MacMahon B. Risk factors for endometrial cancer. Gynecol Oncol 1974; 14:122–129.
208. Peterson EP. Endometrial carcinoma in young women a clinical profile. Obstet Gyncol 1968; 31:702–707.
209. Nyholm HC, Nielsen AL, Lyndrop J, Thorpe SM. Progesterone receptor content in endometrial carcinoma correlates with serum levels of free estradiol. Acta Obstet Gynecol Scand 1993; 72:565–569.
210. Pettersson B, Adami HO, Bergstrom R, Johansson ED. Menstruation span—a time-limited risk factor for endometrial carcinoma. Acta Obstet Gynecol Scand 1986; 65:247–255.
211. Benjamin F, Deutsch S. Plasma levels of fractionated estrogens and pituitary hormones in endometrial carcinoma. Am J Obstet Gynecol 1976; 126:638–647.
212. Judd HL, Davidson BJ, Frumar AM, Shamonki IM, Lagasse LD, Ballon SC. Serum androgens and estrogens in postmenopausal women with and without endometrial cancer. Am J Obstet Gynecol 1980; 136(7):859–871.
213. Potischman N, Hoover RN, Brinton LA, Siiteri P, Dorgan JF, Swanson CA, Berman ML, Mortel R, Twiggs LB, Barrett RJ, Wilbanks GD, Persky V, Lurain JR. Case–control study of endogenous steroid hormones and endometrial cancer. J Natl Cancer Inst 1996; 88(16):1127–1135.
214. Kaufman DW, Shapiro S, Slone D, Rosenberg L, Miettinen OS, Stolley PD, Knapp RC, Leavitt T Jr, Watring WG, Rosenshein NB, Lewis JL Jr, Schottenfeld D, Engle RL Jr. Decreased risk of endometrial cancer among oral-contraceptive users. New Engl J Med 1980; 303:1045–1047.
215. Weiss NS, Sayvetz TA. Incidence of endometrial cancer in relation to the use of oral contraceptives. New Engl J Med 1980; 302:551–554.

216. Hulka BS, Chambless LE, Kaufman DG, Fowler WC Jr, Greenberg BG. Protection against endometrial carcinoma by combination-product oral contraceptives. J Am Med Assoc 1982; 247:475–477.

217. Henderson BE, Casagrande JT, Pike MC, Mack T, Rosario I, Duke A. The epidemiology of endometrial cancer in young women. Br J Cancer 1983; 47:749–756.

218. La Vecchia C, Decarli A, Fasoli M, Franceschi S, Gentile A, Negri E, Parazzini F, Tognoni G. Oral contraceptives and cancers of the breast and of the female genital tract. Interim results from a case–control study. Br J Cancer 1986; 54:311–317.

219. Levi F, La Vecchia C, Gulie C, Negri E, Monnier V, Franceschi S, Delaloye JF, De Grandi P. Oral contraceptives and the risk of endometrial cancer. Cancer Causes Control 1991; 2(2):99–103.

220. Jick SS, Walker AM, Jick H. Oral contraceptives and endometrial cancer. Obstet Gynecol 1993; 82:931–935.

221. Stanford JL, Brinton LA, Berman ML, Mortel R, Twiggs LB, Barrett RJ, Wilbanks GD, Hoover RN. Oral contraceptives and endometrial cancer: do other risk factors modify the association? Int J Cancer 1993; 54:243–248.

222. Beral V, Hermon C, Kay C, Hannaford P, Darby S, Reeves G. Mortality associated with oral contraceptive use: 25 year follow-up of cohort of 46,000 women from Oral Contraception study. Br Med J 1999; 318:96–100.

223. Rosenblatt KA, Thomas DB. Hormonal content of combined oral contraceptives in relation to the reduced risk of endometrial carcinoma. The WHO Collaborative Study of Neoplasia and Steroid Contraceptives. Int J Cancer 1991; 49:870–874.

224. Voigt LF, Deng Q, Weiss NS. Recency, duration, and progestin content or oral contraceptives in relation to the incidence of endometrial cancer (Washington, USA). Cancer Causes Control 1994; 5:227–233.

225. Lyon FA, Frisch MJ. Endometrial abnormalities occurring in young women on long-term sequential oral contraceptives. Obstet Gynecol 1976; 47:639–643.

226. Cohen CJ, Deppe G. Endometrial carcinoma and oral contraceptive agents. Obstet Gynecol 1977; 49:390–392.

227. Silverberg SG, Makowski EL. Endometrial carcinoma in young women taking oral contraceptive agents. Obstet Gynecol 1975; 46:503–506.

228. Silverberg SG, Makowski EL, Roche WD. Endometrial carcinoma in women under 40 years of age: comparison of cases in oral contraceptive users and non-users. Cancer 1977; 39:592–598.

229. Ziel HK, Finkle WD. Increased risk of endometrial carcinoma among users of conjugated estrogens. New Engl J Med 1975; 293:1167–1170.

230. Mack TM, Pike MC, Henderson BE, Pfeffer RI, Gerkins VR, Arthur M, Brown SE. Estrogens and endometrial cancer in a retirement community. New Engl J Med 1976; 294:1262–1267.

231. Gray LA, Christopherson WM, Hoover RN. Estrogens and endometrial carcinoma. Obstet Gynecol 1977; 49:385–389.

232. McDonald TW, Annegers JF, O'Fallon WM, Dockerty MB, Malkasian GD Jr, Kurland LT. Exogenous estrogen and endometrial carcinoma: case–control and incidence study. Am J Obstet Gynecol 1977; 127:572–580.

233. Hoogerland DL, Buchler DA, Crowley JJ, Carr WF. Estrogen use—risk of endometrial carcinoma. Gynecol Oncol 1978; 6:451–458.

234. Antunes CM, Stolley PD, Rosenshein NB, Davies JL, Tonascia JA, Brown C, Burnett L, Rutledge A, Pokempner M, Garcia R. Endometrial cancer and estrogen use. Report of a large case-control study. N Engl J Med 1979; 300: 9–13.

235. Hulka BS, Fowler WC Jr, Kaufman DG, Grimson RC, Greenberg BG, Hogue CJ, Berger GS, Pulliam CC. Estrogen and endometrial cancer: cases and two control groups from North Carolina. Am J Obstet Gynecol 1980; 137:92–101.

236. Jelovsek FR, Hammond CB, Woodard BH, Draffin R, Lev KL, Creasman WT, Parker RT. Risk of exogenous estrogen therapy and endometrial cancer. Am J Obstet Gynecol 1980; 137:85–91.

237. Shapiro S, Kaufman DW, Slone D, Rosenberg L, Miettinen OS, Stolley PD, Rosenshein NB, Watring WG, Leavitt T, Knapp RC. Recent and past use of conjugated estrogens in relation to adenocarcinoma of the endometrium. New Engl J Med 1980; 303:485–489.

238. Spengler RF, Clarke EA, Woolever CA, Newman AM, Osborn RW. Exogenous estrogens and endometrial cancer: a case-control study and assessment of potential biases. Am J Epidemiol 1981; 114:497–506.

239. Stavraky KM, Collins JA, Donner A, Wells GA. A comparison of estrogen use by women with endometrial cancer, gynecologic disorders, and other illnesses. Am J Obstet Gynecol 1981; 141:547–555.

240. Shapiro S, Kelly JP, Rosenberg L, Kaufman DW, Helmrich SP, Rosenshein NB, Lewis JL Jr, Knapp RC, Stolley PD, Schottenfeld D. Risk of localized and widespread endometrial cancer in relation to recent and discontinued use of conjugated estrogens. N Engl J Med 1985; 313:969–972.

241. Buring JE, Bain CJ, Ehrmann RL. Conjugated estrogen use and risk of endometrial cancer. Am J Epidemiol 1986; 124:434–441.

242. Rubin GL, Peterson HB, Lee NC, Maes EF, Wingo PA, Becker S. Estrogen replacement therapy and the risk of endometrial cancer: remaining controversies. Am J Obstet Gynecol 1990; 162:148–154.

243. Brinton LA, Barrett RJ, Berman ML, Mortel R, Twiggs LB, Wilbanks GD. Cigarette smoking and the risk of endometrial cancer. Am J Epidemiol 1993; 137:281–291.

244. Paganini-Hill A, Ross RK, Henderson BE. Endometrial cancer and patterns of use of oestrogen replacement therapy: a cohort study. Br J Cancer 1989; 59:445–447.

245. Perssen I, Adami H-O, Bergkvist L, Lindgren A, Petterson B, Hoover R, Schairer C. Risk of endometrial cancer after treatment with oestrogens alone or in conjunction with progestogens: results of a prospective study. Br Med J 1989; 298:147–151.

246. Pike MC, Peters RK, Cozen W, Probst-Hensch NM, Felix JC, Wan PC, Mack TM. Estrogen-progestin replacement therapy and endometrial cancer. J Natl Cancer Inst 1997; 89:1110–1116.

247. Green PK, Weiss NS, McKnight B, Voigt LF, Beresford SA. Risk of endometrial cancer following cessation of menopausal hormone use (Washington, United States). Cancer Causes Control 1996; 7:575–580.

248. Levi F, Franceschi S, Negri E, La Vecchia C. Dietary factors and the risk of endometrial cancer. Cancer 1993; 71(11):3575–3581.
249. Finkle WD, Greenland S, Miettinen OS, Ziel HK. Endometrial cancer risk after discontinuing use of unopposed conjugated estrogens (California, United States). Cancer Causes Control 1995; 6:99–102.
250. Grady D, Gebretsadik T, Kerlikowske K, Ernster V, Petitti D. Hormone replacement therapy and endometrial cancer risk: a meta-analysis. Obstet Gynecol 1995; 85:304–313.
251. Hammond CB, Jelovsek FR, Lee KL, Creasman WT, Parker RT. Effects of long-term estrogen replacement therapy. II. Neoplasia. Am J Obstet Gynecol 1979; 133:537–547.
252. Beresford SAA, Weiss NS, Voigt LF, McKnight B. Risk of endometrial cancer in relation to use of oestrogen combined with cyclic progestagen therapy in postmenopausal women. Lancet 1997; 349:458–461.
253. Gambrell RD Jr, Massey FM, Castaneda TA, Ugenas AJ, Ricci CA, Wright JM. Use of the progestogen challenge test to reduce the risk of endometrial cancer. Obstet Gynecol 1980; 55(6):732–738.
253a. Anderson GL, Judd HL, Kaunitz AM, Barad DH, Beresford SA, Petting M, Liu J, McNeely SG, Lopez AM. Effects of estrogen plus progestin on gyneco-logic cancers and associated diagnostic procedures: the Women's Health Initiative randomized trial. JAMA 2003; 290(13):1739–1748.
254. Weiderpass E, Adami HO, Baron JA, Magnusson C, Bergstrom R, Lindgren A, Corfreia N, Persson I. Risk of endometrial cancer following estrogen replace-ment with and without progestins. J Natl Cancer Inst 1999; 91(13):1131–1137.
255. The Writing Group for the PEPI Trial. Effects of hormone replacement therapy on endometrial histology in postmenopausal women. The Postmenopausal Estrogen/Progestin Interventions (PEPI) Trial. J Am Med Assoc 1996; 275: 370–375.
256. Sturdee DW, Wade-Evans T, Paterson ME, Thom M, Studd JW. Relations between bleeding pattern, endometrial histology, and oestrogen treatment in menopausal women. Br Med J 1978; 1(6127):1575–1577.
257. Thom MH, White PJ, Williams RM, Sturdee DW, Paterson ME, Wade-Evans T, Studd JW. Prevention and treatment of endometrial disease in climacteric women receiving oestrogen therapy. Lancet 1979; 2:455–457.
258. Paterson ME, Wade-Evans T, Sturdee DW, Thom MH, Studd JW. Endome-trial disease after treatment with oestrogens and progestogens in the climac-teric. Br Med J 1980; 280:822–824.
259. Speroff L, Rowan J, Symons J, Genant H, Wilborn W. The comparative effect on bone density, endometrium, and lipids of continuous hormones as replace-ment therapy (CHART study). A randomized controlled trial. J Am Med Assoc 1996; 276:1397–1403.
260. Levi F, La Vecchia C, Decarli A. Cigarette smoking and the risk of endome-trial cancer. Eur J Cancer Clin Oncol 1987; 23:1025–1029.
261. Franks AL, Kendrick JS, Tyler CW Jr. The Cancer Steroid Hormone Study Group. Postmenopausal smoking, estrogen replacement therapy, and the risk of endometrial cancer. Am J Obstet Gynecol 1987; 156:20–23.

262. La Vecchia C, Franceschi S, Gallus G, Decarli A, Colombo E, Mangioni C, Tognoni G. Oestrogens and obesity as risk factors for endometrial cancer in Italy. Int J Epidemiol 1982; 11:120–126.

263. Franceschi S. Reproductive factors and cancers of the breast, ovary and endometrium. Eur J Cancer Clin Oncol. 1989; 25(12):1933–1943.

264. Kvale G, Heuch I, Ursin G. Reproductive factors and risk of cancer of the uterine corpus: a prospective study. Cancer Res 1988; 48:6217–6221.

265. La Vecchia C, Negri E, Franceschi S, Parazzini F. Long-term impact of reproductive factors on cancer risk. Int J Cancer 1993; 53:215–219.

266. Plesko I, Preston-Martin S, Day NE, Tzonou A, Dimitrova E, Somogyi J. Parity and cancer risk in Slovakia. Int J Cancer 1985; 36:529–533.

267. Parazzini F, La Vecchia C. Epidemiology of adenocarcinoma of the cervix. Gynecol Oncol 1990; 39:40–46.

268. Villani C, Pucci G, Pietrangeli D, Pace S, Tomao S. Role of diet in endometrial cancer patients. Eur J Gynaecol Oncol 1986; 7(2):139–143.

269. Potischman N, Swanson CA, Brinton LA, McAdams M, Barrett RJ, Berman ML, Mortel R, Twiggs LB, Wilbanks GD, Hoover RN. Dietary associations in a case–control study of endometrial cancer. Cancer Causes Control 1993; 4(3):239–250.

270. Shu XO, Zheng W, Potischman N, Brinton LA, Hatch MC, Gao YT, Fraumeni JF Jr. A population-based case-control study of dietary factors and endometrial cancer in Shanghai, People's Republic of China. Am J Epidemiol 1993; 137(2):155–165.

271. La Vecchia C, Decarli A, Fasoli M, Gentile A. Nutrition and diet in the etiology of endometrial cancer. Cancer 1986; 57:1248–1253.

272. Tzonou A, Lipworth L, Kalandidi A, Trichopoulou A, Gamatsi I, Hsieh CC, Notara V, Trichopoulos D. Dietary factors and the risk of endometrial cancer: a case–control study in Greece. Br J Cancer 1996; 73(10):1284–1290.

273. Longcope C, Gorbach S, Goldin B, Woods M, Dwyer J, Morrill A, Warram J. The effect of a low fat diet on estrogen metabolism. J Clin Endocrinol Metab 1987; 64:1246–1250.

274. Woods M, Schaefer EJ, Morrill A, Goldin BR, Longcope C, Dwyer JD, Gorbach SL. Effect of menstrual cycle phase on plasma lipids. J Clin Endocrinol Metab 1987; 65:321–323.

275. Rose DP, Boyar AP, Cohen C, Strong LE. Effect of a low-fat diet on hormone levels in women with cystic breast disease. I. Serum steroids and gonadotropins. J Natl Cancer Inst 1987; 78(4):623–626.

276. Ingram DM, Bennett FC, Willcox D, de Klerk N. Effect of low-fat diet on female sex hormone levels. J Natl Cancer Inst 1987; 79:1225–1229.

277. La Vecchia C, Decarli A, Fasoli M, Parazzini F, Franceschi S, Gentile A, Negri E. Dietary vitamin A and the risk of intraepithelial and invasive cervical neoplasia. Gynecol Oncol 1988; 30:187–195.

278. Barbone F, Austin H, Partridge EE. Diet and endometrial cancer: a case–control study. Am J Epidemiol 1993; 137:393–403.

279. McCann SE, Freudenheim JL, Marshall JR, Brasure JR, Swanson MK, Graham S. Diet in the epidemiology of endometrial cancer in western New York (United States). Cancer Causes Control 2000; 11:965–974.

280. Bennett FC, Ingram DM. Diet and female sex hormone concentrations: an intervention study for the type of fat consumed. Am J Clin Nutr 1990; 52:808–812.
281. Goldin BR, Adlercreutz H, Gorbach SL, et al. Estrogen excretion patterns and plasma levels in vegetarian and omnivorous women. N Engl J Med 1982; 307:1542–1547.
282. Goodman MT, Wilkens LR, Hankin JH, Lyu L-C, Wu AH, Kolonel LN. Association of soy and fiber consumption with the risk of endometrial cancer. Am J Epidemiol 1997; 146:294–306.
283. Messina M, Barnes S. The role of soy products in reducing risk of cancer. J Natl Cancer Inst 1991; 83:541–546.
284. Setchell KDR, Adlercreutz H. Mammalian lignans phytoestrogens Recent studies on their formation, metabolism, and biological role in health disease. In: Rowland IR, ed. Role of Gut Flora in Toxicity and Cancer. London: Academic Press, 1988:315–345.
285. Rose DP. Dietary fiber and breast cancer. Nutr Cancer 1990; 13:1–8.
286. Rose DP, Goldman M, Connolly JM, et al. High-fiber diet reduces serum estrogen concentrations in premenopausal women. Am J Clin Nutr 1991; 54:520–525.
287. Adlercreutz H, Mousavi Y, Clark J, Hockerstedt K, Hamalainen E, Wahala K, Makela T, Hase T. Dietary phytoestrogens and cancer: in vitro and in vivo studies. J Steroid Biochem Mol Biol 1992; 41:331–337.
288. Kato I, Tominaga S, Terao C. Alcohol consumption and cancers of hormone-related organs in females. Jpn J Clin Oncol 1989; 19:202–207.
289. Webster LA, Weiss NS. Alcoholic beverage consumption and the risk of endometrial cancer. Int J Epidemiol 1989; 18:786–791.
290. Austin H, Drews C, Partridge EE. A case–control study of endometrial cancer in relation to cigarette smoking, serum estrogen levels, and alcohol use. Am J Obstet Gynecol 1993; 169:1086–1091.
291. Swanson CA, Potischman N, Wilbanks GD, et al. Relation of endometrial cancer risk to past and contemporary body size and body fat distribution. Cancer Epidemiol Biomarkers Prev 1993; 2:321–327.
292. Gapstur SM, Potter JD, Sellers TA, Kushi LH, Folsom AR. Alcohol consumption and postmenopausal endometrial cancer: results from the Iowa women's health study. Cancer Causes Control 1993; 4:323–329.
293. Zheng W, Kushi LH, Potter JD, Sellers TA, Doyle TJ, Bostick RM, Folsom AR. Dietary intake of energy and animal foods and endometrial cancer incidence. The Iowa women's health study. Am J Epidemiol 1995; 142(4):388–394.
294. Sturgeon SR, Brinton LA, Berman ML, Mortel R, Twiggs LB, Barrett RJ, Wilbanks GD. Past and present physical activity and endometrial cancer risk. Br J Cancer 1993; 68:584–589.
295. Weiderpass E, Persson I, Hans-Olov A, Magnusson C, Lindgren A, Baron JA. Body size in different periods of life, diabetes mellitus, hypertension, and risk of postmenopausal endometrial cancer (Sweden). Cancer Causes Control 2000; 11:185–192.

296. Terry P, Baron JA, Weiderpass E, Yuen J, Lichtenstein P, Nyren O. Lifestyle and endometrial cancer risk: a cohort study from the Swedish Twin Registry. Int J Cancer 1999; 82:38–42.

297. Tyler CW Jr, Webster LA, Ory HW, Rubin GL. Endometrial cancer: how does cigarette smoking influence the risk of women under age 55 years having this tumor? Am J Obstet Gynecol 1985; 151(7):899–905.

298. Baron JA. Cigarette smoking and endometrial cancer. Am J Obstet Gynecol 1986; 154(4):965.

299. Lawrence C, Tessaro I, Durgerian S, et al. Smoking, body weight, and early-stage endometrial cancer. Cancer 1987; 59:1665–1669.

300. La Vecchia C, Negri E, Parazzini F, Boyle P, D'Avanzo B, Levi F, Gentle A, Franceschi S. Height and cancer risk in a network of case–control studies from northern Italy. Int J Cancer 1990; 45:275–279.

301. Parazzini F, La Vecchia C, Negri E, Riboldi GL, Surace M, Benzi G, Maina A. Diabetes and endometrial cancer: an Italian case–control study. Int J Cancer 1999; 81:539–542.

302. Anderson DC. Sex-hormone-binding globulin. Clin Endocrinol 1974; 3(1):69–96.

303. Kaaks R. Nutrition, hormones, and breast cancer: is insulin the missing link? Cancer Causes Control 1996; 7:605–625.

304. de Waard F, Poortman J, de Pedro-Alvarez FM, Baanders-van Halewijn EA. Weight reduction and oestrogen excretion in obese post-menopausal women. Maturitas 1982; 4(2):155–162.

305. Anderson B, Connor JP, Andrews JI, Davis CS, Buller RE, Sorosky JI, Benda JA. Obesity and prognosis in endometrial cancer. Am J Obstet Gynecol 1996; 174(4):1171–1178.

306. Pike MC, Spicer DV, Dahmoush L, Press MF. Estrogens, progesterones, normal breast proliferation and breast cancer risk. Epidemiol Rev 1993; 15:17–35.

307. Hirose K, Taima K, Hamajima N, et al. Sub-site (cervix endometrium)-specific risk and protective factors in uterus cancer. Jpn J Cancer Res 1996; 87:1001–1009.

308. Dosemeci M, Hayes RB, Vetter R, et al. Occupational physical activity, socioeconomic status, and risks of 15 cancer sites in Turkey. Cancer Causes Control 1993; 4:313–321.

309. Shu XO, Hatch MC, Zheng W, Gao YT, Brinton LA. Physical activity and risk of endometrial cancer. Epidemiology 1993; 4(4):342–349.

310. Zheng W, Shu XO, McLaughlin JK, Chow WH, Gao YT, Blot WJ. Occupational physical activity and the incidence of 0cancer of the breast, corpus uteri, and ovary in Shanghai. Cancer 1993; 71:3620–3624.

311. Moradi T, Weiderpass E, Signorello LB, Persson I, Nyren O, Adami H-O. Physical activity and postmenopausal endometrial cancer risk (Sweden). Cancer Causes Control 2000; 11:829–837.

312. Levi F, La Vecchia C, Negri E, Franceschi S. Selected physical activities and the risk of endometrial cancer. Br J Cancer 1993; 67(4):846–851.

313. Nelson ME, Meredith CN, Dawson-Hughes B, Evans WJ. Hormone and bone mineral status in endurance-trained and sedentary postmenopausal women. J Clin Endocrinol Metab 1988; 66:927–933.

314. Cauley JA, Gutai JP, Kuller LH, LeDonne D, Powell JG. The epidemiology of serum sex hormones in postmenopausal women. Am J Epidemiol 1989; 129:1120–1131.

315. Ellison PT, Lager C. Moderate recreational running is associated with lowered salivary progesterone profiles in women. Am J Obstet Gynecol 1986; 154:1000–1003.

316. Broocks A, Pirke KM, Schweiger U, et al. Cyclic ovarian function in recreational athletes. J Appl Physiol 1990; 68:2083–2086.

317. Bullen BA, Skrinar GS, Beitins IZ, von Mering G, Turnbull BA, McArthur JW. Induction of menstrual disorders by strenuous exercise in untrained women. N Engl J Med 1985; 312:1349–1353.

318. Williams RR, Horm JW. Association of cancer sites with tobacco and alcohol consumption and socioeconomic status of patients: interview study from the Third National Cancer Survey. J Natl Cancer Inst 1977; 58:525–547.

319. Smith EM, Sowers MF, Burns TL. Effects of smoking on the development of female reproductive cancers. J Natl Cancer Inst 1984; 73:371–376.

320. Stockwell HG, Lyman GH. Cigarette smoking and the risk of female reproductive cancer. Am J Obstet Gynecol 1987; 157:35–40.

321. Lesko SM, Rosenberg L, Kaufman DW, Helmrich SP, Miller Dr, Strom B, Schottenfeld D, Rosenshein NB, Knapp RC, Lewis J, et al. Cigarette smoking and the risk of endometrial cancer. N Engl J Med 1985; 313(10):593–596.

322. Jick H, Porter J. Relation between smoking and age of natural menopause. Report from the Boston Collaborative Drug Surveillance Program, Boston University Medical Center. Lancet 1977; 1:1354–1355.

323. Willett W, Stampfer MJ, Bain C, Lipnick R, Speizer FE, Rosner B, Cramer D, Hennekens CH. Cigarette smoking, relative weight, and menopause. Am J Epidemiol 1983; 117:651–658.

324. MacMahon B, Trichopoulos D, Cole P, Brown J. Cigarette smoking and urinary estrogens. N Engl J Med 1982; 307:1062–1065.

325. Killackey MA, Hakes TB, Pierce VK. Endometrial adenocarcinoma in breast cancer patients receiving antiestrogens. Cancer Treat Rep 1985; 69:237–238.

326. Curtis RE, Boice JD Jr, Shriner DA, Hankey BF, Fraumeni JF Jr. Second cancers after adjuvant tamoxifen therapy for breast cancer. J Natl Cancer Inst 1996; 88:832–834.

327. Sasco AJ. Tamoxifen and menopausal status: risks and benefits. Lancet 1996; 347:761.

328. van Leeuwen FE, Benraadt J, Willem J, Coebergh W, Kiemeney LALM, Gimbrere CHF, Otter R, Schouten LJ, Damhuls RAM, Bontenbal M, Diepenhorst FW, van den Belt-Dusebout Harm van Tinteren AW. Risk of endometrial cancer after tamoxifen treatment of breast cancer. Lancet 1994; 343:448–452.

329. Fisher B, Costantino JP, Redmond CK, Fisher ER, Wickerham DL, Cronin WM, other NSABP contributors. Endometrial cancer in tamoxifen-treated breast cancer patients: findings from the National Surgical Adjuvant Breast and Bowel Project (NSABP) B-14. J Natl Cancer Inst 1994; 86:527–537.

330. Rutqvist LE, Johansson H, Signomklao T, Johansson U, Fornander T, Wilking N. Adjuvant Tamoxifen therapy for early stage breast cancer and second primary malignancies. J Natl Cancer Inst 1995; 87:645–651.

331. Bernstein L, Deapen D, Cerhan JR, Schwartz SM, Liff J, McGann-Maloney E, Perlman JA, Ford L. Tamoxifen therapy for breast cancer and endometrial cancer risk. J Natl Cancer Inst 1999; 91:1654–1662.

332. IARC on tamoxifen. Environ Health Perspect 1996; 104:688.

333. Cook LS, Weiss NS, Schwartz SM, White E, McKnight B, Moore DE, Daling JR. Population-based study of Tamoxifen therapy and subsequent ovarian endometrial, and breast cancer. J Natl Cancer Inst 1995; 87:1359–1364.

334. Fisher B, Costantino JP, Wickerham DL, Redmond CK, Kavanah M, Cronin WM, Vogel V, Robidous A, Dimitroy N, Atkins J, Daly M, Wieland S, Tan-Chiu E, Ford L, Wolmark N, and Other National Surgical Adjuvant Breast Bowel Project Investigators Tamoxifen for prevention of breast cancer: report of the National Surgical Adjuvant Breast and Bowel Project P-1 Study. J Natl Cancer Inst 1998; 90:1371–1388.

335. Salazar-Martinez EC, Lazcano-Ponce GG, Lira-Lira P, Escudero-De los Rios J, Salmeron-Castro F, Larrea M, Hernandez-Avila M. Case–control study of diabetes, obesity, physical activity and risk of endometrial cancer among Mexican women. Cancer Causes Control 2000; 11(8):707–711.

336. Damon A. Host factors in cancer of the breast and uterine cervix and corpus. J Natl Cancer Inst 1960; 24:483–516.

337. Marshall J. Personal communication of unpublished data. Department of Social and Preventive Medicine. State University of New York at Buffalo, New York, February 1983.

338. O'Mara BA, Byers T, Schoenfeld E. Diabetes mellitus and cancer risk: a multisite case–control study. J Chron Dis 1985; 38:435–441.

339. Deutsch S, Benjamin F. Effect of diabetic status on fractional estrogen levels in postmenopausal women. Am J Obstet Gynecol 1978; 130(1):105–106.

340. Quinn MA, Ruffe H, Brown JB, Ennis G. Circulating gonadotrophins and urinary estrogens in postmenopausal diabetic women. Aust NZ J Obstet Gynecol 1981; 21:234–236.

341. Glickman AS, Myers WPL, Rawson RW. Diabetes melitus carbohydrate metabolism in patients with cancer. Med Clin N Am 1956; 40:887.

342. Lynch HT, Krush AJ, Larsen AI, Magnuson CW. Endometrial carcinoma, multiple primary malignancies, constitutional factors, and heredity. Am J Med Sci 1966; 252:381–398.

343. Benjamin F, Romney S. Disturbed carbohydrate metabolism in endometrial carcinoma. Cancer 1964; 17:386–390.

344. Dahlgren E, Friberg LG, Johansson S, Lindstrom B, Oden A, Samsoioe G, Janson PO. Endometrial carcinoma: Ovarian dysfunction – a risk factor in young women. Eur J Obstet Gynecol Reprod Biol 1991; 41:143–150.

345. Chamlian DL, Taylor HB. Endometrial hyperplasia in young women. Obstet Gynecol 1970; 36:659–666.

346. Cook GA, Draper GJ. Trends in cervical cancer and carcinoma in situ in Great Britain. Br J Cancer 1984; 50:367–375.

347. Parkin DM, Nguyen-Dinh X, Day NE. The impact of screening on the incidence of cervical cancer in England and Wales. Br J Obstet Gynecol 1985; 92:150–157.

348. Devesa SS, Young JL Jr, Brinton LA, Fraumeni JF Jr. Recent trends in cervix uteri cancer. Cancer 1989; 64:2184–2190.
349. Beral V, Hermon C, Munoz N, Devesa SS,. Cervical Cancer: Cancer Surveys Volume 19/20. Trends in Cancer Incidence and Mortality. Imperial Cancer Research Fund, 1994:265–285.
350. Vizcaino AP, Moreno V, Bosch FX, Munoz N, Barros-Dios XM, Borras J, Parkin DM. International trends in incidence of cervical cancer: II. Squamous-cell carcinoma. Int J Cancer 2000; 86:429–435.
351. Vesterinen E, Forss M, Nieminen U. Increase of cervical adenocarcinoma: a report of 520 cases of cervical carcinoma including 112 tumors with glandular elements. Gynecol Oncol 1989; 33:49–53.
352. Syrjanen KJ. Biological behaviour of cervical intraepithelial neoplasia. In: Franco E, Monsonego J, eds. New Developments in Cervical Cancer Screening and Prevention. Oxford: Blackwell Science, Ltd, 1997:93–108.
353. Papanicolaou GN, Traut HF. The diagnostic value of vaginal smears in carcinoma of the uterus. Arch Pathol Lab Med 1997; 121(3):211–224.
354. Richart RM. Cervical intraepithelial neoplasia. Pathol Annu 1973; 8:301–328.
355. Anonymous. The 1988 Bethesda System for Reporting Cervical/Vaginal Cytological Diagnoses. National Cancer Institute Workshop. J Am Med Assoc 1989; 262:931–934.
356. Schenck U, Planding W. Frequency of endocervical cells in cervical smears and hysterectomy rate of the patients. Gen Diagn Pathol 1998; 143:291–296.
357. Ponten J, Adami HO, Friberg LG, Gustafsson L, Miller AB, Parkin M, Sparen P, Trichopoulos D. HPV and cervical cancer. Int J Cancer 1995; 63:317.
358. Kataja V, Syrjanen K, Syrjanen S, Mantyjarvi R, Yliskoski M, Saarikoski S, Salonen JT. Prospective follow-up of genital HPV infections: survival analysis of the HPV typing data. Eur J Epidemiol 1990; 6:9–14.
359. Boyes DA, Morrison B, Knox EG, Draper GJ, Miller AB. A cohort study of cervical cancer screening in British Columbia. Clin Invest Med 1982; 5:1–29.
360. Miller AB, Anderson G, Brisson J, Laidlaw J, Le Pitre N, Malcolmson P, Mirwaldt P, Stuart G, Sullivan W. Report of a National Workshop on Screening for Cancer of the Cervix. Can Med Assoc J 1991; 145:1301–1325.
361. Ostor AG. Natural history of cervical intraepithelial neoplasia: a critical review. Int J Gynecol Pathol 1993; 12:186–192.
362. de Brux J, Orth G, Croissant O, Cochard B, Ionesco M. Condylomatous lesions of the uterine cervix: their course in 2466 patients. Bull Cancer 1983; 70:410–422.
363. Walboomers JMM, Jacobs MV, Manos MM, Bosch FX, Kummer JA, Shah KV, Snudder PJF, Peto J, Meijer CJLM, Munoz N. Human papillomavirus is a necessary cause of invasive cervical cancer worldwide. J Pathol 1999; 189: 12–19.
364. Reichman RC. Human Papillomavirus infections. In: Fauci AS, Braunwald E, Isselbacher KJ, Wilson JD, Martin JB, Hauser SL, Longo DL, eds. Harrison's Principles of Internal Medicine. 14th ed. New York: McGraw-Hill, 1998: 1098–1100.
365. Stoler MH. Human papillomaviruses and cervical neoplasia: a model for carcinogenesis. Int J Gynecol Pathol 2000; 19(1):16–28.

366. Tilson P. Anal human papillomavirus and anal cancer. J Clin Pathol 1997; 50(8):625–634.
367. Richart RM, Masood S, Syrjanen KJ, Vassilakos P, Kaufman RH, Meisels A, Olszewski WT, Sakamoto A, Stoker MH, Vooijs GP, Wilbur DC. Human papillomavirus. International Academy of Cytology Task Force summary. Diagnostic cytology towards the 21st century: an international expert conference and tutorial. Acta Cytol 1998; 42:50–58.
368. Bosch FX, Manos MM, Munoz N, Sherman M, Jansen AM, Peto J, Schiffman MH, Moreno V, Kurman R, Shah KV. Prevalence of human papillomavirus in cervical cancer: a worldwide perspective. International Biological Study on Cervical Cancer (IBSCC) Study Group. J Natl Cancer Inst 1995; 87:796–802.
369. Moons N. IARC Monographs on the Evaluation of the Carcinogenic Risk of Chemicals to Humans. Vol. 64. Human Papillomaviruses. Lyon: IARC, 1995:381–409.
370. Ho GYF, Kadish AS, Burk RD, Basu J, Palan PR, Mikhail M, Romney SL. HPV 16 and cigarette smoking as risk factors for high-grade cervical intraepithelial neoplasia. Int J Cancer 1998; 78:281–285.
371. Woodman CBJ, Collins S, Winter H, Bailey A, Ellis J, Prior P, Yates M, Rollason TP, Young LS. Natural history of cervical human papillomavirus infection in young women: a longitudinal cohort study. Lancet 2001; 357:1831–1836.
372. Franco EL, Villa LL, Sobrinho JP, Prado JM, Rousseau M-C, Desy M, Rohan TE. Epidemiology of acquisition and clearance of cervical human papillomavirus infection in women from a high-risk area for cervical cancer. J Infect Dis 1999; 180:1415–1423.
373. Hisada M, van den Berg BJ, Strickler HD, Christianson RE, Wright WE, Waters DJ, Rabkin CS. Prospective study of antibody to human papilloma virus type 16 and risk of cervical, endometrial, and ovarian cancers (United States). Cancer Causes Control 2001; 12:335–341.
374. Dillner L, Bekassy Z, Jonsson N, Moreno-Lopez J, Blomberg J. Detection of IgA antibodies against human papillomavirus in cervical secretions from patients with cervical intraepithelial neoplasia. Int J Cancer 1989; 43(10):36–40.
375. Vonka V, Hamsikova E, Kanka J, Ludvikova V, Sapp M, Smahel M. Prospective study on cervical neoplasia IC. Presence of HPV antibodies. Int J Cancer 1999; 80:365–368.
376. Shah KV, Viscidi RP, Alberg AJ, Helzlsouer KJ, Comstock GW. Antibodies to human papillomavirus 16 and subsequent in situ or invasive cancer of the cervix. Cancer Epidemiol Biomarkers Prev 1997; 6:233–237.
377. Koutsky LA, Holmes KK, Critchlow CW, Stevens CE, Paavonen J, Beckmann AM, DeRouen TA, Galloway DA, Vernon D, Kiviat NB. A cohort study of the risk of cervical intraepithelial neoplasia grade 2 or 3 in relation to papillomavirus infection. New Engl J Med 1992; 327:1272–1278.
378. Liaw K-L, Glass AG, Manos MM, Greer CE, Scott DR, Sherman M, Burk RD, Kurman RJ, Wacholder S, Rush BB, Cadell DM, Lawler P, Tabor D, Schiffman M. Detection of human papillomavirus DNA in cytologically normal women and subsequent cervical squamous intraepithelial lesions. J Natl Cancer Inst 1999; 91:954–960.

379. Rousseau M-C, Franco EL, Villa LL, Sobrinho JP, Termini L, Prado JM, Rohan TE. A cumulative case–control study of risk factor profiles for oncogenic and nononcogenic cervical human papillomavirus infections. Cancer Epidemiol Biomarkers Prev 2000; 9:469–476.

380. Sillins I, Kallings I, Dillner J. Correlates of the spread of human papillomavirus infection. Cancer Epidemiol Biomarkers Prev 2000; 9:953–959.

381. Palefsky JM, Minkoff H, Kalish LA, Levine A, Sacks HS, Garcia P, Young M, Melnick S, Miotti P, Buck R. Cervicovaginal human papillomavirus infection in human immunodeficiency virus-1 (HIV)-positive and high-risk HIV-negative women. J Natl Cancer Inst 1999; 91:226–231.

382. Vermund SH, Kelley KF, Klein RS, Feingold AR, Schreiber K, Munk G, Burk RD. High risk of human papillomavirus infection and cervical squamous intraepithelial among women with symptomatic human immunodeficiency virus infection. Am J Obstet Gynecol 1991; 165(2):392–400.

383. Williams AB, Darragh TM, Vranizan K, Ochia C, Moss AR, Palefsky JM. Anal and cervical human papillomavirus infection and risk of anal and cervical epithelial abnormalities in human immunodeficiency virus-infected women. Obstet Gynecol 1994; 83:205–211.

384. Hillemanns P, Ellerbrock TV, McPhillips S, Dole P, Alperstein S, Johnson D, et al. Prevalence of anal human papillomavirus infection and anal cytologic abnormalities in HIV-seropositive women. Aids 1996; 10:1641–1647.

385. Sun X-W, Kuhn L, Ellerbrock TV, Chiasson MA, Bush TJ, Wright TC Jr. Human papillomavirus infection in women infected with the human immunodeficiency virus. N Engl J Med 1997; 337:1343–1349.

386. Nobbenhuis MAE, Walboomers JMM, Helmerhorst TJM, Rozendaal L, Remmink AJ, Risse EKJ, van der Linder HC, Voorhorst FJ, Kenemans P, CJL Meijer. Relation of human papillomavirus status to cervical lesions and consequences for cervical-cancer screening: a prospective study. Lancet 1999; 354:20–25.

387. Ho GY, Palan PR, Basu J, Romney SL, Kadish AS, Mikhail M, Wassertheilsmoller S, Runowicz C, Burk RD. Viral characteristics of human papillomavirus infection and antioxidant levels as risk factors for cervical dysplasia. Int Cancer J 1998; 78(5):594–599.

388. Ylitalo N, Serensen P, Josefsson A, et al. Consistent high viral load of human papillomavirus 16 and risk of cervical carcinoma in situ: a nested case–control study. Lancet 2000; 355:2194–2198.

389. Josefsson AM, Magnusson PKE, Yitalo N, Serensen P, Quaforth-Tubbin P, Andersen PK, Melbye M, Adami H-O, Gyllenstein UB. Viral load of human papilloma virus16 as a determinant for development of cervical carcinoma in situ: a nested case–control study. Lancet 2000; 355:2189–2193.

390. Ahdieh L, Munoz A, Vlahov D, Trimble CL, Timpson LA, Shah K. Cervical neoplasia and repeated positivity of human papillomavirus infection in human immunodeficiency virus-seropositive and -seronegative women. Am J Epidemiol 2000; 151:1148–1157.

391. Klein J, Sato A. The HLA system: first of two parts. In: Mackay I, Rosen FS, eds. Advances in Immunology. New Engl J Med 2000; 343:782–786.

392. Hildesheim A, Schiffman M, Brinton LA, Fraumeni JF Jr, Herrero R, Bratti MC, Schwartz P, Mortel R, Barnes W, Greenberg M, McGowan L, Scott DR, Martin M, Hewrrera JE, Carrington M. "p53 polymorphism and the risk of cervical cancer: (Letter). Nature (Lond) 1998; 396:531–532.

393. Odunsi K, Terry G, Ho L, Bell J, Cuzick J, Ganesan TS. Susceptibility to human papillomavirus-associated cervical intra-epithelial neoplasia is determined by specific HLA DR-DQ alleles. Int J Cancer 1996; 67:595–602.

394. Neuman RJ, Huettner PC, Pi L, Mardis ER, Duffy BF, Wilson RK, Rader JS. Association between DQB1 and cervical cancer in patients with human papillomavirus and family controls. Obstet Gynecol 2000; 95:134–140.

395. Cuzick J, Terry G, Ho L, Monaghan J, Lopes A, Clarkson P, Duncan I. Association between high-risk HPV types, HLA DRB1 and DQB1 alleles and cervical cancer in British women. Br J Cancer 2000; 82:1348–1352.

396. Piyathilake CJ, Macaluso M, Johanning GL, Whiteside M, Heimburger DC, Giuliano A. Methylenetetrahydrofolate reductase (MTHFR) polymorphism increases the risk of cervical intraepithelial neoplasia. Anticancer Res 2000; 20:1751–1758.

397. Frosst P, Blom HJ, Milos R, Goyette P, Sheppard CA, Matthews RG, Boers GH, den Heijer, Kluitjmans LAJ, Van den Heuvel LP, Rozen R. A candidate genetic risk factor for vascular disease: A common mutation in methylenetetrahydrofolate reductase. Nat Genet 1995; 10:111–113.

398. Van der Put NM, Steegers-Theunissen RP, Frosst P, Trijbels FJ, Eskes TK, Van den Heuvel LP, Mariman EC, Den Hyer M, Rozen R, Blom HJ. Mutated methylenetetrahydrofolate reductase as a risk factor for spina bifida. Lancet 1995; 46:1070–1071.

399. Kluijtmans LA, Kastelein JJ, Lindemans J, Boers GH, Heil SG, Brusch AV, Jukema JW, van den Heuvel LP, Trijbels FJ, Boerma GJ, Verheugt FW, Willems F, Blom JH. Thermolabile methylene-tetrahydrofolate reductase in coronary artery disease. Circulation 1997; 96:2573–2577.

400. Strange RC, Spiteri MA, Ramachandran S, Fryer AA. Glutathione-S-transferase family of enzymes. Mutat Res 2001; 482:21–26.

401. Chen C, Madeleine MM, Weiss NS, Daling JR. Glutathione S-transferase M1 genotypes and the risk of squamous carcinoma of the cervix: a population-based case–control study. Am J Epidemiol 1999; 150:568–572.

402. Warwick AP, Redman CW, Jones PW, Fryer AA, Gilford J, Alldersea J, Strange RC. Progression of cervical intraepithelial neoplasia to cervical cancer: interactions of cytochrome P450 CYP2D6 EM and glutathione-s-transferase GSTM1 null genotypes and cigarette smoking. Br J Cancer 1994; 70:704–708.

403. Kim JW, Lee CG, Park YG, Kim KS, Kim I-K, Sohn YW, Min HK, Lee JM, Namkoong SE. Combined analysis of germline polymorphisms of p53, GSTM1, GSTT1, CYP1A1, and CYP2E1. Cancer 2000; 88:2082–2091.

404. Scheffner M, Werness BA, Huibregste JM, Levine AJ, Howley PM. The E6 oncoprotein encoded by human papillomavirus types 16 and 18 promotes the degradation of p53. Cell 1990; 63:1129–1136.

405. Crook T, Tidy JA, Vousden KH. Degradation of p53 can be targeted by HPV E6 sequences distinct from those required for p53 binding and transactivation. Cell 1991; 67(3):547–556.

406. Vogelstein B, Kinzler KW. P53 function and dysfunction. Cell 1992; 70: 523–526.

407. Matlashewski GJ, et al. Primary structure polymorphism at amino acid residue 72 of human p53. Mol Cell Biol 1987; 7:961–963.

408. Madeleine MM, Shera K, Schwartz SM, Daling R, Galloway DA, Wipf GC, Carter JJ, McKnight B, McDougall JK. The p53 Arg72Pro polymorphism, human papillomavirus, and invasive squamous cell cervical cancer. Cancer Epidemiol Biomarkers Prev 2000; 9:225–227.

409. Rosenthal AN, Ryan A, Al-Jehani RM, Storey A, Harwood CA, Jacobs IJ. P53 codon 72 *polymorphism and risk of cervical cancer in UK. Lancet 1998; 352:871–872.

410. Giannoudis A, Graham D, Southern S, Herrington C. P53 codon 72ARG/PRO polymorphism is not related to HPV type or lesion grade in low- and high-grade squamous intra-epithelial lesions and invasive squamous carcinoma of the cervix. Int J Cancer 1999; 83:66–69.

411. Lanham S, Campbell I, Watt P, Gornall R. P53 polymorphism and risk of cervical cancer. Lancet 1998; 352:1631.

412. Helland A, Olsen AO, Gjoen K, Akselsen HE, Sauer T, Magnus P, Borresen-Dale AL, Ronningen KS. An increased risk of cervical intra-epithelial neoplasia grade II-III among human papillomavirus positive patients with the HLA-DQA1*0102-DQB1*0602 haplotype: a population-based case–control study of Norwegian women. Int J Cancer 1998; 76:19–24.

413. Josefsson AM, Magnusson PKE, Ylitalo N, Quafort-Tubbin P, Ponten J, Adami HO, Gyllesten UB. P53 polymorphism and the risk of cervical cancer (Letter). Nature (Lond) 1998; 396:531.

414. Bertorelle R, Chieco-Bianchi L, Del Mistro A. Papillomavirus and p53 codon 72 polymorphism. Int J Cancer 1999; 82(4):616–617.

415. Klaes R, Ridder R, Schaefer U, Benner A, von Knebel Doeberitz M. No evidence of p53 allele-specific predisposition in human papillomavirus-associated cervical cancer. J Mol Med 1999; 77(2):299–302.

416. Minaguchi T, Kanamori Y, Matsushima M, Yoshikawa H, Taketani Y, Nakamura Y. No evidence of correlation between polymorphism at codon 72 of p53 and risk of cervical cancer in Japanese patients with human papillomavirus 16/18 infection. Cancer Res 1998; 58(20):4585–4586.

417. Ylitalo N, Sorensen P, Josefsson A, Frisch M, Sparen P, Ponten J, Gyllensten U, Melbye M, Adami HO. Smoking and oral contraceptives as risk factors for cervical carcinoma in situ. Int J Cancer 1999; 81(3):357–365.

418. Kruger-Kjaer S, van den Brule AJC, Svare EI, Engholm G, Sherman ME, Poll PA, Walboomers JMM, Bock JE, Meuer CJLM. Different risk factor patterns for high-grade and low-grade intraepithelial lesions on the cervix among HPV-positive and HPV-negative young women. Int J Cancer 1998; 76:613–619.

419. Lacey JV Jr, Brinton LA, Abbas FM, Barnes WA, Gravitt PE, Greenberg MD, Greene SM, Hadjimichael OC, McGowan L, Mortel R, Schwartz PE, Silverberg SG, Hildesheim A. Oral contraceptives as risk factors for cervical adenocarcinomas and squamous cell carcinomas. Cancer Epidemiol, Biomarkers Prev 1999; 8:1079–1085.

420. Munoz N, Bosch FX, de Sanjose S, Vergara A, del Moral A, Munoz MT, Tafur L, Gili M, Izarzugaza I, Viladiu P, Navarro C, de Ruiz PA, Aristizabal N, Santamaria M, Orfila J, Daniel RW, Guerrero E, Shah KV. Risk factors for cervical intraepithelial neoplasia grade III/carcinoma in situ in Spain and Colombia. Cancer Epidemiol Biomarkers Prev 1993; 2:423–431.
421. Cavalcanti SM, Zardo LG, Passos MR, Oliveira LH. Epidemiological aspects of human papillomavirus infection and cervical cancer in Brazil. J Infect 2000; 40:80–87.
422. Ngelangel C, Munoz N, Bosch FX, Limson GM, Festin MR, Deacon J, Jacobs MV, Santamaria M, CJMeijer LM, Walboomers JMM. Causes of cervical cancer in the Philippines: A case–control study. J Natl Cancer Inst 1998; 90:43–49.
423. Roteli-Martins CM, Panetta K, Alves VA, Siqueira SA, Syrjanen KJ, Derchain SF. Cigarette smoking and high-risk HPV DNA as predisposing factors for high-grade cervical intraepithelial neoplasia (CIN) in young Brazilian women. Acta Obstet Gynecol Scand 1998; 77:678–682.
424. Kjellberg L, Hallmans G, Ahren A-M, Johansson R, Bergman F, Wadell G, Angstrom T, Dillner J. Smoking, diet, pregnancy and oral contraceptive use as risk factors for cervical intra-epithelial neoplasia in relation to human papillomavirus infection. Br J Cancer 2000; 82:1332–1338.
425. Herrero R, Brinton LA, Reeves WC, Brenes MM, de Britton RC, Gaitan E, Tenorio F. Screening for cervical cancer in Latin America: a case–control study. Int J Epidemiol 1992; 21:1050–1056.
426. Parazzini F, Negri E, Ricci E, Franceschi S, La Vecchia C. Correlates of oral contraceptive use in Italian women, 1991–93. Contraception 1996; 54:101–106.
427. Whitehead N, Reyner F, Lindenbaum J. Megaloblastic changes in the cervical epithelium. J Am Med Assoc 1973; 226:1421–1424.
428. Butterworth CE, Hatch KD, Gore H, Mueller H, Krumdieck CL. Improvement in cervical dysplasia associated with folic acid therapy in users of oral contraceptives. Am J Clin Nutr 1982; 35:73–82.
429. Schiffman MH, Brinton LA. The epidemiology of cervical carcinogenesis. Cancer 1995; 76:1888–1901.
430. Schiffman MH, Bauer HM, Hoover RN, Glass AG, Cadell DM, Rush BB, Scott DR, Sherman ME, Kurman RJ, Wacholder S, Stanton CK, Manos MM. Epidemiologic evidence showing that human papillomavirus infection causes most cervical intraepithelial neoplasia. J Natl Cancer Inst 1993; 85:958–964.
431. Alberg AJ, Selhub J, Shah KV, Viscidi RP, Comstock GW, Helzlsouer KJ. The risk of cervical cancer in relation to serum concentrations of folate, vitamin B12, and homocysteine. Cancer Epidemiol Biomarkers Prev 2000; 761–764.
432. Ziegler RG, Brinton LA, Hamman RF, Lehman HF, Levine RS, Mallin K, Normal SA, Rosenthal JF, Trumble AC, Hoover RN. Diet and the risk of invasive cervical cancer among white women in the United States. Am J Epidemiol 1990; 132:432–444.

433. Slattery ML, Abbott TM, Overall JC, Robison LM, French TK, Jolles C, Gardner JW, West DW. Dietary vitamins A, C, and E and selenium as risk factors for cervical cancer. Epidemiol 1990; 1:8–15.
434. McPherson RS. Nutritional factors and the risk of cervical dysplasia. Diss Abst Int 1990; 51:1769-B.
435. Cheeseman KH, Burton GW, Ingold KU, Slater TF. Lipid preoxidation and lipid antioxidants in normal and tumorcells. Toxicol Pathol 1984; 12(3): 235–239.
436. Harris RWC, Forman D, Doll R, Vessey MP, Wald NJ. Cancer of the cervix uteri and vitamin A. Br J Cancer 1986; 53:653–659.
437. Orr JW, Wilson K, Bodiford C, Cornwell A, Soong SJ, Hones KL, Hatch KD, Shingleton HM. Nutritional status of patients with untreated cervical cancer. II. Vitamin assessment. Am J Obstet Gynecol 1985; 151:632–635.
438. Palan PR, Romney SL, Mikhail M, Basu J. Decreased plasma β-carotene levels in women with uterine cervical dysplasias and cancer. J Natl Cancer Inst 1988; 80:454–456.
439. Baticha AM, Armenian HK, Norkus EP, Morris JS, Spate VE, Comstock GW. Serum micronutrients and the subsequent risk of cervical cancer in a population-based nested case–control study. Cancer Epidemiol Biomarkers Prev 1993; 2:335–339.
440. Giuliano AR. The role of nutrients in the prevention of cervical dysplasia and cancer. Nutrition 2000; 16:570–573.
441. Preston AM. Cigarette smoking-nutritional implications. Prog Food Nutr Sci 1991; 15:183–217.
442. Palan PR, Mikhail MS, Goldberg GL, Basu J, Runowicz CD, Romney SL. Plasma levels of beta-carotene, lycopene, canthaxanthin, retinol, and alpha- and tau-tocopherol in cervical intraepithelial neoplasia and cancer. Clin Cancer Res 1996; 2:181–185.
443. Nagata C, Shimizu H, Higashiiwai H, Sugahara N, Morita N, Komatsu S, Hisamichi S. Serum retinol level and risk of subsequent cervical cancer in cases with cervical dysplasia. Cancer Invest 1999; 17:253–258.
444. Verreault R, Chu J, Mandelson M, Shy K. A case–control study of diet and invasive cervical cancer. Int J Cancer 1989; 43:1050–1054.
445. Herrero R, Potischman N, Brinton LA, Reeves WC, Brenes MM, Tenorio F, de Britton RC, Gaitan E. A case–control study of nutrient status and invasive cervical cancer. I. Dietary indicators. Am J Epidemiol 1991; 134:1335–1346.
446. Potischman N. Nutritional epidemiology of cervical neoplasia. J Nutr 1993; 123:424–429.
447. VanEenwyk J, Davis FG, Bowen PE. Dietary and serum carotenoids and cervical intraepithelial neoplasia. Int J Cancer 1991; 48:34–38.
448. Basu J, Palan PR, Vermund SH, Goldberg GL, Burk RD, Romney SL. Plasma ascorbic acid and beta-carotene levels in women evaluated for HPV infection, smoking, and cervix dysplasia. Cancer Detect Prev 1991; 15:165–170.
449. Nagata C, Shimizu H, Yoshikawa H, Noda K, Nozawa S, Yajima A, Sekiya S, Sugimori H, Hirai Y, Kanazawa K, Sugase M, Kawana T. Serum carotenoids and vitamins and risk of cervical dysplasia from a case–control study in Japan. Br J Cancer 1999; 81:1234–1237.

450. Peng YM, Peng YS, Childers JM, Hatch KD, Roe DJ, Lin Y, Lin P. Concentrations of carotenoids, tocopherols, and retinol in paired plasma and cervical tissue of patients with cervical cancer, precancer, and noncancerous diseases. Cancer Epidemiol Biomarkers Prev 1998; 7:347–350.

451. Wassertheil-smoller S, Romney SL, Wylie-Rosett J, Slagle S, Miller G, Lucido D, Duttagupta C, Palan PR. Dietary vitamin C and uterine cervical dyplasia. Am J Epidemiol 1981; 114(5):714–724.

452. VanEenwyk J, Davis FG, Colman N. Folate, vitamin C and cervical intraepithelial neoplasia. Cancer Epidemiol Biomarkers Prev 1992; 1(2):119–124.

453. Brock KE, Berry G, Mock PA, MacLennan R, Truswell AS, Brinton LA. Nutrients in diet and plasma and risk of in situ cervical cancer. J Natl Cancer Inst 1988; 80(8):580–585.

454. Romney SL, Duttagupta C, Basu J, Palan PR, Karp S, Slagle NS, Dwyer A, Wassertheil-Smoller S, Wylie-Rosett J. Plasma vitamin C and uterine cervical dysplasia. Am J Obstet Gynecol 1985; 151:976–980.

455. Ziegler RG, Jones CJ, Brinton LA, Norman SA, Mallin K, Levine RS, Lehman HF, Hamman RF, Trumble AC, Rosenthal JF. Diet and the risk of in situ cervical cancer among white women in the United States. Cancer Causes Control 1991; 2(1):17–29.

456. Sinha R, Frey CM, Kammerer WG, McAdams MJ, Norkus EP, Ziegler RG. Importance of supplemental vitamin C in determining serum ascorbic acid in controls from a cervical cancer case–control study: implications for epidemiological studies. Nutr Cancer 1994; 22:207–217.

457. Ho GY, Bierman R, Beardsley L, Chang CJ, Burk RD. Natural history of cervicovaginal papillomavirus infection in young women. N Engl J Med 1998; 338:423–428.

458. Lehtinen M, Luostarinen T, Youngman LD, Anttila T, Dillner J, Hakulinen T, Koskela P, Lenner P, Hallmans G. Low levels of serum vitamins A and E in blood and subsequent risk for cervical cancer: Interaction with HPV seropositivity. Nutr Cancer 1999; 34:229–234.

459. Kanetsky PA, Gammon MD, Mandelblatt J, Zhang ZF, Ramsey E, Wright TC Jr, Thomas L, Matseoane S, Lazaro N, Felton HT, Sachdev RK, Richart RM, Curtin JP. Cigarette smoking and cervical dysplasia among non-Hispanic black women. Cancer Detect Prev 1998; 22:109–119.

460. Potischman N, Herrero R, Brinton LA, Reeves WC, Stacewicz-Sapuntzakis M, Jones CJ, Brenes MM, Tenorio F, de Britton RC, Gaitan E. A case–control study of nutrient status and invasive cervical cancer. II. Serologic indicators. Am J Epidemiol 1991; 134:1347–1355.

461. Kwasniewska A, Tukendorf A, Semczuk M. Folate deficiency and cervical intraepithelial neoplasia. Eur Gynaecol J Oncol 1997; 18:526–530.

462. Sellors JW, Mahony JB, Kaczorowski J, Lytwyn A, Bangura H, Chong S, Lorincz A, Dalby DM, Janjusevic V, Keller JL. Prevalence and predictors of human papillomavirus infection in women in Ontario, Canada. Survey of HPV in Ontario Women (SHOW) Group. CMAJ 2000; 163:503–508.

463. Olsen AO, Dillner J, Skrondal A, Magnus P. Combined effect of smoking and human papillomavirus type 16 infection in cervical carcinogenesis. Epidemiology 1998; 9:346–349.

464. Kjaer SK, Engholm G, Dahl C, Bock JE. Case–control study of risk factors for cervical squamous ell neoplasia in Denmark IV: role of smoking habits. Eur J Cancer Prev 1996; 5:359–365.

465. Gram IT, Austin H, Stalsberg H. Cigarette smoking and the incidence of cervical intraepithelial neoplasia, grade III, and cancer of the cervix uteri. Am J Epidemiol 1992; 135:341–346.

466. Duggan MA, McGregor SE, Stuart GC, Morris S, Chang-Poon V, Schepansky A, Honore L. Predictors of co-incidental CIN II/III amongst a cohort of owmen with CIN I detected by a screening Pap test.

467. Brisson J, Morin C, Fortier M, Roy M, Bouchard C, Leclerc J, Christen A, Guimont C, Penault F, Meisels A. Risk factors for cervical intraepithelial neoplasia: differences between low- and high-grade lesions. Am J Epidemiol 1994; 140:700–710.

468. Holly EA, Petrakis NL, Friend NF, Sarles DL, Lee RE, Flander LB. Mutagenic mucus in the cervix of smokers. J Natl Cancer Inst 1986; 76:983–986.

469. Prokopczyk B, Cox JE, Hoffmann D, Waggoner SE. Identification of tobacco-specific carcinogen in the cervical mucus of smokers and nonsmokers. J Natl Cancer Inst 1997; 89:868–873.

470. Melikian AA, Sun P, Prokopczyk B, El-Bayoumy K, Hoffmann D, Wang X, Waggoner S. Identification of benzo[a]pyrene metabolites in cervical mucus and DNA adducts in cervical tissues in humans by gas chromatography-mass spectrometry. Cancer Lett 1999; 146:127–134.

471. Barton SE, Maddox PH, Jenkins D, Edwards R, Cuzick J, Singer A. Effect of cigarette smoking on cervical epithelial immunity: a mechanism for neoplastic change? Lancet 1988; 2:652–654.

472. Szarewski A, Jarvis MJ, Sasteni P, Anderson M, Edwards R, Steele SJ, Guillebaud J, Cuzick J. Effect of smoking cessation on cervical lesion size. Lancet 1996; 347:941–943.

473. Koskela P, Anttila T, Bjorge T, Brunsvig A, Dillner J, Hakama M, Hakulinen T, Jellum E, Lehtinen M, Lenner P, Luostarinen T, Pukkala E, Saikku P, Thoresen S, Youngman L, Paavonen J. Chlamydia trachomatis infection as a risk factor for invasive cervical cancer. Int J Cancer 2000; 85:35–39.

474. Bosch FX, Castellsague X, Munoz N, Sanjose S, Ghaffari AM, Gonzalez LC, Gill M, Izarzugaza I, Viladiu P, Navarro C, Vergara A, Ascunce N, Guerrero E, Shah KV. Male sexual behaviour and human papillomavirus DNA: key risk factors for cervical cancer in Spain. J Natl Cancer Inst 1996; 88(15):1060–1067.

475. Schachter JJ, Hill EC, King EB, Heilbron DC, Ray RM, Margolis AJ, Greenwood SA. Chlamydia trachomatis and cervical neoplasia. J Am Med Assoc 1982; 248:2134–2138.

476. Antila T, Saikku P, Koskela P, Bloigu A, Dillner J, Ikaheimo I, Jellum E, Lehtinen M, Lenner P, Hakulinen T, Naranen A, Pukkala E, Thoresen S, Youngman L, Paavonen J. Serotypes of *Chlamydia trachomatis* and risk for development of cervical squamous cell carcinoma. J Am Med Assoc 2001; 285:47–51.

477. Ratnam S, Franco EL, Ferenczy A. Human papillomavirus testing for primary screening of cervical cancer precursors. Cancer Epidemiol Biomarkers Prev 2000; 9:945–951.

478. Clavel C, Masure M, Bory JP, Putaud I, Mangeonjean C, Lorenzato M, Gabriel R, Quereux C, Birebaut P. Hybrid capture II-based human papillomavirus detection, a sensitive test to detect in routine high-grade cervical lesions: a preliminary study on 1518 women. Br J Cancer 1999; 80:1306–1311.
479. Manos MM, Kinney WK, Hurley LB, Sherman ME, Shieh-Ngai J, Kurman RJ, Ransley JE, Fetterman BJ, Hartinger JS, McIntosh KM, Pawlick GF, Hiatt RA. Identifying women with cervical neoplasia: using human papillomavirus DNA testing for equivocal papanicolaou results. J Am Med Assoc 1999; 281: 1605–1610.
480. Rader JS, Rosenzweig BA, Spirtas R, et al. Atypical squamous cells: a case-series study of the association between Papanicolaou smear results and human papillomavirus DNA genotype. J Reproduc Med 1991; 36:291–297.
481. Maier RC, Schultenover SJ. Evaluation of the atypical squamous cell Papanicolaou smear. Int J Gynecol Pathol 1986; 5:242–248.
482. Noumoff JS. Atypia in cervical cytology as a risk factor for intraepithelial neoplasia. Am J Obstet Gynecol 1987; 156:628–631.
483. Davis GL, Hernandez E, Davis JL, Miyazawa K. Atypical squamous cells in Papanicolaou smears. Obstet Gynecol 1987; 69:43–46.
484. Slawson DC, Bennett JH, Herman JM. Follow-up Papanicolaou smear for cervical atypia. Are we missing significant disease? J Fam Pract 1993; 36:289–293.
485. Cecchini S, Iossa A, Ciatto S, et al. Routine colposcopic survey of patients with squamous atypia. A method for identifying cases with false negative smears. Acta Cytol 1990; 34:778–780.
486. Schiffman M, Hildesheim A, Herrero R, Bratti C. Human papillomavirus testing as a screening tool for cervical cancer. J Am Med Assoc 2000; 283(19): 2525–2526.

23

The Natural History of Esophageal Cancer

Philippe Tanière, Ruggero Montesano, and Pierre Hainaut
International Agency for Research on Cancer, Lyon, France

1. INTRODUCTION

Esophageal cancer is the sixth most frequent cancer worldwide. It is estimated that in 1996 the number of deaths due to esophageal cancer amounted to some 286,000 out of a total of 5.2 million cancer deaths (1). Two distinct types of primitive epithelial neoplasm, squamous cell carcinoma (SCCE) and adenocarcinoma (ADCE), represent more than 95% of all esophageal cancers. Since these cancers are usually detected at a late stage, and current therapy is rather ineffective, the 5-year survival rate is very poor (~10%), with no significant difference observed between developed and developing countries.

More than 80% of esophageal cancers occur in developing countries, where the great majority are SCCE. The incidence varies greatly in different parts of the world (2), with areas of extremely high rates in north-eastern Iran (Turkoman plain) and central China (Henan province) (Fig. 1). In these areas, incidence rates higher than 100 per 100,000 have been reported in both males and females. Other less clearly defined high-incidence areas are found in parts of South America and in South and East Africa. In most parts of Europe and the United States, the age-standardized annual mortality from SCCE is no more than five in males and one in females (per 100,000). However, there are areas in Europe, particularly in Normandy and Brittany in France and north-eastern Italy, where the incidence rates

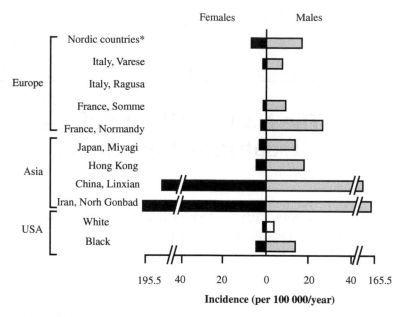

Figure 1   Incidence of squamous cell carcinoma of the esophagus in various populations and geographic areas. Examples of high- and low-incidence areas and/or populations are shown in Europe, Asia, and the United States. * includes Scandinavian countries, Iceland, and Finland. *Source*: Data from Muñoz and Day, 1996.

are much higher in males (up to 30 per 100,000), although still relatively low in females (Fig. 1).

Adenocarcinoma has a very different geographical distribution to SCCE. First, in contrast to SCCE, it occurs mainly in industrialized countries. Recent epidemiological data show that ADCE incidence is steadily increasing in Europe and the United States at a rate of 5 to 10% per year (3). This type of cancer now accounts for more than 50% of all esophageal cancers in the United States and in some European countries (e.g., England) (4).

The cellular and molecular natural history of esophageal cancers is still poorly understood. In particular, there are no reliable markers for assessment of exposure to specific risk factors, or for early diagnosis and prognosis. In this chapter, we discuss the data currently available on the molecular pathology of esophageal cancers and their temporal sequence. We present data suggesting that ADC arising in the cardia and ADC of the lower part of the esophagus with Barrett's mucosa may represent two independent pathological entities. We also show how analysis of mutation patterns in the *TP53* gene may help to unravel the complexity of the epidemiology of SCCE. Finally, we discuss how these various lines of research may contribute to better management of the worldwide challenge posed by esophageal cancers.

2. RISK FACTORS AND PRENEOPLASTIC LESIONS

Epidemiological studies have clearly shown that tobacco smoking and consumption of alcohol, associated with a low intake of fresh fruit, vegetables and meat, is causally associated with SCCE. However, the relative contributions of these risk factors may vary between geographical areas. In industrialized countries, it is estimated that 90% of this cancer is attributable to tobacco and alcohol consumption, with a multiplicative effect in individuals exposed to both factors. In the Japanese population, a polymorphism in the gene encoding aldehyde dehydrogenase 2 (ALDH2) has been shown to be significantly associated with several cancers of the upper digestive tract, including SCCE (5–7). This suggests that acetaldehyde, one of the main carcinogenic metabolites of alcohol, may play a role in the development of esophageal cancer. The consumption of scalding hot beverages is a proposed risk factor, as are betel chewing in South-East Asia and consumption of pickled vegetables and oral consumption of opium by-products in the Caspian Sea area. Conflicting reports have proposed a role for human papilloma viruses in SCCE (8).

Squamous cell carcinoma develops from squamous epithelium according to a classical dysplasia–carcinoma sequence. Esophagitis, a benign, chronic inflammatory disease, seems to represent a risk factor for dysplasia. Esophagitis occurs frequently in response to various types of physical and chemical stress that may harm the esophagus. A hereditary basis of esophageal cancer has been described in the case of an extremely rare syndrome, tylosis, characterized by acute palmoplantar hypekeratosis. The gene responsible for this disease has been mapped to a locus (TOC, Tylosis and Esophageal Cancer) on 17q25, but has not been cloned so far (9,10). Apart for this very rare disease, there is no clear evidence for inherited susceptibility to SCCE, although some familial clustering has been reported in high-risk areas of China. In India, a recent study showed an association between a particular polymorphism in the *CDKN1A* gene and SCCE (11).

Adenocarcinomas of the esophagogastric junction include both adenocarcinomas of the esophagus with Barrett's mucosa (ADCE) and adenocarcinomas of the cardia (ADCC). Barrett's mucosa is a glandular metaplastic mucosa of the normal squamous epithelium. The origin of this metaplasia is not clearly understood. It is often associated with chronic gastroesophageal acid reflux. However, it also occurs in a context of chronic biliary alkaline reflux, as well as, in some cases, in the absence of a detectable reflux (12). Recent evidence suggests that polymorphic expression of glutathione *S*-transferase P1 may determine a genetic susceptibility for developing Barrett's mucosa (13). Barrett's mucosa is reported to occur in more than 10% of the general population in Western countries. Its risk of occurrence may be increased in obese individuals and by the use of muscle-relaxing drugs.

The origin of glandular cells of Barrett's mucosa is not clear. Some evidence suggests that these cells derive from pluripotent cells in the basal cell layer of the normal esophageal epithelium, which can differentiate into either squamous or glandular cells. This hypothesis is consistent with the observation that epithelial cells of Barrett's mucosa show a hybrid pattern of cytokeratin expression, of both squamous and glandular origins (14), as well as of ultrastructural features in both cell types (15). Some authors believe that the metaplastic mucosa originates from the ducts of the normal esophageal glands of the submucosa. Barrett's mucosa can be further classified into different morphological subtypes (intestinal, fundic, and cardiac). Only the intestinal type is thought to be a preneoplastic lesion for ADCE. The estimated risk of developing an adenocarcinoma among patients with Barrett's metaplasia is 30–125 times greater than in the general population (16).

The cardia is the anatomical region at the transition between the esophagus and the stomach. It cannot be identified at the macroscopic level but at the microscopic level, it is characterized by a thin mucosa with clear glandular cells and one of the acid-secreting cells that are present in the fundic mucosa. There are no preneoplastic lesions identified as leading to ADCC. The contributions of gastroesophageal reflux disease and *Helicobacter pylori* infection as risk factors for ADCC remain uncertain (12,17).

There are no exogenic risk factors identified for tumors of the esophagogastric junction. Evidence on the role of tobacco smoking is still controversial (18–21).

3. SEQUENCE OF GENETIC EVENTS IN ESOPHAGEAL CANCERS

Table 1 provides a list of genetic changes that consistently occur in esophageal cancers. Mutation of the *TP53* gene is the most frequent alteration described to date, occurring in both ADCE and SCCE at a prevalence of between 35% and 70%, depending on the study and on the geographical origin of the tumors. However, the two tumor types show widely different mutation patterns (see below). In both cancers, mutation of *TP53* occurs at relatively early stages (22,23) (Fig. 2**A** and **B**). Prospective studies have shown the presence of a *TP53* mutation in Barrett's mucosa and in the dysplasia that precedes the development of ADCE (24). In high-grade dysplasia, a prevalence of *TP53* mutation of approximately 60% is found, similar to that in ADCE (25,26). In squamous lesions, mutations have been observed in dysplasia, in normal mucosa adjacent to cancer lesions and in mucosa with esophagitis without any evidence of cancer (27–31).

Recently, two genes encoding p53 homologues, *TP73* and *P63* (*p40,p73L,p51*), have been identified (32). The *P63* gene plays an essential role in the development of squamous epithelia, since mice lacking this gene

Table 1 List of Genes, Loci, or Markers of Interest in Squamous Cell Carcinoma and/or Adenocarcinoma of the Esophagus[a]

Gene, locus, or marker	Locus	Comments
APC	5q	LOH in ADC
CCND1	Ilql3	Amplification and overexpression in SCC and in ADC
CDKN2A, CDKN2B	9p22	LOH, promoter methylation, mutations in exon 2 in SCC and ADC
CDKN1A	6p21.2	Overexpression in ADC
CDH1	16q22.1	Loss of expression in intraepithelial and invasive ADC
COX2	1q25	Overexpression in SCC and in ADC
DLC1	3p21.3	Transcription shutdown in SCC
DEC1	9q32	LOH in SCC
EGFR	17pl3	Amplification and overexpression in SCC
FAS	10q24	Decrease of expression in SCC and in ADC
FAS-L	1q23	Expression in preneoplastic and neoplastic lesions in SCC and ADC
FEZ1	8p22	Transcription shutdown in SCC
FHIT	3pl4.2	Loss of expression in SCC and ADC, promoter methylation in SCC
GATA-4,Cathepsin B	8p	Amplification in ADC
HST1	Ilql3,	Amplification in SCC
HST2	12pl3	Amplification in SCC
IRF-1	5q31.1	LOH in SCC
MLHI	3p21.3	LOH in SCC and ADC
MSH2	2p22	LOH in SCC and ADC
MYC	8q24.1	Amplification in SCC
NOS2	17cen-q11	Overexpression
P63	3q27-28	Amplification in SCC
Proteases UPA		Prognostic factor in ADC
RAB11 (membrane trafficking)		High expression in low-grade intraepithehal neoplasia
RB1	13q14	LOH, absence of expression in SCC
TOC	17q25	LOH in SCC
TP53	17pl3	Point mutations, LOH in SCC and in ADC
Unknown	4q	LOH in ADC
Unknown	5pI5	LOH in SCC
Unknown	5q31.1	LOH in SCC
Unknown	8p	Amplification in ADC
TSHR?	14q31-32.1	LOH in ADC
Unknown	20q	Amplification in ADC

[a]For full gene names and synonyms, see Tumor Suppressor and Oncogene Directory at http://www.ncbi.nlm.nih.gov/CGAP/hTGI/tso/cgaptso.cgi

(A)

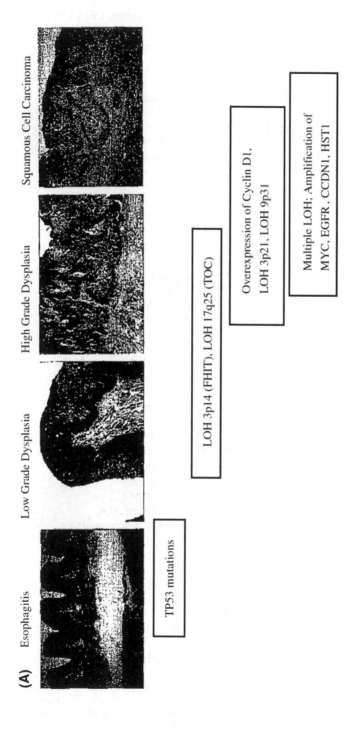

Esophagitis   Low Grade Dysplasia   High Grade Dysplasia   Squamous Cell Carcinoma

TP53 mutations

LOH 3p14 (FHIT), LOH 17q25 (TOC)

Overexpression of Cyclin D1,
LOH 3p21, LOH 9p31

Multiple LOH; Amplification of
MYC, EGFR, CCDN1, HST1

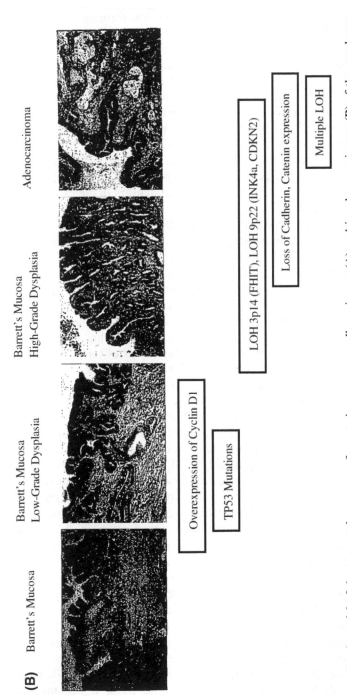

Figure 2 A model of the temporal sequence of events in squamous cell carcinoma (**A**) and in adenocarcinoma (**B**) of the esophagus. A representative picture of the histopathological steps is shown, and the timing of common genetic changes is indicated by arrows. See Table 1 and text for further description.

die at birth from multiple defects due to improper skin formation (33). This gene, as well as *TP73* is expressed in multiple splice-variant forms. Recent results show that the *P63* gene and its variants are often amplified in primary human squamous carcinomas of the lung and the head and neck (34,35). Hibi et al. (2000) (34) have proposed to term this gene (and its expression variants) AIS (amplified in human squamous cell carcinomas). Recent studies in our laboratory have shown that P63 was frequently amplified in esophageal SCC (36). Moreover, by immunohistochemistry, the P63 protein appears to be strongly expressed in all SCC. In contrast, this expression is virually absent in ADC as well as in Barrett's mucosa. These observations suggest that P63 is a key gene for the differentiation of the esophageal mucosa and that its deregulation may be an essential event in the pathogenesis of esophageal cancers.

Other commonly mutated genes include those involved in the control of the Gl/S cell-cycle checkpoint. Amplification of *CCDN1* (encoding cyclin Dl on 11ql3) occurs in 20–40% of SCCE and is frequently detected in cancers that retain expression of the Rb protein, in agreement with the notion that these two factors cooperate within the same signalling cascade (37). Amplification of *CCDN1* has also been detected in Barrett's mucosa and in ADCE (38,39). Inactivation of the *CDKN2A* gene (9p22) is likely to have an important role, since this locus appears to be frequently altered by several distinct mechanisms in both types of esophageal cancer (40–44). This gene encodes two totally distinct proteins, pl6mtsl and pl4arf. The former is a cyclin-kinase inhibitor that suppresses the activities of the cyclin D- and cylin E-dependent kinase complexes which regulate the phosphorylation of Rb in G1 (45). The latter binds to mdm2, a protein that regulates p53 protein levels. By this indirect mechanism, pl4arf acts as a tumor suppressor that utilizes a p53-dependent pathway. Deletion of the short arm of chromosome 9 has been observed in esophageal SCCE and ADCE. Homologous deletions have been reported in both cancer types. However, the most prevalent inactivation mechanism may be specific hypermethylation of the promoter of exon 1, resulting in the silencing of p16 protein expression. Mutations of the gene can also contribute to inactivation of this locus, although they appear to occur in only 10–20% of the tumors. Most of the mutations described to date affect exon 2, which contains coding sequences for both pl6mtsl and pl4arf. In a recent study, we have analyzed the expression of mRNA specific for pl6mtsl and pl4arf in ADCE, and compared it with that seen in matched, normal esophageal mucosa. Our results indicate that tumors frequently show an imbalance in the relative levels of the two transcripts, suggesting that deregulation of expression may also be a mechanism of alteration of pathways controlled by *CDKN2A* (46).

In SCCE, other potentially important genetic alterations include transcriptional inactivation of *FHIT* (fragile histidine triad, a presumptive tumor suppressor on 3pl4) by methylation of 5'-CpG islands (47,48), and deletion of the *TOC* gene on 17q25 (49,50). Recent evidence suggests that loss of heterozygosity (LOH) at a new putative tumor-suppressor locus on 5p15 (51) and 9q32 (52) may occur in a majority of SCCE. Amplification of several proto-oncogenes has also been reported (*HST-1, HST-2, EGFR, MYC*) (53).

In Barrett's mucosa, alteration of the transcription of *FHIT* may also be an early event (48,54). In contrast, a number of other loci are altered relatively late during the development of ADCE, with no obligate sequence of events. Prevalent changes (>50%) include LOH on 4q (55–57), 5q (several loci including *APC*) (56,57), 17q (58) and amplification of *ERBB2* (60) and of 14q (61). Molecules involved in membrane trafficking, such as rab11, have been reported to be specific for the loss of polarity seen in low-grade dysplasia (62,63). In invasive ADCE, reduced expression of the cadherin/catenin complex and increased expression of various proteases are detectable (64).

In both SCCE and ADCE, loss of alleles at loci such as those containing the mismatch repair genes *MLH1* (3p21) and *MSH2* genes (2p22) has been reported in several studies. It is not known whether these losses are accompanied by inactivation of the remaining allele. The fact that microsatellite instability is relatively rare in SCCE and ADCE (65–68) suggests that inactivation of this DNA repair pathway does not play an important role.

Several studies have shown that the expression of Fas, a cell surface receptor for pro-apoptic signals, is downregulated and that Fas-L is upregulated in the tumoral cells in SCCE. This could represent a way to evade the immune surveillance of the host (68). In Barrett's mucosa, Fas-L expression has been shown to be increasingly expressed during the progression to ADC through dysplasia (70,71).

Recently, frequent overexpression of Cox2 in SCCE (72,73) and in ADCE (74) has been reported. Since this molecule is a mediator of inflammation and a regulator of cell proliferation through the synthesis of prostaglandins, it has been suggested that this overexpression could be directly involved in the tumorigenesis of both types of esophageal cancers (72). Whether this overexpression is a cause or a consequence of tumor progression is not known.

Figure 2 proposes a temporal sequence for genetic events in SCCE and in ADCE. Although the two tumors progress through distinct genetic pathways, they have in common the fact that genes regulating the G/S transition of cell cycle are often altered before the detection of an overt tumor. The functions of the products of these genes are complex, with much cross-talk, redundancy and complementarity between pathways. Therefore, it is not surprising that none of these genes, taken alone, represents a reliable marker for risk assessment, early detection or prognosis. The only noticeable exception to this rule is overexpression of cyclin D1 in Barrett's mucosa.

It is very tempting to speculate that alterations in these genes all converge to upset a critical control point for the maintenance of the integrity of the esophageal mucosa. Indeed, G/S regulation is essential for the delicate balance between proliferation and differentiation which controls the formation and renewal of the esophageal mucosa. Further studies are necessary to elucidate the concerted action of these genes in the development of esophageal cancers.

4. ADENOCARCINOMA OF THE CARDIA: A SPECIFIC GENETIC ENTITY

Until now, it has been difficult to clearly distinguish between adenocarcinomas of the gastric cardia (ADCC) and adenocarcinomas of the esophagus (ADCE) at the histopathological level.

In a recent prospective study (75), we used strict anatomopathological criteria to distinguish between these two types of lesion. Adenocarcinoma of the cardia was defined as a tumor developing at the esophagogastric junction, extending essentially to the stomach for which no Barrett's mucosa could be identified even by microscopic analysis of the whole junction. Adenocarcinoma of the esophagus was defined as a tumor developing at the lower part of the esophagus or as a tumor developing at the esophago-gastric junction with a Barrett's mucosa identified at the macroscopic or at the microscopic level.

We found that ADCE and ADCC differ in the prevalence of *TP53* mutations, which is lower in ADCC (35%) than in ADCE (50%). We also found several other molecular differences, in particular in *MDM2* amplification. Amplification of *MDM2* is a common phenomenon in several types of cancer, in particular in tumors expressing wild-type TP53. The mdm2 protein binds and down-regulates the p53 protein, and amplification of *MDM2* has been proposed to represent an alternative mechanism to inactivate p53 (39,76). *MDM2* gene amplification has been observed in 19 tumor types, with the highest frequency observed in soft-tissue tumors (20%), osteosarcomas (16%), and esophageal carcinomas (13%) (76). *MDM2* amplification has been reported to be present in SCCE from Europe (39) and Japan (18%) (77). In our series, amplification of the *MDM2* gene was detected in 22% of ADCC, but in only one of the ADCE tested. Furthermore, the two tumor types showed different patterns of cytokeratin 7 expression. This expression was seen in 100% of our ADCE, but only in 37% of ADCC. These results suggest that ADCC and ADCE are distinct pathological entities at the molecular level. This hypothesis is supported by clinical data showing that the two groups of patients differ in sex ratio (male/female ratio of 0.65 in ADCC vs. 0.97 in ADCE) and in the frequency of secondary neoplasms in patients with ADCC.

5. LESSONS FROM *TP53* MUTATION ANALYSIS

Mutations in *TP53* are distributed throughout the central portion of the gene (mostly in exons 5–8) and differ in their chemical nature. In several cancers, specific mutation patterns have been shown to exist. These patterns can often be interpreted as "fingerprints" of the agents or events involved in *TP53* mutagenesis, either exogenous (such as chemical carcinogens) or endogenous (such as spontaneous mutations) (78).

The pattern of mutations in ADCE differs greatly from that in SCCE. Whereas the latter shows a very mixed pattern of mutations, almost half of the mutations found in ADCE are C to T transitions at dipyrimidine sites (CpG). This type of mutation represents about 25% of all known *TP53* mutations in human cancers. To date, ADCE is among the pathologies showing the highest prevalence of CpG mutations. Transitions at CpG sites are known to be related to endogenous mutation mechanisms. A common pathway involves methylation of cytosine and spontaneous deamination to thymine. The latter step is enhanced by exposure to nitric oxide (NO). Several recent studies have shown overexpression of the nitric oxide synthase gene *NOS2* in ADCE, that could be responsible for a high level of exposure to NO.

In SCCE, the pattern of mutations shows wide variations according to the geographical origin of the tumor. In SCCE from the high-incidence area of western Europe, a high prevalence of mutations at A:T base pairs has been observed. These mutations, which are relatively infrequent in other cancers, may reflect a contribution of metabolites of alcohol. This hypothesis has received recent support from studies by Noori et al. (79), who have shown that the mutation spectrum induced by acetaldehyde in the reporter gene hypoxanthine phosphoribosyl transferase (HPRT) resembled that in the TP53 gene in esophageal cancers. In SCCE from eastern Asia, mutations at A:T base pairs are less common but transversions at G:C base pairs occur at a higher rate than in western Europe (80) (Fig. 3). These differences are consistent with the notion that alcohol may not be a major contributor to esophageal carcinogenesis in eastern Asia, where specific exogenous factors may cause a higher rate of G to T transversions. The search for correlations between epidemiological data and *TP53* mutation patterns may reveal further clues as to the nature of the agents involved in the etiology of esophageal cancers.

6. GENETIC BIOMARKERS OF EARLY TUMORIGENESIS OR PROGNOSIS

To date, the use of genetic markers and immunohistochemistry has been of little use for the identification, diagnosis, or prognosis of esophageal cancers. However, several recent studies have indicated that overexpression of cyclin D1 in Barrett's mucosa could be associated with a higher risk of evolution into a carcinoma (38,81). Since Barrett's mucosa is common in

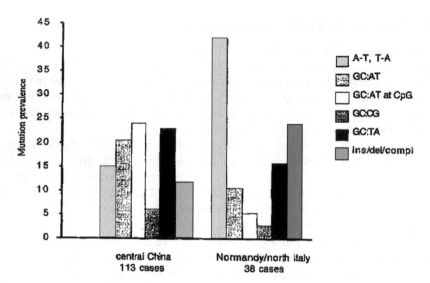

Figure 3 TP53 mutation spectrum in tumors from areas of high incidence of SCCE in Asia (Lixian country, Henan Province) and in western Europe (Normandy and Brittany, France, and northern Italy). *Source*: Data from Ref. 80.

the general population, the availability of a predictive marker would be a crucial contribution to the identification of patients at high risk of developing ADCE. Other markers which correlate with the neoplastic transformation of Barrett's mucosa are hyperexpression of P21 (82,83) and mutation of *TP53*. Although these changes may be useful for the detection of cancer, their predictive value remains to be ascertained.

Several genetic and expression changes have been identified as possible markers of poor prognosis. In ADCE, a significantly worse outcome has been shown to be associated with the presence of *TP53* mutations (26). Limited evidence also suggests that downregulation of expression of CD44v4 (83) or amplification of *ERBB2* (85) may be predictive of poor survival. Other useful markers may include microvessel density and expression of *vEGF* (86,87). For SCCE, predictors of poor prognosis include expression of P21 (83,88) as well as of cyclin D1. *TP53* mutations and loss of p16 expression may also be markers of poor prognosis (43). Other possible, independent factors may include overexpression of metalloproteinase 7, high levels of the proliferation antigen Ki67, high microvessel density (89), and expression of vEGF (90) and Ki67 (90). In contrast, expression of heat-shock proteins 27 and 70 was found to be reduced in SCCE and to correlate negatively with depth of tumor invasion and distant metastasis (92,93). Moreover, the Fas antigen was shown to be expressed in the upper portion of the squamous epithelium (69). Its presence in cancer lesions correlates with good histological differentiation and may represent an independent marker of favorable outcome (77). It is interesting to note that expression of the Fas ligand (FasL) is restricted to the basal layer of normal squamous epithelium (69). However, the prognostic relevance of FasL expression remains to be evaluated.

7. CONCLUSIONS AND PERSPECTIVES

Despite significant progress in the description of genetic alterations, our knowledge of the sequence of events leading to esophageal cancer remains limited. A major challenge for the years to come is to exploit recent advances in high-throughput genetic analysis to better identify patterns of gene expression during the progression of these cancers. Such studies may help in further dissecting the genetic heterogeneity of these cancers and to identify new genes involved in esophageal carcinogenesis. In the long term, this knowledge may help in designing and selecting adequate therapeutic strategies, taking into account the specific nature of the genetic alterations observed in the tumor.

Over the past 10 years, it has been shown that SCCE and ADCE develop through different genetic mechanisms. A crucial aspect of the natural history of these two cancers is what cellular and molecular factors induce esophageal stem cells to switch from a squamous to a glandular differentiation pathway in the pathogenesis of Barrett's mucosa. Adenocarcinoma of the esophagus is mostly a tumor prevalent in developed, industrialized countries. One of the main problems raised by these cancers is the development of adequate screening assays to identify patients with Barrett's mucosa or early dysplasias which are at high risk of neoplastic evolution. These patients may benefit from more intensive intervention, including local or systemic therapies. It will also be essential to determine the reasons for the rapid increase observed in the incidence of ADCE throughout Western countries.

In contrast to ADCE, SCCE is most prevalent in developing countries. Major efforts should be primarily aimed at better identification of risk factors as well as possible genetic susceptibility factors. Molecular epidemiological studies should be performed in order to identify the causes of the high incidences observed in regions such as northern Iran, central China, and South Africa. This will require careful, prospective tissue collection. Knowledge of the specific geographical risk factors causing these cancers will allow better primary prevention, as well as possible chemopreventive intervention. It is hoped that a combination of these approaches may lead to a significant decrease in the tumor burden and reduction of mortality in these populations.

REFERENCES

1. Pisani P, Parkin DM, Bray F, Ferlay J. Estimates of the worldwide mortality from 25 cancers in 1990. Int J Cancer 1999; 83:18.
2. Munoz N. Esophageal cancer. In: Schottenfeld D, Fraumeni JF, eds. Cancer Epidemiology and Prevention. Oxford, New York: Oxford University Press, 1996.
3. Devesa SS, Blot WJ, Fraumeni JF Jr. Changing patterns in the incidence of esophageal and gastric carcinoma in the United States. Cancer 1998; 83:2049.
4. Parkin D, Whelan S, Ferlay J, Raymond L, Young J. Cancer Incidence in Five Continents. Cancer Incidence in Five Continents Vol. VII. Lyon, France: IARC Scientific Publications, 1997:143.
5. Tian D, Feng Z, Hanley NM, Setzer RW, Mumford JL, DeMarini DM. Multifocal accumulation of p53 protein in esophageal carcinoma: evidence for field cancerization. Int J Cancer 1998; 78:568.
6. Yokoyama A, Muramatsu T, Ohmori T, Yokoyama T, Okuyama K, Takahashi H, Hasegawa Y, Higuchi S, Maruyama K, Shirakura K, Ishii H. Alcohol-related cancers and aldehyde dehydrogenase-2 in Japanese alcoholics. Carcinogenesis 1998; 19:1383.
7. Yokoyama A, Muramatsu T, Omori T, Matsushita S, Yoshimizu H, Higuchi S, Yokoyama T, Maruyama K, Ishii H. Alcohol and aldehyde dehydrogenase gene polymorphisms influence susceptibility to esophageal cancer in Japanese alcoholics. Alcohol Clin Exp Res 1999; 23:1705.
8. de Villiers EM, Lavergne D, Chang F, Syrjanen K, Tosi P, Cintorino M, Santopietro R, Syrjanen S. An interlaboratory study to determine the presence of human papillomavirus DNA in esophageal carcinoma from China. Int J Cancer 1999; 81:225.
9. Kelsell DP, Risk JM, Leigh LM, Stevens HP, Ellis A, Hennies HC, Reis A, Weissenbach J, Bishop DT, Spurr NK, Field JK. Close mapping of the focal non-epidermolytic palmoplantar keratoderma (PPK) locus associated with oesophageal cancer (TOC). Hum Mol Genet 1996; 5:857.
10. Risk JM, Field EA, Field JK, Whittaker J, Fryer A, Ellis A, Shaw JM, Friedmann PS, Bishop DT, Bodmer J. Tylosis oesophageal cancer mapped. Nat Genet 1994; 8:319.
11. Bahl R, Arora S, Nath N, Mathur M, Shukla NK, Ralhan R. Novel polymorphism in p21(waf1/cip1) cyclin dependent kinase inhibitor gene: association with human esophageal cancer. Oncogene 2000; 19:323.
12. Spechler SJ. The role of gastric carditis in metaplasia and neoplasia at the gastroesophageal junction. Gastroenterology 1999; 117:218.
13. van Lieshout EM, Roelofs HM, Dekker S, Mulder CJ, Wobbes T, Jansen JB, Peters WH. Polymorphic expression of the glutathione S-transferase P1 gene and its susceptibility to Barrett's esophagus and esophageal carcinoma. Cancer Res 1999; 59:586.
14. Boch JA, Shields HM, Antonioli DA, Zwas F, Sawhney RA, Trier JS. Distribution of cytokeratin markers in Barrett's specialized columnar epithelium. Gastroenterology 1997; 112:760.
15. Shields HM, Zwas F, Antonioli DA, Doos WG, Kim S, Spechler SJ. Detection by scanning electron microscopy of a distinctive esophageal surface cell at the junction of squamous and Barrett's epithelium. Dig Dis Sci 1993; 38:97.

16. Pera M. Epidemiology of esophageal cancer, especially adenocarcinoma of the esophagus and esophagogastric junction. Recent Results Cancer Res 2000; 155:1.
17. Chow WH, Blaser MJ, Blot WJ, Gammon MD, Vaughan TL, Risch HA, Perez-Perez GI, Schoenberg JB, Stanford JL, Rotterdam H, West AB, Fraumeni JF Jr. An inverse relation between cagA + strains of *Helicobacter pylori* infection and risk of esophageal and gastric cardia adenocarcinoma. Cancer Res 1998; 58:588.
18. Zhang ZF, Kurtz RC, Sun M, Karpeh M Jr, Yu GP, Gargon N, Fein JS, Georgopoulos SK, Harlap S. Adenocarcinomas of the esophagus and gastric cardia: medical conditions, tobacco, alcohol, and socioeconomic factors. Cancer Epidemiol Biomarkers Prev 1996; 5:761.
19. Gammon MD, Schoenberg JB, Ahsan H, Risch HA, Vaughan TL, Chow WH, Rotterdam H, West AB, Dubrow R, Stanford JL, Mayne ST, Farrow DC, Niwa S, Blot WJ, Fraumeni JF Jr. Tobacco, alcohol, and socioeconomic status and adenocarcinomas of the esophagus and gastric cardia. J Natl Cancer Inst 1997; 89:1277.
20. Ye W, Ekstrom AM, Hansson LE, Bergstrom R, Nyren O. Tobacco, alcohol and the risk of gastric cancer by sub-site and histologic type. Int J Cancer 1999; 83:223.
21. Lagergren J, Bergstrom R, Lindgren A, Nyren O. The role of tobacco, snuff and alcohol use in the aetiology of cancer of the oesophagus and gastric cardia. Int J Cancer 2000; 85:340.
22. Gao H, Wang LD, Zhou Q, Hong JY, Huang TY, Yang CS. p53 tumor suppressor gene mutation in early esophageal precancerous lesions and carcinoma among high-risk populations in Henan, China. Cancer Res 1994; 54:4342.
23. Neshat K, Sanchez CA, Galipeau PC, Blount PL, Levine DS, Joslyn G, Reid BJ. p53 mutations in Barrett's adenocarcinoma and high-grade dysplasia. Gastroenterology 1994; 106:1589.
24. Montesano R, Hainaut P. Molecular precursor lesions in oesophageal cancer. Cancer Surv 1998; 32:53.
25. Campomenosi P, Conio M, Bogliolo M, Urbini S, Assereto P, Aprile A, Monti P, Aste H, Lapertosa G, Inga A, Abbondandolo A, Fronza G. p53 is frequently mutated in Barrett's metaplasia of the intestinal type. Cancer Epidemiol Biomarkers Prev 1996; 5:559.
26. Ireland AP, Clark GW, DeMeester TR. Barrett's esophagus. The significance of p53 in clinical practice. Ann Surg 1997; 225:17.
27. Bennett WP, Hollstein MC, Metcalf RA, Welsh JA, He A, Zhu SM, Kusters I, Resau JH, Trump BF, Lane DP. p53 mutation and protein accumulation during multistage human esophageal carcinogenesis. Cancer Res 1992; 52:6092.
28. Bennett WP, von Brevern MC, Zhu SM, Bartsch H, Muehlbauer KR, Hollstein MC. p53 mutations in esophageal tumors from a high incidence area of China in relation to patient diet and smoking history. Cancer Epidemiol Biomarkers Prev 1997; 6:963.
29. Sarbia M, Porschen R, Borchard F, Horstmann O, Willers R, Gabbert HE. p53 protein expression and prognosis in squamous cell carcinoma of the esophagus. Cancer 1994; 74:2218.

30. Mandard AM, Hainaut P, Hollstein M. Genetic steps in the development of squamous cell carcinoma of the esophagus. Mutat Res 2000; 462:335.
31. Mandard AM, Marnay J, Lebeau C, Benard S, Mandard JC. Expression of p53 in oesophageal squamous epithelium from surgical specimens resected for squamous cell carcinoma of the oesophagus, with special reference to uninvolved mucosa. J Pathol 1997; 181:153.
32. Kaelin WG Jr. The emerging p53 gene family. J Natl Cancer Inst 1999; 91:594.
33. Yang A, Schweitzer R, Sun D, Kaghad M, Walker N, Bronson RT, Tabin C, Sharpe A, Caput D, Crum C, McKeon F. p63 is essential for regenerative proliferation in limb, craniofacial and epithelial development. Nature 1999; 398:714.
34. Hibi K, Trink B, Patturajan M, Westra WH, Caballero OL, Hill DE, Ratovitski EA, Jen J, Sidransky D. AIS is an oncogene amplified in squamous cell carcinoma. Proc Natl Acad Sci USA 2000; 97:5462.
35. Yamaguchi K, Wu L, Caballero OL, Hibi K, Trink B, Resto V, Cairns P, Okami K, Koch WM, Sidransky D, Jen J. Frequent gain of the p40/p5l/p63 gene locus in primary head and neck squamous cell carcinoma. Int J Cancer 2000; 86:684.
36. Taniere P, Martel-Planche G, Saurin JC, Lombard-Bohas C, Berger F, Scoazec JY, Hainaut P. TP53 mutations, amplification of P63 and expression of cell cycle proteins in squamous cell carcinoma of the oesophagus from a low incidence area in Western Europe. Br J Cancer 2001; 85:721.
37. Jiang W, Zhang YJ, Kahn SM, Hollstein MC, Santella RM, Lu SH, Harris CC, Montesano R, Weinstein IB. Altered expression of the cyclin Dl and retinoblastoma genes in human esophageal cancer. Proc Natl Acad Sci USA 1993; 90: 9026.
38. Arber N, Gammon MD, Hibshoosh H, Britton JA, Zhang Y, Schonberg JB, Roterdam H, Fabian I, Holt PR, Weinstein LB. Overexpression of cyclin D1 occurs in both squamous carcinomas and adenocarcinomas of the esophagus and in adenocarcinomas of the stomach. Hum Pathol 1999; 30:1087.
39. Morgan RJ, Newcomb PV, Hardwick RH, Alderson D. Amplification of cyclin D1 and MDM-2 in oesophageal carcinoma. Eur J Surg Oncol 1999; 25:364.
40. Esteve A, Martel-Planche G, Sylla BS, Hollstein M, Hainaut P, Montesano R. Low frequency of pl6/CDKN2 gene mutations in esophageal carcinomas. Int J Cancer 1996; 66:301.
41. Galipeau PC, Prevo LJ, Sanchez CA, Longton GM, Reid BJ. Clonal expansion and loss of heterozygosity at chromosomes 9p and 17p in premalignant esophageal (Barrett's) tissue. J Natl Cancer In 1999; 91:2087.
42. Klump B, Hsieh CJ, Holzmann K, Gregor M, Porschen R. Hypermethylation of the CDKN2/pl6 promoter during neoplastic progression in Barrett's esophagus. Gastroenterology 1998; 115:1381.
43. Takeuchi H, Ozawa S, Ando N, Shih CH, Koyanagi K, Ueda M, Kitajima M. Altered pl6/MTS1/CDKN2 and cyclin D1/PRAD-1 gene expression is associated with the prognosis of squamous cell carcinoma of the esophagus. Clin Cancer Res 1997; 3:2229.
44. Xing EP, Nie Y, Song Y, Yang GY, Cai YC, Wang LD, Yang CS. Mechanisms of inactivation of p14ARF, p15INK4b, and p1 6INK4a genes in human esophageal squamous cell carcinoma. Clin Cancer Res 1999; 5:2704.

45. Sarbia M, Stahl M, Fink U, Heep H, Dutkowski P, Willers R, Seeber S, Gabbert HE. Prognostic significance of cyclin D1 in esophageal squamous cell carcinoma patients treated with surgery alone or combined therapy modalities. Int J Cancer 1999; 84:86.

46. Hardie LJ, Darnton SJ, Wallis YL, Chauhan A, Hainaut P, Wild CP, Casson AG. p16 expression in Barrett's esophagus and esophageal adenocarcinoma: association with genetic and epigenetic alterations. Cancer Lett 2005; 217:221.

47. Mori M, Mimori K, Shiraishi T, Alder H, Inoue H, Tanaka Y, Sugimachi K, Huebner K, Croce CM. Altered expression of Fhit in carcinoma and precarcinomatous lesions of the esophagus. Cancer Res 2000; 60:1177.

48. Tanaka H, Shimada Y, Harada H, Shinoda M, Hatooka S, Imamura M, Ishizaki K. Methylation of the 5' CpG island of the FHIT gene is closely associated with transcriptional inactivation in esophageal squamous cell carcinomas. Cancer Res 1998; 58:3429.

49. von Brevern M, Hollstein MC, Risk JM, Garde J, Bennett WP, Harris CC, Muehlbauer KR, Field JK. Loss of heterozygosity in sporadic oesophageal tumors in the tylosis oesophageal cancer (TOC) gene region of chromosome 17q. Oncogene 1998; 17:2101.

50. Iwaya T, Maesawa C, Ogasawara S, Tamura G. Tylosis esophageal cancer locus on chromosome 17q25.1 is commonly deleted in sporadic human esophageal cancer. Gastroenterology 1998; 114:1206.

51. Peralta RC, Casson AG, Wang RN, Keshavjee S, Redston M, Bapat B. Distinct regions of frequent loss of heterozygosity of chromosome 5p and 5q in human esophageal cancer. Int J Cancer 1998; 78:600.

52. Nishiwaki T, Daigo Y, Kawasoe T, Nakamura Y. Isolation and mutational analysis of a novel human cDNA, DEC1 (deleted in esophageal cancer 1), derived from the tumor suppressor locus in 9q32. Genes Chromosomes Cancer 2000; 27:169.

53. Montesano R, Hollstein M, Hainaut P. Genetic alterations in esophageal cancer and their relevance to etiology and pathogenesis: a review. Int J Cancer 1996; 69:225.

54. Michael D, Beer DG, Wilke CW, Miller DE, Glover TW. Frequent deletions of FHIT and FRA3B in Barrett's metaplasia and esophageal adenocarcinornas. Oncogene 1997; 15:1653.

55. Hammoud ZT, Kaleem Z, Cooper JD, Sundaresan RS, Patterson GA, Goodfellow PJ. Allelotype analysis of esophageal adenocarcinomas: evidence for the involvement of sequences on the long arm of chromosome 4. Cancer Res 1996; 56:4499.

56. Rumpel CA, Powell SM, Moskaluk CA. Mapping of genetic deletions on the long arm of chromosome 4 in human esophageal adenocarcinomas. Am J Pathol 1999; 154:1329.

57. Walch AK, Zitzelsberger HF, Bruch J, Keller G, Angeimeier D, Aubele MM, Mueller J, Stein H, Braselmann H, Siewert JR, Hofler H, Werner M. Chromosomal imbalances in Barrett's adenocarcinoma and the metaplasia–dysplasia–carcinoma sequence. Am J Pathol 2000; 156:555.

58. Wu TT, Watanabe T, Heitmiller R, Zahurak M, Forastiere AA, Hamilton SR. Genetic alterations in Barrett esophagus and adenocarcinomas of the esophagus and esophagogastric junction region. Am J Pathol 1998; 153:287.

59. Swift A, Risk JM, Kingsnorth AN, Wright TA, Myskow M, Field JK. Frequent loss of heterozygosity on chromosome 17 at 17q11.2-q12 in Barrett's adenocarcinoma. Br J Cancer 1995; 71:995.

60. Polkowski W, van Sandick JW, Offerhaus GJ, ten Kate FJ, Mulder J, Obertop H, van Lanschot JJ. Prognostic value of Lauren classification and c-erbB-2 oncogene overexpression in adenocarcinoma of the esophagus and gastroesophageal junction. Ann Surg Oncol 1999; 6:290.

61. van Dekken H, Geelen E, Dinjens WN, Wijnhoven BP, Tilanus HW, Tanke HJ, Rosenberg C. Comparative genomic hybridization of cancer of the gastroesophageal junction: deletion of 14Q31–32.1 discriminates between esophageal (Barrett's) and gastric cardia adenocarcinomas. Cancer Res 1999; 59:748.

62. Ray GS, Lee JR, Nwokeji K, Mills LR, Goldenring JR. Increased immunoreactivity for Rab11, a small GTP-binding protein, in low-grade dysplastic Barrett's epithelia. Lab Invest 1997; 77:503.

63. Goldenring JR, Ray GS, Lee JR. Rab11 in dysplasia of Barrett's epithelia. Yale J Biol Med 1999; 72:113.

64. Tselepis C, Perry I, Jankowski J. Barrett's esophagus: disregulation of cell cycling and intercellular adhesion in the metaplasia-dysplasia-carcinoma sequence. Digestion 2000; 61:1.

65. Gleeson CM, Sloan JM, McGuigan JA, Ritchie AJ, Weber JL, Russell SE. Widespread microsatellite instability occurs infrequently in adenocarcinoma of the gastric cardia. Oncogene 1996; 12:1653.

66. Kagawa Y, Yoshida K, Hirai T, Toge T, Yokozaki H, Yasui W, Tahara E. Microsatellite instability in squamous cell carcinomas and dysplasias of the esophagus. Anticancer Res 2000; 20:213.

67. Meltzer SJ, Yin J, Manin B, Rhyu MG, Cottrell J, Hudson E, Redd JL, Krasna MJ, Abraham JM, Reid BJ. Microsatellite instability occurs frequently and in both diploid and aneuploid cell populations of Barrett's-associated esophageal adenocarcinomas. Cancer Res 1994; 54:3379.

68. Muzeau F, Flejou JF, Belghiti J, Thomas G, Hamelin R. Infrequent microsatellite instability in oesophageal cancers. Br J Cancer 1997; 75:1336.

69. Gratas C, Tohma Y, Barnas C, Taniere P, Hainaut P, Ohgaki H. Up-regulation of Fas (APO-1/CD95) ligand and down-regulation of Fas expression in hitman esophageal cancer. Cancer Res 1998; 58:2057.

70. Coppola D, Schreiber RH, Mora L, Dalton W, Karl RC. Significance of Fas and retinoblastoma protein expression during the progression of Barrett's metaplasia to adenocarcinoma. Ann Surg Oncol 1999; 6:298.

71. Younes M, Schwartz MR, Finnie D, Younes A. Overexpression of Fas ligand (FasL) during malignant transformation in the large bowel and in Barrett's metaplasia of the esophagus. Hum Pathol 1999; 30:1309.

72. Zimmermann KC, Sarbia M, Weber AA, Borchard F, Gabbert HE, Schror K. Cyclooxygenase-2 expression in human esophageal carcinoma. Cancer Res 1999; 59:198.

73. Ratnasinghe D, Tangrea J, Roth MJ, Dawsey S, Hu N, Anver M, Wang QH, Taylor PR. Expression of cyclooxygenase-2 in human squamous cell carcinoma of the esophagus; an immunohistochemical survey. Anticancer Res 1999; 19:171.

74. Wilson KT, Fu S, Ramanujam KS, Meltzer SJ. Increased expression of inducible nitric oxide synthase and cyclooxygenase-2 in Barrett's esophagus and associated adenocarcinomas. Cancer Res 1998; 58:2929.

75. Taniere P, Martel-Planche G, Maurici D, Lombard-Bohas C, Scoazec JY, Montesano R, Berger F, Hainaut P. Molecular and clinical differences between adenocarcinomas of the esophagus and of the gastric cardia. Am J Pathol 2001; 158:33.

76. Momand J, Jung D, Wilczynski S, Niland J. The MDM2 gene amplification database. Nucleic Acids Res 1998; 26:3453.

77. Shibakita M, Tachibana M, Dhar DK, Kotoh T, Kinugasa S, Kubota H, Masunaga R, Nagasue N. Prognostic significance of Fas and Fas ligand expressions in human esophageal cancer. Clin Cancer Res 1999; 5:2464.

78. Hainaut P, Hollstein M. p53 and human cancer: the first ten thousand mutations. Adv Cancer Res 2000; 77:81.

79. Noori P, Hou SM. Mutational spectrum induced by acetaldehyde in the HPRT gene of human T lymphocytes resembles that in the p53 gene of esophageal cancers. Carcinogenesis 2001; 22:1825.

80. Taniere P, Martel-Planche G, Puttawibul P, Casson A, Montesano R, Chanvitan A, Hainaut P. TP53 mutations and MDM2 gene amplification in squamous-cell carcinomas of the esophagus in south Thailand. Int J Cancer 2000; 88:223.

81. Kohmura T, Hasegawa Y, Ogawa T, Matsuura H, Takahashi M, Yanagita N, Nakashima T. Cyclin D1 and p53 overexpression predicts multiple primary malignant neoplasms of the hypopharynx and esophagus. Arch Otolaryngol Head Neck Surg 1999; 125:1351.

82. Hanas JS, Ler MR, Lightfoot SA, Raczkowski C, Kastens DJ, Brackett DJ, Postier RG. Expression of the cyclin-dependent kinase inhibitor p21(WAF1/CIP1) and p53 tumor suppressor in dysplastic progression and adenocarcinoma in Barrett esophagus. Cancer 1999; 86:756.

83. Hirai T, Kuwahara M, Yoshida K, Osaki A, Toge T. The prognostic significance of p53, p21 (Waf1/Cip1), and cyclin D1 protein expression in esophageal cancer patients. Anticancer Res 1999; 19:4587.

84. Bottger TC, Youssef V, Dutkowski P, Maschek H, Brenner W, Junginger T. Expression of CD44 variant proteins in adenocarcinoma of Barrett's esophagus and its relation to prognosis. Cancer 1998; 83:1074.

85. Brien TP, Odze RD, Sheehan CE, McKenna BJ, Ross JS. HER-2/neu gene amplification by FISH predicts poor survival in Barrett's esophagus-associated adenocarcinoma. Hum Pathol 2000; 31:35.

86. Igarashi M, Dhar DK, Kubota H, Yamamoto A, El Assal O, Nagasue N. The prognostic significance of microvessel density and thymidine phosphorylase expression in squamous cell carcinoma of the esophagus. Cancer 1998; 82:1225.

87. Koide N, Nishio A, Kono T, Yazawa K, Igarashi J, Watanabe H, Nimura Y, Hanazaki K, Adachi W, Amano J. Histochemical study of vascular endothelial growth factor in squamous cell carcinoma of the esophagus. Hepatogastroenterology 1999; 46:952.

88. Natsugoe S, Nakashima S, Matsumoto M, Xiangming C, Okumura H, Kijima F, Ishigami S, Takebayashi Y, Baba M, Takao S, Aikou T. Expression of p21WAF1/Cip1 in the p53-dependent pathway is related to prognosis in patients with advanced esophageal carcinoma. Clin Cancer Res 1999; 5:2445.

89. Torres C, Wang H, Turner J, Shahsafaei A, Odze RD. Prognostic significance and effect of chemoradiotherapy on microvessel density (angiogenesis) in esophageal Barrett's esophagus-associated adenocarcinoma and squamous cell carcinoma. Hum Pathol 1999; 30:753.

90. Yamashita K, Mori M, Shiraishi T, Shibuta K, Sugimachi K. Clinical significance of matrix metalloproteinase-7 expression in esophageal carcinoma. Clin Cancer Res 2000; 6:1169.

91. Ikeda G, Isaji S, Chandra B, Watanabe M, Kawarada Y. Prognostic significance of biologic factors in squamous cell carcinoma of the esophagus. Cancer 1999; 86:1396.

92. Kawanishi K, Shiozaki H, Doki Y, Sakita I, Inoue M, Yano M, Tsujinaka T, Shamma A, Monden M. Prognostic significance of heat shock proteins 27 and 70 in patients with squamous cell carcinoma of the esophagus. Cancer 1999; 85:1649.

93. Shamma A, Doki Y, Tsujinaka T, Shiozaki H, Inoue M, Yano M, Kawanishi K, Monden M. Loss of p27(KIP1) expression predicts poor prognosis in patients with esophageal squamous cell carcinoma. Oncology 2000; 58:152.

24

Liver Cancer: Risk Factors and Prevention

Christopher Loffredo

Cancer Genetics and Epidemiology Program, Department of Oncology, Georgetown University School of Medicine, Washington, D.C., U.S.A.

Christina Frank

Department of Epidemiology, University of Maryland School of Medicine, Baltimore, Maryland, U.S.A.

1. OVERVIEW

Hepatocellular carcinoma (HCC), is the most common primary malignancy affecting the liver, accounting for 75% of all liver cancers (1,2). Benign types of liver tumors, which occur very rarely, include hepatocellular adenoma, hemangioma, and mixed or mesenchymal hamartomas. Primary malignancies of the liver involve a wide variety of cell types, from angiosarcoma to hepatoblastoma and bile duct carcinoma, but HCC is by far the most common of these malignant tumors. Hepatocellular carcinoma is characterized histologically by well, moderately, or poorly differentiated parenchymal cells, with trabeculae ranging in thickness from two to eight cells and separated by sinusoids. Grossly, HCC is more likely to occur in the right lobe than in the left, and may present as a single mass, multiple diffuse nodules, or in a slow-growing fibrolamellar pattern.

Despite rapid advances in knowledge of tumor biology, HCC remains one of the most serious and challenging malignancies in terms of mortality and survival. Early detection and effective treatments are major problems, with most patients coming to medical attention in late stages of the disease. In the United States in the year 2000, for example, the ratio of liver cancer deaths to new cases was expected to be 0.90 (3), indicating the poor prognosis of this disease and highlighting the need for prevention.

Worldwide, HCC is a serious public health problem with wide geographic variation in its prevalence. It affects many more males than females, for reasons not yet well understood but probably related in part to differences in exposure histories and partly to patterns of sex hormone levels at different life stages (4,5). Several viruses, most importantly hepatitis B (HBV) and hepatitis C (HCV), are major risk factors for HCC in different parts of the world (6) and in certain susceptible subgroups within populations (7). A recent model of future morbidity and mortality, anticipated from the growing prevalence of HCV in the United States, predicts that between 2010 and 2019 there will be 27,200 deaths from HCC and $10.7 billion in direct medical expenditures for HCV-related diseases (8). Fortunately, the wide availability of an existing vaccine for HBV and the anticipated development of a vaccine for HCV offer hope of the primary prevention of viral hepatitis-associated HCC, especially as childhood vaccination against these viral diseases becomes routine around the world (9).

Several environmental risk factors for HCC are known: definitely alcohol abuse, aflatoxin, and certain herbicides and industrial solvents, and perhaps tobacco in susceptible individuals. Public health strategies to reduce the impacts of these risk factors will continue to evolve as new information from basic research and epidemiological studies clarifies the role of these agents in HCC causality. Finally, as new molecular tools are being applied to study human genetic susceptibility to viral and environmental risk factors of HCC, medical science is poised to understand more fully the biology and natural history of HCC, and ways to diagnose, treat, and prevent this serious disease.

2. PREVALENCE OF HEPATOCELLULAR CARCINOMA

The prevalence of HCC exhibits striking geographical prevalence, suggesting possible etiologic differences in genetic, environmental, or social risk factors. Hepatocellular carcinoma ranks eighth among the world's most common cancers, and is particularly common in parts of Africa and eastern Asia (Table 1). The incidence of HCC per 100,000 persons is extremely high in China and in Eastern, Middle, and Western Africa, and varies considerably by sex (10,11). Rates as high as 113 among males and 31 among females in Mozambique, and 65 among males and 25 among females in Zimbabwe have been reported (12). In comparison, HCC rates in Europe and in North America are generally reported to be below 6 per 100,000 persons, with consistently higher rates among males than among females (Table 1).

Not surprisingly, the highest rates of HCC tend to occur in areas of the world with high rates of chronic HBV and/or HCV infections (13–15). These viral risk factors are discussed below.

Table 1 Age-Standardized Rates of Liver Cancer Incidence (Per 100,000 Persons) by Sex and Area, 1990

	Male	Female
Eastern Africa	21.8	9.5
Middle Africa	20.7	10.6
Northern Africa	5.9	2.7
Southern Africa	14.7	4.8
Western Africa	22.6	7.7
Central America	2.3	1.4
South America	3.1	3.3
China	3.7	3.2
Southeast Asia	18.7	6.7
Southern Asia	3.1	1.7
Western Asia	5.3	2.9
Melanesia	21.3	9.3
Micronesia and Polynesia	8.5	2.6
United States	3.5	1.5
Europe	5.8	2.0

3. GENDER DIFFERENCES

The consistent pattern of higher rates in males compared to females suggests that HCC might be influenced by environmental or hormonal factors. For example, males might experience higher levels of exposures to carcinogens, or tend to be exposed earlier in life, compared to females. This hypothesis is supported by evidence of different rates of alcohol consumption and heavy cigarette smoking between men and women, particularly in Asian societies in which fewer women than men drink or smoke cigarettes regularly (4,16). Male–female variations in liver cancer incidence may also reflect hormonal influences. Some case–control studies have reported an association between oral contraceptive use in women and the risk of HCC. For example, Yu et al. (17) reported an odds ratio (OR) of 3.0 (95% CI 1.0–8.8) for this exposure, and an even higher risk among those who used oral contraceptives for 5 or more years (OR=5.5; 95% CI 1.2–24.8). Lui et al. (5) proposed that the growth of HCC tumors is significantly delayed among females compared to males, due to high levels of estradiol metabolized in the livers of women during their reproductive years. Supporting this hypothesis is the observation that 2-methoxyestradiol, a metabolite of estradiol produced in the liver, inhibits the growth of various tumors in situ. Also, a prospective study of nearly 10,000 men in Taiwan (18) found that elevated testosterone levels were associated with increased risk of HCC, even after adjusting for viral markers, age, and other risk factors, suggesting a role for androgens in the etiology of primary liver tumors. The clinical implications of these observations is not yet clear.

The relative contributions of the male and female sex hormones to HCC risk may also depend on other patient characteristics, such as HBV status and cirrhosis, as suggested in a recent prospective study of male cirrhotic patients at risk for HCC (19). In this study, serially collected serum samples were analyzed for levels of free testosterone, estradiol, and other markers in relation to the risk of developing HCC during 5 years of follow-up. The results indicated significant associations of increasing free testosterone level and elevated testosterone:estradiol ratio with increased risk of HCC, even after statistical adjustment for age, viral markers, and other clinical factors. This suggests that male sex hormones may promote the oncogenesis of HCC in male patients with cirrhosis. It remains to be seen whether a more general phenomenon of hormone-associated HCC risk exists among noncirrhotic individuals.

4. INFECTIOUS AGENTS
4.1. Hepatitis B Virus

Hepatitis B virus is a DNA virus with a circular genome of approximately 3.2 kilobases. Four open reading frames code for the different viral antigens. Hepatitis B virus is the only known human hepadnavirus. Six genotypes, A–F, have been identified. It is host-specific for humans and has a high affinity for infecting hepatocytes.

Hepatitis B virus infection occurs worldwide, but the highest population prevalence of chronic HBV infection is found in Southeast Asia (East of India and excluding Japan), sub-Saharan Africa, north-central South America, and the North American Arctic. Presence of antibodies to the hepatitis B core antigen (anti-HBc) reliably identifies any previous HBV infection. HBV surface antigen (HBsAg), the foremost marker for active HBV infection, was discovered in 1965 by Blumberg (20). HBsAg in serum becomes measurable at the end of a 4–12-week incubation period and typically persists in chronic HBV infection. However, the occurrence of occult HBV infection, defined as the presence of HBV DNA in liver tissue or serum in the absence of measurable HBsAg, has been described as well (21,22). This situation is particularly common in cases of dual HBV and HCV infection, hinting at viral interference and at least partial suppression of HBV replication by HCV (23).

Hepatitis B virus can be isolated from most body fluids of infected individuals. It is quite stable in the environment (24), and is effectively transmitted parenterally, sexually, and vertically. In industrialized countries, sexual transmission and transmission through needle sharing among drug users predominate. In hyperendemic areas of the developing world, perinatal transmission is very common. Healthcare workers are at risk of HBV infection through needle stick injuries, and healthcare clients through the reuse of nonsterile medical equipment.

Based on the considerable time lag between initial HBV viremia and the manifestation of acute symptoms, HBV itself is considered a noncytopathic virus. Its associated hepatocellular destruction is mainly a function of the HBV-directed immune response (25). HBV usually causes only mild clinical disease upon infection (26). The rate of symptomatic infections increases with age, and approximately 25% of adults with HBV show signs of hepatic dysfunction, including fatigue and jaundice. Cases of fulminant hepatitis with an associated high mortality are rare and also most common in older individuals.

Almost all (90–95%) infected adults clear the virus within a few months. Only a minority of cases develops chronic HBV infection. The rate of chronicity is inversely associated with age—younger age at the time of infection confers higher risk of chronic infection. For vertical transmission from mother to child (either at birth or in early childhood), the rate of chronic infections is as high as 80%. In those subjects who are chronically infected, the annual rate of HBsAg clearance is approximately 1% (27). Over time, approximately 10–30% of those chronically infected show some clinical signs of active hepatitis. The symptoms reflect inflammatory and necrotic histology in the liver, which can progress to cirrhosis and HCC. Hepatitis B virus infection acquired early in life carries the highest risk of HCC (15,28). There is some evidence that the HBV associated risk of HCC may also depend on the viral genotype (29).

The risk of HCC in Taiwan is almost 200 times higher in HBV-infected persons than in those not infected. It has been estimated that approximately 40% of chronic HBV-infected Chinese males die of cirrhosis or HCC (15). In Western countries, this risk ratio is significantly lower, probably due to a higher average age at infection and competing risk factors for mortality: In Italy, for example, Donato et al. (30) found an odds ratio of 11.4 for HBsAg-positivity (95% CI 5.7–22.8) in 172 HCC cases compared to 332 matched hospital controls.

Multiple studies have measured disease progression. In 66 Italian HBsAg-positive (anti-HCV negative) patients with cirrhosis followed for an average of 64.5 months, Chiramonte et al. (31) observed an annual rate of progression to HCC of 2% (95% CI 0.4–3.6). Male gender and age over 50 years were independent predictors of HCC development. In Japan, Ikeda et al. (32) measured 2.1%, 4.8%, and 18.8% of HCC development in a cohort of 645 cirrhotic patients with HBsAg (and no HCV markers) at 5, 10, and 15 years of follow-up, respectively.

Hepatitis B virus-associated hepatocarcinogenesis is thought to occur through both direct and indirect pathways: indirectly, malignant cell transformations can be a result of decades of immune-mediated hepatocellular injury and mitogenic regeneration in response to HBV infection. This process allows for the accumulation of mutations and can give rise to the formation of hyperplastic nodules and subsequent HCC. A high hepatocyte proliferation rate, as well as signs of irregular regeneration in liver biopsy samples, have been found to be predictive for the development of HCC (33,34).

In addition to this indirect oncogenic action of HBV, HBV DNA fragments coding for *trans*-activating proteins can integrate into the host genome and directly interfere with host gene expression (35,36). Chimeric HBV sequences are found in about 80% of HBV-associated HCC (37) and have been shown to transform cell lines in vitro (38). Sequences coding for the hepatitis X antigen (HBxAg) are especially implicated in HCC development, particularly if integrated in proximity to oncogenes or tumor-suppressor protein-encoding genes (39–41). Studies have demonstrated that inserted HBV DNA can indirectly inactivate the p53 tumor-suppressor gene (42,43) and inhibit negative growth regulatory pathways that normally prevent unchecked cell proliferation (44). Any impairment of the cellular DNA repair and growth regulatory systems also opens the door to potential co-carcinogens (45,46). Recent research has identified highly complex viral–host–environment interactions involved in HBV-related carcinogenesis (47,48).

A safe and effective recombinant vaccine for HBV is available (49). A high cost still precludes its general use in some of the most affected populations in industrialized and developing countries alike. However, studies in Taiwan have demonstrated the spectacular preventive effect that general HBV vaccination can have in a high prevalence population with high rates of perinatal transmission: the incidence of HCC in children aged 6–9 was reduced by three quarters, in those born after the implementation of nationwide HBV childhood vaccination in 1984, compared to children born before universal HBV vaccination (50). The World Health Organization's "Expanded Programme of Immunizations" (EPI) has recommended inclusion of the HBV vaccine into national vaccination programs (51).

Regrettably, the vaccine is of no help to those estimated 350 million people worldwide (52) already chronically infected and ultimately at risk for HCC. Treatment with interferon-alpha (IFN-alpha) until recently was the only option for therapy of chronic HBV infection (53). However, this form of therapy is expensive, has considerable side effects and is only successful in certain populations of patients. More recently, the better tolerated nucleoside-analogue lamivudine has been approved for therapy of chronic HBV infections. The drug has shown reduction of hepatic inflammation in 38–52% of treated patients, as well as sustained clearance of HBV DNA from serum in 65% (54,55). The successful combination of therapy with IFN-alpha and lamivudine has been described by Schalm et al. (56).

Aside from vaccination, prevention of HBV infection relies on education about the risks and prevention of sexually transmitted diseases, addiction treatment, and needle exchange programs for intravenous (IV) drug users, and the introduction and upkeep of good hygiene practices in medicine and alternative medicine.

4.2. Hepatitis C Virus

Hepatitis C virus is an RNA virus, taxonomically grouped into the family *Flaviviridae*. Its positive-stranded RNA is 9.4 kilobases long and constitutes a single open reading frame. Hepatitis C virus was first cloned by Choo et al. in 1989 (57) and subsequently shown to be the most common etiologic agent for what had been previously labeled "non-A, non-B hepatitis." Serological testing methods for HCV antibodies were published in 1989 (58); polymerase chain reaction (PCR) protocols for the detection of viral RNA in serum became available shortly thereafter (59,60).

Humans are the only natural host of HCV, though chimpanzees can be experimentally infected. The virus displays a marked hepatotropism and replicates primarily in hepatocytes (61–63). There are currently six genotypic groups of virus isolates, encompassing multiple subtypes. Immunity against one strain may not confer immunity against another (64,65), and infections of mixed genotypes are possible. Moreover, the virus has a tendency to produce quasispecies within the infected host, probably as a response to immune pressure (66).

Transmission of HCV occurs mainly through blood contact, resulting in a high potential for iatrogenic transmission of the virus. In developed countries, population subgroups at risk of HCV infection are those who received blood or blood products that were either not screened for HCV or did not undergo viral inactivation (67,68), injection drug users who share injection equipment (69,70), patients with renal failure undergoing dialysis (71), and healthcare workers at risk for needle stick injuries (72,73). Household, sexual, and perinatal transmission of HCV are known to occur (74), but the risk of transmission via these routes of exposure is considered low. A small percentage of persons with antibody to HCV have no known risk factor for HCV infection (75). However, it has been found that stigmatized risk factors like IV drug use are likely to be denied by study participants in risk factor studies, even if present (76).

In developing countries, the major routes of HCV transmission are apt to be medical and dental procedures carried out with nonsterile equipment, skin-breaking practices in traditional medicine, and injection drug use (77,78).

Hepatitis C virus is found worldwide, but published antibody prevalence in the general population varies widely between less than 1% and more than 20%. Prevalence in developing countries is typically higher than in industrialized countries. Within populations, prevalence typically rises with age and is inversely related with socioeconomic status (75,79). Genoytpes 1a, 1b, 2a, and 2b are most common in Europe and the Americas; types 1a, 2a, and 2b in East Asia; type 3 in Southeast Asia; type 4 in the Middle East and type 5 in Southern Africa (80). In some areas, genotypes show distinctive age profiles, suggesting cohort-specific waves of epidemics (81). Chronic infection with HCV is considered carcinogenic to humans by the IARC (82).

Little acute hepatitis, and very little fulminant hepatitis (<1%) is associated with HCV infection. Instead, approximately 70% of incident infections are asymptomatic during the early phase of infection. Within months, 15–30% of newly infected persons clear the virus permanently. The other 70–85% remain HCV infected. Approximately 50% will progress to some level of chronic hepatitis 10–15 years after infection, often with progressive fibrotic changes in the liver. The most serious long-term sequelae of HCV infection, cirrhosis and HCC, develop in only a minority of chronic carriers decades after infection. Approximately 15% of those initially infected will become cirrhotic. Only 1–4% will develop HCC—typically through the intermediary step of cirrhosis.

The association between HCV infection and HCC was established by a series of epidemiological studies: Kiyosawa et al. (83) retrospectively evaluated a group of transfusion HCV-infected patients with chronic non-A, non-B hepatitis. Serial liver biopsies in some patients described a progression from inflammation of varying severity, via fibrosis and cirrhosis, to HCC. The time between presumed infection and development of HCC was 17–60 years, most commonly more than 30 years. To investigate the effect of HCV on HCC aside from HBV infections in the United States, Hasan et al. (84) studied the prevalence of anti-HCV in a group of 59 HBsAg negative cases of HCC. The study found 66% of the HCC cases to have evidence of HCV infection, compared to 0.5% in blood donors. In Japan, a study of 105 HBsAg-negative HCC cases and blood donor controls found 76% anti-HCV prevalence in the cases compared to 1% in the controls (85). A meta-analysis by Resnick and Koff (86) calculated an OR of 25 for anti-HCV positivity in HCC cases compared to controls.

Progression of chronic HCV to HCC was studied in multiple cohorts of patients with cirrhosis. Fattovich et al. (87) observed 384 European patients with compensated HCV-related cirrhosis. In over 11 years of follow-up, 29 patients developed HCC, with an average yearly incidence of 1.4%. In Japan, Ikeda et al.(32) found HCC progression rates of 4.8%, 13.6%, and 26% among 1500 anti-HCV positive (HBsAg-negative) cirrhotics after 5, 10, and 15 years of follow-up, respectively. Degos et al. (88) followed 416 patients with HCV-related uncomplicated Child–Pugh A cirrhosis and found an even higher rate of HCC, with 13.4% of patients developing liver cancer within 5 years. Tong et al. (89) followed a cohort of patients presumably infected through unscreened blood transfusions for a specified time before being referred to their hospital for chronic hepatitis. In this cohort, the average time from infection to development of symptomatic chronic hepatitis was 13.7 years, to cirrhosis 20.6 years, and to HCC 28.3 years. Moreover, HCV-associated disease apparently progressed faster in those infected over the age of 50 compared to those infected earlier in life (mean time to HCC: 14.7 and 31.5 years, respectively).

The epidemiological evidence for a causal relationship between chronic HCV infection, cirrhosis and HCC is compelling. In contrast to HBV, the mechanism of HCV carcinogenesis seems to indirect, through the intermediate step of cirrhosis: the accelerated cell cycle of constant compensatory regeneration as a response to chronic viral and immune-mediated hepatocellular injury carries an increased risk of malignant transformations. The exact molecular oncogenic mechanism associated with HCV is still unclear (90).

The etiology of HCC cases without underlying cirrhosis (approximately 10%) and their relation to HCV infection also remains obscure (91). Possibly their etiology is fundamentally different despite the occasional presence of HCV markers. Kubo et al. (92) showed that HCC without cirrhosis was more common in HCV-positive patients also having anti-HBc evidence of a previous HBV infection, than in those with markers for HCV only.

There are few data on chronicity rates and clinical course of chronic HCV infection in children. Two studies of transfusion-infected children in Germany and Japan found low rates of clinical and morphological liver disease, and no cases of HCC after up to 27 years of follow-up (93,94). Results from other studies concur that children seem to experience a comparatively mild course of chronic HCV infection compared to adults (95,96). For persons infected early in their lifetime, a slow and mild course of chronic HCV infection may confer a lower risk of HCC development per year or decade compared to those infected as adults. However, their cumulative risk of HCC development may be higher, reflecting longer durations of lifelong chronic infections.

Currently there is no vaccination available for HCV. The main impediment for the development of a vaccine is the highly variable nature of the virus. Due to the existence of multiple genotypes, a multivalent vaccine approach will likely be needed. The isolation of stable viral epitopes that elicit a protective immune response is complicated by the existence of quasispecies within individual hosts. Additional obstacles are the lack of an in vitro culture system for HCV and an animal model aside from chimpanzees.

The main focus of primary prevention of HCV infection thus lies in the interruption of transmission via iatrogenic and accidental exposure to infected blood. In the developed world, HCV transmission through contaminated blood and blood products has been all but eliminated since the advent of anti-HCV screening in the early 1990s. An area of great concern is the continued spread of HCV in populations of illicit drug users. Programs aimed at fighting addiction as well as needle exchange projects are the most promising avenues to curb further spread of HCV and other blood borne viruses in these populations.

In the developing world, low levels of infection control in the medical and traditional medicine establishments continue to provide ample opportunity for the spread of blood borne viruses like HCV. Lack of awareness often goes hand in hand with a chronic shortage of funds for the most basic supplies needed for standard precautions. While large-scale vaccination campaigns are generally conducted in a safe manner due to international involvement and monitoring, other medical procedures may carry a substantial risk of HCV transmission—especially where HCV prevalence in the population is already high. Programs need to be instituted guaranteeing the safety of the blood supply, the single-use of nonsterilizable syringes, the sterilization of medical instruments and the safe disposal of medical wastes.

Chronic HCV infection can be treated with a combination therapy of IFN-alpha and ribavirin (97,98). Sustained biochemical and virological response to this drug combination is achieved in around 40–50% of the cases and depends, among other factors, on viral genotype (99,100). High cost and considerable side effects preclude widespread use of this form of therapy in the most severely HCV-affected countries in the developing world.

Multiple studies of cohorts of interferon-treated patients with chronic HCV infection have reported reduced incidence of HCC in patients with sustained virological or even just transient biochemical response to treatment (101–106). Possibly the treatment is able to slow or halt the cirrhotic process and thus interrupt HCV's carcinogenic mechanism. However, it has also been suggested that those who respond to therapy may also be the cirrhotic patients at lower risk from HCC in the first place (107).

4.3. Viral Interactions

Multiple studies have shown at least additive and potentially multiplicative effects of dual, or even triple, infections with hepatitis viruses on the risk of HCC (30,108–112). Chiramonte et al. (31) described an annual rate of progression from cirrhosis of 2% in HBsAg-positive patients, 3.7% in anti-HCV positive patients, and 6.4% in patients with both markers present. The risk of HCC in dually infected patients was 2.3 times (95% CI 1.1–4.6) as high as that in patients infected with only HBV. The mechanism behind this phenomenon may be an increased level (or duration) of fibrotic and cirrhotic activity associated with such at least partially concomitant infections. As in simple HCV infection, the resultant accelerated process of tissue regeneration may bear an increased risk of cell transformation and malignancy.

Hepatitis D virus (HDV) is an RNA virus dependent on HBV as a helper virus, co-infecting or super-infecting varying proportions of HBV carriers worldwide. Dual infection with HBV and HDV has been implicated in more rapid progression of chronic liver disease to HCC (113,114).

Some reports from high prevalence areas in Japan indicate at a potential interaction between HCV and the human T-lymphotropic virus type I (HTLV-1) with regard to the development of HCC (115–118). In dual infections with HCV and the human immunodeficiency virus (HIV) higher levels of HCV viremia (119) and more rapidly progressing clinical liver disease

(120,121) have been described. The effect of these possible viral interactions on HCC development remains unclear.

5. ENVIRONMENTAL AND GENETIC FACTORS
5.1. Alcohol

Chronic alcohol abuse is associated with an increased risk for both cirrhosis and HCC (122,123). Cirrhosis of the liver is the primary mechanism by which alcohol exposure predisposes to HCC, although some researchers believe that alcohol itself may be carcinogenic either by affecting the metabolism and distribution of other carcinogens (124) or through nutritional imbalances often associated with alcoholism (125).

Most HCC tumors are found in cirrhotic livers, and the epidemiology of HCC supports the view that alcohol is an independent risk factor for HCC as well as an exacerbating influence on other risk factors such as chronic HBV infection, depending on the prevalence of these factors in the population under study. In areas of low HCC incidence, for example, where HBV and HCV are rare, alcohol-induced cirrhosis may be the major risk factor associated with HCC, with a much higher attributable risk in the population relative to other factors (126,127). In high-incidence areas, it has been observed that alcohol consumption alters the natural history of HCV infection, leading to a more rapid histological and clinical progression to HCC compared to nonalcoholic HCV carriers (2,128). Thus, it has been often recommended that HCV-infected persons avoid excessive alcohol consumption in order to reduce the risks of progressive liver disease and cancer.

Genetic variations among individuals in their capacity to detoxify ethanol may play an additional role in susceptibility to HCC. Ethanol metabolism is mediated by several enzymes, including alcohol dehydrogenase and cytochrome p450 2E1, both of which are encoded by genes known to be polymorphic in populations. Individuals with mutations in one or both of these genes may be at greater or lesser risk from ethanol toxicity depending on the phenotypic consequences of the mutations. A meta-analysis of the RsaI polymorphism in the CYP2E1 gene revealed no association with alcoholic liver disease nor with HCC, while the TaqI allele was significantly less prevalent in persons with alcoholic liver disease compared to healthy subjects (129), suggesting a protective effect. However, there is no direct evidence that the TaqI allele alters the metabolism of ethanol, and the apparent protective effect might be due to linkage disequilibrium with other, unidentified protective genes or factors. More research is clearly needed on this topic.

5.2. Aflatoxin and *p*53

Aflatoxins are substances produced by the ubiquitous fungi *Aspergillis flavis* and *A. parasiticus* which can infect improperly stored grains, such as peanuts and corn. Aflatoxin B1 (AFB1) is metabolized in the human body to form potent epoxide compounds capable of damaging the DNA; measurable macromolecule adducts are detectable in biological samples, such as AFB1–albumin adducts in serum and AFB1–N7-guanine adducts in urine (130). Considerable research has documented the unique molecular dosimetry of aflatoxin exposure markers, with the development and validation of these biomarkers representing a tremendous advance over the use of dietary questionnaires to estimate the dose.

The metabolism of AFB1 is complex and involves several different enzymatic pathways, with recent discovery of new mechanisms by which the compound is bioactivated and subsequently detoxified (131). Genetic variations in the enzymes responsible for detoxifying AFB1 appear to mediate the risk of HCC, as suggested by a study of epoxide hydrolase genotypes (132). Aflatoxin–albumin adduct levels have been shown to vary according to environmental factors (rural vs. urban, season) and host factors (HBV status, GSTM1 genotype), notably in a study conducted in Gambia, West Africa (133). Aflatoxin B1 is also associated with a mutation at codon 249 of the tumor suppressor gene, p53, indicating that the effects of AFB1 on liver cells may include both direct toxicity of the epoxide metabolites and DNA mutations. Other aflatoxins, such as AFM1, are also cytotoxic and undergo complex metabolic reactions in the liver (134), and are probably associated with increased liver cancer risk.

In some populations, dietary exposure to AFB1 is a major risk factor for HCC (135–137); however, analysis of cancer risk is complicated by the dependence of alfatoxin biomarkers on factors such as cigarette smoking, alcohol consumption, age, HBV status, and plasma levels of antioxidant vitamins (138,139). Studies of HBV and AFB1 interactions in populations where both risk factors are prevalent reveal a supra-multiplicative effect on HCC risk. Qian et al. (140) reported from their prospective study of over 18,000 men in Shanghai the following risk estimates for HCC: relative to subjects with neither risk factor, those with HBV only had an OR of 7.3, those with AFB1 only had an OR of 3.4, and those with both factors had an OR of 59.4.

There may be hope for chemoprevention of aflatoxin toxicity due to expanding knowledge of its biotransformation pathways. A randomized, placebo-controlled, double-blind clinical trial is underway in Qidong, China, to test whether oltipraz, an antischistosomal drug with significant effects in reducing hepatocarcinogenesis in animal models, can prevent human hepatocarcinogenesis by inhibiting the bioactivation of aflatoxins (141). Early results indicate that 1 month of weekly dosing of 500 g of this drug resulted in a 51% decrease in urinary levels of a phase I metabolite of AFM1, relative to placebo, while sustained low-dose administration led to a 2.6-fold increase in the urinary excretion of a phase II metabolite (142). The authors of that report concluded that it "highlights the feasibility of inducing phase 2 enzymes as a chemopreventive strategy in humans."

5.3. Solvents and Pesticides

A wide variety of industrial chemicals and commonly used pesticides has been shown to cause liver cancer in laboratory animals. Among hepatocarcinogenic chemicals that have a high potential for human exposures are: organic solvents (such as vinyl chloride), fumigants (such as ethylene oxide), and pesticides (including arsenic-containing sprays, organochlorine compounds, and chlorophenoxy herbicides). Highly elevated risks of HCC have been associated with occupational exposures to the solvents vinyl chloride and carbon tetrachloride (143,144), which are still used in a wide variety of industrial processes and in certain household products. Vinyl chloride contamination of ground water and landfill sites, partly due to its origin as a breakdown product of other chlorinated hydrocarbon compounds, is a continuing public health problem in some areas (145). Organochlorine pesticides such as chlordecone (Kepone) are known liver carcinogens (146). Selected solvents and pesticides that appear to increase the risks for human HCC, listed by the IARC as Group I or Group II carcinogens (12), are listed in Table 2.

Epidemiological studies of human pesticide exposures and HCC suggest a positive association. Hayashi and Zeldis (147) reported that exposure to organochlorine compounds by Chinese rice workers increased their risk for HCC. Sterling and Arundel (148) reviewed studies of cancer and birth defects among Vietnamese populations exposed to herbicides, and reported an OR of 5.2 for liver cancer. Another epidemiological study in Vietnam (149) reported that agricultural workers exposed to organophosphorus pesticides were at increased risk for HCC. In addition to pesticide exposures and agricultural occupations, elevated risks for HCC were also associated with highway construction occupations using asphalt in the United States (150). Finally, concern over potential associations of chemical exposures and HCC may be especially urgent in less-developed parts of the world where occupational levels are still too high: a pilot study recently conducted in rural areas of Egypt (151) reported that serum measurements of organochlorine pesticides, including DDE and DDT, in cancer patients were 50–300 times higher than levels measured in U.S. rural populations.

Table 2 Selected Solvents and Pesticides Implicated as Human Liver Carcinogens

Group I (carcinogenic)	Group II-A (probably carcinogenic)	Group II-B (possibly carcinogenic)
Arsenical compounds	Ethylene dibromide	Chlorophenoxy herbicides
Vinyl chloride	Ethylene oxide	Kepone, Mirex, TCDD
DDT		

5.4. Smoking

Cigarette smoking may also increase the risk for HCC but the evidence is
not consistent, and the risk may be confined to certain subgroups such as
heavy drinkers and HBV carriers. Probably in some of the earlier epidemiological studies the role of smoking was obscured due to the comparison of
HCC cases to hospital controls, who might be similar on smoking history
compared to persons in the general population, and therefore more likely
to be hospitalized than members of the general population. Several such
case–control studies using hospital controls as the comparison group, but
not all, for example, (152) have reported no association between levels of
cigarette smoking and HCC (126,153–155), in contrast to studies using
population-based controls which have tended to report positive associations
between cigarette smoking and HCC risk (17,156). In the case–control study
of Yu et al. in California, the OR was 2.1 (95% CI 1.1–4.0) for any positive
cigarette smoking history, while in a larger study in Taiwan there was a
dose-dependent association with odds ratios of 1.1, 1.5, and 2.6 for men
who smoked 1–10, 11–20, and > 20 cigarettes per day, respectively (156).
Prospective studies of the smoking–HCC association are often limited by
small numbers of incident cancers, possibly accounting for the lack of significant associations with smoking in many such studies (157,158).

Some studies have found that cigarette smoking can enhance the risk
of HCC, when assessed by careful dosimetry or in susceptible subgroups. A
case–control study that measured smoking-related DNA adducts in surgical
liver samples (159) detected a significant dose-related increase in the risk of
HCC among cigarette smokers. Yu et al. (47) examined the risk of HCC in
relation to several risk factors, including interactions between HBV, cigarette smoking, and the *N*-acetyltransferase 2 gene (NAT2) which mediates
the toxicity of certain carcinogenic compounds in cigarette smoke. In that
study, the risk of HCC among HBV carriers who smoked was elevated
(OR 2.67, 95% CI 1.15–6.22) among subjects who were heterozygous for
the NAT2*4 functional allele, relative to those who lacked this allele, and
no association with NAT2 was found among HBV carriers who were
nonsmokers. The use of sensitive biomarkers of exposure and of genetic
susceptibility in these two studies may explain their strongly positive results,
which are in contrast to weaker associations with cigarettes reported in
previous studies.

Finally, the question arises of whether smoking and alcohol both contribute to the risk of HCC, and in what manner: independently, additively,
synergistically, or otherwise. A recent case–control study by Kuper et al.
(160) examined this question in a comparison of 333 HCC cases (including
both men and women) to a group of 360 cancer-free hospital controls in
Athens, Greece. In age-adjusted descriptive analyses, both smoking and
alcohol showed dose-dependent associations with increased risk of HCC,

Table 3 Interaction of Smoking and Drinking in Association with the Risk of HCC

Alcohol consumption	Never smoked	<2 packs per day	≥2 packs per day
<40 glasses per week	1.0 (reference)	1.7 (0.9–3.2)	1.5 (0.6–3.9)
≥40 glasses per week	2.0 (0.4–11.0)	2.5 (1.0–5.9)	9.6 (3.4–27.5)

Odds ratios and 95% confidence intervals shown here are adjusted for age, gender, education, coffee drinking, HbsAg, and anti-HCV. *Source*: Ref. 160.

with similar trends in men and women. Adjusted for both gender and age, as well as educational level and HBV and HCV markers, the OR for smoking ≥2 packs per day was 2.5 (95% CI 1.1–5.5) and the OR for heavy drinking (≥40 glasses per week) was 1.9 (95% CI 0.9–3.9). The synergistic (i.e., supramultiplicative) effects of these two exposures are shown in Table 3, in which the OR for heavy drinking and heavy smoking combined is 9.6. When the analysis was restricted to subjects without HbsAg or anti-HCV, similar results were observed for the combination of heavy smoking and drinking (OR=10.9, 95% CI 3.5–33.8). At least one other case–control study (161) has reported a similar interaction between heavy smoking and heavy drinking, suggesting that both factors may be important in the etiology of HCC.

6. SUMMARY AND CONCLUSIONS

The major risk factors for HCC today are HBV, HCV, aflatoxin, alcohol, and smoking, with additional risks from certain occupational exposures to pesticides and vinyl chloride. The combinations and attributable risks of these risk factors varies globally, with profound implications for risk assessment and risk reduction strategies. It has been suggested, for example, that in the developed nations of North America and western Europe, the population impacts of HBV and HCV on liver cancer rates are relatively low due to the rarity of those infections (even though the relative risks from HBV and HCV are quite high), whereas more HCC cases in those regions may be attributable to heavy smoking and chronic alcohol abuse even though these factors are nonspecific and have low relative risks (152). The situation in other areas may be quite different. Egypt, with a large proportion of nondrinkers and high rates of HCV, may be illustrative of a population with a high attributable risk from chronic HCV infection, with additional risk inputs from HBV and cigarette smoking. In parts of the world where dietary aflatoxin exposure is prevalent, constellations of risk factors may be present, encompassing not only aflatoxin but HBV, HCV, alcohol, and smoking as well. This is why studies designed to examine different combinations of risk factors are urgently needed to help clarify their impacts on HCC, and to ultimately aid in designing effective prevention strategies at the local level.

REFERENCES

1. Niederhuber J. Tumors of the liver. In: Murphy G, Lawrence WJ, Lenhard R, eds. Amerian Cancer Society Textbook of Clinical Oncology. Atlanta, GA: American Cancer Society, 1995:269–280.
2. London W, McGlynn K. Liver cancer. In: Schottenfeld D, Fraumeni JJ, eds. Cancer Epidemiology and Prevention. 2nd ed. New York: Oxford University Press, 1996:772–793.
3. American Cancer Society. Cancer Facts and Figures 2000. Atlanta, GA: American Cancer Society Inc., 2000.
4. Tanaka K, Hirohata T, Fukuda K, Shibata A, Tsukuma H, Hiyama T. Risk factors for hepatocellular carcinoma among Japanese women. Cancer Causes Control 1995; 6:91–98.
5. Lui W, Lin H, Chau G, Liu T, Chi C. Male predominance in hepatocellular carcinoma: new insight and a possible therapeutic alternative. Med Hypotheses 2000; 55:348–350.
6. Purcell RH. Hepatitis viruses: changing patterns of human disease. Proc Natl Acad Sci USA 1994; 91:2401–2406.
7. Harsch HH, Pankiewicz J, Bloom AS, et al. Hepatitis C virus infection in cocaine users—a silent epidemic [In Process Citation]. Community Ment Health J 2000; 36:225–233.
8. Wong JB, McQuillan GM, McHutchison JG, Poynard T. Estimating future hepatitis C morbidity, mortality, and costs in the United States. Am J Public Health 2000; 90:1562–1569.
9. Stuver SO. Towards global control of liver cancer? Semin Cancer Biol 1998; 8:299–306.
10. Parkin DM, Pisani P, Ferlay J. Estimates of the worldwide incidence of eighteen major cancers in 1985. Int J Cancer 1993; 54:594–614.
11. Parkin D, Ziegler J. Malignant diseases. In: Strickland G, ed. Hunter's Tropical Medicine and Emerging Infectious Diseases. Part 1. Clinical Practice in the Tropics. 8th ed. Philadelphia: W.B. Saunders Co., 2000:94–107.
12. Higginson J, Muir CS, Munoz N. Human Cancer: Epidemiology and Environmental Causes. Cambridge: Cambridge University Press, 1992.
13. Kew MC. Hepatitis B and C viruses and hepatocellular carcinoma. Clin Lab Med 1996; 16:395–406.
14. Sallie R, Di Bisceglie AM. Viral hepatitis and hepatocellular carcinoma. Gastroenterol Clin North Am 1994; 23:567–579.
15. Beasley RP, Hwang LY, Lin CC, Chien CS. Hepatocellular carcinoma and hepatitis B virus. A prospective study of 22 707 men in Taiwan. Lancet 1981; 2:1129–1133.
16. Lai CL, Gregory PB, Wu PC, Lok AS, Wong KP, Ng MM. Hepatocellular carcinoma in Chinese males and females. Possible causes for the male predominance. Cancer 1987; 60:1107–1110.

17. Yu MC, Tong MJ, Govindarajan S, Henderson BE. Nonviral risk factors for hepatocellular carcinoma in a low-risk population, the non-Asians of Los Angeles County, California. J Natl Cancer Inst 1991; 83:1820–1826.
18. Yu MW, Chen CJ. Elevated serum testosterone levels and risk of hepatocellular carcinoma. Cancer Res 1993; 53:790–794.
19. Tanaka K, Sakai H, Hashizume M, Hirohata T. Serum testosterone:estradiol ratio and the development of hepatocellular carcinoma among male cirrhotic patients. Cancer Res 2000; 60:5106–5110.
20. Blumberg BS, Gerstley BJ, Hungerford DA, London WT, Sutnick AI. A serum antigen (Australia antigen) in Down's syndrome, leukemia, and hepatitis. Ann Intern Med 1967; 66:924–931.
21. Chazouilleres O, Mamish D, Kim M, et al. "Occult" hepatitis B virus as source of infection in liver transplant recipients. Lancet 1994; 343:142–146.
22. Cacciola I, Pollicino T, Squadrito G, Cerenzia G, Orlando ME, Raimondo G. Occult hepatitis B virus infection in patients with chronic hepatitis C liver disease. N Engl J Med 1999; 341:22–26.
23. Sagnelli E, Coppola N, Scolastico C, et al. Virologic and clinical expressions of reciprocal inhibitory effect of hepatitis B, C, and delta viruses in patients with chronic hepatitis. Hepatology 2000; 32:1106–1110.
24. Bond WW, Favero MS, Petersen NJ, Gravelle CR, Ebert JW, Maynard JE. Survival of hepatitis B virus after drying and storage for one week [letter]. Lancet 1981; 1:550–551.
25. Mondelli M, Vergani GM, Alberti A, et al. Specificity of T lymphocyte cytotoxicity to autologous hepatocytes in chronic hepatitis B virus infection: evidence that T cells are directed against HBV core antigen expressed on hepatocytes. J Immunol 1982; 129:2773–2778.
26. Ganem D. Persistent infection of humans with hepatitis B virus: mechanisms and consequences. Rev Infect Dis 1982; 4:1026–1047.
27. Alward WL, McMahon BJ, Hall DB, Heyward WL, Francis DP, Bender TR. The long-term serological course of asymptomatic hepatitis B virus carriers and the development of primary hepatocellular carcinoma. J Infect Dis 1985; 151:604–609.
28. Buendia MA. Hepatitis B viruses and hepatocellular carcinoma. Adv Cancer Res 1992; 59:167–226.
29. Kao JH, Chen PJ, Lai MY, Chen DS. Hepatitis B genotypes correlate with clinical outcomes in patients with chronic hepatitis B. Gastroenterology 2000; 118:554–559.
30. Donato F, Tagger A, Chiesa R, et al. Hepatitis B and C virus infection, alcohol drinking, and hepatocellular carcinoma: a case–control study in Italy. Brescia HCC Study. Hepatology 1997; 26:579–584.
31. Chiaramonte M, Stroffolini T, Vian A, et al. Rate of incidence of hepatocellular carcinoma in patients with compensated viral cirrhosis. Cancer 1999; 85:2132–2137.
32. Ikeda K, Saitoh S, Suzuki Y, et al. Disease progression and hepatocellular carcinogenesis in patients with chronic viral hepatitis: a prospective observation of 2215 patients. J Hepatol 1998; 28:930–938.

33. Borzio M, Trere D, Borzio F, et al. Hepatocyte proliferation rate is a powerful parameter for predicting hepatocellular carcinoma development in liver cirrhosis. Mol Pathol 1998; 51:96–101.

34. Shibata M, Morizane T, Uchida T, et al. Irregular regeneration of hepatocytes and risk of hepatocellular carcinoma in chronic hepatitis and cirrhosis with hepatitis-C-virus infection. Lancet 1998; 351:1773–1777.

35. Caselmann WH. Transactivation of cellular gene expression by hepatitis B viral proteins: a possible molecular mechanism of hepatocarcinogenesis. J Hepatol 1995; 22:34–37.

36. Henkler FF, Koshy R. Hepatitis B virus transcriptional activators: mechanisms and possible role in oncogenesis. J Viral Hepat 1996; 3:109–121.

37. Buendia MA, Pineau P. The complex role of hepatitis B virus in human hepatocarcinogenesis. In: Barbanti-Brodano G, Bendinelli M, Friedman H, eds. DNA Tumor Viruses. New York: Plenum Press, 1995:171–193.

38. Luber B, Arnold N, Sturzl M, et al. Hepatoma-derived integrated HBV DNA causes multi-stage transformation in vitro. Oncogene 1996; 12:1597–1608.

39. Butel JS, Lee TH, Slagle BL. Is the DNA repair system involved in hepatitis-B-virus-mediated hepatocellular carcinogenesis? Trends Microbiol 1996; 4: 119–124.

40. Becker SA, Lee TH, Butel JS, Slagle BL. Hepatitis B virus X protein interferes with cellular DNA repair. J Virol 1998; 72:266–272.

41. Jia L, Wang XW, Harris CC. Hepatitis B virus X protein inhibits nucleotide excision repair. Int J Cancer 1999; 80:875–879.

42. Feitelson MA, Zhu M, Duan LX, London WT. Hepatitis B x antigen and p53 are associated in vitro and in liver tissues from patients with primary hepatocellular carcinoma. Oncogene 1993; 8:1109–1117.

43. Slagle BL, Zhou YZ, Butel JS. Hepatitis B virus integration event in human chromosome 17p near the p53 gene identifies the region of the chromosome commonly deleted in virus-positive hepatocellular carcinomas. Cancer Res 1991; 51:49–54.

44. Koike K, Moriya K, Yotsuyanagi H, Iino S, Kurokawa K. Induction of cell cycle progression by hepatitis B virus HBx gene expression in quiescent mouse fibroblasts. J Clin Invest 1994; 94:44–49.

45. Shibata Y, Nakata K, Tsuruta S, et al. Detection of hepatitis B virus X-region DNA in liver tissue from patients with hepatitis C virus-associated cirrhosis who subsequently developed hepatocellular carcinoma. Int J Oncol 1999; 14:1153–1156.

46. Poussin K, Dienes H, Sirma H, et al. Expression of mutated hepatitis B virus X genes in human hepatocellular carcinomas. Int J Cancer 1999; 80:497–505.

47. Yu MW, Pai CI, Yang SY, et al. Role of N-acetyltransferase polymorphisms in hepatitis B related hepatocellular carcinoma: impact of smoking on risk. Gut 2000; 47:703–709.

48. Jaitovitch-Groisman I, Fotouhi-Ardakani N, Schecter RL, Woo A, Alaoui-Jamali MA, Batist G. Modulation of glutathione S-transferase alpha by hepatitis B virus and the chemopreventive drug oltipraz. J Biol Chem 2000; 275:33395–33403.

49. Van Damme P, Tormans G, Beutels P, Van Doorslaer E. Hepatitis B prevention in Europe: a preliminary economic evaluation. Vaccine 1995; 13: S54–S57.
50. Chang MH, Chen CJ, Lai MS, et al. Universal hepatitis B vaccination in Taiwan and the incidence of hepatocellular carcinoma in children. Taiwan Childhood Hepatoma Study Group. N Engl J Med 1997; 336:1855–1859.
51. Kane MA. World-wide status of hepatitis B vaccination 1998. Soz Praventivmed 1998; 43:S44–S46, S118–S120.
52. Zuckerman AJ. More than third of world's population has been infected with hepatitis B virus. Br Med J 1999; 318:1213.
53. Vail BA. Management of chronic viral hepatitis. Am Fam Physician 1997; 55:2749–2756, 2759–2761.
54. Lai CL, Ching CK, Tung AK, et al. Lamivudine is effective in suppressing hepatitis B virus DNA in Chinese hepatitis B surface antigen carriers: a placebo-controlled trial. Hepatology 1997; 25:241–244.
55. Dusheiko G. Lamivudine therapy for hepatitis B infection. Scand J Gastroenterol Suppl 1999; 230:76–81.
56. Schalm SW, Heathcote J, Cianciara J, et al. Lamivudine and alpha interferon combination treatment of patients with chronic hepatitis B infection: a randomised trial [see comments]. Gut 2000; 46:562–568.
57. Choo QL, Kuo G, Weiner AJ, Overby LR, Bradley DW, Houghton M. Isolation of a cDNA clone derived from a blood-borne non-A, non-B viral hepatitis genome. Science 1989; 244:359–362.
58. Kuo G, Choo QL, Alter HJ, et al. An assay for circulating antibodies to a major etiologic virus of human non-A, non-B hepatitis. Science 1989; 244:362–364.
59. Okamoto H, Okada S, Sugiyama Y, et al. Detection of hepatitis C virus RNA by a two-stage polymerase chain reaction with two pairs of primers deduced from the 5'-noncoding region. Jpn J Exp Med 1990; 60:215–222.
60. Cha TA, Kolberg J, Irvine B, et al. Use of a signature nucleotide sequence of hepatitis C virus for detection of viral RNA in human serum and plasma. J Clin Microbiol 1991; 29:2528–2534.
61. Krawczynski K, Beach MJ, Bradley DW, et al. Hepatitis C virus antigen in hepatocytes: immunomorphologic detection and identification. Gastroenterology 1992; 103:622–629.
62. Cho SW, Hwang SG, Han DC, et al. In situ detection of hepatitis C virus RNA in liver tissue using a digoxigenin-labeled probe created during a polymerase chain reaction. J Med Virol 1996; 48:227–233.
63. Fong TL, Shindo M, Feinstone SM, Hoofnagle JH, Di Bisceglie AM. Detection of replicative intermediates of hepatitis C viral RNA in liver and serum of patients with chronic hepatitis C. J Clin Invest 1991; 88:1058–1060.
64. Farci P, Alter HJ, Govindarajan S, et al. Lack of protective immunity against reinfection with hepatitis C virus. Science 1992; 258:135–140.
65. Lai ME, Mazzoleni AP, Argiolu F, et al. Hepatitis C virus in multiple episodes of acute hepatitis in polytransfused thalassaemic children. Lancet 1994; 343:388–390.

66. Martell M, Esteban JI, Quer J, et al. Hepatitis C virus (HCV) circulates as a population of different but closely related genomes: quasispecies nature of HCV genome distribution. J Virol 1992; 66:3225–3229.

67. Alter HJ, Purcell RH, Shih JW, et al. Detection of antibody to hepatitis C virus in prospectively followed transfusion recipients with acute and chronic non-A, non-B hepatitis. N Engl J Med 1989; 321:1494–1500.

68. Pistello M, Ceccherini-Nelli L, Cecconi N, Bendinelli M, Panicucci F. Hepatitis C virus seroprevalence in Italian haemophiliacs injected with virus-inactivated concentrates: five year follow-up and correlation with antibodies to other viruses. J Med Virol 1991; 33:43–46.

69. Murphy EL, Bryzman SM, Glynn SA, et al. Risk factors for hepatitis C virus infection in United States blood donors. NHLBI Retrovirus Epidemiology Donor Study (REDS). Hepatology 2000; 31:756–762.

70. Garfein RS, Vlahov D, Galai N, Doherty MC, Nelson KE. Viral infections in short-term injection drug users: the prevalence of the hepatitis C, hepatitis B, human immunodeficiency, and human T-lymphotropic viruses. Am J Public Health 1996; 86:655–661.

71. Moyer AL, Alter MJ. Hepatitis C virus in the hemodialysis setting: a review with recommendations for control. Sem Dial 1994; 7:124–127.

72. Mitsui T, Iwano K, Masuko K, et al. Hepatitis C virus infection in medical personnel after needlestick accident. Hepatology 1992; 16:1109–1114.

73. Kiyosawa K, Sodeyama T, Tanaka E, et al. Hepatitis C in hospital employees with needlestick injuries. Ann Intern Med 1991; 115:367–369.

74. Dienstag JL. Sexual and perinatal transmission of hepatitis C. Hepatology 1997; 26:66S–70S.

75. Alter MJ. Epidemiology of hepatitis C. Hepatology 1997; 26:62S–65S.

76. Conry-Cantilena C, VanRaden M, Gibble J, et al. Routes of infection, viremia, and liver disease in blood donors found to have hepatitis C virus infection. N Engl J Med 1996; 334:1691–1696.

77. Abdel-Aziz F, Habib M, Mohamed MK, et al. Hepatitis C virus (HCV) infection in a community in the nile delta: population description and HCV prevalence. Hepatology 2000; 32:111–115.

78. Khan AJ, Luby SP, Fikree F, et al. Unsafe injections and the transmission of hepatitis B and C in a periurban community in Pakistan. Bull World Health Organ 2000; 78:956–963.

79. World Health Organisation. Hepatitis C—global prevalence (update). Wkly epidemial Rec 2000; 75:18–19.

80. Bendinelli M, Vatteroni ML, Maggi F, Pistello M. Hepatitis C virus. In: Specter S, ed. Viral Hepatitis. Totowa, NJ: Humana Press, 1999:65–127.

81. Nousbaum JB, Pol S, Nalpas B, Landais P, Berthelot P, Brechot C. Hepatitis C virus type 1b (II) infection in France and Italy. Collaborative Study Group. Ann Intern Med 1995; 122:161–168.

82. IARC. Hepatitis viruses. IARC Monogr Eval Carcinog Risks Hum 1994; 59:1–255.

83. Kiyosawa K, Sodeyama T, Tanaka E, et al. Interrelationship of blood transfusion, non-A, non-B hepatitis and hepatocellular carcinoma: analysis by detection of antibody to hepatitis C virus. Hepatology 1990; 12:671–675.

84. Hasan F, Jeffers LJ, De Medina M, et al. Hepatitis C-associated hepatocellular carcinoma. Hepatology 1990; 12:589–591.
85. Nishioka K, Watanabe J, Furuta S, et al. A high prevalence of antibody to the hepatitis C virus in patients with hepatocellular carcinoma in Japan. Cancer 1991; 67:429–433.
86. Resnick RH, Koff R. Hepatitis C-related hepatocellular carcinoma. Prevalence and significance. Arch Intern Med 1993; 153:1672–1677.
87. Fattovich G, Giustina G, Degos F, et al. Morbidity and mortality in compensated cirrhosis type C: a retrospective follow-up study of 384 patients. Gastroenterology 1997; 112:463–472.
88. Degos F, Christidis C, Ganne-Carrie N, et al. Hepatitis C virus related cirrhosis: time to occurrence of hepatocellular carcinoma and death. Gut 2000; 47:131–136.
89. Tong MJ, el-Farra NS, Reikes AR, Co RL. Clinical outcomes after transfusion-associated hepatitis C. N Engl J Med 1995; 332:1463–1466.
90. Butel JS. Viral carcinogenesis: revelation of molecular mechanisms and etiology of human disease. Carcingenesis 2000; 21:405–426.
91. De Mitri MS, Poussin K, Baccarini P, et al. HCV-associated liver cancer without cirrhosis. Lancet 1995; 345:413–415.
92. Kubo S, Nishiguchi S, Hirohashi K, et al. Clinical significance of prior hepatitis B virus infection in patients with hepatitis C virus-related hepatocellular carcinoma. Cancer 1999; 86:793–798.
93. Hoshiyama A, Kimura A, Fujisawa T, Kage M, Kato H. Clinical and histologic features of chronic hepatitis C virus infection after blood transfusion in Japanese children. Pediatrics 2000; 105:62–65.
94. Vogt M, Lang T, Frosner G, et al. Prevalence and clinical outcome of hepatitis C infection in children who underwent cardiac surgery before the implementation of blood-donor screening. N Engl J Med 1999; 341:866–870.
95. Luban N, Post J, Glymph C. Transfusion associated hepatitis C and G in pediatric patients identified through a universal look-back approach. Transfusion 1999; 106 (suppl.):110S.
96. Locasciulli A, Testa M, Pontisso P, et al. Prevalence and natural history of hepatitis C infection in patients cured of childhood leukemia. Blood 1997; 90:4628–4633.
97. Chemello L, Cavalletto L, Bernardinello E, Guido M, Pontisso P, Alberti A. The effect of interferon alfa and ribavirin combination therapy in naive patients with chronic hepatitis C. J Hepatol 1995; 23:8–12.
98. Brillanti S, Garson J, Foli M, et al. A pilot study of combination therapy with ribavirin plus interferon alfa for interferon alpha-resistant chronic hepatitis C. Gastroenterology 1994; 107:812–817.
99. Davis GL, Lau JY. Factors predictive of a beneficial response to therapy of hepatitis C. Hepatology 1997; 26:122S–127S.
100. Pozzato G, Kaneko S, Moretti M, et al. Different genotypes of hepatitis C virus are associated with different severity of chronic liver disease. J Med Virol 1994; 43:291–296.
101. Yabuuchi I, Imai Y, Kawata S, et al. Long-term responders without eradication of hepatitis C virus after interferon therapy: characterization

of clinical profiles and incidence of hepatocellular carcinoma. Liver 2000; 20:290–295.

102. Yoshida H, Shiratori Y, Moriyama M, et al. Interferon therapy reduces the risk for hepatocellular carcinoma: national surveillance program of cirrhotic and noncirrhotic patients with chronic hepatitis C in Japan. IHIT Study Group. Inhibition of Hepatocarcinogenesis by Interferon Therapy. Ann Intern Med 1999; 131:174–181.

103. Tanaka H, Tsukuma H, Kasahara A, et al. Effect of interferon therapy on the incidence of hepatocellular carcinoma and mortality of patients with chronic hepatitis C: a retrospective cohort study of 738 patients. Int J Cancer 2000; 87:741–749.

104. Toyoda H, Kumada T, Nakano S, et al. The effect of retreatment with interferon-alpha on the incidence of hepatocellular carcinoma in patients with chronic hepatitis C. Cancer 2000; 88:58–65.

105. Kasahara A, Hayashi N, Mochizuki K, et al. Clinical characteristics of patients with chronic hepatitis C showing biochemical remission, without hepatitis C virus eradi-cation, as a result of interferon therapy. J Viral Hepat 2000; 7:343–351.

106. Nishiguchi S, Kuroki T, Nakatani S, et al. Randomised trial of effects of interferon-alpha on incidence of hepatocellular carcinoma in chronic active hepatitis C with cirrhosis. Lancet 1995; 346:1051–1055.

107. Aizawa Y, Shibamoto Y, Takagi I, Zeniya M, Toda G. Analysis of factors affecting the appearance of hepatocellular carcinoma in patients with chronic hepatitis C. A long term follow-up study after histologic diagnosis.. Cancer 2000; 89:53–59.

108. Tagger A, Donato F, Ribero ML, et al. Case–control study on hepatitis C virus (HCV) as a risk factor for hepatocellular carcinoma: the role of HCV genotypes and the synergism with hepatitis B virus and alcohol. Brescia HCC Study. Int J Cancer 1999; 81:695–699.

109. Kew MC, Yu MC, Kedda MA, Coppin A, Sarkin A, Hodkinson J. The relative roles of hepatitis B and C viruses in the etiology of hepatocellular carcinoma in southern African blacks. Gastroenterology 1997; 112:184–187.

110. Yu MC, Yuan JM, Ross RK, Govindarajan S. Presence of antibodies to the hepatitis B surface antigen is associated with an excess risk for hepatocellular carcinoma among non-Asians in Los Angeles County, California. Hepatology 1997; 25:226–228.

111. Tanaka K, Ikematsu H, Hirohata T, Kashiwagi S. Hepatitis C virus infection and risk of hepatocellular carcinoma among Japanese: possible role of type 1b (II) infection. J Natl Cancer Inst 1996; 88:742–746.

112. Donato F, Boffetta P, Puoti M. A meta-analysis of epidemiological studies on the combined effect of hepatitis B and C virus infections in causing hepatocellular carcinoma. Int J Cancer 1998; 75:347–354.

113. Fattovich G, Giustina G, Christensen E, et al. Influence of hepatitis delta virus infection on morbidity and mortality in compensated cirrhosis type B. Gut 2000; 46:420–426.

114. Tamura I, Kurimura O, Koda T, et al. Risk of liver cirrhosis and hepatocellular carcinoma in subjects with hepatitis B and delta virus infection: a study from Kure, Japan. J Gastroenterol Hepatol 1993; 8:433–436.

115. Boschi-Pinto C, Stuver S, Okayama A, et al. A follow-up study of morbidity and mortality associated with hepatitis C virus infection and its interaction with human T lymphotropic virus type I in Miyazaki, Japan. J Infect Dis 2000; 181:35–41.

116. Okayama A, Maruyama T, Tachibana N, et al. Increased prevalence of HTLV-I infection in patients with hepatocellular carcinoma associated with hepatitis C virus. Jpn J Cancer Res 1995; 86:1–4.

117. Kamihira S, Yamada Y, Sohda H, et al. Human T-lymphotropic virus type-I influence on hepatotropic virus infections and the subsequent development of hepatocellular carcinoma. Cancer Detect Prev 1994; 18:329–334.

118. Stuver SO, Okayama A, Tachibana N, Tsubouchi H, Mueller NE, Tabor E. HCV infection and liver cancer mortality in a Japanese population with HTLV-I. Int J Cancer 1996; 67:35–37.

119. Cribier B, Rey D, Schmitt C, Lang JM, Kirn A, Stoll-Keller F. High hepatitis C viraemia and impaired antibody response in patients coinfected with HIV. AIDS 1995; 9:1131–1136.

120. Lesens O, Deschenes M, Steben M, Belanger G, Tsoukas CM. Hepatitis C virus is related to progressive liver disease in human immunodeficiency virus-positive hemophiliacs and should be treated as an opportunistic infection. J Infect Dis 1999; 179:1254–1258.

121. Soto B, Sanchez-Quijano A, Rodrigo L, et al. Human immunodeficiency virus infection modifies the natural history of chronic parenterally-acquired hepatitis C with an unusually rapid progression to cirrhosis. J Hepatol 1997; 26:1–5.

122. IARC. Alcohol drinking. Biological data relevant to the evaluation of carcinogenic risk to humans. IARC Monogr Eval Carcinog Risks Hum 1988; 44: 101–152.

123. Yu H, Harris RE, Kabat GC, Wynder EL. Cigarette smoking, alcohol consumption and primary liver cancer: a case–control study in the USA. Int J Cancer 1988; 42:325–328.

124. Lieber CS, Baraona E, Leo MA, Garro A. International Commission for Protection against Environmental Mutagens and Carcinogens. ICPEMC Working Paper No. 15/2. Metabolism and metabolic effects of ethanol, including interaction with drugs, carcinogens and nutrition. Mutat Res 1987; 186:201–233.

125. Lieber CS, Seitz HK, Garro AJ, Worner TM. Alcohol-related diseases and carcinogenesis. Cancer Res 1979; 39:2863–2886.

126. Austin H, Delzell E, Grufferman S, et al. A case–control study of hepatocellular carcinoma and the hepatitis B virus, cigarette smoking, and alcohol consumption. Cancer Res 1986; 46:962–966.

127. Mirkin IR, Remington PL, Moss M, Anderson H. Liver cancer in Wisconsin: the potential for prevention. Wis Med J 1990; 89:49–53.

128. Khan KN, Yatsuhashi H. Effect of alcohol consumption on the progression of hepatitis C virus infection and risk of hepatocellular carcinoma in Japanese patients. Alcohol Alcohol 2000; 35:286–295.

129. Wong NA, Rae F, Simpson KJ, Murray GD, Harrison DJ. Genetic polymorphisms of cytochrome p4502E1 and susceptibility to alcoholic liver disease and hepatocellular carcinoma in a white population: a study and literature review, including meta-analysis. Mol Pathol 2000; 53:88–93.

130. Groopman JD, Wild CP, Hasler J, Junshi C, Wogan GN, Kensler TW. Molecular epidemiology of aflatoxin exposures: validation of aflatoxin-N7-guanine levels in urine as a biomarker in experimental rat models and humans. Environ Health Perspect 1993; 99:107–113.

131. Knight LP, Primiano T, Groopman JD, Kensler TW, Sutter TR. cDNA cloning, experssion activity of a second human aflatoxin B1-metabolizing member of the aldo-keto reductase superfamily AKR7A3. Carcinogenesis 1999; 20:1215–1223.

132. McGlynn KA, Rosvold EA, Lustbader ED, et al. Susceptibility to hepatocellular carcinoma is associated with genetic variation in the enzymatic detoxification of aflatoxin B1. Proc Natl Acad Sci USA 1995; 92:2384–2387.

133. Wild CP, Yin F, Turner PC, et al. Environmental and genetic determinants of aflatoxin-albumin adducts in the Gambia. Int J Cancer 2000; 86:1–7.

134. Neal GE, Eaton DL, Judah DJ, Verma A. Metabolism and toxicity of aflatoxins M1 and B1 in human-derived in vitro systems. Toxicol Appl Pharmacol 1998; 151:152–158.

135. Bosch F, Munoz N. Prospects for epidemiological studies on hepatocellular cancer as a model for assessing viral and chemical interactions. In: Bartsch H, Hemminki K, O'Neill I, eds. Methods for Detecting DNA Damaging Agents in Humans: Applications in Cancer Epidemiology and Prevention. IARC Scientific Publications No. 89. Lyon: International Agency for Research on Cancer, 1988:427–438.

136. Chen CJ, Wang LY, Lu SN, et al. Elevated aflatoxin exposure and increased risk of hepatocellular carcinoma. Hepatology 1996; 24:38–42.

137. Ross RK, Yuan JM, Yu MC, et al. Urinary aflatoxin biomarkers and risk of hepatocellular carcinoma [see comments]. Lancet 1992; 339:943–946.

138. Yu MW, Lien JP, Liaw YF, Chen CJ. Effects of multiple risk factors for hepatocellular carcinoma on formation of aflatoxin B1-DNA adducts. Cancer Epidemiol Biomarkers Prev 1996; 5:613–619.

139. Yu MW, Chiang YC, Lien JP, Chen CJ. Plasma antioxidant vitamins, chronic hepatitis B virus infection and urinary aflatoxin B1-DNA adducts in healthy males. Carcinogenesis 1997; 18:1189–1194.

140. Qian GS, Ross RK, Yu MC, et al. A follow-up study of urinary markers of aflatoxin exposure and liver cancer risk in Shanghai, People's Republic of China [see comments]. Cancer Epidemiol Biomarkers Prev 1994; 3:3–10.

141. Zhang BC, Zhu YR, Wang JB, et al. Oltipraz chemoprevention trial in Qidong, Jiangsu Province, People's Republic of China. J Cell Biochem Suppl 1997; 29:166–173.

142. Wang JS, Shen X, He X, et al. Protective alterations in phase 1 and 2 metabolism of aflatoxin B1 by oltipraz in residents of Qidong, People's Republic of China. J Natl Cancer Inst 1999; 91:347–354.

143. Pirastu R, Comba P, Reggiani A, Foa V, Masina A, Maltoni C. Mortality from liver disease among Italian vinyl chloride monomer/polyvinyl chloride manufacturers. Am J Ind Med 1990; 17:155–161.

144. Lelbach WK. A 25-year follow-up study of heavily exposed vinyl chloride workers in Germany. Am J Ind Med 1996; 29:446–458.

145. Kielhorn J, Melber C, Wahnschaffe U, Aitio A, Mangelsdorf I. Vinyl chloride: still a cause for concern. Environ Health Perspect 2000; 108:579–588.

146. Sirica AE, Wilkerson CS, Wu LL, Fitzgerald R, Blanke RV, Guzelian PS. Evaluation of chlordecone in a two-stage model of hepatocarcinogenesis: a significant sex difference in the hepatocellular carcinoma incidence. Carcinogenesis 1989; 10:1047–1054.

147. Hayashi PH, Zeldis JB. Molecular biology of viral hepatitis and hepatocellular carcinoma. Compr Ther 1993; 19:188–196.

148. Sterling TD, Arundel A. Review of recent Vietnamese studies on the carcinogenic and teratogenic effects of phenoxy herbicide exposure. Int J Health Serv 1986; 16:265–278.

149. Cordier S, Le TB, Verger P, et al. Viral infections and chemical exposures as risk factors for hepatocellular carcinoma in Vietnam. Int J Cancer 1993; 55:196–201.

150. Austin H, Delzell E, Grufferman S, et al. Case–control study of hepatocellular carcinoma, occupation, and chemical exposures. J Occup Med 1987; 29: 665–669.

151. Soliman AS, Smith MA, Cooper SP, et al. Serum organochlorine pesticide levels in patients with colorectal cancer in Egypt. Arch Environ Health 1997; 52:409–415.

152. Trichopoulos D, Day NE, Kaklamani E, et al. Hepatitis B virus, tobacco smoking and ethanol consumption in the etiology of hepatocellular carcinoma. Int J Cancer 1987; 39:45–49.

153. La Vecchia C, Negri E, Decarli A, D'Avanzo B, Franceschi S. Risk factors for hepatocellular carcinoma in northern Italy. Int J Cancer 1988; 42:872–876.

154. Mohamed AE, Kew MC, Groeneveld HT. Alcohol consumption as a risk factor for hepatocellular carcinoma in urban southern African blacks. Int J Cancer 1992; 51:537–541.

155. Peters M, Wellek S, Dienes HP, et al. Epidemiology of hepatocellular carcinoma. Evaluation of viral and other risk factors in a low-endemic area for hepatitis B and C. Z Gastroenterol 1994; 32:146–151.

156. Chen CJ, Liang KY, Chang AS, et al. Effects of hepatitis B virus, alcohol drinking, cigarette smoking and familial tendency on hepatocellular carcinoma. Hepatology 1991; 13:398–406.

157. Tanaka K, Sakai H, Hashizume M, Hirohata T. A long-term follow-up study on risk factors for hepatocellular carcinoma among Japanese patients with liver cirrhosis. Jpn J Cancer Res 1998; 89:1241–1250.

158. Mori M, Hara M, Wada I, et al. Prospective study of hepatitis B and C viral infections, cigarette smoking, alcohol consumption, and other factors associated with hepatocellular carcinoma risk in Japan. Am J Epidemiol 2000; 151:131–139.

159. Wang LY, Chen CJ, Zhang YJ, et al. 4-Aminobiphenyl DNA damage in liver tissue of hepatocellular carcinoma patients and controls. Am J Epidemiol 1998; 147:315–323.

160. Kuper H, Tzonou A, Kaklamani E, et al. Tobacco smoking, alcohol consumption and their interaction in the causation of hepatocellular carcinoma. Int J Cancer 2000; 85:498–502.

161. Mukaiya M, Nishi M, Miyake H, Hirata K. Chronic liver diseases for the risk of hepatocellular carcinoma: a case–control study in Japan. Etiologic association of alcohol consumption, cigarette smoking and the development of chronic liver diseases. Hepatogastroenterology 1998; 45:2328–2332.

25

Brain Cancer

**Randa El-Zein, Yuri Minn, Margaret Wrensch, and
Melissa L. Bondy**

*Department of Epidemiology, M. D. Anderson Cancer Center,
University of Texas, Houston, Texas, U.S.A.*

1. INTRODUCTION

Brain cancer accounts for approximately 1.4% of all cancers and 2.3% of all
cancer-related deaths. The dangerous aspect of these tumors is that they can
interfere with normal brain function that is essential for life (1). The American Cancer Society estimates that 18,500 individuals will be diagnosed with
malignant brain tumors in 2005, and 12,760 of them will die (1). Despite
the high lethality and inescapable traumatic impact, brain tumors rarely
metastasize outside the central nervous system.

   Despite the recent increase in the number of epidemiological studies
on brain cancer, there is little consensus on the nature and magnitude of
the risk factors for it. Contributing to the confusion, in addition to the
methodological differences in eligibility and the representativeness of the
patients studied, are the variable use of proxies to report information about
the case subjects; the choices of control groups; the substantial heterogeneity of primary brain tumors; the inconsistencies in histological diagnoses;
definitions and groupings; and the difficulties of measuring exposure
retrospectively.

2. HISTOLOGY AND MOLECULAR GENETICS OF BRAIN TUMORS

Any central nervous system cell can become cancerous. Primary brain tumors are currently classified in a manner that reflects their histological appearance and location. Some brain tumors contain a mixture of cell types. Gliomas are the most common primary brain tumors and account for more than 40% of all central nervous system neoplasms (2). Glioma is a general category that includes astrocytomas, oligodendrogliomas, and ependymomas. According to the World Health Organization (WHO) (3), there are four major grades of astrocytoma.

2.1. Astrocytomas

Astrocytomas, the most frequent and most invasive brain tumors in children and adults, arise and take their name from the astrocyte cells.

1. WHO Grade I or pilocytic astrocytomas are the most frequent brain tumors in children. These tumors rarely undergo neoplastic transformation.
2. WHO Grade II or low-grade astrocytomas account for 25% of all gliomas and are infiltrative in nature.
3. WHO Grade III or anaplastic malignant astrocytomas are highly malignant gliomas and have an increased tendency to progress to glioblastoma.
4. WHO Grade IV or glioblastoma multiforme is a highly malignant brain tumor and typically affects adults. This type of glioma has poor prognosis, largely because the tumor rapidly spreads to other regions of the brain.

The identification of the genetical alterations found in astrocytomas led to the recognition that the nonrandom series of genetical changes that take place reflects increase of malignancy and clinical grade (4). Several common chromosomal alterations are observed and lead to changes in the expression of several genes. For example, mutations in the *p53* gene (located on chromosome 17p) have been reported in 40% of astrocytic tumors of all grades. These mutations are primarily found in gliomas in young adults and not in supratentorial astrocytic tumors in children (5). Another tumor suppressor gene frequently inactivated in astrocytic neoplasms is cyclin-dependent kinase N2 (*CDKN2*) or *p16*. The *CDKN2* gene is located on chromosome 9p and is inactivated by deletion of both copies of the gene. Loss of CDKN2 occurs rarely in low-grade astrocytomas but frequently in high-grade astrocytomas (6). Deletions of chromosome 10 commonly occur in astrocytic tumors, and there is considerable evidence for the presence of several tumor suppressor genes on chromosome 10 (7). Loss of heterozygosity at 10q23 has been reported to occur in approximately

70% of glioblastomas. Mutated in multiple advanced cancers (*MMAC1*) or phosphatase tensin homolog, also know as *PTEN,* is a tumor suppressor gene located on 10q and mutated in 40% of glioblastomas. Because *MMAC1* mutations are rarely found in low-grade gliomas, *MMAC1* is assumed to play an important role in progression from low-grade to high-grade tumors (8).

In contrast to loss of tumor suppressor genes, activation of oncogenes increases cell proliferation. The epidermal growth factor receptor (*EGFR*) gene is the gene most frequently amplified in malignant astrocytomas. The EGFR protein is a receptor for epidermal growth factor, an important stimulant for astrocytes. Amplification of a mutated *EGFR* allele has been found in approximately one-third of glioblastomas but not in low-grade astrocytomas (9).

2.2. Oligodendrogliomas

Accounting for less than 10% of intracranial tumors, oligodendrogliomas take their name and arise from the oligodendrocytes in the brain. Oligodendrogliomas are less aggressive than astrocytomas but are invasive and can traverse the cerebral spinal fluid (CSF). The ability of oligodendrogliomas to metastasize complicates their surgical removal, but because they are limited to the brain and CSF, some patients have a better prognosis and longer survival. Oligodendrogliomas characteristically exhibit loss of chromosomal regions on 1p and 19q13, and less frequently 9q and 22 (10).

2.3. Ependymomas

Ependymomas are tumors arising from the cell lining of the brain ventricles or ependymal cells. Their growth may block the flow of CSF, causing notable swelling of the ventricle or hydrocephalus. Although ependymomas may move along the CSF, they characteristically do not infiltrate normal brain tissue and are sometimes amenable to surgical treatment, especially surgery of the spinal cord. The most commonly described genetical alterations in ependymomas are deletions of 17p and monosomy 22 (4). Although believed to be derived from astrocytomas, oligodendrocytes, or ependymal cells, gliomas display a broad spectrum of histological features. The variation in the behavior of the gliomas probably reflects the genes involved in their transformation (2).

2.4. Meningiomas

Meningiomas arise from the sheaths surrounding the brain. The growth of meningiomas and the pressure they produce lead to the symptoms of brain tumors. Meningiomas are quite common, accounting for about 50% of primary central nervous system tumors. Because meningiomas are usually near the surface of the brain, they are often operable and are usually benign. Malignant meningiomas are associated with deletions of loci on chromosome 1 and, to a lesser extent, deletions on 6p, 9q, and 17p (4). Mutations in the *p53* gene have also been reported in malignant meningioma.

2.5. Medulloblastomas

Medulloblastomas are primitive neuroectodermal tumors that arise in the cerebellum. Medulloblastomas replicate quickly but can be treated with radiation because of their site specificity and early age of onset. They occur most commonly in children and frequently spread throughout the CSF. Chromosome 17p is a frequent site of deletions in medulloblastomas. Other, less frequent, sites of deletions are 2p, 6q 10q, 11p, 11q, and 16q (4).

2.6. Ganglioglioma

Gangliogliomas are tumors containing both neurons and glial cells. They have a high rate of cure by surgery alone or surgery combined with radiation therapy.

2.7. Schwannomas (Neurilemomas)

Schwannomas arise from Schwann cells, which surround cranial and other nerves. Schwannomas are usually benign tumors and often form near the cerebellum and in the cranial nerves responsible for hearing and balance (5).

2.8. Chordomas

These spinal tumors preferentially arise at the extremities of the spinal column and usually do not invade brain tissues and other organs. They are amenable to treatment but stubbornly recur over a span of 10–20 years.

3. ETIOLOGY AND RISK FACTORS OF BRAIN TUMORS
3.1. Ionizing Radiation

There is reasonable consensus of research that therapeutic ionizing radiation is a strong risk factor for intracranial tumors (11–13). Even the relatively low doses (averaging 1.5 Gy) used to treat ringworm of the scalp (tinea capitis) have been associated with relative risks of 18, 10, and 3 for nerve sheath tumors, meningiomas, and gliomas respectively (11,12,14). Other studies showed a high (17%) prevalence of prior therapeutic radiation among patients with glioblastoma or glioma and increased risk of brain tumors in children after radiation for acute lymphoblastic leukemia.

On the other hand, diagnostic radiation does not seem to play a role in glioma; three case–control studies of history of dental x-rays reported relative risks of 0.4, 1.2, and 3.0 for exposure to dental x-rays. The evidence is slightly stronger for meningioma, for which three of four studies have shown relative risks exceeding 2 for exposure to dental x-rays. All of the positive studies were conducted in Los Angeles (12,15) and so these findings should be replicated in other geographical areas.

The role of prenatal exposure to radiation in the etiology of childhood brain tumors is unclear. Japanese studies of individuals exposed in utero to atomic bomb radiation revealed no increase in brain tumor incidence (12). Other studies that reported increased relative risks of 1.2–1.6 for those exposed prenatally were statistically insignificant because of the small sample size. Furthermore, relative risks of this low magnitude associated with a comparatively uncommon exposure cannot account for many childhood brain tumors. Parental exposure to ionizing radiation before conception of the affected child has not been shown to be a risk factor for childhood brain tumors (12).

Occupational findings from atomic energy and airline employees are equivocal. A small but statistically significant elevated risk of 1.2 for brain tumors in nuclear facility employees and nuclear materials production workers has been reported (16). However, confounding or effect modification by chemical exposures complicates the interpretation of causality. A large cohort of U.S. nuclear workers was recently re-examined and again shown to have about 15% increased risk of brain tumors (17). There is no consensus about the risk of malignant brain tumor among pilots, although some believe that exposure to cosmic radiation at high altitudes may contribute to a brain tumor risk (18,19). However, a recent study of British Airway flight deck workers did not show statistically significant mortality from brain tumors (20).

3.2. Electromagnetic Fields

The debate on the impact of electromagnetic fields (EMFs) on brain cancer continues, despite largely negative findings. The debate has been prolonged by methodological difficulties with some studies. In 1979, Wertheimer and Leeper reported increased risks of brain tumors and leukemia in children living in homes in Denver near high-current vs. low-current wiring. This triggered widespread public and scientific interest in the potential health effects of electromagnetic fields. One meta-analysis revealed a nonsignificant 50% increased risk of childhood brain tumors with residence in high vs. low wire-coded homes (21). In a meta-analysis of 29 studies of adult brain tumors in relation to occupational exposures to electrical and magnetic fields, Kheifets et al. (22) found a significant 10–20% increased risk for brain cancer among electrical workers. However, they found no evidence for a consistent dose–response relationship with jobs considered to have higher vs. lower exposure. Three recent occupational studies reported an association among EMF exposed workers (23–25) and others did not (26,27).

Studies have not found an association between maternal EMF exposures and brain tumors in children (28,29). Although one meta-analysis has shown a nonstatistically significant 50% increased risk of brain tumors for children living in high as opposed to low wire-coded homes (21), a comprehensive assessment of childhood brain tumors in relation to residential EMF concluded that the evidence did not support an association (30). Another epidemiological study of adult brain tumors [reviewed in Ref. (31)] and a recent large population-based study of adult glioma in the San Francisco Bay area did not provide strong support for the hypothesis that electromagnetic fields in homes may increase the risk of brain tumors (32). In the San Francisco study, 492 adults with glioma and 463 controls were equally likely to have lived in homes with high wire codes during the 7 years before diagnosis. Spot measurements taken in homes also showed no pattern of higher residential electromagnetic field exposures for cases compared to controls (32).

However, measurements of electromagnetic fields are not precise. Wire codes of electrical distribution to homes and spot measurements of electromagnetic fields in and around homes can lead to incorrect exposure estimates (33). Wire codes also do not reflect exposures from internal wiring or sources such as appliances. Spot measurements change over time and do not always reflect the overall measurement in homes. The spot measurements can also be made at places where the subjects spend little or no time. Such assessments also neglect exposures outside the home, which may exceed those inside the home. A positive Swedish study of adult leukemia and central nervous system tumors found increased risks in those exposed both residentially and occupationally but not in those with neither exposure or with only residential or only occupational exposure (33). The Swedish study also was able to calculate residential magnetic field exposures over time because of detailed information available from Swedish power suppliers, which is not available in the United States (34).

Although there is no proof that EMF does not influence the risk of brain tumors, no causal connection has been established either. Methodological and conceptual issues of equivalency make it especially difficult (and perhaps impossible) to prove the existence of no association between power-frequency EMF and brain tumors. Apart from the lack of information about total electromagnetic field exposure and its duration, a more basic limitation in assessing the relative risk is the failure, thus far, to show that electromagnetic fields induce mutations that in turn might promote tumorigenesis and brain tumors (35).

3.3. Diet
3.3.1. *N*-Nitroso Compounds, Vitamins, Alcohol, Tobacco

Several observations have led to studies of diet and brain tumors. First, in experimental animal studies, *N*-nitroso compounds have been clearly identified as neurocarcinogens (36). Other investigators have suggested several mechanisms involving DNA damage through which *N*-nitroso compounds might cause brain tumors (37,38). These compounds can initiate neurocarcinogenesis through both prenatal and postnatal exposure, although in animals more tumors result from fetal than from postnatal exposures (36). Because there can be a substantial lag between exposure and tumor formation it is conceivable that early exposure could produce adult tumors. Animal studies showed that a wide variety of primates and other mammals are susceptible to chemically induced brain tumors.

In humans, the ubiquity of *N*-nitroso compounds has complicated their epidemiological evaluation as carcinogens. About half of all human exposures in the digestive system occur when common amino compounds produced from fish, other foods, or drugs contact a nitrosating agent (such as nitrites from cured meats) in the right enzymatic milieu (37). Equally common external exposures include agents such as tobacco smoke, cosmetics, auto interiors, and cured meats. To complicate matters further, some vegetables have nitrates convertible to nitrites but also contain a high level of vitamins that block formation of *N*-nitroso compounds.

A comprehensive assessment of exposure to dietary and environmental compounds is thus difficult. Despite this, many studies have tried to examine major dietary sources of these chemicals and to assess the safeguards against formation of nitrosoureas presented by vitamins such as C and E, which are thought to inhibit *N*-nitroso formation.

No consensus has been achieved in human studies. Diet and vitamin supplementation investigations have provided only partial support for the hypothesis that dietary *N*-nitroso compounds increase the risk of both childhood and adult brain tumors (37–41). However, increased consumption of foods cured with nitrosamines has been observed among brain tumor cases (or their mothers) compared with controls (42). Also, lower rates after increased consumption of fruits and vegetables or vitamins that might block nitrosation or the harmful effects of nitrosamines have been observed in some, but not all, studies.

Lee et al. (43) found that adults with glioma were more likely than controls to consume diets high in cured foods or nitrites and low in fruits and vegetables rich in vitamin C. The effect was more pronounced and only achieved statistical significance in men. Although the finding is compatible with the hypothesis that *N*-nitroso compounds might play a role in human neuro-oncogenesis, the observed patterns also support the hypothesis of oxidative burden and antioxidant protection.

After a comprehensive survey of nitrosamines in food and beverages, beer contamination with the nitrosamine derivative (NDMA) was considered a serious matter, especially in Germany. The source of the contamination was traced to oxidation of malt (44). Beer in several countries was a major source of exposure to carcinogenic nitrosamines, because of the very large quantities consumed. Nitrosamine derivative was also present in whiskies of various kinds but at lower concentrations than in beer and therefore posing a lower cancer risk probably because of the smaller amounts consumed. In spite of much research, particularly in connection with pediatric brain tumors, alcoholic products have not been implicated in brain tumors (39).

Since tobacco smoke contains polycyclic aromatic hydrocarbons and nitroso compounds, many studies have sought connections between brain tumors and cigarette smoke. No significant effect has been established from smoke, although two studies report increased risk of adult glioma with smoking unfiltered but not filtered cigarettes [reviewed in Refs. (39,43)]. Both a meta-analysis and a review (45,46) found no clear association between a mother's smoking tobacco during pregnancy and risk of brain tumor in the child. The suspected role of secondary or passive smoking has more support. Several studies found slightly increased relative risks, generally lower than 1.5, i.e., the order of magnitude associated with some recognized hazards of exposure to passive smoking (1.2–1.3 for adult lung cancer and cardiovascular diseases) (47,48). Tumors most often found associated with maternal smoking in pregnancy or passive smoke exposures are childhood brain tumors and leukemia-lymphoma, with risks of up to 2 or greater in selected studies (49,50). A few studies have found elevated risk more closely associated with paternal smoking rather than the maternal smoking (51). Even in the absence of the definitive findings on the impact of the secondary smoke, the evidence from human studies coupled with demonstration of genotoxic effects on the fetus exposed to metabolites of tobacco smoke, and the demonstrable presence of adducts, should lead to strong recommendations aiming at fully protecting fetuses, newborns, and infants from exposure to tobacco smoke (52).

3.4. Industry and Occupation

Attempts to link specific chemicals to human brain tumors in occupationally or industrially exposed groups have proved inconclusive. In 1986, Thomas and Waxweiler (53) published a comprehensive review of occupational risk factors for brain tumors and established a group of suspect chemicals and occupations. Additional studies in the intervening 13 years have not established a conclusive link between any of these factors and brain tumor risk. Many occupational and industrial studies focused on individuals exposed to carcinogenic and/or neurotoxic substances such as organic solvents, lubricating oils, acrylonitrile, formaldehyde, polycyclic aromatic hydrocarbons, and phenols and phenolic compounds, which are part of workplace exposures and induce brain tumors in experimental animals. Animal neurocarcinogenicity studies, mainly in rats, have shown that susceptibility is significantly influenced by strain, gestational age, and fetal vs. adult status, factors that cannot be accounted for in or generalized to human occupational cohort exposure studies.

Animal studies can also test exposures that cannot be tested in human studies. For instance, some compounds such as polycyclic aromatic hydrocarbons generally induce brain tumors only through direct placental implantation, not through inhalation or dermal exposure as in worker populations. Workers also are rarely exposed to a single chemical but rather are exposed to many chemicals that probably interact to affect risk. Follow-up studies of occupationally induced brain cancer usually consist of too few affected subjects to permit pinpointing the causal chemicals, physical agents, work processes, or interactions.

Thus, no definitive link has been established between brain tumors and specific chemicals or strongly suspected carcinogens. For example, organochlorides, alkyl ureas, and copper sulfate compounds reliably induce cancer in laboratory animals. Yet studies of agricultural workers using these chemicals have about equally often produced negative and positive findings with regard to brain tumor risk. Nor have studies shown excess risk for workers involved in manufacturing these pesticides or fertilizers. In the meta-analysis of brain malignancies and farming by Khuder et al. (54), the 33 studies yielded a relative risk of 1.3 (95% CI 1.1–1.6). Although studies of workers in pesticide or fertilizer manufacturing have not shown an unusual risk of brain tumors, four of five studies of pesticide applicators have shown an increased risk of brain tumors with a nearly threefold median relative risk (55). In an occupational study of women in the United States, insecticide and fungicide exposure was associated with a small but statistically significant increased risk of brain tumors [odds ratio (OR) 1.3; 95% CI 1.1–1.5] (56). A recent study reported a positive association between wheat producing acreage and brain tumor mortality in Minnesota, Montana, and the Dakotas, suggesting a possible role of chlorophynoxy herbicides employed in wheat agriculture (57).

Because they involve production of many suspect carcinogens, synthetic rubber production and processing have received careful scrutiny by investigators who generally found a median increase in brain tumors of as much as 90% (36,38). A recent study also showed increased risks (58). The by-products of synthetic rubber processing, such as coal tars, carbon tetrachloride, N-nitroso compounds, and carbon disulfide, might appear to account for this increased risk of brain tumors. However, several studies showed no increased risk or a decreased risk of brain tumors in this industry, and studies have usually failed to show a link with a single chemical.

The picture seems clearer with vinyl chloride. Vinyl chloride induces brain tumors in rats, and nine of 11 studies of polyvinyl chloride production workers have shown a median twofold increased relative risk of dying from brain tumors. Some argue, however, that the small number of brain tumor cases and statistical insignificance cast doubt on causality. A recent review of the association between vinyl chloride and cancers indicated that the role of vinyl chloride in the development of brain tumors is still inconclusive (59). A large cohort study supports this notion, stating that mortality from brain cancer has attenuated, but the role of vinyl chloride is still unclear (60). Another study also did not demonstrate a relationship of brain tumors to the extent of vinyl chloride exposure (61). However, in reviews of animal studies that indicated neurocarcinogenicity of vinyl chloride, there have been difficulties in determining whether the tumors were primary or metastatic (62). Future plans for trying to understand the role, if any, of vinyl chloride in causing human brain tumors need to reconsider the biological plausibility of the association.

With formaldehyde, another long-suspected compound, conclusions for carcinogenesis are elusive. Formaldehyde produces cancer in laboratory animals, and nearly two million workers in the United States are occupationally exposed to it. Thirty epidemiological studies of segments of this large group were evaluated by Blair et al. (63). The unclear result was that the risk was elevated about 50% for those exposed in professional roles such as embalmers, pathologists, and anatomists (63). However, Blair et al., did not find a similar risk for industrial workers with formaldehyde exposure, and therefore rejected a causal role for formaldehyde in human brain tumorigenesis. Other unknown cofactors may obscure the true risk in industrially exposed workers and create a skewed estimate of risk in occupational groups.

3.5. Viruses

Certain viruses, like the suspect chemicals, have been found to induce brain tumors in animal studies. As in the chemical studies, small numbers and negative findings hinder epidemiological evaluation. Repeatedly, calls have been made for aggressive studies of the role of viruses (and other infectious agents), in causing human brain tumors (39,41). The putative cancer–virus connection has been supported by several studies of animal tumor induction by viral exposure. Unfortunately, very few epidemiological studies have addressed the virus–tumor relationship, probably because of the difficulties in designing meaningful studies.

Between 1955 and 1963, 92 million U.S. residents received Salk polio vaccine that may have been contaminated with simian virus 40 (SV40) (64,65). The levels of the SV40 varied among lots and manufacturers. The vaccine was treated with formalin, but because SV40 is less susceptible to formalin inactivation than poliovirus is, the IPV contained infectious SV40. Early cohort studies of cancer in SV40-contaminated poliovirus vaccine recipients generally demonstrated no association between SV40 exposure and cancer mortality among children in the United States (66–68) and in Germany (69). A recently published cohort study specifically examined the risk of ependymoma, osteosarcoma, and mesothelioma among Americans who as children received SV40-contaminated poliovirus vaccine. The study indicated that exposure was not associated with significantly increased rates of brain cancers, osteosarcomas, mesotheliomas, or medulloblastomas (70,71). Another study also showed no association between poliovirus immunization and childhood cancer among children in England, while yet another study showed a small association between poliovirus immunization and cancer among Australian children (72). Studies of maternal vaccination with the SV40-contaminated vaccines have shown a possible risk between vaccine-related exposure and childhood cancer [and brain cancers in particular (73,67)], but interpreting these reports is difficult because of the small number of cases and methodological limitations. As with other brain tumor investigations, studies of SV40 often resemble case reports and follow-ups, offering hints, clues, or perhaps merely coincidences that must be further tested.

Another virus investigated in a small number of studies is the JC virus, which is commonly excreted in urine, particularly by immunosuppressed, immunodeficient, and pregnant women. JC virus—a polyoma virus similar to SV40—induces brain tumors in experimental animals (74) and infects more than 70% of the human population worldwide (75). Khalili et al. (76) recently detected JC virus in paraffin-embedded tissues from children with medulloblastoma. JC virus was also found in a rare case of pleomorphic xanthoastrocytoma (77) and in oligodendrogliomas (78). However, JC virus exists in cancer-free subjects and its connection, if any, to tumorigenesis is only speculation at this time.

Contradicting studies have found that more mothers of children with medulloblastoma than mothers of children without it were exposed to chicken pox during pregnancy. Wrensch et al. (79) found that adults in the San Francisco Bay area with glioma were significantly less likely to report having had either chicken pox or shingles than controls were. This observation was supported by serological evidence that cases were less likely than controls to have antibody to varicella zoster virus, the agent for chicken pox and shingles (80). There is some plausibility that viruses and infectious agents could be an explanation for a proportion of brain tumors, and therefore intriguing results addressing this issue are preliminary.

3.6. Drugs and Medications

The need for research on drugs and medications is also evident, as very few studies have examined the effects of medications and drugs on the risk of adult brain tumors. A nonsignificant protective association was observed for headache, sleep, and pain medications [reviewed in Ref. (40)]. Ryan et al. (81) found that diuretics have a nonsignificant protective association against meningioma but the opposite for adult glioma. They also found essentially no association between antihistamine use and adult glioma but a 60% increased relative risk for meningioma. Three studies have assessed childhood brain tumors and prenatal exposures to some or all of the following drugs: fertility drugs, oral contraceptives, sleeping pills or tranquilizers, pain medications, antihistamines, and diuretics. These studies showed few significant findings. Prenatal exposure to diuretics was half as common among children with brain tumors as among controls in two studies, but twice as common in one study. Prenatal exposure to barbiturates has not been consistently or convincingly linked to childhood brain tumors. As nonsteroidal anti-inflammatory drugs may be protective against certain cancers, the role of these drugs in brain tumors should be investigated.

4. SUSCEPTIBILITY TO BRAIN TUMORS

The most generally accepted current model of carcinogenesis holds that cancers develop through accumulation of genetical alterations which allow the cells to grow out of control of normal regulatory mechanisms and/or escape destruction by the immune system. Some inherited alterations in crucial cell-cycle control genes, such as *p53*, as well as chemical, physical, and biological agents that damage DNA, are therefore considered candidate carcinogens. Although rapid advances in molecular biology, genetics, and virology promise to help elucidate the molecular causes of brain tumors, continued epidemiological work will be necessary to clarify the relative roles of different mechanisms in the full scope of human brain tumors. Genetical and familial factors implicated in brain tumors have been the subject of many studies and were previously reviewed by us (82).

4.1. Familial Aggregation

Because only a small proportion of brain tumors are due solely to heredity, most are probably due to gene–environment interactions. Although findings of familial cancer aggregation may suggest a genetical etiology, such aggregations can be the result of common familial exposure to environmental agents. Some epidemiological studies that compare family medical histories of brain tumor cases with those of controls find significantly increased family histories both of brain tumors and of other cancers. Other studies find no increase for any cancer, with a relative risk ranging from 1 to 1.8 and from 1 to 9 for brain tumors (82–85). These contradictions might be explained by differences in study methodologies, sample size, types of relatives included in the study, how cancers were ascertained and validated, and the country where the study was conducted.

Also supporting a genetical role in etiology are studies of cases reporting a high frequency of siblings with brain tumors, although twin studies have not. In a family study of 250 childhood brain tumor patients, we

(82) showed by segregation analysis that familial aggregation, although small, supported multifactorial inheritance, not chance alone. Segregation analyses of the families of more than 600 adult glioma patients revealed that a polygenic environment-interactive model best explained the pattern of occurrence of brain tumors (86). Segregation analyses of 2,141 first-degree relatives of 297 glioma families did not reject a multifactorial model, but an autosomal recessive model provided the best fit (87). The study estimated that 5% of all glioma cases were familial. Grossman et al. (88) showed that brain tumors can occur in families without a known predisposing hereditary disease and that the pattern of occurrence in many families suggests environmental causes. Given the previously described complexities of environmental impact and the multiplicity of possible heritable factors, more work will be required to delineate how genetical susceptibility affects brain cancer risk.

4.2. Hereditary Syndromes

A few rare genes and chromosomal abnormalities can greatly increase the chances of developing brain tumors. Numerous case reports have associated central nervous system tumors with gross malformations, including medulloblastoma with gastrointestinal and genitourinary system abnormalities, ependymoma with multisystem abnormalities, astrocytoma with arteriovenus malformation of the overlying meninges, and glioblastoma multiforme with adjacent arteriovenous angiomatous malformation and pulmonary arteriovenous fistula. Central nervous system tumors may also be associated with Down's syndrome, a disorder involving chromosome 21. Three epidemiological studies have found that brain tumor cases are two to five times more likely than controls to have a mentally retarded relative although the result was statistically significant in only one study [reviewed in Ref. (82)]. The heritability of brain tumors is also suggested by many reports of these tumors in individuals with hereditary syndromes such as tuberous sclerosis, neurofibromatosis types 1and 2, nevoid basal cell carcinoma syndrome, and syndromes involving adenomatous polyps [reviewed in Ref. (82)].

Although there is convincing evidence that genetics plays a role in most cancers, including brain tumors, inherited predisposition through high penetrant genetical traits to brain tumors probably accounts for only a very small percentage (5–10%) of these tumors (89). In a review of 16,564 cases of childhood cancers diagnosed from 1971 to 1983, and reported to the National Registry of Childhood Tumors in Great Britain, Narod et al. (89) estimated that the heritable fraction of childhood brain tumors was about 2%. In a population-based study of nearly 500 adults with glioma, only four individuals (less than 1%), all of whom were diagnosed in their thirties, reported having a known heritable syndrome (three had neurofibromatosis and one had tuberous sclerosis) (83).

Another class of heritable conditions are the cancer family syndromes [such as the Li–Fraumeni syndrome (LFS)], so called because individuals in affected families have an increased risk of developing certain types of cancers. In LFS, the cancers include brain tumors, sarcomas, breast cancer, and cancer of the adrenal gland. Individuals with LFS have inherited at least one copy of a defective gene—which can be passed from parent to child.

In some families, LFS has been linked to a gene mutation in *p53* on chromosome 17p (82). In addition, germline *p53* mutations were found to be more frequent in patients with multifocal glioma, glioma and another primary malignancy, and a family history of cancer. In a population-based study of malignant glioma, Li et al. (90) reported that *p53* mutation-positive patients were more likely to have a first-degree relative affected with cancer (58% vs. 42%) or a personal history of a previous cancer (17% vs. 8%). Further research needs to be done to determine the role of heredity, the frequency of *p53* mutations, and whether specific *p53* mutations correlate with specific exposures.

4.3. Metabolic Susceptibility

Genetic traits involved in susceptibility refer to more common genetic alterations that influence oxidative metabolism, carcinogen detoxification, and DNA stability and repair. The role of genetic polymorphisms (alternative states of genes established in the population) in modulating susceptibility to carcinogenic exposures has been explored in some detail for tobacco-related neoplasms but much less so for other neoplasms including gliomas. Due to rapid developments in genetic technology, an increasing number of potentially relevant polymorphisms are available for epidemiological evaluation, including genes involved in carcinogen detoxification, oxidative metabolism, and DNA repair. The first study to report the role of metabolic polymorphisms in brain tumor risk found that the variants of cytochrome P450 2D6 (*CYP2D6*) and glutathione transferase (*GSTT1*) were significantly associated with increased risk of brain tumors (91). Kelsey et al. (92) were unable to find an association of adult onset glioma with either the *GSTT1* null genotype or homozygosity for the *CYP2D6* variant poor-metabolizer genotype. However, when they stratified the data by histological subtype, there was a significant threefold increased risk for oligodendroglioma associated with the *GSTT1* null genotype. Trizna et al. (93) found no statistically significant associations between the null genotypes of glutathione transferase µ, *GSTT1*, and *CYP1A1* and the risk of adult gliomas. However, they observed an intriguing pattern with *N*-acetyltransferase acetylation status, with a nearly twofold increased risk for rapid acetylation and a 30% increased risk for intermediate acetylation.

It is unlikely that any single polymorphism will be sufficiently predictive of brain tumor risk. Therefore, a panel of relevant markers integrated with epidemiological data should be assessed in a large number of study participants to clarify the role of genetic polymorphisms and brain tumor risk.

4.4. Mutagen Sensitivity

Cytogenetical assays of peripheral blood lymphocytes have been extensively used to determine response to genotoxic agents. The basis for these cytogenetical assays is that genetical damage reflects critical events in carcinogenesis in the affected tissue. To test this hypothesis, Hsu et al. (94) developed a mutagen sensitivity assay in which the frequency of in vitro bleomycin-induced breaks in short-term lymphocyte cultures is used to measure genetical susceptibility. We (95) have modified the assay by using gamma radiation to induce chromosome breaks because radiation is a risk factor for brain tumors and can produce double-stranded DNA breaks and mutations. It is believed that mutagen sensitivity indirectly assesses the effectiveness of one or more DNA repair mechanisms. The following observations support this hypothesis. First, the relationship between chromosome instability syndromes and cancer susceptibility is well established (96). Patients with these syndromes also have defective DNA repair systems (97). Furthermore, patients with ataxia telangiectasia, who are extremely sensitive to the clastogenic effects of x-irradiation and bleomycin, differ from normal people in the speed with which aberrations induced by these agents are repaired but not in the number of aberrations produced (98).

Gamma-radiation-induced mutagen sensitivity is one of the few significant independent risk factors for brain tumors (95). DNA repair capability and predisposition to cancer are hallmarks of rare chromosome instability syndromes, and are related to differences in radiosensitivity. An in vitro study showed that individuals vary in lymphocyte radiosensitivity, which correlates with DNA repair capacity (95). Therefore, it is biologically plausible that increased sensitivity to gamma radiation results in increased risk of developing brain tumors because of individuals' inability to repair radiation damage. However, this finding needs to be tested in a larger study to determine the roles of mutagen sensitivity and radiation exposure in the risk of developing gliomas. The mutagen sensitivity assay has been shown to be an independent risk factor for other cancers including head and neck and lung, suggesting that the phenotype is constitutional (99). The breaks are not affected by smoking status or dietary factors (micronutrients) (100).

4.5. Chromosome Instability

A number of chromosomal loci have been reported to play a role in brain tumorigenesis because of the numerous gains and losses in those loci. For example, Bigner et al., (101) reported gain of chromosome 7 and loss of chromosome 10 in malignant gliomas and structural abnormalities involving chromosomes 1, 6p, 9p, and 19q; Bello et al. (102) reported involvement of chromosome 1 in oligodendrogliomas and meningiomas; and Magnani et al. (103) demonstrated involvement of chromosomes 1, 7, 10, and 19 in anaplastic gliomas and glioblastomas. Loss of heterozygosity for loci on chromosome 17p (104) and 11p15 (105) has also been reported.

There are few data on chromosomal alterations in the peripheral blood lymphocytes of brain tumor patients. Information on such changes might shed light on premalignant changes that lead to tumor development. We (95) demonstrated that compared with controls, glioma cases have less efficient DNA repair, measured by increased chromosome sensitivity to gamma radiation in stimulated peripheral blood lymphocytes. This inefficiency was shown to be an independent risk factor for glioma (95). Recently, we investigated whether glioma patients have increased chromosomal instability that could account for their increased susceptibility to cancer (106). Using fluorescent in situ hybridization methods, background instability in these patients was measured at hyper-breakable regions in the genome. Reports indicate that the human heterochromatin regions are frequently involved in stable chromosome rearrangements (107,108). Smith and Grosovsky (109) and Grosovsky et al. (110) reported that breakage affecting the centromeric and pericentromeric heterochromatin regions of human chromosomes can lead to mutations and chromosomal rearrangements and increase genomic instability. Our (106) study demonstrated that individuals with a significantly higher level of background chromosomal instability have a 15-fold increased risk of development of gliomas. A significantly higher level of hyperdiploidy was also detected. Chromosome instability leading to aneuploidy has been observed in many cancer types (111). Although previous studies have demonstrated the presence of chromosomal instability in brain tumor tissues (112–115), our (105) study was the first study to investigate the role of background chromosomal instability in the peripheral blood lymphocytes of patients with gliomas. This suggests that accumulated chromosomal damage in peripheral blood lymphocytes may be an important biomarker for identifying individuals at risk of developing gliomas.

5. SUMMARY

In summary, the etiology of brain tumors remains largely unknown. Biologically intensive studies incorporating new molecular genetical techniques have the potential to increase our understanding of the etiology of gliomas. Use of more consistent applied histopathological classification systems, and greater understanding and use of molecular and genetical markers to classify tumors, should help to create a more complete picture of the natural history and pathogenesis of brain tumors. We now know that primary brain tumors have many causes. Because not one cause thus far identified accounts for a very large proportion of cases, many possibilities remain that will enable us to discover important risk factors. Moreover, in the continuing search for explanations for this devastating disease, new concepts about neuro-oncogenesis might emerge, making the study of brain tumor epidemiology particularly exciting.

REFERENCES

1. American Cancer Society. Cancer Facts and Figures—2005. Atlanta, GA: American Cancer Society, Inc., 2005.
2. Kleihues P, Soylememzoglu F, Schauble B, et al. Histopathology, classification and grading of gliomas. Glio 1995; 15:11–221.
3. Kleihues P, Cavenee WK, eds. Tumors of the Central Nervous System: Pathology and Genetics. Lyon, France: International Agency for Research on Cancer, 1997.
4. Hill JR, Kuriyama N, Kuriyama H, Israel MA. Molecular genetics of brain tumors. Arch Neurol 1999; 56(4):439–441.
5. Hass-Kogan DA, Kogan SS, Yount G, Hsu J, Haas M, Deen DF, Israel MA. P53 function influences the effect of fractionated radiotherapy on glioblastoma tumors. Int J Radiat Oncol Biol Phys 1999; 43(2):399–403.
6. Ueki K, Ono Y, Henson JW, Efird JT, von Deimling A, Louis DN. CDKN2/p16 or RB alterations occur in the majority of glioblastomas and are inversly correlated. Cancer Res 1996; 56:150–153.
7. Ichimura K, Schmidt EE, Miyakawa A, Goike HM, Collins VP. Distinct patterns of deletion on 10p and 10q suggest involvement of multiple tumor suppressor genes in the development of astrocytic gliomas of different malignancy grades. Genes Chromosomes Cancer 1998; 22:9–15.
8. Biernat W, Tohma Y, Yonekawa Y, Kleihues P, Ohgaki H. Alterations of cell cycle regulatory genes in primary (de novo) and secondary glioblastomas. Acta Neuropathol 1997; 94:303–309.
9. Hunter SB, Abbot K, Varma VA, Olson JJ, Barnett DW, James CD. Reliability of differential PCR for the detection of EGFR and MDM2 gene amplification in DNA extracted from FFPE glioma tissues. J Neuropathol Exp Neurol 1995; 54:57–64.
10. Ritland SR, Ganju V, Jenkins RB. Region-specific loss of heterozygosity on chromosome 19 is related to the morphologic type of human glioma. Genes Chromosomes Cancer 1995; 12:277–282.
11. Bondy M, Wiencke J, Wrensch M, et al. Genetics of primary brain tumors: a review Neurooncology 1994; 18:69–81.
12. Hodges LC Smith JL, Garrett A, Tate S. Prevalence of glioblastoma multiforme in subjects with prior therapeutic radiation. J Neurosci Nurs 1992; 24:79–83.
13. Socie G, Curtis RE, Deeg HJ, Sobocinski KA, Filipovich AH, Travis LB, Sullivan KM, Rowlings PA, Kingma DW, Banks PM, Travis WD, Witherspoon

RP, Sanders J, Jaffe ES, Horowitz MM. New malignant diseases after allogeneic marrow transplantation for childhood acute leukemia. J Clin Oncol 2000; 18:348–357.

14. Karlsson P, Holmberg E, Lundell M, Mattsson A, Holm LE, Wallgren A. Intracranial tumors after exposure to ionizing radiation during infancy: a pooled analysis of two Swedish cohorts of 28,008 infants with skin hemangioma. Radiat Res 1998; 150:357–364.

15. Wrensch M, Miike R, Lee M, Neuhaus J. Are prior head injuries or diagnostic X-rays associated with glioma in adults? The effects of control selection bias. Neuroepidemiology 2000; 19:234–244.

16. Loomis DP, Wolf SH. Mortality of workers at a nuclear materials production plant at Oak Ridge, Tennessee, 1947–1990. Am J Ind Med 1996; 29:131–141.

17. Alexander V DiMarco JH. Reappraisal of brain tumor risk among U.S. nuclear workers: a 10-year review. Occup Med 2001; 16:289–315.

18. Wrensch M, Bondy ML, Wiencke J, Yost M. Environmental risk factors for primary malignant brain tumors: a review. J Neurooncol 1993; 17:47–64.

19. Gundestrup M, Storm HH. Radiation-induced acute myeloid leukaemia other cancers in commercial jet cockpit crew: a population-based cohort study. Lancet 1999; 354:2029–2031.

20. Irvine D, Davies DM. British Airways flightdeck mortality study 1950–1992. Aviat Space Environ Med 1999; 70:548–555.

21. Minert R, Michaelis J. Meta-anaylsis of studies on the association between electromagnetic fields and childhood cancer. Radiat Environ Biophys 1996; 35:11–18.

22. Kheifets LI, Afifi AA, Buffler PA, et al. Occupational electric and magnetic field exposure and brain cancer: a meta analysis. J Occup Environ Med 1995; 37:1327–1341.

23. Savitz DA, Cai J, van Wijngaarden E, Loomis D, Mihlan G, Dufort V, Kleckner RC, Nylander-French L, Kromhout H, Zhou H. Case-cohort analysis of brain cancer and leukemia in electric utility workers using a refined magnetic field job-exposure matrix. Am J Ind Med 2000; 38:417–425.

24. Robinson CF, Petersen M, Palu S. Mortality patterns among electrical workers employed in the U.S. construction industry, 1982–1987. Am J Ind Med 1999; 36:630–637.

25. Minder CE, Pfluger DH. Leukemia, brain tumors, and exposure to extremely low frequency electromagnetic fields in Swiss railway employees. Am J Epidemiol 2001; 153(9): 836–838.

26. Johansen C, Olsen JH. Risk of cancer among Danish electricity workers. A cohort study. Ugeskr Laeger 1999; 161:2079–2085.

27. Floderus B, Stenlund C, Persson T. Occupational magnetic field exposure and site-specific cancer incidence: a Swedish cohort study. Cancer Causes Control 1999; 10:323–332.

28. Feychting M, Floderus B, Ahlbom A. Parental occupational exposure to magnetic fields and childhood cancer (Sweden). Cancer Causes Control 2000; 11:151–156.

29. Sorahan T, Hamilton L, Gardiner K, Hodgson JT, Harrington, JM. Maternal occupational exposure to electromagnetic fields before, during, and after

pregnancy in relation to risks of childhood cancers: findings from the Oxford Survey of Childhood Cancers, 1953–1981 deaths. Am J Ind Med 1999; 35: 348–357.

30. Kheifets LI, Sussman SS, Preston-Martin S. Childhood brain tumors and residential electromagnetic fields (EMF). Rev Environ Contam Toxicol 1999; 159:111–129.

31. Wrensch M, Minn Y, Bondy ML. Epidemiology. In: Bernstein M, Berger M, eds. Neuro-oncology: The Essentials. New York: Thieme, 1999:1–17.

32. Wrensch M, Yost M, Mike R, Lee G, Touchstone J, et al. Adult glioma in relation to residential power frequency electromagnetic filed exposures in the San Francisco Bay Area. Epidemiology 1999; 10(5):523–527.

33. EMF Science Review Symposium. Breakout Group Reports for Epidemiological Research Findings. Symposium, San Antonio, TX, Jan 12–14, 1998. Research Triangle, NC: National Institute of Environmental Health Sciences, National Institute of Health 1998:121.

34. Floderus B, Tornqvist S, Stenlund C. Incidence of selected cancers in Swedish railway workers, 1961–1979. Cancer Causes Control 1994; 5(2):189–194.

35. Gurney JG, van Wijnagaarden E. Extremely low frequency electromagnetic fields (EMF) and brain cancer in adults and children: review and comment. Neuro-Oncology 1999; 1:212–220.

36. Preston-Martin S. Epidemiological studies of perinatal carcinogeneis. In: Napalkov NP, Rice JM, Tomatis L, et al., eds. Perinatal and Multigenerational Carcinogenesis. Lyon: IARC, 1989:289–314.

37. Magnani I, Guerneri S, Pollo B, Cirenei N, Colombo BM, Broggie G, Galli C, Bugiani O, DiDonato S, Finocchiaro G. Increasing complexity of the karyotype in 50 human gliomas: progressive evolution and de novo occurrence of cytogenetic alterations. Cancer Genet Cytogenet 1994; 75:77–89.

38. Bondy M, Wiencke J, Wrensch M, et al. Genetics of primary brain tumors: a review. J Neurooncol 1994; 18:69–81.

39. Wrensch M, Bondy ML, Wiencke J, et al. Environmental risk factors for primary malignant brain tumors: a review. J Neurooncol 1993; 17:47–64.

40. Preston-Martin S, Mack WJ. Neoplasms of the nervous system. In: Schottenfeld D, Fraumeni JF, eds. Cancer Epidemiology and Prevention. 2nd ed. New York: Oxford University Press, 1996:1231–1281.

41. Berleur MP, Cordier S. The role of chemical, physical, or viral exposures and health factors in neurocarcinogenesis: implications for epidemiologic studies of brain tumors. Cancer Causes Control 1995; 6:240–256.

42. Preston-Martin S, Pogoda JM, Mueller BA, et al. Results from an international case–control study of childhood brain tumors: the role of prenatal vitamin supplementation. Environ Health Perspect 1998; 106(suppl 3): 887–892.

43. Lee M, Wrensch M, Miike R. Dietary and tobacco risk factors for adult onset glioma in the San Francisco Bay Area (California, USA). Cancer Causes Control 1997; 8:13–24.

44. Mangino M, Scalan SR, O'Brien TJ. N-Nitrosamines in beer. In: Scalan RA, Tannenbaum SR, eds. N-Nitroso Compounds. American Chemical Society Symposium Series 1981; 174:229–245.

45. Norman MA, Holly EA, Preston-Martin S. Childhood brain tumors and exposure to tobacco smoke. Cancer Epidemiol Biomarkers Prev 1996; 5: 85–91.
46. Boffetta P, Tredaniel J, Greco A. Risk of childhood cancer and adult lung cancer after childhood exposure to passive smoke: a meta-analysis. Environ Health Perspect 2000; 108:73–82.
47. Scheidt S. Changing mortality from coronary heart disease among smokers and nonsmokers over a 20-year interval. Prev Med 1997; 26:441–446.
48. Schwarz B, Schmeiser-Rieder A. Epoidemiology of health problems caused by passive smoking. Wien Klin Wochenschr 1996; 108:565–569.
49. Cordier S, Iglesias MJ, Le Goaster C, Guyot MM, Mandereau L, Hemon D. Incidence and risk factors for childhood brain tumors in the le de France. Int J Cancer 1994; 59:776–782.
50. Filippini G, Farinotti M, Lovicu G, Maisonneuve P, Boyle P. Mothers' active and passive smoking during pregnancy and risk of brain tumors in children. Int J Epdemiol 1994; 57:769–774.
51. Magnani C, Pastore G, Luzzatto L, Carli M, Lubrano P, Terracini B. Risk factors for soft tissue sarcomas in childhood cancer: a case–control study. Tumori 1989; 75:396–400.
52. Sasco A, Vainio H. From in utero and childhood exposure to parental smoking to childhood cancer: a possible link and the need for action. Hum Exp Toxicol 1999; 18:192–201.
53. Thomas TL, Waxweiler RJ. Brain tumors and occupational risk factors. Scand J Work Environ Health 1986; 12:1–15.
54. Khuder SA, Mutgi AB, Schaub ES. Meta-analysis of brain cancer and farming. Am J Ind Med 1998; 34:252–260.
55. Bohnen NL, Kurland LT. Brain tumor and exposure to pesticides in humans: a review of the epidemiologic data. J Neurol Sci 1995; 132:110–121.
56. Cocco P, Heineman EF, Dosemeci M. Occupational risk factors for cancer of the central nervous system (CNS) among US women. Am J Ind Med 1999; 36:70–74.
57. Schreinemachers DM. Cancer mortality in four northern wheat-producing states. Environ Health Perspect 2000; 108:873–881.
58. Straif K, Weiland SK, Bungers M, Holthenrich D, Taeger D, Yi S, Keil U. Exposure to high concentrations of nitrosamines and cancer mortality among a cohort of rubber workers. Occup Environ Med 2000; 57:180–187.
59. McLaughlin JK, Lipworth L. A critical review of the epidemiologic literature on health effects of occupational exposure to vinyl chloride. J Epidemiol Biostat 1999; 4:253–275.
60. Mundt KA, Dell LD, Austin RP, Luippold RS, Noess R, Bigelow C. Historical cohort study of 10 109 men in the North American vinyl chloride industry, 1942–72: update of cancer mortality to 31 December 1995. Occup Environ Med 2000; 57:774–781.
61. Simonato L, L'Abbe' KA, Andersen A, Belli S, Comba P, Engholm G, Ferro G, Hagmar L, Langard S, Lundberg I, et al. A collaborative study of cancer incidence and mortality among vinyl chloride workers. Scand J Work Environ Health 1991; 17:159–169.

62. Rice JM, Wilbourn JD. Tumors of the nervous system in carcinogenic hazard identification. Toxicol Pathol 2000; 28:202–214.
63. Blair A, Saracci R, Stewart PA, Hayes RB, Shy C. Epidemiologic evidence on the relationship between formaldehyde exposure and cancer. Scand J Work Environ Health 1990; 16:381–393.
64. Shah KV. SV40 infections in simians and humans. Dev Biol Stand 1998; 94: 9–12.
65. Fisher SG, Weber L, Carbone M. Cancer risk associated with simian virus 40 contaminated polio vaccine. Anticancer Res 1999; 19:2173–2180.
66. Fraumeni JF Jr, Stark CR, Gold E, Lepow ML. Simian virus 40 in polio vaccine: follow-up of newborn recipients. Science 1970; 167:59–60.
67. Heinonen OP, Shapiro S, Monson RR, Hartz SC, Rosenberg L, Slone D. Immunization during pregnancy against poliomyelitis and influenza in relation to childhood malignancy. Int J Epidemiol 1973; 2:229–235.
68. Mortimer EA Jr, Lepow ML, Gold E, Robbins FC, Burton GJ, Fraumeni JF Jr. Long term follow-up of persons inadvertently inocualted with SV40 as neonates. N Engl J Med 1981; 305:1517–1518.
69. Geissler E. SV40 and human brain tumors. Prog Med Virol 1990; 37:211–222.
70. Strickler HD, Goedert JJ. Exposure to SV40-contaminated poliovirus vaccine and the risk of cancer—a review of the epidemiological evidence. Dev Biol Stand 1998; 94:235–244.
71. Strickler HD, Rosenberg PS, Devesa SS, Fraumeni JF Jr, Goedert JJ. Contamination of poliovirus vaccine with SV40 and the incidence of medulloblastoma. Med Pediatr Oncol 1999; 32:77–78.
72. Innis MD. Oncogenesis and poliomyelitis vaccine. Nature 1968; 219:972–973.
73. Farwell JR, Dohrmann GJ, Marrett LD, Meigs JW. Effect of SV49 virus-contaminated poliovaccine on the incidence of and type of CNS neoplasms in children: a population-based study. Trans Am Neurol Assoc 1979; 104:261–264.
74. Inskip PD, Linet MS, Heineman EF. Etiology of brain tumors in adults. Epidemiol Rev 1995; 17:382–414.
75. Del Valle L, Gordon J, Assimakopoulou M, Enam S, Geddes JF, Varakis JN, Katsetos CD, Croul S, Khalili K. Detection of JC virus DNA sequences and expression of the viral regulatory protein T-antigen in tumors of the central nervous system. Cancer Res. 2001; 61:4287–4293.
76. Khalili K, Krynska B, del Valle L, Katstos CD, Croul S. Medulloblastomas and the human neurotropic polymavirus JC virus. Lancet 1999; 353: 1152–1153.
77. Martin JD, King DM, Slauch JM, Frisque RJ. Differences in regulatory sequences of naturally occuring JC virus variants. J Virol 1985; 53:306–311.
78. Rencic A, Gordon J, Otte J, Curtis M, Kovatich A, Zoltick P, Khalili K, Andrews D. Detection of JC virus DNA sequence and expression of the viral oncoprotein, tumor antigen, in brain of immunocompetent patients with oligoastrocytoma. Proc Natl Acad Sci USA 1996; 93:7352–7357.
79. Wrensch M, Weinberg A, Wiencke J, Masters H, Miike R, Lee M. Does prior infection with varicella zoster virus influence risk of adult glioma?Am J Epidemiol 1997; 145:594–597.

80. Wrensch M, Weinberg A, Wiencke J, Miike R, Barger G, Kelsey K. Prevalence of antibodies to four herpesviruses among adults with glioma and controls. Am J Epidemiol 2001; 154:161–165.
81. Ryan P, Lee MW, North JB, et al. Risk factors for tumors of the brain and meninges: results from the adelaide adult brain tumor study. Int J Cancer 1992; 51:20–27.
82. Bondy M, Wiencke J, Wrensch M, et al. Genetics of primary brian tumors: a review. J Neurooncol 1994; 18:69–81.
83. Wrensch M, Lee M, Miike R, Newman B, Barger G, Davis R, West D, Glaser S, Wiencke J, Neuhaus J. Family and personal medical history of cancer and nervous system conditions among adults with glioma and controls. Am J Epidemiol 1997; 145:581–593.
84. Malmer B, Gronberg H, Bergenheim AT, Lenner P, Henriksson R. Familial aggregation of astrocytoma in northern Sweden: an epidemiological cohort study. Int J Cancer 1999; 81:366–370.
85. Hemminki K, Li X, Vaittinen P, Dong C. Cancers in the first-degree relatives of children with brain tumours. Br J Cancer 2000; 83:407–411.
86. de Andrade M, Barnholtz JS, Amos CI, Adatto P, Spencer C, Bondy ML. Segregation analysis of cancer in families of glioma patients. Genet Epidemiol 2001; 20:258–270.
87. Malmer B, Iselius L, Holmberg E, Collins A, Henriksson R, Gronberg H. Genetic epidemiology of glioma. Br J Cancer 2001; 84:429–434.
88. Grossman SA, Osman M, Hruban R, Piantadosi S. Central nervous system cancers in first-degree relatives and spouses. Cancer Invest 1999; 17:299–308.
89. Narod SA, Stiller C, Lenoir GM. An estimate of the heritable fraction of childhood cancer. Br J Cancer 1991; 63(6):993–999.
90. Li Y, Millikan RC, Carozza S, et al. p53 mutations in malignant gliomas. Cancer Epidemiol Biomarkers Prev 1998; 7:303–308.
91. Elexpuru-Camiruaga J, Buxton N, Kandula V, et al. Susceptibility to astrocytoma and meningioma: influence of allelism at glutathione S-transferase (GSTT1 and GSTM1) and cytochrome P-450 (CYP2D6) loci. Cancer Res 1995; 55:4237–4239.
92. Kelsey KT, Wrensch M, Zuo ZF, et al. A population-based case–control study of the CYP2D6 and GSTT1 polymorphisms and malignant brain tumors. Pharmacogenetics 1997; 7:463–468.
93. Trizna Z, de Andrade M, Kryitsis AP, et al. Genetic polymorphisms in glutathione S-transferase μ and θ N-acetyltransferase, and CYP1A1 and risk of gliomas. Cancer Epidemiol Biomarkers Prev 1998; 7:553–555.
94. Hsu TC, Johnston DA, Cherry LM, Ramkisson D, Schantz SP, Jessup JM, Winn RJ, Shirely L, Furlong C. Sensitivity to genotoxic effect of bleomycin in humans: possible relationship to environmental carcinogenesis. Int J Cancer 1989; 43:403–409.
95. Bondy ML, Kryitsis AP, Gu J, de Andrade M, Cunningham J, Levin VA, Bruner JM, Wei Q. Mutagen sensitivity and risk of gliomas: a case–control study. Cancer Res 1996; 56:1484–1486.
96. Busch D. Genetic susceptibility to radiation and chemotherapy injury: diagnosis and management. Int J Radiat Oncol Biol Phys 1994; 30:997–1002.

97. Wei Q, Spitz MR, Gu J, Cheng L, Xu X, Strom SS, Kripke ML, Hsu TC. DNA repair capacity correlates with mutagen sensitivity in lymphoblastoid cell lines. Cancer Epidemiol Biomarkers Prev 1996; 5:199–204.

98. Hittelman WN, Sen P. Heterogeneity in chromosome damage and repair rates after bleomycin in ataxia telangiectasia cells. Cancer Res 1988; 48: 276–279.

99. Caporaso N. Genetics of smoking-related cancer and mutagen sensitivity. J Natl Cancer Inst 1999; 91:1097.

100. Spitz MR, McPherson RS, Jiang H, Hsu TC, Trizna Z, Lee JJ, Lippman SM, Khuri RF, Steffen Batey L, Chamberlain RM, Schantz SP, Hong WK. Correlates of mutagen sensitivity in patients with upper aerodigestive tract cancer. Cancer Epidemiol Biomarkers Prev 1997; 6:687–692.

101. Bigner SH, Mark J, Burger PC, Mahaley MS, Bullard DE, Muhlbaier LH, Bigner DD. Specific chromosomal abnormalities in malignant gliomas. Cancer Res 1988; 88:405–411.

102. Bello MJ, De Campos JM, Kusak ME, Sarasa JL, Saez-Castresana J, Pestana A, Rey JA. Molecular analysis of chromosome 1 abnormalities in human gliomas reveals frequent loss of 1p in oligodendroglial tumors. Int J Cancer 1994; 57:172–175.

103. Magnani I, Guerneri S, Pollo B, Cirenei N, Colombo BM, Broggie G, Galli C, Bugiani O, DiDonato S, Finocchiaro G. Increasing complexity of the karyotype in 50 human gliomas: progressive evolution and de novo occurrence of cytogenetic alterations. Cancer Genet Cytogenet 1994; 75: 77–89.

104. Fults D, Tippets RH, Thomas GA, Nakamura Y, White R. Loss of heterozygosity for loci on chromosome 17p in human malignant astrocytoma. Cancer Res 1989; 49:6572–6577.

105. Sonoda Y, Iizuka M, Yasuda J, Makino R, Ono T, Kayama T, Yoshimoto T, Sekiya T. Loss of heterozygosity at 11p15 in malignant gliomas. Cancer Res 1995; 55:2166–2168.

106. El-Zein R, Bondy ML, Wang Li-E, de Andrade M, Sigurdson A, Kyritsis A, Levin V, Wei Q. Increased chromosomal instability in peripheral lymphocytes and risk of human gliomas. Carcinogenesis 1999; 20(5):811–815.

107. Larizza L, Doneda L, Ginelli E, Fossati G. C-heterochromatin vartiation and transposition in tumor progression. In: Prodi G, et al., eds. Cancer Metastasis: Biological and Biochemical Mechanisms and Clinical Aspects. New York: Plenum Publishing Corp., 1988:309–318.

108. Doneda L, Ginelli E, Agresti A, Larizza L. In situ hybridization analysis of interstitial C-heterochromatin in marker chromosomes of two human melanomas. Cancer Res 1989; 49:433–438.

109. Smith LE, Grosovsky AJ. Genetic instability on chromosome 16 in a human B lymphoblastoid cell line. Somat Cell Mol Genet 1993; 19:515–527.

110. Grosovsky AJ, Parks KK, Giver CR, Nelson SL. Clonal analysis of delayed karyotypic abnormalities and gene mutations in radiation-induced genetic instability. Mol Cell Biol 1996; 16:6252–6262.

111. Lengauer C, Kinzler KW, Vogelstein B. Genetic instability in colorectal cancers. Nature 1997; 386:623–627.

112. Arnoldus EPJ, Walters LBT, Voormolen JHC, van Duinen SG, Raap AK, van Der Ploeg M, Peters ACB. Interphase cytogenetics: a new tool for the study of genetic changes in brain tumors. J. Neurosurg 1992; 76:997–1003.
113. Mohapatra G, Kim DH, Feuerstein BG. Detection of multiple gains and losses of genetic material in ten glioma cell lines by comparative genomic hybridization. Genes Chromosomes Cancer 1995; 13:86–93.
114. Wernicke C, Thiel G, Lozanova T, Vogel S, Witkowski R. Numerical aberrations of chromosomes 1,2 and 7 in astrocytomas studied by interphase cytogenetics. Genes Chromosomes Cancer 1997; 19:6–13.
115. Rosso SM, Van Dekken H, Krishnadath KK, Alers JC, Kros JM. Detection of chromosomal changes by interphase cytogenetics in biopsies of recurrent astrocytomas and oligodendrogliomas. J Neuropathol Exp Neurol 1997; 56: 1125–1131.

26

New Perspectives on the Epidemiology of Hematological Malignancies and Related Disorders

Martha S. Linet and Susan S. Devesa

Division of Cancer Epidemiology and Genetics, National Cancer Institute, Bethesda, Maryland, U.S.A.

Gareth J. Morgan

Department of Hematology, Institute of Pathology, University of Leeds, Leeds, U.K.

1. INTRODUCTION

Hematological malignancies originate in the bone marrow, lymph nodes, and/or other lymphoid tissue with immune function. For decades, hematological malignancies were classified morphologically, culminating in an international effort that systematized the approach (1–5). Recently, a classification was adopted, under the auspices of the World Health Organization (WHO) (6), that incorporated information about normal development and function of cells according to lineage, pathogenesis, prognostic indicators, cytogenetic, and immunophenotypic characteristics (7–10). The epidemiology of hematological disorders is presented within two major sections in this chapter that correspond to the myeloid and lymphoid lineage origins of the entities.

2. MYELOID MALIGNANCIES AND MYELODYSPLASIA

Myeloid malignancies originate in pluripotential precursor cells that normally give rise to red blood cells, polymorphonuclear neutrophils, monocytes, and platelets. Acute myeloid leukemia (AML) may arise de novo or following a myelodysplastic or myeloproliferative state. Myelodysplastic syndromes (MDS) and myeloproliferative disorders (MPD), in contrast, are the clinical consequences of disordered, but relatively complete, maturation (11).

Acute myeloid leukemia comprises four categories in the WHO classification, including: (1) AML with recurrent cytogenetic abnormalities, (2) AML with multilineage dysplasia, (3) AML not otherwise categorized, and (4) AML/MDS that is therapy or occupation related (10). Nonrandomly occurring cytogenetic abnormalities characterizing the myeloid disorders include the Philadelphia (Ph) chromosome, which results from a reciprocal translocation in which the ABL oncogene from chromosome 9 is transposed to chromosome 22 within the breakpoint cluster region (BCR) of a gene, balanced translocations [such as t(8; 21)], partial deletions or loss of whole chromosomes (such as 5q or 7q), and numerical forms (such as trisomy 21). Acute myeloid leukemia is usually preceded by MDS among elderly and Fanconi's anemia patients, but not in 85–90% of younger patients. Myelodysplastic syndromes are characterized by bone marrow hyperplasia, peripheral cytopenias, and morphologically recognizable abnormal differentiation.

Myeloproliferative disorders, which are associated with bone marrow hyperplasia and an excess of differentiated progeny, include polycythemia vera (comprising progenitors of red blood cells), primary (essential) thrombocythemia (comprising the progeny of platelets), chronic myeloid leukemia (CML, comprising the progeny of myeloid cells), and chronic myelomonocytic leukemia (comprising the progeny of monocytes,) (12,13). Chronic myeloid leukemia results from transformation of a hemopoietic stem cell, is initially manifest by an excess of committed precursors and their differentiated progeny, and, after a typical interval of 4 years, transforms, following a "blast crisis," into acute leukemia.

Figure 1 depicts the international variation in age-adjusted incidence rates for AML and CML by gender. In general, for both AML and CML, age-adjusted incidence rates are lower for females than for males, although the geographic patterns are similar for both sexes. The highest AML rates occur in Caucasians in northern and western Europe, North America, and Oceania; midlevel rates in African-Americans, U.S. Hispanics, southern Europeans, and Israeli Jews; and the lowest rates in Asians (14). Chronic myeloid leukemia incidence varies less than the incidence for all other myeloid and lymphopoietic disorders, with only a fourfold gradient between the highest and the lowest age-standardized incidence rates.

International variation in age-adjusted rates, 1988–1992: Myeloid Disorders

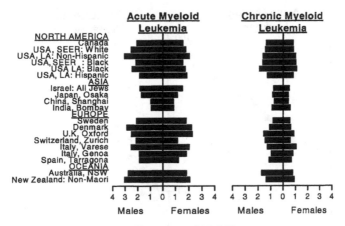

Rates per 100,000 person-years

Figure 1 International incidence rates for myeloid disorders (acute myeloid leukemia and chronic myeloid leukemia) per 100,000 (age-adjusted, World Standard) by continent and sex, 1988–1992. *Source*: From Parkin DM, et al. Cancer Incidence in Five Continents. Vol. 7. Lyon, France: IARC Scientific Publication Number 143, 1997.

As shown in Figure 2, AML incidence in the nine U.S. Surveillance, Epidemiology, and End Results (SEER) program registries peaks slightly in infancy, then declines until age 10 when incidence begins to rise slowly; after age 40, incidence rates rise more rapidly, with a slower rate of increase after age 70 (15). In late middle age, AML rates begin rising more rapidly in males than in females of both races, and in U.S. Caucasians than in African-Americans for persons of both sexes (Fig. 2). Chronic myeloid leukemia rates are consistently higher in males than in females, and higher in African-Americans than in U.S. Caucasians of both sexes until age 70; among the elderly, rates for African-Americans begin to flatten with increasing age, whereas rates for elderly Caucasians continue to increase linearly (Fig. 2).

2.1. Causes of Myeloid Malignancies and Myelodysplasia

Since few epidemiological studies focus solely on MDS, the literature is summarized for both AML and MDS in this section. Known risk factors explain a very small proportion of the leukemias, but more is known about the causes of AML than of other leukemia subtypes.

Ionizing radiation, consistently linked with increased risk of AML and other leukemias except CLL, induces DNA strand breaks (16). The most

SEER age-specific rates by race and sex,
1973-1997 Myeloid Disorders

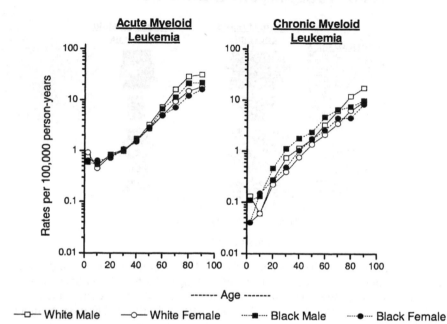

Figure 2 Age-specific incidence rates for myeloid disorders (acute myeloid leukemia and chronic myeloid leukemia) per 100,000 in the nine SEER areas by race and sex, 1973–1997. □, white male; ■, black male; o, white female; •, black female. *Source*: From Ries LAG, et al. SEER Cancer Statistics Review, 1973–1997. NIH Pub. No. 00–2789. Bethesda, MD: National Cancer Institute, 2000.

important epidemiological investigation quantifying cancer risks associated with radiation exposures is the long-term follow-up of the Japanese atomic bomb survivors. While the bombings of Hiroshima and Nagasaki occurred in 1945, follow-up studies of the survivors did not begin until 1950, so cancer incidence and mortality are unknown during 1945–1950 (17,18). A significant dose–response pattern was observed for AML incidence during 1950–1987. Males had twofold higher absolute excess risks than females, and those exposed before age 10 had substantially higher average absolute excess risks than persons who were older at exposure (19,20). Patients treated with radiotherapy for non-Hodgkin lymphoma, Ewing's sarcoma, and breast, uterine cervix, or uterine corpus cancers consistently experience two- to threefold excess risks of secondary AML 5–15 years after exposure (21–29). Increased AML risk has been observed following radiation treatment for ankylosing spondylitis (30), benign gynecological disorders (31), menorrhagia not associated with malignancy (32,33), peptic ulcers (34), and tinea capitis (35). In the occupational setting, relative risks of leukemia mortality were 6- to 8.8-fold increased among British (36) and U.S. (37,38) radiologists joining specialty societies during 1897–1921 and 1920–1929, but not in those joining later. Leukemia mortality was modestly increased in U.S. (39) and Japanese (40) radiological technologists who first worked before 1950 or 1960, respectively, and incidence was significantly elevated among Chinese technologists during 1950–80 (41). There is debate on whether diagnostic x-rays are etiologically associated with adult AML (42,43), or merely statistically linked because x-rays are used to evaluate early symptoms of AML (44). In contrast to ionizing radiation, there is insufficient evidence to link AML with nonionizing radiation, such as extremely low-frequency (ELF) residential magnetic field levels (45,46). Also, the data are inconsistent for AML and ELF magnetic fields in the occupational setting (47–56).

Chronic myelogenous leukemia also has been extensively studied in the context of radiation. Japanese atomic bomb survivors experienced a significantly elevated risk of CML (17,19). Radiotherapy for selected malignant and benign conditions, including histiocytosis X (58), uterine bleeding treated with intrauterine radiation (33), and metastatic papillary and follicular thyroid cancer treated with low-dose ^{131}I (59), has been associated with increased risk of CML in some clinical reports (60,61) and a few epidemiological studies (19,33). Thorotrast, has been linked with increased risk of CML (62).

Benzene-exposed painters, printers, and workers employed in chemical, rubber, Pliofilm, and shoe manufacturing and in petroleum refining (63–68) industries have consistently shown 1.9- to 10-fold increased risks of AML and aplastic anemia. Chronic myeloid leukemia has been reported among benzene-exposed workers in China (69,70) and the United States (64), but the small numbers of cases preclude precise quantification of risk. Excesses of myelomonocytic leukemia (71) and myelofibrosis (72) have been identified among pressmen and printers. Risks were also elevated for MDS, CML, ALL, CLL, or non-Hodgkin lymphoma (NHL) in a few studies (64,66,67,73–79). Much debated aspects of the findings of U.S. (64) and Chinese (67) studies of benzene workers are risk estimates, dose–response, and latency at low benzene exposure levels (80–85).

Treatment of Hodgkin lymphoma, non-Hodgkin lymphoma, multiple myeloma (MM), polycythemia vera, and breast, ovarian, or testicular cancers with alkylating agents is associated with increased risk of therapy-related MDS (t-MDS) and AML. The risk is related to cumulative dose and is characterized by a typical latency of 5–7 years, a preleukemic phase in 70% of patients developing t-MDS/AML, trilineage dysplasia, and partial deletions of chromosomes 5 and 7 (86). Some alkylating agents (e.g., melphalan), pose higher risks than others (e.g., cyclophosphamide) (24,26,87–92). Treatment with topoisomerase II inhibitors (specifically epipodophyllotoxins) has also been linked with elevated risk of t-AML, which is generally not related to cumulative dose and typically develops after a 2 year latency, not preceded by a preleukemic phase, characterized by the t(11q23) translocation (93–95). Platinum-based chemotherapy used to treat ovarian (92) and testicular cancers (96) has been associated with elevated risks of t-MDS/AML, as have treatments with mitoxantrone and methotrexate or methotrexate and mitomycin C for breast cancer (97), and pretransplantation chemotherapy (e.g., mechlorethamine) (98) and/or conditioning treatments (e.g., total body irradiation) (99), particularly at doses >12 Gy, or VP-16 (91) in preparation for autologous stem cell transplantation for lymphoma or other malignant diseases (98). Predisposing genetic factors are currently under study (100,101).

Several large studies (102–104), but not all (105,106), have linked cigarette smoking with small 1.2- to 1.5-fold excesses of AML (107). Thus, the evidence linking smoking and AML is less convincing than data linking smoking with many other cancers. Limited data link smoking with MDS (108).

Many other exposures have been tested for an increased AML or MDS risk, but there are limited data to support them, inconsistencies, or no measurable association. These include painters (109,110); machine operators and assemblers (111); embalmers (112,113); garage and transport workers (114,115); shoe workers (116); hairdressers and cosmetologists (117,118); seamen on tankers (119); and laboratory and science technicians (120). There are inconsistent findings for AML/MDS risk in farmers (121–124), which may reflect the variation in agricultural workers' exposure to pesticides, fertilizers, diesel fuel and exhaust, or infectious agents (125–130). But increased risk of myeloid leukemia occurred within 10 years in 20,000 persons under age 19 who resided in Seveso, Italy, after an industrial accident contaminated the region with 2,3,7,8-tetrachlorobibenzo-*p*-dioxin (TCDD) (131).

2.2. Familial Aggregation

Families with multiple members in different generations who develop AML, MDS, or both are rare, but data support the contribution of highly penetrant mutations in leukemia susceptibility genes (132). Some familial AML cases are characterized by monosomy 7 (133,134), others demonstrate loss of the long arm of chromosome 5 (135,136), while yet a third group have other or no karyotypic abnormalities (137). Approximately 5% of AML/MDS may be associated with inherited genetical syndromes (138), such as Down syndrome (139), the bone marrow failure syndromes of Fanconi's anemia (140), Bloom's (141,142) and Schwachman–Diamond syndromes (143), amegakaryocytic thrombocytopenia, dyskeratosis congenita, and Kostmann's syndrome (144).

2.3. Genetic Polymorphisms

Because the etiology of most hematological malignancies is believed to be multifactorial, common genetical variants, including single-nucleotide polymorphisms, may influence susceptibility.

The metabolizer enzymes *GST T1*, *GST M1*, and *GST P1* detoxify environmental carcinogens associated with AML/MDS, such as chemicals in cigarette smoke, ethylene oxide, and certain cytotoxic drugs (145–148). It was postulated that homozygosity for null alleles for one or more *GST*s might predispose to increased risk of AML/MDS, due to the inability to detoxify specific leukemogens (149,150). Persons with null alleles for *GST T1* were at modestly increased risk of developing de novo MDS/AML in some (145,149,151,152), but not all (153,154), case–control studies. However, three studies showed that null alleles for *GST T1* were not related to risk of t-AML (153–155). Individuals with null alleles for *GST M1* were at elevated risk of developing de novo AML (151,152) or MDS (156), but not t-AML (154,155), whereas persons with null alleles for both *GST T1* and *GST M1* experienced an excess risk of developing t-AML (157). Risks of t-AML were increased among patients previously treated with chemotherapy agents that are known substrates of *GST P1*; the *GST P1* codon 105 Val allele occurred more often in the t-AML cases than in those with de novo AML (155). The null genotype of *GST T1* was not associated with increased risk of developing t-AML among children treated with epipodophyllotoxins for ALL (100).

The potential predisposing nature of the slow acetylator *N*-acetyl transferase (NAT) status to leukemogenesis was suggested by increased DNA adduct levels in peripheral blood lymphocytes (158), but adult AML was not linked with *NAT2* metabolizer status in the large U.K. case–control study (159).

Roddam et al. (2000) (159a) found that the *CYP2C19* PM phenotype, but not the *CYP1A1*3* allele, was associated with an increased risk of both AML and sAML; there were no interactions with age, gender, or smoking status for either of these alleles. Among 447 patients with an abnormal karyotype treated in the U.K. Medical Research Council AML clinical trials, the *CYP1A1*2B (Val)* variant allele was overrepresented in patients with *NRAS* mutation compared with no mutation in both the entire population and the poor-risk karyotype group of patients with partial or complete deletion of chromosomes 5 or 7 or abnormalities of chromosome 3 (160). There were no differences in the frequencies for the *CYP3A5*3* or the *CYP3A4*1B* alleles between childhood ALL patients who developed t-AML and those who did not develop t-AML (161).

NQO1, an enzyme induced by synthetic antioxidants and cruciferous vegetables, detoxifies quinones, derivatives, and other natural and synthetic compounds, and protects cells against oxidative stress (162,163). Individuals who are homozygous for the variant allele completely lack *NQO1* activity, while heterozygotes have low-to-intermediate activity compared to individuals with the wild-type alleles. Disruption of the *NQO1* gene in mice has been shown to cause myeloid hyperplasia of bone marrow (164). Occupational benzene poisoning (e.g., hematotoxicity, particularly leukopenia), which was strongly linked with development of hematopoietic neoplasms in Chinese benzene-exposed workers, was associated with polymorphisms in genotypes of enzymes that activate (i.e., *CYP2E1*) and detoxify (i.e., *NQO1*) benzene and its metabolites (165). The *NQO1* variant allele also appears to be significantly over-represented in therapy-related myeloid leukemias in adults (154,166). In addition, null alleles for *NQO1* predisposed to increased risk of de novo AML in adults (167). Infants with leukemia characterized by *MLL* gene rearrangements were eightfold more likely to have low *NQO1* function than healthy children or childhood leukemia patients with *TEL-AML1* gene fusions or with hyperdiploidy (168). Low *NQO1* function was not more common in childhood ALL patients treated with chemotherapy who developed tAML than in those who did not develop tAML (161).

Limited data suggest that variant alleles and/or mutations in genes involved in DNA repair may be important in the etiology of t-AML and genetic syndromes that predispose to increased risk of myeloid leukemias (169). At least one copy of the variant allele XRCC1 399Glu conferred a protective effect against t-AML in a small case–control study (170). Families with individuals homozygous for mutations in mismatch repair genes are at increased risk for developing hematological malignancies and/or neurofibromatous, type 1, at an early age (171,172). Patients with Fanconi's anemia, a condition characterized by cells that are sensitive to DNA cross-linking, are at increased risk of developing AML (173,174).

3. DISEASES OF LYMPHOID LINEAGE

The WHO classification (6) recognizes: (1) precursor disease lymphoid disorders comprising stem or immature precursor cells, including pediatric and adult forms of acute lymphocytic leukemia (ALL), and (2) peripheral disease lymphoid disorders comprising functional peripheral B-cells and T-cells, which include non-Hodgkin lymphoma (NHL), Hodgkin lymphoma (HL), chronic lymphocytic leukemia (CLL), and multiple myeloma (MM) (6,8). Peripheral diseases are further classified according to B-cell (further categorized by stage of differentiation of the cells compared to the germinal center) or T-cell lineage. Understanding of etiology requires recognition of the characteristic genetic instability and highly variable history of the normal life cycle of lymphocytes, which undergo genetic recombination and mutation to generate high-affinity antibodies (175,176).

3.1. Acute Lymphoblastic Leukemia

Acute lymphoblastic leukemia (ALL) includes three subtypes: (1) precursor B-cell ALL, (2) precursor T-cell ALL, and (3) Burkitt-cell leukemia (6). Acute lymphoblastic leukemia is the most common cancer in children, comprising about 30% of all pediatric cancers in most populations internationally except in Africa and the Middle East (177). Patterns for childhood ALL, similar to those for adults, demonstrate highest incidence in Hispanics (pediatric ALL is highest in Costa Rica and in Latinos in Los Angeles), and lowest rates in African-Americans, the Middle East, and India (Fig. 3). Pediatric ALL is notably higher in U.S. Caucasians than in African-Americans of both sexes. The age-specific incidence pattern for ALL is quite distinctive, with a peak at ages 2–4, followed by a declining incidence rate throughout the remainder of childhood, adolescence, and early adulthood to a nadir at age 40; subsequently, incidence of ALL rises with increasing age to a second, albeit lower, peak among the elderly (Fig. 4). Incidence rates of ALL are consistently highest in males than in females at all ages.

Ionizing radiation is among the best documented causes of ALL. Exposed Japanese atomic bomb survivors who were less than 10 years old at exposure experienced the highest excess absolute risks for ALL. Risks decreased by 5% for each 1-year increase in-age, and peaked at less than 10 years after exposure (178). The pattern of risk following adult exposure was similar, but with a substantially lower peak also occurring less than 10 years after exposure, the excess absolute risk declining rapidly at 14% per year. Females had a risk less than half of that for males.

While it has been hypothesized that children of radiation workers are at an increased risk of ALL (179), risks are probably very small or not increased. A large record linkage U.K. study revealed a small increase in childhood leukemia and NHL of children of nuclear workers, but no dose–response trend (180). There was no association in a case–control record linkage study in Ontario, Canada (181). Small clusters of childhood leukemia cases in geographical proximity to nuclear plants in the United Kingdom in the mid-1980s prompted large surveys, which revealed excess leukemia and lymphoma in persons under age 25 living near nuclear fuel reprocessing or weapons production plants (particularly the Sellafield and Dounreay plants) (182), but no excess among populations residing close to nuclear plants generating electricity (183–185). Environmental radiation levels measured in proximity to Sellafield and other nuclear facilities were too low to be etiologically related.

Exposure to pesticides also has been extensively studied for ALL risk, where the overall evidence is consistent with an association. In California, excess risks of childhood leukemia were linked with mothers' and fathers' use of pesticides and herbicides in gardens and residences during pregnancy

(186,187), with the use of indoor insecticides from the beginning of pregnancy until diagnosis (188), and with the use of a professional pest control service (187). Childhood leukemia in Denver was associated with the use of pest strips in the home during the last 3 months of pregnancy and postnatally (189). Pesticide application on farms was linked with a modest increase in childhood leukemia in Germany (190), as was preconception paternal exposure to pesticides in Quebec (191). Frequent use of pesticides in the garden or on interior plants during pregnancy was associated with elevated risk of childhood ALL in offspring who were carriers of the *CYP1A1m1* and *CYP1A1m2* polymorphisms in Quebec (192). In contrast, childhood ALL was not associated with pesticide use density at the residence at diagnosis in California (193), nor in relation to parental occupational exposure to pesticides in the Netherlands (194) or Sweden (195), or paternal exposure to chlorophenate fungicides in British Columbia sawmills (196).

Lifestyle exposures also are implicated in ALL risk. Paternal smoking during the preconception period was associated with significantly elevated risks of childhood ALL in Shanghai, China (197), and in the United Kingdom, the latter based on two investigations (198,199), but not in Italy (200). Paternal preconception smoking was linked with an excess of leukemia among children less than 18 months old in the United States and Canada (201). Most investigations have shown 20–30% reduced risks of ALL among children who were *breastfed* during infancy (202–205), with a declining risk observed for prolonged breastfeeding in two investigations (205,206). Other studies have shown a smaller reduction in risk (207) or no clear relationship (208).

A large literature on childhood leukemia clusters (209–211) suggests an infectious etiology for childhood ALL. Some of the supportive studies utilize such measures as maternal infection during pregnancy (212,213); the type (214–217) and timing (217–220) of childhood vaccinations; daycare attendance (204,205,221,222), household crowding (223); household pets (221,224); and seasonal variation in diagnosis (225–227), temporal trends in incidence among the youngest children (228,229), and ecological investigations assessing correlations of childhood ALL birth and diagnosis data with mycoplasma pneumonia surveillance data (210). The specific infectious agents, however, have not been identified. Screening studies have shown no novel herpesvirus genomes (230,231), or evidence of genomes of the JC and BK polyoma viruses (232) in childhood ALL cases.

Two- to threefold excesses of childhood leukemia were observed in children residing in homes with high levels of extremely low-frequency 60 Hz magnetic field (EMF) exposures induced by nearby power lines based on proxy (233,234) or measured levels in the United States (188) and Sweden (235). Larger studies, however, characterized by more extensive and direct measures of children's exposures (236–239), and pooled analyses (240,241) revealed no increase in risks for children residing in homes with magnetic field

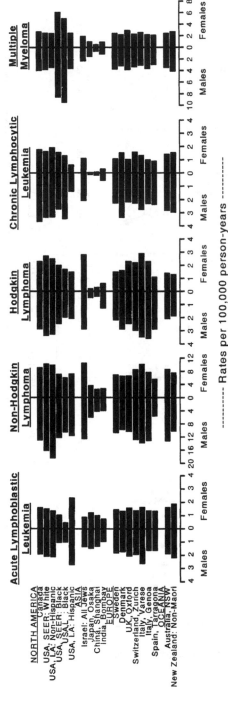

Figure 3 International incidence rates for lymphoid disorders (acute lymphoblastic leukemia, non-Hodgkin lymphoma, Hodgkin lymphoma, chronic lymphocytic leukemia, and multiple myeloma) per 100,000 (age-adjusted, World Standard) by continent and sex, 1988–1992. *Source:* From Parkin DM, et al. Cancer Incidence in Five Continents. Vol. 7. Lyon, France: IARC Scientific Publication Number 143, 1997.

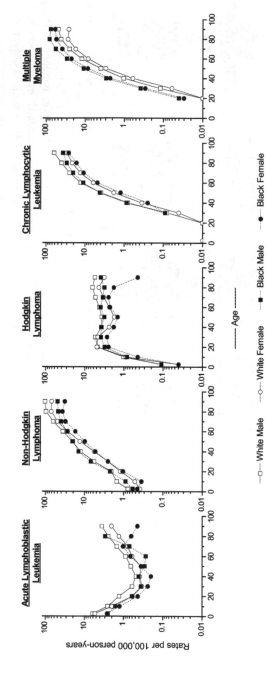

Figure 4 Age-specific incidence rates for lymphoid disorders (acute lymphoblastic leukemia, non-Hodgkin lymphoma, Hodgkin lymphoma, chronic lymphocytic leukemia, and multiple myeloma) per 100,000 in the nine SEER areas by race and sex, 1973–1997. □, white male; ■, black male; o, white female; •, black female. *Source:* From Ries LAG, et al. SEER Cancer Statistics Review, 1973–1997. NIH Pub. No. 00-2789. Bethesda, MD: National Cancer Institute, 2000.

exposures less than 0.3 or 0.4 μT, but a twofold excess among the very small percentage exposed to 0.3 or 0.4 μT or greater.

Individuals with specific polymorphisms in the methylenetetrahydrofolate reductase gene (*MTHFR*) have been found to be at reduced risk of adult ALL (242). Folic acid is essential in the transfer of methyl groups to various biochemical targets in mammalian tissues involved in amino acid metabolism and in the synthesis of the purine and pyrimidine components of DNA and RNA (243). The *MTHFR* and ALL relationship was found for a common polymorphism (677 C → T) that results in reduced specific activity of the enzyme, thus affecting folate metabolism (244,245). Up to 15% of individuals are homozygous (677TT) for this allelic variant (244–246); homozygotes have significantly reduced levels of enzyme activity (245).

3.2. Hodgkin Lymphoma

The two major forms are classical Hodgkin lymphoma (including nodular sclerosis, mixed cellularity, and lymphocyte depleted) and lymphocyte-predominant nodular HL (8). At least 95% of the pathognomonic Reed–Sternberg (RS) cells of classic HL are clonally derived malignant cells of germinal center B-cell origin, characterized by crippling mutations due to functional defects in the immunoglobulin gene regulatory elements (247–251). Approximately 2% of RS cells appear to be derived from T-cells (250).

Hodgkin lymphoma is characterized by a bimodal age-specific incidence pattern in most western populations, with rates low in early childhood, rising to a peak early in the third decade, then declining to a nadir at age 40, and subsequently rising until age 70. In developing countries there is a small peak in childhood among boys, low rates among young adults, and a second peak among the elderly (14). Incidence rates for HL are higher in U.S. Caucasians than in African-Americans in early adulthood. From ages 25 to age 60, rates are higher in males of both races than in females; subsequent to age 70, rates are highest in U.S. Caucasian males, somewhat lower although overlapping in U.S. Caucasian females and African-American males, but decline precipitously in African-American females (Fig. 4).

The differing incidence patterns of HL in economically advantaged vs. disadvantaged populations and the relationship of HL subtypes with social class suggest that HL may develop as a rare consequence of a common infection. Risk is believed to increase if occurrence of infections typically encountered in early childhood is delayed until adolescence or young adulthood (252). Growing evidence, including the presence of Epstein–Barr virus (EBV) genomes in RS cells and the expression of viral proteins and other evidence of EBV latent infections in up to 50% of HL tumors, suggests that EBV is etiologically related to HL (253–255). Infectious mononucleosis, a common viral disorder caused by EBV, has been linked with HL in numerous case–control and cohort studies [reviewed in Mueller (252)]. In large cohorts of infectious mononucleosis patients in Denmark and Sweden followed for cancer occurrence, significantly elevated risks were seen only for Hodgkin lymphoma and skin cancer. The excess risk for HL persisted for up to two decades, but declined with time since diagnosis (256). Glaser et al. (253) examined data from 14 studies that had applied EBV assays to HL tumors, and found that EBV-associated HL was notably higher in Hispanics than in whites, in those with mixed cellularity than in those with nodular sclerosis histology, in children from economically less developed than in those from more developed geographical regions, and in young adult males than in females. Recently, investigators found a stronger association of a reported history of infectious mononucleosis with DNA evidence for EBV in the RS cells of young adults with HL who typed positive for HLA-DPB1*0301 than in cases who did not type positive for this HLA subtype, which may implicate an inherited component to susceptibility to EBV in the etiology of Epstein–Barr DNA-positive HL (257).

Some occupational studies have implicated exposures to HL. These include employment in agriculture, particularly among those exposed to livestock and meat processing, farming (258,259), and woodworking (260,261).

Familial HL has been estimated to occur in approximately 4–5% of all HL cases, with a male-to-female ratio of 1.5 in the familial HL population similar to that of sporadic HL (263). In a linked registry study in Israel, the interval between lymphoma occurring among siblings was 1–4 years for siblings with concordant types of HL or NHL, whereas the interval ranged from 16 to 21 years for HL/NHL among sibling pairs (264). Elevated risks of NHL and HL have been observed among subjects who had a sibling with lymphoma (265,264) and among first-degree relatives of children with NHL (266). Lymphoma was 2.5-fold increased among siblings of lymphoma probands and the risk of HL in siblings was even higher for identical twins (267), whereas the risk was lower for HL among family members other than siblings. The difference may reflect the greater likelihood of familial HL concordance generally occurring among siblings in the 15- to 34-year age group (263), whereas familial concordant NHL may be more common in parent/childpairs (268).

3.3. Non-Hodgkin Lymphoma

The classification of NHL is complex. Follicular lymphoma is characterized by the translocation t(14;18). Occurrence of this translocation in the peripheral blood of normal individuals (269–271) suggests that additional genetic abnormalities are required in the pathogenesis of follicular lymphoma. Large-cell lymphoma in the new WHO classification is clinically distinct (272), combining the previously differentiated immunoblastic and centroblastic NHL and nonendemic Burkitt's lymphoma (e.g., those occurring outside Africa) (273). Marginal-zone lymphoma, characterized by an indolent natural history, often presents at extranodal sites (including thyroid, salivary glands, and stomach) that were closely associated with chronic inflammatory conditions.

Internationally, NHL is highest among non-Hispanic whites in the U.S., followed in declining order by rates in Italians, Canadians, Israeli Jews, Australians and Africans-Americans; lowest rates occur in China, India, and other parts of Asia and in Spain (Fig. 3). Incidence of NHL, all types combined, rises dramatically with increasing age, beginning in early childhood among U.S. boys and in early adolescence among girls, to age 70, when the rate of the increase slows down (Fig. 4). While incidence rates are higher in males than in females at all ages in the United States (Fig. 4), internationally the male excess is most marked among children [274]. Before age 70 there is little racial difference in U.S. incidence rates, whereas after age 70, rates are higher in whites than in African-Americans of either gender (Fig. 4).

There are several known associations for exposures and NHL. Severe immunosuppression from medication, with or without organ transplantation, may dramatically increase the risk of developing NHL (275,276). Post-transplantation lymphoproliferative disorders (PTLD) occur following renal (associated with 20- to- 59-fold increases) (275,277–279), heart, or bone marrow transplants (associated with 48- to 336-fold increases) (278,280). Risks of PTLD appear to be lower in recent years (281), but some persons transplanted recently experienced higher PTLD risks, including patients with graft- vs. -host disease and recipients of HLA-mismatched or T-cell depleted bone marrow transplants (282,283).

Autoimmune or connective tissue disorders that have been linked with 2- to 44-fold increased risks of NHL include systemic lupus erythematosus (284–287), rheumatoid arthritis (288–290), Felty syndrome (291), Sjogren's disease (276,292), and celiac disease and/or dermatitis herpetiformis (293–296). The highest relative risks often derive from hospital-based epidemiological investigations, while lower relative risks generally characterize population-based studies. Subtype information is limited. In patients with an autoimmune disorders treated with an immunosuppressive drug, it is not clear whether an excess of NHL occurring among these patients is due to the autoimmune disorders per se or to one or more immunosuppressive drugs sometimes used to treat the disorder (284).

There are several viral etiologies to NHL. Epidemiological, serological, and molecular data have consistently linked early EBV infection with African Burkitt's lymphoma, in conjunction with malaria as a cofactor, the latter implicated because of the overlapping geographical distribution of malaria and Burkitt's lymphoma, high rates of both in the same population, and reduction in the occurrence of both conditions following malarial prophylaxis (297).

Non-Hodgkin lymphoma may be one of the presenting manifestations of the acquired immunodeficiency disorder (AIDS) and is the most frequent malignancy associated with the human immunodeficiency virus (HIV) (the relative risks range from 60 to 100, and the cumulative incidence is as high as 29%) (298–300). AIDS patients with the CCR5-delta 32 allele experience a threefold lower risk of developing NHL (301).

Gastric mucosal-associated lymphoid tissue (MALT) lymphomas, low-grade B-cell lymphomas, are usually preceded by infection with *Helicobacter pylori*, which is often not clinically recognized (302,303). Eradication of *H. pylori* following treatment with antibiotics often results in complete remission of the gastric B-cell MALT lymphoma, which appears to be stable, although PCR sometimes reveals residual evidence of monoclonal B cells (304).

Numerous studies have reported small increases in the risk of NHL among farmers in the United States and elsewhere (121,305), pesticide applicators (306,307), and grain workers (308,309). Higher risks were observed among farmers who reported using any pesticides, 2,4-dichlorophenoxyacetic acid (2,4-D) pesticides, or organophosphate insecticides more than 20 days per year (310,311); using dichloro-diphenyl-trichloroethane (DDT) at least 5 days per year (312); or mixing and applying herbicides themselves (310). Herbicides increased risk of follicular large-cell NHL, and farmers using dieldrin, toxaphene, lindane, atrazine, and fungicides had significantly elevated risks of t(14;18)-positive, but not 5(14;18)-negative, NHL (313). Small excesses of NHL, particularly follicular NHL, have been observed in meat packaging and processing workers (313a). Not all studies of farmers (124) pesticide applicators (125), or persons agriculturally exposed to 2,4-D, phenoxy acids, and the associated contaminant TCDD, have found elevated risks. Risks of NHL were also not associated with measured levels of DDT (313b), individual organochlorine compounds, or summed chlordane related compounds in serum obtained years prior to diagnosis of NHL, although there was a strong dose–response relation between measured serum PCB concentrations and NHL (313b).

Studies of chemical manufacturing workers exposed to TCDD have been inconsistent for NHL (314–316). A pooled analysis of 21,863 workers exposed to phenoxy herbicides, chlorophenols, and dioxins from 36 cohorts in 12 countries showed a nonsignificant modest excess risk of NHL [standardized mortality ratio (SMR) = 1.39, 95% CI = 0.89–2.06, based on 24 deaths] (317). In 1997, the International Agency for Research on Cancer classified TCDD as a Group 1 human carcinogen, based on excesses for all cancers combined observed in four cohort studies (317a). Significant excess risks of NHL (and/or CLL) have been reported among rubber manufacturing and processing workers in one U.S. cohort (318–320). Non-Hodgkin lymphoma (321) and sometimes CLL were significantly increased among some, but not most, workers manufacturing styrene or butadiene

(322,323) (see section on CLL below). Similarly, occupational exposure to ethylene oxide has also not been conclusively linked with NHL (324,324a). Other occupational solvent exposures sometimes linked with elevated risk of NHL include benzene (67), carbon tetrachloride, xylene, carbon disulfide, and hexane (325). These results require further investigation.

A few case–control (326,327) and cohort investigations (328,329) have reported increased risks for high-grade and follicular NHL, respectively, associated with cigarette smoking, but the majority of large studies found no relationship (105,106,329a). The small epidemiological literature evaluating diet includes studies linking red meat (330,331) particularly if broiled or barbecued (332), beef, pork, lamb (332), and butter, liver, ham, milk, and dietary products containing transunsaturated fat (332) with elevated risks, while fruit (330), carrots, and whole-grain products (332a) reduced risks of NHL. Alcohol consumption by women was associated with reduced NHL in two studies (330,331). Small increases in risk were associated with the use of black or brown hair dyes for 10 or more years in two studies (333,334), but not in others (335).

3.4. Chronic Lymphocytic Leukemia

Chronic lymphocytic leukemia can be classified into two major subtypes based on the pattern of immunoglobulin gene mutations of pre- and postgerminal center CLL (336). Molecular pathogenesis remains largely unknown, but common cytogenetic abnormalities include interstitial deletions of 13q, trisomy 12, deletions of 11q at the AT gene locus, and 6p and 6q rearrangements.

CLL shows greater international variation (ranging from 26- to 38-fold differences) in age-adjusted incidence than other lymphoid neoplasms. Rates are consistently higher in males than in females, although the male:female ratio varies from 1.4 in Zurich, Switzerland to 3.2 in Shanghai, China. Rates are highest among Caucasians in North America, Denmark, and Oceania, whereas rates are lowest in China, India, Japan, and Israeli Jews (Fig. 3). Chronic lymphocytic leukemia is uncommon before age 30, then increases exponentially until age 60, when the rate of the increase becomes slower. At all ages, rates are higher in males than in females in the United States; in the United Kingdom, the greatest male excess is observed among persons in their 40s and 60s (337). Incidence rates of CLL are similar in U.S. Caucasians and African-Americans until age 50, when the Caucasian: African-American ratio increases (Fig. 4).

There are studies to suggest a relationship between CLL risk and occupation, but the data allow for only limited conclusions. Several studies have implicated farming and related exposures in risk of CLL (338–340), including DDT (341), animal breeding (127), and working in flourmills (308). While some case–control studies have suggested a link between benzene exposure and CLL (325,342), cohort studies of benzene-exposed workers show little evidence of increased risk of CLL (64,67,80). A few studies have described excesses of lymphocytic leukemia or CLL (343,344) among petroleum industry workers, but no excess risk was found for CLL in other studies (74,345–348) or in a leukemia type-specific meta-analysis of 208,000 workers (349). A retrospective cohort study of 40,683 workers in the reinforced plastics industry from Denmark, Finland, Italy, Norway, Sweden, and the United Kingdom (350) revealed no excesses of neoplasms of the lymphatic and hematopoietic system overall or increasing risk with longer duration of exposure, but mortality from leukemia and lymphoma rose two-fold 20 years after first exposure. Elevated risks were observed in workers employed in the 1960s in companies producing reinforced plastics in Denmark. Interpretation of much of the literature on occupation and risk of CLL is complicated by lack of homogeneity of the lymphopoietic disorders studied and lack of validation of diagnosis in most studies. An International Agency for Research on Cancer (IARC) committee concluded that there was a small excess of CLL after a detailed review of 12 cohort studies of the rubber industry (351). Chronic lymphocytic leukemia has not been associated with exposure to ionizing radiation (43,352).

Smoking was linked with elevated risk of lymphocytic leukemia in three cohort investigations (102,353,354) and one case–control study (355), but not in other large cohort studies (106,356). There is little information on diet or alcohol consumption and CLL.

Familial clustering of CLL, recognized for more than 50 years (357), is one of the strongest risk factors for development of CLL (358). First-degree relatives with leukemia were more frequent in families of CLL cases than in CML cases (359), but only a small percentage of CLL cases have affected close family members (132,360). The proportion may be higher among families of CLL cases among Ashkenazi Jews of Eastern European or Russian descent (361). Within a family with two or more cases of leukemia among close family members, the subtypes of leukemia are generally concordant, particularly for CLL (265,329). Postulated genetical mechanisms for familial leukemia include inherited germline mutations, primary immunological alterations, sharing of common haplotypes, and/or consanguinity.

3.5. Multiple Myeloma

Multiple myeloma, comprising 10% of all hematological malignancies, is characterized by an accumulation of malignant plasma cells in the bone marrow (13). Genetic changes include a rearrangement involving the IgH gene at 14q32, with reciprocal translocations involving 11q13 or 4p16 (seen in 60–75% of patients), aneuploidy (seen in almost all cases), and interstitial deletion of chromosome 13q (which appears to be a poor prognostic feature).

Internationally, incidence of MM is highest among African-Americans, while mid-level rates occur among Caucasians in North America, Europe, and Oceania, and lowest rates are apparent in China, India, Japan, and Israeli Jews (Fig.3). Multiple myeloma like CLL, is rare before age 30, then increases exponentially with age, until age 70 when the rate of increase steadies in all groups. Incidence rates are higher at all ages among African-Americans than among U.S. Caucasians. Rates are similar for both men and women of each race in young and middle-aged adults, but at age 60 rates diverge, with higher rates apparent for males than for females of each race (Fig. 4).

Radiation treatment was linked with small but significantly elevated risk, which remained elevated 35 years since the first treatment and a dose–response trend for MM among patients with ankylosing spondylitis (estimated mean total body dose was 2.64 Gy, with the heaviest dose to the vertebrae) (362). A trend analysis revealed significantly increased risks of MM 10 years following the first radiation treatment in a large cohort of women treated for cervical cancer, but no overall excess risk for all time periods combined (363). Women in Scotland treated with radiotherapy for metropathia hemorrhagica developed significantly elevated risk of MM 5 or more years after receiving a mean bone marrow dose of 1.3 Gy (364). Thorotrast was associated with a significantly increased risk of MM among Danish women (365).

Several epidemiological studies have reported positive associations between employment in agriculture and risk of MM (121,366–369). Multiple myeloma was significantly elevated among 140,208 Swedish farmers, even in those parts of Sweden where the use of pesticides has been less frequent (370); 246,104 Norwegian farmers, particularly those cultivating potatoes (371); and 205,000 Finnish farmers, particularly those on pig or poultry farms (259). A meta-analysis of 32 studies published between 1981 and 1996 revealed a modest increase in MM (369). Specific agricultural exposures implicated include triazine herbicides (123,347), (DDT, used in application or inspection jobs (372), grain dusts (308,373), and farm animals (374).

Mortality studies of atomic bomb survivors have reported a radiation effect (17,57), with an estimated excess risk of 0.17 per 10^4 person-years per sievert (PY Sv) PY Sv (95% CI = 0.02–0.40) for both sexes combined, that was slightly higher for females (0.19 per 10^4 PY Sv, based on 35 cases) than for males (0.15 per 10^4 PY Sv, based on 16 cases). However, incidence analyses for 1950–1987 show no evidence of a significant dose–response relationship (178). The estimated absolute risk was 0.08 cases per 10^4 PY Sv (95% CI < 0–0.3), with no variation by gender, age at exposure, or time since exposure (178). Reasons for the apparent differences between mortality and incidence risks included poorer agreement (only 59%) between tumor registry and death certificate diagnoses for MM than for other hematological malignancies, and exclusion of a relatively large proportion

(8.4% of MM cases which were second primaries) from the incidence analyses. Because of the small numbers of exposed persons who developed MM, more years of follow-up and continued monitoring of the atomic bomb survivors will be required to clarify the nature of the relationship. An excess of deaths from MM among American radiologists was first reported 40 years ago (375). Subsequently, risk of MM was found to be two times higher among U.S. radiologists than among physicians in other specialties (38), but risk was not increased in British radiologists (376), or among Chinese (41), Japanese (40), or U.S. (39) radiological technologists. In a combined analysis of cancer mortality data for 95,673 nuclear industry workers in the United States, the United Kingdom, and Canada, the relative risk of MM was almost twofold increased and the excess relative risk was 4.2 per sievert for MM (377). The authors concluded that the excess most likely reflected the increase in MM previously reported for two of the nuclear plants (e.g., Hanford and Sellafield). Among 124,743 workers included in the National Registry for Radiation Workers in the United Kingdom, there was some evidence of an increasing trend in the risk of multiple myeloma with increasing estimated external radiation dose, although the rising trend disappeared after the investigators excluded workers monitored for exposure to internal radiation emitters (377a). Increases in MM mortality and incidence were observed among British military participants in above-ground nuclear weapons tests (378), but not in New Zealand (379) or U.S. soldiers participating in nuclear tests (380,381). In contrast, no association has been found between risk of myeloma and diagnostic x-rays in most case–control (382,383) or cohort (384,385) studies, although a positive dose–response and a significant excess risk was observed among members of a prepaid health plan who had had a mean of 35 or more x-ray procedures (386).

One of the most contentious topics is whether or not benzene exposure is linked with elevated risk of multiple myeloma (387–389). A U.S. study initially described four workers with MM and nine with myeloid leukemia in a population of approximately 1100 workers manufacturing Pliofilm (64), but an updated follow-up revealed no association of benzene with MM (68). In a study reported in 1996, shoe workers in Florence with the highest exposure to solvents developed an elevated risk of MM (390). Nonsignificant modest excesses of MM occurred among chemical manufacturing workers 20 or more years after their first exposure to low levels of benzene (77), workers in the crude and fluid catalytic cracking units within the research and petrochemical units of Texaco (348), and workers at Texas oil refineries (391,392), but were not supported in studies of Canadian petroleum distribution workers (74) or in a meta-analysis of 22 cohort mortality studies of petroleum workers (393).

Cigarette smoking has not been found to be a risk factor for multiple myeloma (106,107,327,328,356,373,384,394–397), except in a single study of

Seventh Day Adventists (397a). There is little evidence about the possible role of diet in the etiology of MM, although increased risks were found for liver and butter intake, and animal fat (332a); reduced risks for fish consumption (398), whole-grain intake (399), and diets rich in green vegetables (332a); and elevated risks in overweight and obese persons (400). Alcohol consumption has not been linked with MM (373,384,397). Women who used permanent darkening hair dyes had increased risk of MM in one case–control (397b) and one cohort study (334,401), but these findings were not confirmed in other case–control (402), or large cohort (335) studies.

Multiple myeloma is three- to sixfold elevated among persons with a history of a first-degree relative with multiple myeloma (262,403,404). Risks of familial occurrence of lymphoproliferative malignancies in families of probands with MM were higher for African-Americans than for Caucasians, although the difference was not statistically significant (404).

ACKNOWLEDGMENTS

The authors are grateful to the staff of the NCI Surveillance Epidemiology and End Results registries for the high quality of data collection and preparation, and to John Lahey of Information Management Systems, Inc. for preparation of the figures.

REFERENCES

1. Bennett JM, Catovsky D, Daniel MT, Flandrin G, Galton DA, Gralnick HR, et al. Proposals for the classification of the acute leukaemias. French-American-British (FAB) Cooperative group. Br J Haematol 1976; 33:451–458.
2. Bennett JM, Catovsky D, Daniel MT, Flandrin G, Galton DA, Gralnick HR, et al. Proposals for the classification of the myelodysplastic syndromes. Br J Haematol 1982; 51:189–199.
3. Bennett JM, Catovsky D, Daniel MT, Flandrin G, Galton DA, Gralnick HR, et al. Criteria for the diagnosis of acute leukemia of megakaryocyte lineage (M7). A report of the French-American-British Cooperative Group. Ann Intern Med 1985; 103:460–462.
4. Bennett JM, Catovsky D, Daniel MT, Flandrin G, Galton DA, Gralnick HR, et al. Proposals for the classification of chronic (mature) B and T lymphoid leukaemias. French-American-British (FAB) Cooperative Group. J Clin Pathol 1989; 42: 567–584.
5. Bennett JM, Catovsky D, Daniel MT, Flandrin G, Galton DA, Gralnick H, et al. The chronic myeloid leukaemias: guidelines for distinguishing chronic granulocytic, atypical chronic myeloid, and chronic myelomonocytic leukaemia. Proposals by the French-American-British Cooperative Leukaemia Group. Br J Haematol 1994; 87:746–754.
6. Jaffe ES, Harris NL, Stein H, Vardiman JW. Pathology and Genetics of Tumours of Haematopoietic and Lymphoid Tissues. Lyon: IARC Press, 2001.

7. Head DR. Revised classification of acute myeloid leukemia. Leukemia 1996; 10:1826–1831.
8. Harris NL. Hodgkin's lymphomas: classification, diagnosis, and grading. Semin Hematol 1999; 36:220–232.
9. McKenna RW. Multifaceted approach to the diagnosis and classification of acute leukemias. Clin Chem 2000; 46:1252–1259.
10. Bennett JM. World Health Organization classification of the acute leukemias and myelodysplastic syndromes. Int J Hematol 2000; 72:131–133.
11. Hayashi Y. The molecular genetics of recurring chromosome abnormalities in acute myeloid leukemia. Semin Hematol 2000; 37:368–380.
12. Gordon MY, Dazzi F, Marley SB, Lewis JL, Nguyen D, Grand FH, et al. Cell biology of CML cells. Leukemia 1999; 13(suppl 1):S65–S71.
13. Hoffman R, Benz EJ, Shattil S, Furie B, Cohen H, Silberstein S, et al. Hematology. Basic Principles and Practice. 3rd ed. New York: Church Livingston, 2000:979–1416.
14. Parkin DM, Muir CS. Cancer incidence in five continents. Comparability and quality of data. IARC Sci Publ 1992; 45–173.
15. Ries LAG, Eisner MP, Kosary CL, Hankey BF, Miller BA, Clegg LX, Edwards BF. Cancer Statistics Review, 1973–1996. NIH Publication Number 00-2789. Bethesda, MD: National Cancer Institute, 2000.
16. Little JB. Cellular, molecular, and carcinogenic effects of radiation. Hematol Oncol Clin North Am 1993; 7:337–352.
17. Shimizu Y, Schull WJ, Kato H. Cancer risk among atomic bomb survivors. The RERF Life Span Study. Radiation Effects Research Foundation. J Am Med Assoc 1990; 264:601–604.
18. UNSCEAR. Sources and Effects of Ionizing Radiation. Epidemiological Studies of Radiation Carcinogenesis. New York: United Nations Scientific Committee of the Effects of Atomic Radiation 1994:11–183.
19. Preston DL, Kusumi S, Tomonaga M, Izumi S, Ron E, Kuramoto A, et al. Cancer Incidence in atomic bomb survivors. Part III. Leukemia, lymphoma, and multiple myeloma, 1950–87. Radiat Res 1994; 137:568–597.
20. Little MP, Weiss HA, Boice JD Jr, Darby SC, Day NE, Muirhead CR. Risks of leukemia in atomic bomb survivors, in women treated for cervical cancer and in patients treated for ankylosing spondylitis. Radiat Res 1999; 152:280–292.
21. Li FP, Yan JC, Sallan S, Cassady JR Jr, Danahy J, Fine W, et al. Second neoplasms after Wilms' tumor in childhood. J Natl Cancer Inst 1983; 71:1205–1209.
22. Greene M. Interaction between radiotherapy and chemotherapy in human leukemogenesis. In: Boice J, Fraumeni JJ, eds. Radiation Carcinogenesis: Epidemiology and Biological Significance. New York: Raven press, 1984: 199–210.
23. Boice JD Jr, Blettner M, Kleinerman RA, Stovall M, Moloney WC, Engholm G, et al. Radiation dose and leukemia risk in patients treated for cancer of the cervix. J Natl Cancer Inst 1987; 79:1295–1311.
24. Curtis RE, Boice JD Jr, Stovall M, Bernstein L, Greenberg RS, Flannery JT, et al. Risk of leukemia after chemotherapy and radiation treatment for breast cancer [see comments]. N Engl J Med 1992; 326:1745–1751.

25. Curtis RE, Boice JD Jr, Stovall M, Bernstein L, Holowaty E, Karjalainen S, et al. Relationship of leukemia risk to radiation dose following cancer of the uterine corpus. J Natl Cancer Inst 1994; 86:1315–1324.

26. Travis LB, Curtis RE, Stovall M, Holowaty EJ, Van Leeuwen FE, Glimelius B, et al. Risk of leukemia following treatment for non-Hodgkin's lymphoma. J Natl Cancer Inst 1994; 86:1450–1457.

27. Travis LB, Weeks J, Curtis RE, Chaffey JT, Stovall M, Banks PM, et al. Leukemia following low-dose total body irradiation and chemotherapy for non-Hodgkin's lymphoma. J Clin Oncol 1996; 14:565–571.

28. Kuttesch JF Jr, Wexler LH, Marcus RB, Fairclough D, Weaver-McClure L, White M, et al. Second malignancies after Ewing's sarcoma: radiation dose-dependency of secondary sarcomas. J Clin Oncol 1996; 14:2818–2825.

29. Inskip PD. Second cancers following radiotherapy. In: Neugut AI, Meadows AT, eds. Multiple Primary Cancers. Philadelphia, PA: Lippincott Williams & Wilkins, 1999:91–135.

30. Weiss HA, Darby SC, Fearn T, Doll R. Leukemia mortality after X-ray treatment for ankylosing spondylitis. Radiat Res 1995; 142:1–11.

31. Inskip PD, Kleinerman RA, Stovall M, Cookfair DL, Hadjimichael O, Moloney WC, et al. Leukemia, lymphoma, and multiple myeloma after pelvic radiotherapy for benign disease. Radiat Res 1993; 135:108–124.

32. Smith PG, Doll R. Late effects of x irradiation in patients treated for metropathia haemorrhagica. Br J Radiol 1976; 49:224–232.

33. Inskip PD, Monson RR, Wagoner JK, Stovall M, Davis FG, Kleinerman RA, et al. Leukemia following radiotherapy for uterine bleeding. Radiat Res 1990; 122:107–119.

34. Griem ML, Kleinerman RA, Boice JD Jr, Stovall M, Shefner D, Lubin JH. Cancer following radiotherapy for peptic ulcer. J Natl Cancer Inst 1994; 86:842–849.

35. Ron E, Modan B, Boice JD Jr. Mortality after radiotherapy for ringworm of the scalp. Am J Epidemiol 1988; 127:713–725.

36. Smith PG, Doll R. Mortality from cancer and all causes among British radiologists. Br J Radiol 1981; 54:187–194.

37. Seltser R, Sartwell PE. The influence of occupational exposure on the mortality of American radiologists and other medical specialists. Am J Epidemiol 1965; 101:188–198.

38. Matanoski GM, Sartwell P, Elliott E, et al. Cancer risks in radiologists and radiation workers. In: Boice JD Jr, Fraumeni JF Jr, eds. Radiation Carcinogenesis: Epidemiology and Biological Significance. New York: Raven Press, 1984:83–96.

39. Mohan AK, Hauptmann M, Freedman DM, Ron E, Matanoski GM, Lubin JH, et al. Cancer and other causes of mortality among radiologic technologists in the United States. Int J Cancer 2003; 103:259–267.

40. Yoshinaga S, Aoyama T, Yoshimoto Y, Sugahara T. Cancer mortality among radiological technologists in Japan: updated analysis of follow-up data from 1969 to 1993. J Epidemiol 1999; 9:61–72.

41. Wang JX, Inskip PD, Boice JD Jr, Li BX, Zhang JY, Fraumeni JF Jr. Cancer incidence among medical diagnostic X-ray workers in China, 1950 to 1985. Int J Cancer 1990; 45:889–895.

42. Gunz FW, Atkinson H. Medical radiation and leukemia: a retrospective survey. Br Med J 1964; 5380:389–396.
43. UNSCEAR. Sources and effects of ionizing radiation. Epidemiological Evaluation of Radiation-Induced Cancer. New York: United Nations Committee on the Effects of Atomic Radiation, 2000:297–431.
44. Boice JD Jr, Morin MM, Glass AG, Friedman GD, Stovall M, Hoover RN, et al. Diagnostic x-ray procedures and risk of leukernia, lymphoma, and multiple myeloma. JAMA 1991; 265:1290–1294.
45. Severson RK, Stevens RG, Kaune WT, Thomas DB, Heuser L, Davis S, et al. Acute nonlymphocytic leukemia and residential exposure to power frequency magnetic fields. Am J Epidemiol 1988; 128:10–20.
46. Feychting M, Ahlbom A. Magnetic fields, leukemia, and central nervous system tumors in Swedish adults residing near high-voltage power lines. Epidemiology 1994; 5:501–509.
47. Kheifets LI, Afifi AA, Buffler PA, Zhang ZW, Matkin CC. Occupational electric and magnetic field exposure and leukemia. A meta-analysis. J Occup Environ Med 1997; 39:1074–1091.
48. Floderus B, Persson T, Stenlund C, Wennberg A, Ost A, Knave B. Occupational exposure to electromagnetic fields in relation to leukemia and brain tumors: a case–control study in Sweden. Cancer Causes Control 1993; 4:465–476.
49. Matanoski GM, Elliott EA, Breysse PN, Lynberg MC. Leukemia in telephone linemen. Am J Epidemiol 1993; 137:609–619.
50. Sahl JD, Kelsh MA, Greenland S. Cohort and nested case–control studies of hematopoietic cancers and brain cancer among electric utility workers. Epidemiology 1993; 4:104–114.
51. London SJ, Bowman JD, Sobel E, Thomas DC, Garabrant DH, Pearce N, et al. Exposure to magnetic fields among electrical workers in relation to leukemia risk in Los Angeles County. Am J Ind Med 1994; 26:47–60.
52. Theriault G, Goldberg M, Miller AB, Armstrong B, Guenel P, Deadman J, et al. Cancer risks associated with occupational exposure to magnetic fields among electric utility workers in Ontario and Quebec, Canada, and France: 1970–1989. Am J Epidemiol 1994; 139:550–572. [Published erratum appears in Am J Epidemiol 1994; 139(10):1053.].
53. Savitz DA, Loomis DP. Magnetic field exposure in relation to leukemia and brain cancer mortality among electric utility workers. Am J Epidemiol 1995; 141:123–134. [Published erratum appears in Am J Epidemiol 1996; 144(2):205.
54. Miller AB, To T, Agnew DA, Wall C, Green LM. Leukemia following occupational exposure to 60-Hz electric and magnetic fields among Ontario electric utility workers. Am J Epidemiol 1996; 144:150–160.
55. Feychting M, Forssen U, Floderus B. Occupational and residential magnetic field exposure and leukemia and central nervous system tumors. Epidemiology 1997; 8:384–389.
56. Johansen C, Olsen JH. Risk of cancer among Danish utility workers—a nationwide cohort study. Am J Epidemiol 1998; 147:548–555.
57. Pierce DA, Shimizu Y, Preston DL, Vaeth M, Mabuchi K. Studies of the mortality of atomic bomb survivors. Report 12, part I. Cancer: 1950–1990. Radiat Res 1996; 146:1–27.

58. Chap L, Nimer SD. Chronic myelogenous leukemia following repeated radiation therapy for histiocytosis X. Leuk Lymphoma 1994; 12:315–316.
59. Shimon I, Kneller A, Olchovsky D. Chronic myeloid leukaemia following 131I treatment for thyroid carcinoma: a report of two cases and review of the literature. Clin Endocrinol (Oxf) 1995; 43:651–654.
60. Iurlo A, Foa P, Maiolo AT, Polli EE. Chronic myelogenous leukemia following radiation therapy for testicular seminoma. Blut 1989; 59:503–504.
61. Beaty O III, Hudson MM, Greenwald C, Luo X, Fang L, Wilimas JA, et al. Subsequent malignancies in children and adolescents after treatment for Hodgkin's disease. J Clin Oncol 1995; 13:603–609.
62. Visfeldt J, Andersson M. Pathoanatomical aspects of malignant haematological disorders among Danish patients exposed to thorium dioxide. APMIS 1995; 103:29–36.
63. Ott MG, Townsend JC, Fishbeck WA, Langner RA. Mortality among individuals occupationally exposed to benzene. Arch Environ Health 1978; 33:3–10.
64. Rinsky RA, Smith AB, Hornung R, Filloon TG, Young RJ, Okun AH, et al. Benzene and leukemia. An epidemiologic risk assessment. N Engl J Med 1987; 316:1044–1050.
65. Wong O. An industry wide mortality study of chemical workers occupationally exposed to benzene. II. Dose response analyses. [Published erratum appears in Br J Ind Med 1987; 44(11):776]. Br J Ind Med 1987; 44:382–395].
66. Yin SN, Li GL, Tain FD, Fu ZI, Jin C, Chen YJ, et al. Leukaemia in benzene workers: a retrospective cohort study. Br J Ind Med 1987; 44:124–128.
67. Hayes RB, Yin SN, Dosemeci M, Li GL, Wacholder S, Travis LB, et al. Benzene and the dose-related incidence of hematologic neoplasms in China. Chinese Academy of Preventive Medicine—National Cancer Institute Benzene Study Group. J Natl Cancer Inst 1997; 89:1065–1071.
68. Rinsky RA, Hornung RW, Silver SR, Tseng CY. Benzene exposure and hematopoietic mortality: a long-term epidemiologic risk assessment. Am J Ind Med 2002; 42: 474–480.
69. Yin SN, Li GL, Tain FD, Fu ZI, Jin C, Chen YJ, et al. A retrospective cohort study of leukemia and other cancers in benzene workers. Environ Health Perspect 1989; 82:207–213.
70. Yin SN, Hayes RB, Linet MS. A cohort study among workers exposed to benzene in China III. Mortality and incidence findings. Am J Ind Med 1996; 29: 227–235.
71. Paganini-Hill A, Glazer E, Henderson BE, Ross RK. Cause-specific mortality among newspaper web pressmen. J Occup Med 1980; 22:542–544.
72. Zoloth SR, Michaels DM, Villalbi JR, Lacher M. Patterns of mortality among commercial pressmen. J Natl Cancer Inst 1986; 76:1047–1051.
73. Schnatter AR, Theriault G, Katz AM, Thompson FS, Donaleski D, Murray N. A retrospective mortality study within operating segments of a petroleum company. Am J Ind Med 1992; 22:209–229.
74. Schnatter AR, Armstrong TW, Nicolich MJ, Thompson FS, Katz AM, Huebner WW, et al. Lymphohaematopoietic malignancies and quantitative estimates of exposure to benzene in Canadian petroleum distribution workers. Occup Environ Med 1996; 53:773–781.

75. Schnatter AR, Armstrong TW, Thompson LS, Nicolich MJ, Katz AM, Huebner WW, et al. The relationship between low-level benzene exposure and leukemia in Canadian petroleum distribution workers. Environ Health Perspect 1996; 104(suppl 6):1375–1379.

76. Huebner WW, Schnatter AR, Nicolich MJ, Jorgensen G. Mortality experience of a young petrochemical industry cohort. 1979–1992 follow-up study of US-based employees. J Occup Environ Med 1997; 39:970–982.

77. Ireland B, Collins JJ, Buckley CF, Riordan SG. Cancer mortality among workers with benzene exposure. Epidemiology 1997; 8:318–320.

78. Rushton L, Romaniuk H. A case–control study to investigate the risk of leukaemia associated with exposure to benzene in petroleum marketing and distribution workers in the United Kingdom. Occup Environ Med 1997; 54:152–166.

79. Savitz DA, Andrews KW. Review of epidemiologic evidence on benzene and lymphatic and hematopoietic cancers. Am J Ind Med 1997; 31:287–295.

80. Utterback DF, Rinsky RA. Benzene exposure assessment in rubber hydrochloride workers: a critical evaluation of previous estimates. Am J Ind Med 1995; 27:661–676.

81. Crump KS. Risk of benzene-induced leukemia predicted from the Pliofilm cohort. Environ Health Perspect 1996; 104(suppl 6):1437–1441.

82. Irons RD. Molecular models of benzene leukemogenesis. J Toxicol Environ Health A 2000; 61:391–397.

83. Eastmond DA, Schuler M, Frantz C, Chen H, Parks R, Wang L, et al. Characterization and mechanisms of chromosomal alterations induced by benzene in mice and humans. Res Rep Health Eff Inst 2001; 1–68.

84. Hayes RB, Songnian Y, Dosemeci M, Linet M. Benzene and lymphohematopoietic malignancies in humans. Am J Ind Med 2001; 40:117–126.

85. Zhang L, Eastmond DA, Smith MT. The nature of chromosomal aberrations detected in humans exposed to benzene. Crit Rev Toxicol 2002; 32:1–42.

86. Giles FJ, Koeffler HP. Secondary myelodysplastic syndromes and leukemias. Curr Opin Hematol 1994; 1:256–260.

87. Kaldor JM, Day NE, Clarke EA, Van Leeuwen FE, Henry-Amar M, Fiorentino MV, et al. Leukemia following Hodgkin's disease. N Engl J Med 1990; 322:7–13.

88. Kaldor JM, Day NE, Pettersson F, Clarke EA, Pedersen D, Mehnert W, et al. Leukemia following chemotherapy for ovarian cancer. N Engl J Med 1990; 322:1–6.

89. Van Leeuwen FE, Chorus AM, Belt-Dusebout AW, Hagenbeek A, Noyon R, van Kerkhoff EH, et al. Leukemia risk following Hodgkin's disease: relation to cumulative dose of alkylating agents, treatment with teniposide combinations, number of episodes of chemotherapy, and bone marrow damage. J Clin Oncol 1994; 12:1063–1073.

90. Riedel DA, Pottern LM. The epidemiology of multiple myeloma. Hematol Oncol Clin North Am 1992; 6:225–247.

91. Krishnan A, Bhatia S, Slovak ML, Arber DA, Niland JC, Nademanee A, et al. Predictors of therapy-related leukemia and myelodysplasia following autologous transplantation for lymphoma: an assessment of risk factors. Blood 2000; 95:1588–1593.

92. Travis LB, Holowaty EJ, Bergfeldt K, Lynch CF, Kohler BA, Wiklund T, et al. Risk of leukemia after platinum-based chemotherapy for ovarian cancer. N Engl J Med 1999; 340:351–357.

93. Felix CA. Secondary leukemias induced by topoisomerase-targeted drugs. Biochim Biophys Acta 1998; 1400:233–255.

94. Smith MA, Rubinstein L, Anderson JR, Arthur D, Catalano PJ, Freidlin B et al. Secondary leukemia or myelodysplastic syndrome after treatment with epipodophyllotoxins. J Clin Oncol 1999; 17:569–577.

95. Andersen MK, Pedersen-Bjergaard J. Increased frequency of dicentric chromosomes in therapy-related MDS and AML compared to de novo disease is significantly related to previous treatment with alkylating agents and suggests a specific susceptibility to chromosome breakage at the centromere. Leukemia 2000; 14:105–111.

96. Travis LB, Andersson M, Gospodarowicz M, Van Leeuwen FE, Bergfeldt K, Lynch CF, et al. Treatment-associated leukemia following testicular cancer. J Natl Cancer Inst 2000; 92:1165–1171.

97. Saso R, Kulkarni S, Mitchell P, Treleaven J, Swansbury GJ, Mehta J, et al. Secondary myelodysplastic syndrome/acute myeloid leukaemia following mitoxantrone-based therapy for breast carcinoma. Br J Cancer 2000; 83: 91–94.

98. Metayer C, Curtis RE, Vose J, Sobocinski KA, Horowite MM, Bhatia S, et al. Myelodysplastic syndrome and acute myeloid leukemia after autotransplantation for lymphoma: a multicenter case-control study. Blood 2003; 101: 2015–2033.

99. Pedersen-Bjergaard J, Andersen MK, Christiansen DH. Therapy-related acute myeloid leukemia and myelodysplasia after high-dose chemotherapy and autologous stem cell transplantation. Blood 2000; 95:3273–3279.

100. Woo MH, Shuster JJ, Chen C, Bash RO, Behm FG, Camitta B, et al. Glutathione S-transferase genotypes in children who develop treatment-related acute myeloid malignancies. Leukemia 2000; 14:232–237.

101. Perentesis JP. Genetic predisposition and treatment-related leukemia. Med Pediatr Oncol 2001; 36:541–548.

102. Garfinkel L, Boffetta P. Association between smoking and leukemia in two American Cancer Society prospective studies. Cancer 1990; 65:2356–2360.

103. Sandler DP, Shore DL, Anderson JR, Davey FR, Arthur D, Mayer RJ, et al. Cigarette smoking and risk of acute leukemia: associations with morphology and cytogenetic abnormalities in bone marrow. J Natl Cancer Inst 1993; 85:1994–2003.

104. Kane EV, Roman E, Cartwright R, Parker J, Morgan G. Tobacco and the risk of acute leukaemia in adults. Br J Cancer 1999; 81:1228–1233.

105. Engeland A, Andersen A, Haldorsen T, Tretli S. Smoking habits and risk of cancers other than lung cancer: 28 years' follow-up of 26,000 Norwegian men and women. Cancer Causes Control 1996; 7:497–506.

106. Adami J, Nyren O, Bergstrom R, Ekbom A, Engholm G, Englund A et al. Smoking and the risk of leukemia, lymphoma, and multiple myeloma (Sweden). Cancer Causes Control 1998; 9:49–56.

107. Brownson RC, Novotny TE, Perry MC. Cigarette smoking and adult leukemia. A meta-analysis. Arch Intern Med 1993; 153:469–475.

108. Bjork J, Albin M, Mauritzson N, Stromberg U, Johansson B, Hagmar L. Smoking and myelodysplastic syndromes. Epidemiology 2000; 11:285–291.

109. Matanoski GM, Stockwell HG, Diamond EL, Haring-Sweeney M, Joffe RD, Mele LM, et al. A cohort mortality study of painters and allied tradesmen. Scand J Work Environ Health 1986; 12:16–21.

110. Chen R, Seaton A. A meta-analysis of painting exposure and cancer mortality. Cancer Detect Prev 1998; 22:533–539.

111. Nisse C, Lorthois C, Dorp V, Eloy E, Haguenoer JM, Fenaux P. Exposure to occupational and environmental factors in myelodysplastic syndromes. Preliminary results of a case–control study. Leukemia 1995; 9:693–699.

112. Hayes RB, Blair A, Stewart PA, Herrick RF, Mahar H. Mortality of U.S. embalmers and funeral directors. Am J Ind Med 1990; 18:641–652.

113. Linos A, Blair A, Cantor KP, Burmeister L, VanLier S, Gibson RW, et al. Leukemia and non-Hodgkin's lymphoma among embalmers and funeral directors. J Natl Cancer Inst 1990; 82:66.

114. Hunting KL, Longbottom H, Kalavar SS, Stern F, Schwartz E, Welch LS. Haematopoietic cancer mortality among vehicle mechanics. Occup Environ Med 1995; 52:673–678.

115. Hotz P, Lauwerys RR. Hematopoietic and lymphatic malignancies in vehicle mechanics. Crit Rev Toxicol 1997; 27:443–494.

116. Bulbulyan MA, Changuina OV, Zaridze DG, Astashevsky SV, Colin D, Boffetta P. Cancer mortality among Moscow shoe workers exposed to chloroprene (Russia). Cancer Causes Control 1998; 9:381–387.

117. Lynge E. Danish Cancer Registry as a resource for occupational research. J Occup Med 1994; 36:1169–1173.

118. Miligi L, Seniori CA, Crosignani P, Fontana A, Masala G, Nanni O, et al. Occupational, environmental, and life-style factors associated with the risk of hematolymphopoietic malignancies in women. Am J Ind Med 1999; 36:60–69.

119. Nilsson RI, Nordlinder R, Horte LG, Jarvholm B. Leukaemia, lymphoma, and multiple myeloma in seamen on tankers. Occup Environ Med 1998; 55:517–521.

120. Burnett C, Robinson C, Walker J. Cancer mortality in health and science technicians. Am J Ind Med 1999; 36:155–158.

121. Blair A, Zahm SH. Agricultural exposures and cancer. Environ Health Perspect 1995; 103(suppl 8):205–208.

122. Keller-Byrne JE, Khuder SA, Schaub EA. Meta-analysis of leukemia and farming. Environ Res 1995; 71:1–10.

123. Pearce NE, Smith AH, Howard JK, Sheppard RA, Giles HJ, Teague CA. Case-control study of multiple myeloma and farming. Br J Cancer 1986; 54:493–500.

124. Zahm SH, Ward MH, Blair A. Pesticides and cancer. Occup Med 1997; 12:269–289.

125. Wiklund K, Holm LE. Trends in cancer risks among Swedish agricultural workers. J Natl Cancer Inst 1986; 77:657–664.

126. Dean G. Deaths from primary brain cancers, lymphatic and haematopoietic cancers in agricultural workers in the Republic of Ireland. J Epidemiol Community Health 1994; 48:364–368.

127. Amadori D, Nanni O, Falcini F, Saragoni A, Tison V, Callea A, et al. Chronic lymphocytic leukaemias and non-Hodgkin's lymphomas by histological type in farming-animal breeding workers: a population case–control study based on job titles. Occup Environ Med 1995; 52:374–379.

128. Kristensen P, Andersen A, Irgens LM, Bye AS, Sundheim L. Cancer in offspring of parents engaged in agricultural activities in Norway: incidence and risk factors in the farm environment. Int J Cancer 1996; 65:39–50.

129. Nanni O, Amadori D, Lugaresi C, Falcini F, Scarpi E, Saragoni A, et al. Chronic lymphocytic leukaemias and non-Hodgkin's lymphomas by histological type in farming-animal breeding workers: a population case–control study based on a priori exposure matrices. Occup Environ Med 1996; 53:652–657.

130. Avnon L, Oryan I, Kordysh E, Goldsmith J, Sobel R, Friger M. Cancer incidence and risks in selected agricultural settlements in the Negev of Israel. Arch Environ Health 1998; 53:336–343.

131. Pesatori AC, Consonni D, Tironi A, Zocchetti C, Fini A, Bertazzi PA. Cancer in a young population in a dioxin-contaminated area. Int J Epidemiol 1993; 22:1010–1013.

132. Horwitz M. The genetics of familial leukemia. Leukemia 1997; 11:1347–1359.

133. Gilchrist DM, Friedman JM, Rogers PC, Creighton SP. Myelodysplasia and leukemia syndrome with monosomy 7: a genetic perspective. Am J Med Genet 1990; 35:437–441.

134. Kwong YL, Ng MH, Ma SK. Familial acute myeloid leukemia with monosomy 7: late onset and involvement of a multipotential progenitor cell. Cancer Genet Cytogenet 2000; 116: 170–173.

135. Grimwade DJ, Stephenson J, De Silva C, Dalton RG, Mufti GJ. Familial MDS with 5q-abnormality. Br J Haematol 1993; 84:536–538.

136. Olopade OI, Roulston D, Baker T, Narvid S, Le Beau MM, Freireich EJ, et al. Familial myeloid leukemia associated with loss of the long arm of chromosome 5. Leukemia 1996; 10:669–674.

137. Mandla SG, Goobie S, Kumar RT, Hayne O, Zayed E, Guernsey DL, et al. Genetic analysis of familial myelodysplastic syndrome: absence of linkage to chromosomes 5q31 and 7q22. Cancer Genet Cytogenet 1998; 105: 113–118.

138. Taylor G, Birch J. The hereditary basis of human leukemia. In: Henderson E, Lister T, Greaves M, eds. Leukemia. 6th ed. Philadelphia: WB Saunders, 1996:210–245.

139. Hill DA, Gridley G, Cnattingius S, Mellemkjaer L, Linet M, Adami HO, et al. Mortality and cancer incidence among individuals with Down syndrome. Arch Intern Med 2003; 163: 705–711.

140. Alter BP. Cancer in Fanconi anemia, 1927–2001. Cancer 2003; 97:425–440.

141. Bloom GE, Warner S, Gerald PS, Diamond LK. Chromosome abnormalities in constitutional aplastic anemia. N Engl J Med 1966; 274:8–14.

142. German J. Bloom's syndrome. XX. The first 100 cancers. Cancer Genet Cytogenet 1997; 93:100–106.

143. Dror Y, Freedman MH. Shwachman–Diamond syndrome marrow cells show abnormally increased apoptosis mediated through the Fas pathway. Blood 2001; 97:3011–3016.

144. Alter BP. Fanconi's anemia and malignancies. Am J Hematol 1996; 53:99–110.

145. Chen H, Sandler DP, Taylor JA, Shore DL, Liu E, Bloomfield CD, et al. Increased risk for myelodysplastic syndromes in individuals with glutathione transferase theta 1 (GSTT1) gene defect. Lancet 1996; 347:295–297.

146. Basu T, Gale RE, Langabeer S, Linch DC. Glutathione S-transferase theta 1 (GSTT1) gene defect in myelodysplasia and acute myeloid leukaemia. Lancet 1997; 349:1450.

147. Atoyebi W, Kusec R, Fidler C, Peto TE, Boultwood J, Wainscoat JS. Glutathione S-transferase gene deletions in myelodysplasia. Lancet 1997; 349:1450–1451.

148. Strange RC, Fryer AA. The glutathione S-transferases: influence of Polymorphisms on cancer susceptability. In: IARC. Metabolic Polymorphisms and Suceptibility to Cancer 148th ed. Oxford: Oxford University Press, 1999:231–249.

149. Sasai Y, Horiike S, Misawa S, Kaneko H, Kobayashi M, Fujii H, et al. Genotype of glutathione S-transferase and other genetic configurations in myelodysplasia. Leuk Res 1999; 23:975–981.

150. Davies SM, Robison LL, Buckley JD, Radloff GA, Ross JA, Perentesis JP. Glutathione S-transferase polymorphisms in children with myeloid leukemia: a Children's Cancer Group study. Cancer Epidemiol Biomarkers Prev 2000; 9:563–566.

151. Arruda VR, Lima CS, Grignoli CR, de Melo MB, Lorand-Metze I, Alberto FL, et al. Increased risk for acute myeloid leukaemia in individuals with glutathione S-transferase mu 1 (GSTM1) and theta 1 (GSTT1) gene defects. Eur J Haematol 2001; 66:383–388.

152. Rollinson S, Roddam P, Kane E, Roman E, Cartwright RA, Jack A, Morgan GJ. Polymorphic variation within the glutathione S-transferase genes and risk of adult acute leukemia. Carcinogenesis 2000; 21:43–47.

153. Crump C, Chen C, Appelbaum FR, Kopecky KJ, Schwartz SM, Willman CL, et al. Glutathione S-transferase theta 1 gene deletion and risk of acute myeloid leukemia. Cancer Epidemiol Biomarkers Prev 2000; 9:457–460.

154. Naoe T, Takeyama K, Yokozawa T, Kiyoi H, Seto M, Uike N, et al. Analysis of genetic polymorphism in NQO1, GST-M1, GST-T1, and CYP3A4 in 469 Japanese patients with therapy-related leukemia/myelodysplastic syndrome and de novo acute myeloid leukemia. Clin Cancer Res 2000; 6:4091–4095.

155. Allan JM, Wild CP, Rollinson S, Willett EV, Moorman AV, Dovey GJ, et al. Polymorphism in glutathione S-transferase P1 is associated with susceptibility to chemotherapy-induced leukemia. Proc Natl Acad Sci USA 2001; 98: 11592–11597.

156. Tsabouri SE, Georgiou I, Alamanos I, Bourantas KL. Increased prevalence of GSTM(1) null genotype in patients with myelodysplastic syndrome: a case–control study. Acta Haematol 2000; 104:169–173.

157. Haase D, Binder C, Bunger J, Fonatsch C, Streubel B, Schnittger S, et al. Increased risk for therapy-associated hematologic malignancies in patients

with carcinoma of the breast and combined homozygous gene deletions of glutathione transferases M1 and T1. Leuk Res 2002; 26: 249–254.

158. Millikan RC, Pittman GS, Newman B, Tse CK, Selmin O, Rockhill B, et al. Cigarette smoking, N-acetyltransferases 1 and 2, and breast cancer risk. Cancer Epidemiol Biomarkers Prev 1998; 7:371–378.

159. Rollinson S, Roddam P, Willett E, Roman E, Cartwright R, Jack A, et al. NAT2 acetylator genotypes confer no effect on the risk of developing adult acute leukemia: a case–control study. Cancer Epidemiol Biomarkers Prev 2001; 10:567–568.

159a. Roddam PL, Rollinson S, Kane E, Moorman A, Cartwright R, Morgan GJ. Poor metabolizers at the cytochrome P450 2D6 and 2C19 loci are at increased risk of developing acute leukaemia. Pharmacogenetics 2000;10:605–615. Pharmacogenetics 2000; 10:605–615.

160. Bowen DT, Frew ME, Rollinson S, Roddam PL, Dring A, Smith MT, et al. CYP1A1*2B (Val) allele is overrepresented in a subgroup of acute myeloid leukemia patients with poor-risk karyotype associated with NRAS mutation, but not associated with FLT3 internal tandem duplication. Blood 2003; 101:2770–2774.

161. Blanco JG, Edick MJ, Hancock ML, Winick NJ, Dervieux T, Amylon MD, et al. Genetic polymorphisms in CYP3A5, CYP3A4 and NQO1 in children who developed therapy-related myeloid malignancies. Pharmacogenetics 2002; 12: 605–611.

162. Joseph P, Xie T, Xu Y, Jaiswal AK. NAD(P)H:quinone oxidoreductase1 (DT-diaphorase): expression, regulation, and role in cancer. Oncol Res 1994; 6:525–532.

163. Traver RD, Horikoshi T, Danenberg KD, Stadlbauer TH, Danenberg PV, Ross D, et al. NAD(P)H:quinone oxidoreductase gene expression in human colon carcinoma cells: characterization of a mutation which modulates DT-diaphorase activity and mitomycin sensitivity. Cancer Res. 1992; 52:797–802.

164. Long DJ, Gaikwad A, Multani A, Pathak S, Montgomery CA, Gonzalez FJ, et al. Disruption of the NAD(P)H: quinone oxidoreductase 1 (NQO1) gene in mice causes myelogenous hyperplasia. Cancer Res 2002; 62:3030–3036.

165. Rothman N, Smith MT, Hayes RB, Traver RD, Hoener B, Campleman S, et al. Benzene poisoning, a risk factor for hematological malignancy, is associated with the NQO1 609C→T mutation and rapid fractional excretion of chlorzoxazone. Cancer Res 1997; 57:2839–2842.

166. Larson RA, Wang Y, Banerjee M, Wiemels J, Hartford C, Le Beau MM, et al. Prevalence of the inactivating 609C→T polymorphism in the NAD(P)H: quinone oxidoreductase (NQO1) gene in patients with primary and therapy-related myeloid leukemia. Blood 1999; 94:803–807.

167. Smith MT, Wang Y, Kane E, Rollinson S, Wiemels JL, Roman E, et al. Low NAD(P)H:quinone oxidoreductase 1 activity is associated with increased risk of acute leukemia in adults. Blood 2001; 97:1422–1426.

168. Wiemels JL, Pagnamenta A, Taylor GM, Eden OB, Alexander FE, Greaves MF. A lack of a functional NAD(P)H:quinone oxidoreductase allele is selectively associated with pediatric leukemias that have MLL fusions. United Kingdom Childhood Cancer Study Investigators. Cancer Res 1999; 59: 4095–4099.

169. Hansen WK, Kelley MR. Review of mammalian DNA repair and translational implications. J Pharmacol Exp Ther 2000; 295:1–9.

170. Seedhouse C, Bainton R, Lewis M, Harding A, Russell N, Das-Gupta E. The genotype distribution of the XRCC1 gene indicates a role for base excision repair in the development of therapy-related acute myeloblastic leukemia. Blood 2002; 100:3761–3766.

171. Ricciardone MD, Ozcelik T, Cevher B, Ozdag H, Tuncer M, Gurgey A, et al. Human MLH1 deficiency predisposes to hematological malignancy and neurofibromatosis type 1. Cancer Res 1999; 59:290–293.

172. Whiteside D, McLeod R, Graham G, Steckley JL, Booth K, Somerville MJ, et al. A homozygous germ-line mutation in the human MSH2 gene predisposes to hematological malignancy and multiple cafe-au-lait spots. Cancer Res 2002; 62: 359–362.

173. Folias A, Matkovic M, Bruun D, Reid S, Hejna J, Grompe M, et al. BRCA1 interacts directly with the Fanconi anemia protein FANCA. Hum Mol Genet 2002; 11:2591–2597.

174. Tamary H, Bar-Yam R, Zemach M, Dgany O, Shalmon L, Yaniv I. The molecular biology of Fanconi anemia. Isr Med Assoc J 2002; 4:819–823.

175. Kelsoe G. V(D)J hypermutation and DNA mismatch repair: vexed by fixation. Proc Natl Acad Sci USA 1998; 95:6576–6577.

176. Vanasse GJ, Concannon P, Willerford DM. Regulated genomic instability and neoplasia in the lymphoid lineage. Blood 1999; 94:3997–4010.

177. Parkin DM, Kramarova E, Draper GJ, Masuyer E, Michaelis J, Neglia J, Queresshi S, Stiller CA. International Incidence of Childhood Cancer. Vol. II. IARC Scientific Publication No. 144. Lyon: International Agency for Research on Cancer, 1998.

178. Preston DL, Kusumi S, Tomonaga M, Izumi S, Ron E, Kuramoto A, et al. Cancer incidence in atomic bomb survivors. Part III. Leukemia, lymphoma and multiple myeloma, 1950–1987. Radiat Res 1994; 137:S68–S97

179. Gardner MJ, Snee MP, Hall AJ, Powell CA, Downes S, Terrell JD. Results of case–control study of leukaemia and lymphoma among young people near Sellafield nuclear plant in West Cumbria. Br Med J 1990; 300:423–429.

180. Draper GJ, Little MP, Sorahan T, Kinlen LJ, Bunch KJ, Conquest AJ, et al. Cancer in the offspring of radiation workers: a record linkage study. BMJ 1997; 315:1181–1188.

181. McLaughlin JR, King WD, Anderson TW, Clarke EA, Ashmore JP. Paternal radation posure and leutemia in offspring: the Ontario case-control study. BMJ 1993; 307:959–966.

182. Draper GJ, Stiller CA, Cartwright RA, Craft AW, Vincent TJ. Cancer in Cumbria and in the vicinity of the Sellafield nuclear installation, 1963–1990. Br Med J 1993; 306:89–94.

183. Cook-Mozaffari P, Darby S, Doll R. Cancer near potential sites of nuclear installations. Lancet 1989; 2:1145–1147.

184. Roman E, Beral V, Carpenter L, Watson A, Barton C, Ryder H, et al. Childhood leukaemia in the West Berkshire and Basingstoke and North Hampshire District Health Authorities in relation to nuclear establishments in the vicinity. Br Med J (Clin Res Ed) 1987; 294:597–602.

185. Darby SC, Doll R. Fallout, radiation doses near Dounreay, and childhood leukaemia. Br Med J (Clin Res Ed) 1987; 294:603–607.
186. Lowengart RA, Peters JM, Cicioni C, Buckley J, Bernstein L, Preston-Martin S, et al. Childhood leukemia and parents' occupational and home exposures. J Natl Cancer Inst 1987; 79:39–46.
187. Ma X, Buffler PA, Gunier RB, Dahl G, Smith MT, Reinier K, et al. Critical windows of exposure to household pesticides and risk of childhood leukemia. Environ Health Perspect 2002; 110:955–960.
188. London SJ, Thomas DC, Bowman JD, Sobel E, Cheng TC, Peters JM. Exposure to residential electric and magnetic fields and risk of childhood leukemia. Am J Epidemiol 1991; 134:923–937. [Published erratum appears in Am J Epidemiol 1993; 137(3):381.]
189. Leiss JK, Savitz DA. Home pesticide use and childhood cancer: a case–control study. Am J Public Health 1995; 85:249–252.
190. Meinert R, Schuz J, Kaletsch U, Kaatsch P, Michaelis J. Leukemia and non-Hodgkin's lymphoma in childhood and exposure to pesticides: results of a register-based case–control study in Germany. Am J Epidemiol 2000; 151:639–646.
191. Infante-Rivard C, Sinnett D. Preconceptional paternal exposure to pesticides and increased risk of childhood leukaemia. Lancet 1999; 354:1819.
192. Infante-Rivard C, Labuda D, Krajinovic M, Sinnett D. Risk of childhood leukemia associated with exposure to pesticides and with gene polymorphisms. Epidemiology 1999; 10:481–487.
193. Reynolds P, Von Behren J, Gunier RB, Goldberg DE, Hertz A, Harnly ME. Childhood cancer and agricultural pesticide use: an ecologic study in California. Environ Health Perspect 2002; 110:319–324.
194. Steensel-Moll HA, Valkenburg HA, van Zanen GE. Childhood leukemia and parental occupation. A register-based case–control study. Am J Epidemiol 1985; 121:216–224.
195. Feychting M, Plato N, Nise G, Ahlbom A. Paternal occupational exposures and childhood cancer. Environ Health Perspect 2001; 109:193–196.
196. Heacock H, Hertzman C, Demers PA, Gallagher R, Hogg RS, Teschke K, et al. Childhood cancer in the offspring of male sawmill workers occupationally exposed to chlorophenate fungicides. Environ Health Perspect 2000; 108:499–503.
197. Ji BT, Shu XO, Linet MS, Zheng W, Wacholder S, Gao YT, et al. Paternal cigarette smoking and the risk of childhood cancer among offspring of nonsmoking mothers. J Natl Cancer Inst 1997; 89:238–244.
198. Sorahan T, McKinney PA, Mann JR, Lancashire RJ, Stiller CA, Birch JM, et al. Childhood cancer and parental use of tobacco: findings from the inter-regional epidemiological study of childhood cancer (IRESCC). Br J Cancer 2001; 84:141–146.
199. Sorahan T, Prior P, Lancashire RJ, Faux SP, Hulten MA, Peck IM, et al. Childhood cancer and parental use of tobacco: deaths from 1971 to 1976. Br J Cancer 1997; 76:1525–1531.

200. Magnani C, Pastore G, Luzzatto L, Terracini B. Parental occupation and other environmental factors in the etiology of leukemias and non-Hodgkin's lymphomas in childhood: a case–control study. Tumori 1990; 76:413–419.

201. Shu XO, Ross JA, Pendergrass TW, Reaman GH, Lampkin B, Robison LL. Parental alcohol consumption, cigarette smoking, and risk of infant leukemia: a Childrens Cancer Group study. J Natl Cancer Inst 1996; 88:24–31.

202. Kwan ML, Buffler PA, Abrams B, Kiley VA. Breastfeeding and the risk of childhood leukemia: a meta-analysis. Publ Health Rep 2004; 119:521–535.

203. Bener A, Denic S, Galadori S. Longer breastfeeding and protection against childhood leukaemia and lymphoma. Eur J Cancer 2001; 37:234–238.

204. Infante-Rivard C, Fortier I, Olson E. Markers of infection, breast-feeding and childhood acute lymphoblastic leukaemia. Br J Cancer 2000; 83:1559–1564.

205. Perrillat F, Clavel J, Auclerc MF, Baruchel A, Leverger G, Nelken B, et al. Day-care, early common infections and childhood acute leukaemia: a multi-centre French case–control study. Br J Cancer 2002; 86:1064–1069.

206. Shu XO, Linet MS, Steinbuch M, Wen WQ, Buckley JD, Neglia JP, et al. Breast-feeding and risk of childhood acute leukemia. J Natl Cancer Inst 1999; 91:1765–1772.

207. UK Childhood Cancer Study Investigators. Breastfeeding and childhood cancer. Br J Cancer 2001; 85:1685–1694.

208. Schuz J, Kaletsch U, Meinert R, Kaatsch P, Michaelis J. Association of child-hood leukaemia with factors related to the immune system. Br J Cancer 1999; 80:585–590.

209. Linet MS, Cartwright RA. The leukemias. In: Schottenfeld DM, Fraumeni JF Jr eds. Cancer Epidemiology Prevention. 2nd ed. New York: Oxford University Press, 1996:841–892.

210. Alexander FE. Is mycoplasma pneumonia associated with childhood acute lymphoblastic leukemia? Cancer Causes Control 1997; 8:803–811

211. Birch JM, Alexander FE, Blair V, Eden OB, Taylor GM, McNally RJ. Space–time clustering patterns in childhood leukaemia support a role for infection. Br J Cancer 2000; 82:1571–1576.

212. Till M, Rapson N, Smith PG. Family studies in acute leukaemia in childhood: a possible association with autoimmune disease. Br J Cancer 1979; 40:62–71.

213. Roman E, Ansell P, Bull D. Leukaemia and non-Hodgkin's lymphoma in chil-dren and young adults: are prenatal and neonatal factors important determi-nants of disease? Br J Cancer 1997; 76:406–415

214. Comstock GW. Leukaemia and BCG. A controlled trial. Lancet 1971; 2:1062–1063.

215. Comstock GW, Martinez I, Livesay VT. Efficacy of BCG vaccination in prevention of cancer. J Natl Cancer Inst 1975; 54:835–839.

216. Snider DE, Comstock GW, Martinez I, Caras GJ. Efficacy of BCG vaccination in prevention of cancer: an update. J Natl Cancer Inst 1978; 60:785–788.

217. Groves FD, Gridley G, Wacholder S, Shu XO, Robison LL, Neglia JP, et al. Infant vaccinations and risk of childhood acute lymphoblastic leukaemia in the USA. Br J Cancer 1999; 81:175–178.

218. Auvinen A, Hakulinen T, Groves F. Haemophilus influenzae type B vaccination and risk of childhood leukaemia in a vaccine trial in Finland. Br J Cancer 2000; 83:956–958.

219. Groves F, Auvinen A, Hakulinen T. Haemophilus influenzae type b vaccination and risk of childhood leukemia in a vaccine trial in Finland. Ann Epidemiol 2000; 10:474.

220. Groves FD, Sinha D, Kayhty H, Goedert JJ, Levine PH. Haemophilus influenzae type b serology in childhood leukaemia: a case–control study. Br J Cancer 2001; 85:337–340.

221. Petridou E, Trichopoulos D, Kalapothaki V, Pourtsidis A, Kogevinas M, Kalmanti M, et al. The risk profile of childhood leukaemia in Greece: a nationwide case–control study. Br J Cancer 1997; 76:1241–1247.

222. Neglia JP, Linet MS, Shu XO, Severson RK, Potter JD, Mertens AC, et al. Patterns of infection and day care utilization and risk of childhood acute lymphoblastic leukaemia. Br J Cancer 2000; 82:234–240.

223. Murray L, McCarron P, Bailie K, Middleton R, Davey SG, Dempsey S, et al. Association of early life factors and acute lymphoblastic leukaemia in childhood: historical cohort study. Br J Cancer 2002; 86:356–361.

224. Swensen AR, Ross JA, Shu XO, Reaman GH, Steinbuch M, Robison LL. Pet ownership and childhood acute leukemia (USA and Canada). Cancer Causes Control 2001; 12:301–303.

225. Westerbeek RM, Blair V, Eden OB, Kelsey AM, Stevens RF, Will AM, et al. Seasonal variations in the onset of childhood leukaemia and lymphoma. Br J Cancer 1998; 78:119–124.

226. Higgins CD, dos-Santos-Silva I, Stiller CA, Swerdlow AJ. Season of birth and diagnosis of children with leukaemia: an analysis of over 15 000 UK cases occurring from 1953–95. Br J Cancer 2001; 84:406–412.

227. Sorensen HT, Pedersen L, Olsen J, Rothman K. Seasonal variation in month of birth and diagnosis of early childhood acute lymphoblastic leukemia. J Am Med Assoc 2001; 285: 168–169.

228. Linet MS, Ries LA, Smith MA, Tarone RE, Devesa SS. Cancer surveillance series: recent trends in childhood cancer incidence and mortality in the United States. J Natl Cancer Inst 1999; 91:1051–1058.

229. McNally RJ, Cairns DP, Eden OB, Kelsey AM, Taylor GM, Birch JM. Examination of temporal trends in the incidence of childhood leukaemias and lymphomas provides aetiological clues. Leukemia 2001; 15:1612–1618.

230. MacKenzie J, Gallagher A, Clayton RA, Perry J, Eden OB, Ford AM, et al. Screening for herpesvirus genomes in common acute lymphoblastic leukemia. Leukemia 2001; 15: 415–421.

231. Smith MA, Strickler HD, Granovsky M, Reaman G, Linet M, Daniel R, et al. Investigation of leukemia cells from children with common acute lymphoblastic leukemia for genomic sequences of the primate polyomaviruses JC virus, BK virus, and simian virus 40. Med Pediatr Oncol 1999; 33:441–443.

232. MacKenzie J, Perry J, Ford AM, Jarrett RF, Greaves M. JC and BK virus sequences are not detectable in leukaemic samples from children with common acute lymphoblastic leukaemia. Br J Cancer 1999; 81:898–899.

233. Wertheimer N, Leeper E. Electrical wiring configurations and childhood cancer. Am J Epidemiol 1979; 109:273–284.
234. Savitz DA, Wachtel H, Barnes FA, John EM, Tvrdik JG. Case–control study of childhood cancer and exposure to 60-Hz magnetic fields. Am J Epidemiol 1988; 128:21–38.
235. Feychting M, Ahlbom A. Magnetic fields and cancer in children residing near Swedish high-voltage power lines. Am J Epidemiol 1993; 138:467–481.
236. Michaelis J, Schuz J, Meinert R, Menger M, Grigat JP, Kaatsch P, et al. Childhood leukemia and electromagnetic fields: results of a population-based case–control study in Germany. Cancer Causes Control 1997; 8:167–174.
237. Linet MS, Hatch EE, Kleinerman RA, Robison LL, Kaune WT, Friedman DR, et al. Residential exposure to magnetic fields and acute lymphoblastic leukemia in children. N Engl J Med 1997; 337:1–7.
238. McBride ML, Gallagher RP, Theriault G, Armstrong BG, Tamaro S, Spinelli JJ, et al. Power-frequency electric and magnetic fields and risk of childhood leukemia in Canada. Am J Epidemiol 1999; 149:831–842. [Published erratum appears in Am J Epidemiol 1999; 150(2):223.].
239. UK Childhood Study Investigators. Exposure to power-frequency magnetic fields and the risk of childhood cancer. Lancet 1999; 354:1925–1931.
240. Ahlbom A, Day N, Feychting M, Roman E, Skinner J, Dockerty J, et al. A pooled analysis of magnetic fields and childhood leukaemia. Br J Cancer 2000; 83:692–698.
241. Greenland S, Sheppard AR, Kaune WT, Poole C, Kelsh MA. A pooled analysis of magnetic fields, wire codes, and childhood leukemia. Childhood Leukemia—EMF Study Group. Epidemiology 2000; 11:624–634.
242. Skibola CF, Smith MT, Kane E, Roman E, Rollinson S, Cartwright RA, et al. Polymorphisms in the methylenetetrahydrofolate reductase gene are associated with susceptibility to acute leukemia in adults. Proc Natl Acad Sci U S A 1999; 96:12810–12815.
243. Selhub J. Folate binding proteins. Mechanisms for placental and intestinal uptake. Adv Exp Med Biol 1994; 352:141–149.
244. de Franchis R, Sebastio G, Mandato C, Andria G, Mastroiacovo P. Spina bifida, 677T→C mutation, and role of folate. Lancet 1995; 346:1703.
245. Frosst P, Blom HJ, Milos R, Goyette P, Sheppard CA, Matthews RG, et al. A candidate genetic risk factor for vascular-disease—a common mutation in methylenetetrahydrofolate reductase. Nat Genet 1995; 10:111–113.
246. Nishio H, Lee MJ, Fujii M, Kario K, Kayaba K, Shimada K, et al. A common mutation in methylenetetrahydrofolate reductase gene among the Japanese population. Jpn J Hum Genet 1996; 41:247–251.
247. Kuppers R, Rajewsky K, Zhao M, Simons G, Laumann R, Fischer R, et al. Hodgkin disease: Hodgkin and Reed-Sternberg cells picked from histological sections show clonal immunoglobulin gene rearrangements and appear to be derived from B cells at various stages of development. Proc Natl Acad Sci U S A 1994; 91:10962–10966.
248. Braeuninger A, Kuppers R, Strickler JG, Wacker HH, Rajewsky K, Hansmann ML. Hodgkin and Reed-Sternberg cells in lymphocyte predomi-

nant Hodgkin disease represent clonal populations of germinal center-derived tumor B cells. Proc Natl Acad Sci U S A 1997; 94:9337–9342.

249. Irsch J, Nitsch S, Hansmann ML, Rajewsky K, Tesch H, Diehl V, et al. Isolation of viable Hodgkin and Reed-Sternberg cells from Hodgkin disease tissues. Proc Natl Acad Sci U S A 1998; 95:10117–10122.

250. Seitz V, Hummel M, Marafioti T, Anagnostopoulos I, Assaf C, Stein H. Detection of clonal T-cell receptor gamma-chain gene rearrangements in Reed-Sternberg cells of classic Hodgkin disease. Blood 2000; 95:3020–3024.

251. Marafioti T, Hummel M, Foss HD, Laumen H, Korbjuhn P, Anagnostopoulos I, et al. Hodgkin and Reed-Sternberg cells represent an expansion of a single clone originating from a germinal center B-cell with functional immunoglobulin gene rearrangements but defective immunoglobulin transcription. Blood 2000; 95:1443–1450.

252. Mueller N. Hodgkins disease. In: Schottenfeld DM, Fraumen JF Jr eds. Cancer Epidemiology and Prevention. 2 New York: Oxford University Press, 1996:893–919.

253. Glaser SL, Lin RJ, Stewart SL, Ambinder RF, Jarrett RF, Brousset P, et al. Epstein–Barr virus-associated Hodgkin's disease: epidemiologic characteristics in international data. Int J Cancer 1997; 70:375–382.

254. Jarrett RF, MacKenzie J. Epstein–Barr virus and other candidate viruses in the pathogenesis of Hodgkin's disease. Semin Hematol 1999; 36:260–269.

255. Hsu JL, Glaser SL. Epstein–Barr virus-associated malignancies: epidemiologic patterns and etiologic implications. Crit Rev Oncol Hematol 2000; 34:27–53.

256. Hjalgrim H, Askling J, Sorensen P, Madsen M, Rosdahl N, Storm HH, et al. Risk of Hodgkin's disease and other cancers after infectious mononucleosis. J Natl Cancer Inst 2000; 92:1522–1528.

257. Alexander FE, Jarrett RF, Cartwright RA, Armstrong AA, Gokhale DA, Kane E, et al. Epstein–Barr virus and HLA-DPB1-*0301 in young adult Hodgkin's disease: evidence for inherited susceptibility to Epstein–Barr Virus in cases that are EBV(+ve). Cancer Epidemiol Biomarkers Prev 2001; 10:705–709.

258. Khuder SA, Mutgi AB, Schaub EA, Tano BD. Meta-analysis of Hodgkin's disease among farmers. Scand J Work Environ Health 1999; 25:436–441.

259. Pukkala E, Notkola V. Cancer incidence among Finnish farmers, 1979–93. Cancer Causes Control 1997; 8:25–33.

260. McCunney RJ. Hodgkin's disease, work, and the environment. A review. J Occup Environ Med 1999; 41:36–46.

261. Rix BA, Villadsen E, Engholm G, Lynge E. Hodgkin's disease, pharyngeal cancer, and soft tissue sarcomas in Danish paper mill workers. J Occup Environ Med 1998; 40:55–62.

262. Eriksson M, Hallberg B. Familial occurrence of hematologic malignancies and other diseases in multiple myeloma: a case–control study. Cancer Causes Control 1992; 3:63–67.

263. Ferraris AM, Racchi O, Rapezzi D, Gaetani GF, Boffetta P. Familial Hodgkin's disease: a disease of young adulthood? Ann Hematol 1997; 74:131–134.

264. Paltiel O, Schmit T, Adler B, Rachmilevitz EA, Polliack A, Cohen A, et al. The incidence of lymphoma in first-degree relatives of patients with Hodgkin

disease and non-Hodgkin lymphoma: results and limitations of a registry-linked study. Cancer 2000; 88:2357–2366.

265. Pottern LM, Linet M, Blair A, Dick F, Burmeister LF, Gibson R, et al. Familial cancers associated with subtypes of leukemia and non-Hodgkin's lymphoma. Leuk Res 1991; 15: 305–314.

266. Le Bihan C, Moutou C, Chompret A, Abel A, Poisson N, Brugieres L, et al. Cancers in relatives of children with non-Hodgkin's lymphoma. Leuk Res 1996; 20:181–186.

267. Mack TM, Cozen W, Shibata DK, Weiss LM, Nathwani BN, Hernandez AM, et al. Concordance for Hodgkin's disease in identical twins suggesting genetic susceptibility to the young–adult form of the disease. N Engl J Med 1995; 332: 413–418.

268. Siebert R, Louie D, Lacher M, Schluger A, Offit K. Familial Hodgkin's and non-Hodgkin's lymphoma: different patterns in first-degree relatives. Leuk Lymphoma 1997; 27:503–507.

269. Limpens J, de Jong D, van Krieken JH, Price CG, Young BD, van Ommen GJ, et al. Bcl-2/JH rearrangements in benign lymphoid tissues with follicular hyperplasia. Oncogene 1991; 6:2271–2276.

270. Lipkowitz S, Garry VF, Kirsch IR. Interlocus V-J recombination measures genomic instability in agriculture workers at risk for lymphoid malignancies. Proc Natl Acad Sci USA 1992; 89:5301–5305.

271. Liu Y, Hernandez AM, Shibata D, Cortopassi GA. BCL2 translocation frequency rises with age in humans. Proc Natl Acad Sci USA 1994; 91: 8910–8914.

272. Knowles DM (ed.). Neoplastic hematopathology. 2nd ed. Philadelphia: Lippincott Williams & Wilkins, 2001.

273. Fritz A, Percy C, Jack A, Shanmugaratnam K, Sobin L, Parkin DM, Whelan S. 3rd ed. International Classification of Diseases for Oncology. 3rd ed. U.S. Interim Version 2000: Geneva: World Health Organization, 2000.

274. Cartwright RA, Gurney KA, Moorman AV. Sex ratios and the risks of haematological malignancies. Br J Haematol 2002; 118:1071–1077.

275. Kinlen LJ, Sheil AG, Peto J, Doll R. Collaborative United Kingdom-Australasian study of cancer in patients treated with immunosuppressive drugs. Br Med J 1979; 2:1461–1466.

276. Kinlen LJ, Webster AD, Bird AG, Haile R, Peto J, Soothill JF, et al. Prospective study of cancer in patients with hypogammaglobulinaemia. Lancet 1985; 1:263–266.

277. Hoover R, Fraumeni JF Jr. Risk of cancer in renal-transplant recipients. Lancet 1973; 2:55–57.

278. Opelz G, Henderson R. Incidence of non-Hodgkin lymphoma in kidney and heart transplant recipients. Lancet 1993; 342:1514–1516.

279. Birkeland SA, Storm HH, Lamm LU, Barlow L, Blohme I, Forsberg B, et al. Cancer risk after renal transplantation in the Nordic countries, 1964–1986. Int J Cancer 1995; 60: 183–189.

280. Penn I. Tumors after renal and cardiac transplantation. Hematol Oncol Clin North Am 1993; 7:431–445.

281. Curtis RE, Rowlings PA, Deeg HJ, Shriner DA, Socie G, Travis LB, et al. Solid cancers after bone marrow transplantation. N Engl J Med 1997; 336:897–904.

282. Curtis RE, Travis LB, Rowlings PA, Socie G, Kingma DW, Banks PM, et al. Risk of lymphoproliferative disorders after bone marrow transplantation: a multi-institutional study. Blood 1999; 94:2208–2216.

283. Swinnen LJ. Overview of posttransplant B-cell lymphoproliferative disorders. Semin Oncol 1999; 26:21–25.

284. Kinlen LJ. Malignancy in autoimmune diseases. J Autoimmun 1992; 5(Suppl A):363–371.

285. Pettersson T, Pukkala E, Teppo L, Friman C. Increased risk of cancer in patients with systemic lupus erythematosus. Ann Rheum Dis 1992; 51: 437–439.

286. Mellemkjaer L, Andersen V, Linet MS, Gridley G, Hoover R, Olsen JH. Non-Hodgkin's lymphoma and other cancers among a cohort of patients with systemic lupus erythematosus. Arthritis Rheum 1997; 40:761–768.

287. Bjornadal L, Lofstrom B, Yin L, Lundberg IE, Ekbom A. Increased cancer incidence in a Swedish cohort of patients with systemic lupus erythematosus. Scand J Rheumatol 2002; 31:66–71.

288. Silman AJ, Petrie J, Hazleman B, Evans SJ. Lymphoproliferative cancer and other malignancy in patients with rheumatoid arthritis treated with azathioprine: a 20 year follow up study. Ann Rheum Dis 1988; 47:988–992.

289. Gridley G, McLaughlin JK, Ekbom A, Klareskog L, Adami HO, Hacker DG et al. Incidence of cancer among patients with rheumatoid arthritis. J Natl Cancer Inst 1993; 85: 307–311.

290. Vineis P, Crosignani P, Sacerdote C, Fontana A, Masala G, Miligi L, et al. Haematopoietic cancer and medical history: a multicentre case-control study. J Epidemiol Community Health 2000;54:431–436.

291. Gridley G, Klippel JH, Hoover RN, Fraumeni JF Jr. Incidence of cancer among men with the Felty syndrome. Ann Intern Med 1994; 120:35–39.

292. Kassan SS, Thomas TL, Moutsopoulos HM, Hoover R, Kimberly RP, Budman DR, et al. Increased risk of lymphoma in sicca syndrome. Ann Intern Med 1978; 89:888–892.

293. Holmes GK, Stokes PL, Sorahan TM, Prior P, Waterhouse JA, Cooke WT. Coeliac disease, gluten-free diet, and malignancy. Gut 1976; 17:612–619.

294. Leonard JN, Tucker WF, Fry JS, Coulter CA, Boylston AW, McMinn RM, et al. Increased incidence of malignancy in dermatitis herpetiformis. Br Med J (Clin Res Ed) 1983; 286:16–18.

295. Sigurgeirsson B, Agnarsson BA, Lindelof B. Risk of lymphoma in patients with dermatitis herpetiformis. Br Med J 1994; 308:13–15.

296. Collin P, Pukkala E, Reunala T. Malignancy and survival in dermatitis herpetiformis: a comparison with coeliac disease. Gut 1996; 38:528–530.

297. International Agency for Research on Cancer. IARC Monographs on the Evaluation of the Carcinogenic Risk of Chemicals to Man: Epstein–Barr Virus and Kaposi's Sarcoma Herpesvirus/Human Herpesvirus 8. Vol. 70. IARC: Lyon, 1997:82–127.

298. Beral V, Peterman T, Berkelman R, Jaffe H. AIDS-associated non-Hodgkin lymphoma. Lancet 1991; 337:805–809.

299. Rabkin CS, Biggar RJ, Horm JW. Increasing incidence of cancers associated with the human immunodeficiency virus epidemic. Int J Cancer 1991; 47: 692–696.

300. Goedert JJ, Cote TR, Virgo P, Scoppa SM, Kingma DW, Gail MH, et al. Spectrum of AIDS-associated malignant disorders. Lancet 1998; 351: 1833–1839.

301. Dean M, Jacobson LP, McFarlane G, Margolick JB, Jenkins FJ, Howard OM, et al. Reduced risk of AIDS lymphoma in individuals heterozygous for the CCR5 delta32 mutation. Cancer Res 1999; 59:3561–3564.

302. Wotherspoon AC, Ortiz-Hidalgo C, Falzon MR, Isaacson PG. Helicobacter pylori-associated gastritis and primary B-cell gastric lymphoma. Lancet 1991; 338:1175–1176.

303. Wotherspoon AC. Gastric lymphoma of mucosa-associated lymphoid tissue and Helicobacter pylori. Annu Rev Med 1998; 49:289–299.

304. Neubauer A, Thiede C, Morgner A, Alpen B, Ritter M, Neubauer B, et al. Cure of Helicobacter pylori infection and duration of remission of low-grade gastric mucosa-associated lymphoid tissue lymphoma. J Natl Cancer Inst 1997; 89:1350–1355.

305. Khuder SA, Schaub EA, Keller-Byrne JE. Meta-analyses of non-Hodgkin's lymphoma and farming. Scand J Work Environ Health 1998; 24:255–261.

306. Fleming LE, Bean JA, Rudolph M, Hamilton K. Mortality in a cohort of licensed pesticide applicators in Florida. Occup Environ Med 1999; 56:14–21.

307. Sperati A, Rapiti E, Settimi L, Quercia A, Terenzoni B, Forastiere F. Mortality among male licensed pesticide users and their wives. Am J Ind Med 1999; 36:142–146.

308. Alavanja MC, Blair A, Masters MN. Cancer mortality in the U.S. flour industry. J Natl Cancer Inst 1990; 82:840–848.

309. Gambini GF, Mantovani C, Pira E, Piolatto PG, Negri E. Cancer mortality among rice growers in Novara Province, northern Italy. Am J Ind Med 1997; 31:435–441.

310. Hoar SK, Blair A, Holmes FF, Boysen CD, Robel RJ, Hoover R, et al. Agricultural herbicide use and risk of lymphoma and soft-tissue sarcoma [Published erratum appears in J Am Med Assoc 1986; 256(24):3351.] J Am Med Assoc 1986; 256:1141–1147.

311. Zahm SH, Weisenburger DD, Babbitt PA, Saal RC, Vaught JB, Cantor KP, et al. A case–control study of non-Hodgkin's lymphoma and the herbicide 2,4-dichlorophenoxyacetic acid (2,4-D) in eastern Nebraska. Epidemiology 1990; 1:349–356.

312. Baris D, Zahm SH, Cantor KP, Blair A. Agricultural use of DDT and risk of non-Hodgkin's lymphoma: pooled analysis of three case–control studies in the United States. Occup Environ Med 1998; 55:522–527.

313. Schroeder JC, Olshan AF, Baric R, Dent GA, Weinberg CR, Yount B, et al. Agricultural risk factors for t(14; 18) subtypes of non-Hodgkin's lymphoma. Epidemiology 2001; 12:701–709.

313a. Metayer C, Johnson ES, Rice JC. Nested case-control study of tumors of the hemopoietic and lymphatic systems among workers in the meat industry. Am J Epidemiol 1998; 147:727–738.

313b. Rothman N, Cantor KP, Blair A, Bush D, Brock JW, Helzlsouer K, et al. A nested case-control study of non-Hodgkin lymphoma and serum organochlorine residues. Lancet 1997;350(9073):240–244.

314. Fingerhut MA, Halperin WE, Marlow DA, Piacitelli LA, Honchar PA, Sweeney MH, et al. Cancer mortality in workers exposed to 2,3,7,8-tetrachlorodibenzo-p-dioxin. N Engl J Med 1991; 324:212–218.

315. Becher H, Flesch-Janys D, Kauppinen T, Kogevinas M, Steindorf K, Manz A, et al. Cancer mortality in German male workers exposed to phenoxy herbicides and dioxins. Cancer Causes Control 1996; 7:312–321.

316. Lynge E. Cancer incidence in Danish phenoxy herbicide workers, 1947–1993. Environ Health Perspect 1998; 106(suppl 2):683–688.

317. Kogevinas M, Becher H, Benn T, Bertazzi PA, Boffetta P, Bueno-de-Mesquita HB, et al. Cancer mortality in workers exposed to phenoxy herbicides, chlorophenols, and dioxins. An expanded and updated international cohort study. Am J Epidemiol 1997; 145:1061–1075.

317a. McGregor DB, Partensky C, Wilbourn J, Rice JM. An IARC evaluation of polychlorinated dibenzo-p-dioxins and polychlorinated dibezofurans as risk factors in human carcinogenesis. Environ Health Perspect 1998; 106(Suppl 2):755–760.

318. Monson RR, Fine LJ. Cancer mortality and morbidity among rubber workers. J Natl Cancer Inst 1978; 61:1047–1053.

319. Delzell E, Monson RR. Mortality among rubber workers. III. Cause-specific mortality, 1940–1978. J Occup Med 1981; 23:677–684.

320. Delzell E, Monson RR. Mortality among rubber workers: X. Reclaim workers. Am J Ind Med 1985; 7:307–313.

321. Hodgson JT, Jones RD. Mortality of styrene production, polymerization and processing workers at a site in northwest England. Scand J Work Environ Health 1985; 11:347–352.

322. Cole P, Delzell E, Acquavella J. Exposure to butadiene and lymphatic and hematopoietic cancer. Epidemiology 1993; 4:96–103.

323. Wong O, Trent LS, Whorton MD. An updated cohort mortality study of workers exposed to styrene in the reinforced plastics and composites industry. Occup Environ Med 1994; 51: 386–396.

324. Shore RE, Gardner MJ, Pannett B. Ethylene oxide: an assessment of the epidemiological evidence on carcinogenicity. Br J Ind Med 1993; 50:971–997

324a. Steenland K, Stayner L, Deddens J. Mortality analyses in a cohort of 18 235 ethylene oxide exposed workers: followup extended from 1987 to 1998. Occup Environ Med 2004; 61:2–7.

325. Wilcosky TC, Checkoway H, Marshall EG, Tyroler HA. Cancer mortality and solvent exposures in the rubber industry. Am Ind Hyg Assoc J 1984; 45:809–811.

326. Tavani A, Negri E, Franceschi S, Serraino D, La Vecchia C. Smoking habits and non-Hodgkin's lymphoma: a case-control study in northern Italy. Prev Med 1994; 23:447–452.

327. Brown LM, Everett GD, Gibson R, Burmeister LF, Schuman LM, Blair A. Smoking and risk of non-Hodgkin's lymphoma and multiple myeloma. Cancer Causes Control 1992; 3:49–55.

328. Linet MS, McLaughlin JK, Hsing AW, Wacholder S, Co Chien HT, Schuman LM, et al. Is cigarette smoking a risk factor for non-Hodgkin's lymphoma or multiple myeloma? Results from the Lutheran Brotherhood Cohort Study. Leuk Res 1992; 16:621–624.

329. Linet MS, Pottern LM. Familial aggregation of hematopoietic malignancies and risk of non-Hodgkin's lymphoma. Cancer Res 1992; 52:5468s–5473s.

329a. Scherr PA, Mueller NE. Non-Hodgkin lymphoma. In: Schottenfeld DM, Fraumeni JF Jr eds. Cancer Epidemiology and Prevention. 2nd ed. New York: Oxford University Press, 1996:920–945.

330. Chiu BC, Cerhan JR, Folsom AR, Sellers TA, Kushi LH, Wallace RB, et al. Diet and risk of non-Hodgkin lymphoma in older women. J Am Med Assoc 1996; 275:1315–1321.

331. De Stefani E, Fierro L, Barrios E, Ronco A. Tobacco, alcohol, diet and risk of non-Hodgkin's lymphoma: a case–control study in Uruguay. Leuk Res 1998; 22:445–452.

332. Zhang S, Hunter DJ, Rosner BA, Colditz GA, Fuchs CS, Speizer FE, et al. Dietary fat and protein in relation to risk of non-Hodgkin's lymphoma among women. J Natl Cancer Inst 1999; 91:1751–1758.

332a. Tavani A, Pregnolato A, Negri E, Franceschi S, Serraino D, Carbone A, et al. Diet and risk of lymphoid neoplasms and soft tissue sarcomas. Nutr Cancer 1997;27:256–260.

333. Zahm SH, Weisenburger DD, Babbitt PA, Saal RC, Vaught JB, Blair A. Use of hair coloring products and the risk of lymphoma, multiple myeloma, and chronic lymphocytic leukemia. Am J Public Health 1992; 82:990–997.

334. Altekruse SF, Henley SJ, Thun MJ. Deaths from hematopoietic and other cancers in relation to permanent hair dye use in a large prospective study (United States). Cancer Causes Control 1999; 10:617–625.

335. Grodstein F, Hennekens CH, Colditz GA, Hunter DJ, Stampfer MJ. A prospective study of permanent hair dye use and hematopoietic cancer. J Natl Cancer Inst 1994; 86:1466–1470.

336. Hamblin TJ, Orchard JA, Gardiner A, Oscier DG, Davis Z, Stevenson FK. Immunoglobulin V genes and CD38 expression in CLL. Blood 2000; 95:2455–2457.

337. Cartwright RA, Bernard SM, Bird CC, Darwin CM, O'Brien C, Richards ID, et al. Chronic lymphocytic leukaemia: case–control epidemiological study in Yorkshire. Br J Cancer 1987; 56:79–82.

338. Blair A, White DW. Leukemia cell types and agricultural practices in Nebraska. Arch Environ Health 1985; 40:211–214.

339. Brown LM, Blair A, Gibson R, Everett GD, Cantor KP, Schuman LM, et al. Pesticide exposures and other agricultural risk factors for leukemia among men in Iowa and Minnesota. Cancer Res 1990; 50:6585–6591.

340. Kelleher C, Newell J, MacDonagh-White C, MacHale E, Egan E, Connolly E, et al. Incidence and occupational pattern of leukaemias, lymphomas, and

testicular tumours in western Ireland over an 11 year period. J Epidemiol Community Health 1998; 52:651–656.

341. Flodin U, Fredriksson M, Persson B, Axelson O. Chronic lymphocytic leukaemia and engine exhausts, fresh wood and DDT: a case-referent study. Br J Ind Med 1988; 45:33–38.

342. Arp EW Jr, Wolf PH, Checkoway H. Lymphocytic leukemia and exposures to benzene and other solvents in the rubber industry. J Occup Med 1983; 25: 598–602.

343. Bertazzi PA, Pesatori AC, Zocchetti C, Latocca R. Mortality study of cancer risk among oil refinery workers. Int Arch Occup Environ Health 1989; 61: 261–270.

344. Wongsrichanalai C, Delzell E, Cole P. Mortality from leukemia and other diseases among workers at a petroleum refinery. J Occup Med 1989; 31: 106–111.

345. Rushton L, Alderson MR. An epidemiological survey of eight oil refineries in Britain. Br J Ind Med 1981; 38:225–234.

346. Honda Y, Delzell E, Cole P. An updated study of mortality among workers at a petroleum manufacturing plant. J Occup Environ Med 1995; 37:194–200.

347. Sathiakumar N, Delzell E. A review of epidemiologic studies of triazine herbicides and cancer. Crit Rev Toxicol 1997; 27:599–612.

348. Divine BJ, Hartman CM, Wendt JK. Update of the Texaco mortality study 1947–93: part II. Analyses of specific causes of death for white men employed in refining, research, and petrochemicals. Occup Environ Med 1999; 56: 174–180.

349. Raabe GK, Wong O. Leukemia mortality by cell type in petroleum workers with potential exposure to benzene. Environ Health Perspect 1996; 104(suppl 6):1381–1392.

350. Kogevinas M, Ferro G, Andersen A, Bellander T, Biocca M, Coggon D, et al. Cancer mortality in a historical cohort study of workers exposed to styrene. Scand J Work Environ Health 1994; 20:251–261.

351. Kogevinas M, Sala M, Boffetta P, Kazerouni N, Kromhout H, Hoar-Zahm S. Cancer risk in the rubber industry: a review of the recent epidemiological evidence. Occup Environ Med 1998; 55:1–12.

352. Boice JD Jr, Land CE, Preston DL. Ionizing radiation. In: Schottenfeld D, Fraumeni JF Jr, eds. 2nd ed. New York: Oxford University Press, 1996:319–354.

353. Kinlen LJ, Rogot E. Leukaemia and smoking habits among United States veterans. Br Med J 1988; 297:657–659.

354. Linet MS, McLaughlin JK, Hsing AW, Wacholder S, Co-Chien HT, Schuman LM, et al. Cigarette smoking and leukemia: results from the Lutheran Brotherhood Cohort Study. Cancer Causes Control 1991; 2:413–417.

355. Brown LM, Gibson R, Blair A, Burmeister LF, Schuman LM, Cantor KP, et al. Smoking and risk of leukemia. Am J Epidemiol 1992; 135:763–768.

356. Friedman GD. Cigarette smoking, leukemia, and multiple myeloma. Ann Epidemiol 1993; 3:425–428.

357. Vidabaek A. Familial leukemia. Acta Med Scand 1947; 127: 26–52.

358. Sgambati M, Linet M, Devesa S. Chronic lymphocytic leukemia: epidemiolical, familial, and genetic aspects In: Cheson B Chronic Lymphocytic Leukemia. 2nd ed. New York: Marcel Dekker, 2001:33–62.

359. Gunz FW, Gunz JP, Vincent PC, Bergin M, Johnson FL, Bashir H, et al. Thirteen cases of leukemia in a family. J Natl Cancer Inst 1978; 60:1243–1250.

360. Linet MS, Van Natta ML, Brookmeyer R, Khoury MJ, McCaffrey LD, Humphrey RL, et al. Familial cancer history and chronic lymphocytic leukemia. A case–control study. Am J Epidemiol 1989; 130:655–664.

361. Cuttner J. Increased incidence of hematologic malignancies in first-degree relatives of patients with chronic lymphocytic leukemia. Cancer Invest 1992; 10:103–109.

362. Weiss HA, Darby SC, Doll R. Cancer mortality following X-ray treatment for ankylosing spondylitis. Int J Cancer 1994; 59:327–338.

363. Boice JD Jr, Day NE, Andersen A, Brinton LA, Brown R, Choi NW, et al. Second cancers following radiation treatment for cervical cancer. An international collaboration among cancer registries. J Natl Cancer Inst 1985; 74: 955–975.

364. Darby SC, Reeves G, Key T, Doll R, Stovall M. Mortality in a cohort of women given X-ray therapy for metropathia haemorrhagica. Int J Cancer 1994; 56:793–801.

365. Andersson M, Storm HH. Cancer incidence among Danish Thorotrast-exposed patients. J Natl Cancer Inst 1992; 84:1318–1325.

366. Blair A, Zahm SH, Pearce NE, Heineman EF, Fraumeni JF Jr. Clues to cancer etiology from studies of farmers. Scand J Work Environ Health 1992; 18:209–215.

367. Pottern LM, Linet MS, Devesa SS. Epidemiology of Multiple Myeloma. Neoplastic Diseases of the Blood. 3rd ed. New York: Churchill Livingstone, 1996:441–452.

368. Herrinton LJ, Weiss NS, Olshan AF. Epidemiology of multiple myeloma. In: Malpas JS, Bergsagel DE, Kyle RA, eds. Myeloma-Biology and Management. Oxford: Oxford University Press, 1995:1127.

369. Khuder SA, Mutgi AB. Meta-analyses of multiple myeloma and farming. Am J Ind Med 1997; 32:510–516.

370. Wiklund K, Dich J. Cancer risks among female farmers in Sweden. Cancer Causes Control 1994; 5:449–457.

371. Kristensen P, Andersen A, Irgens LM, Laake P, Bye AS. Incidence and risk factors of cancer among men and women in Norwegian agriculture. Scand J Work Environ Health 1996; 22:14–26.

372. Cocco P, Blair A, Congia P, Saba G, Ecca AR, Palmas C. Long-term health effects of the occupational exposure to DDT. A preliminary report. Ann N Y Acad Sci 1997; 837:246–256.

373. Gallagher RP, Spinelli JJ, Elwood JM, Skippen DH. Allergies and agricultural exposure as risk factors for multiple myeloma. Br J Cancer 1983; 48:853–857.

374. Pahwa P, McDuffie HH, Dosman JA, Robson D, McLaughlin JR, Spinelli JJ, et al. Exposure to animals and selected risk factors among Canadian farm residents with Hodgkin's disease, muldiple myeloma, or soft tissue sarcoma. J Occup Environ Med 2003;45:857–868.

375. Lewis EB. Leukemia, multiple myeloma and aplastic anemia in American radiologists. Science 1963; 142: 1492–1499.
376. Berrington A, Darby SC, Weiss HA, Doll R. 100 years of observation on British radiologists: mortality from cancer and other causes 1897–1997. Br J Radiol 2001; 74:507–519.
377. Cardis E, Gilbert ES, Carpenter L, Howe G, Kato I, Armstrong BK, et al. Effects of low oses and low dose rates of external ionizing radiation: cancer mortality among nuclear industry workers in three countries. Radiat Res 1995; 142:117–132.
377a. Muirhead CR, Goodill AA, Haylock RG, Vokes J, Little MP, Jackson DA, et al. Occupational radiation exposure and mortality: second analysis of the National Registry for Radiation Workers. J Radiol Prot 1999;19:3–26.
378. Darby SC, Kendall GM, Fell TP, O'Hagan JA, Muirhead CR, Ennis JR, et al. A summary of mortality and incidence of cancer in men from the United Kingdom who participated in the United Kingdom's atmospheric nuclear weapon tests and experimental programmes. Br Med J (Clin Res Ed) 1988; 296:332–338.
379. Pearce N, Prior I, Methven D, Culling C, Marshall S, Auld J, et al. Follow up of New Zealand participants in British atmospheric nuclear weapons tests in the Pacific. Br Med J 1990; 300:1161–1166.
380. Caldwell GG, Kelley D, Zack M, Falk H, Heath CW Jr. Mortality and cancer frequency among military nuclear test (Smoky) participants, 1957 through 1979. J Am Med Assoc 1983; 250:620–624.
381. Robinette CD, Jablon S, Preston TL. Mortality of Nuclear Weapons Test Participants. Medical Follow-up Agency. National Research Council. Washington, DC: National Academy Press, 1985.
382. Friedman GD. Multiple myeloma: relation to propoxyphene and other drugs, radiation and occupation. Int J Epidemiol 1986; 15:424–426.
383. Cuzick J, De Stavola B. Multiple myeloma—a case-control study. Br J Cancer 1988; 57:516–520.
384. Boffetta P, Stellman SD, Garfinkel L. A case-control study of multiple myeloma nested in the American Cancer Society prospective study. Int J Cancer 1989; 43:554–559.
385. Davis FG, Boice JD Jr, Hrubec Z, Monson RR. Cancer mortality in a radiation-exposed cohort of Massachusetts tuberculosis patients. Cancer Res 1989; 49:6130–6613.
386. Boice JD Jr, Morin MM, Glass AG, Friedman GD, Stovall M, Hoover RN, et al. Diagnostic x-ray procedures and risk of leukemia, lymphoma, and multiple myeloma. J Am Med Assoc1991; 265:1290–1294. [Published erratum appears in J Am Med Assoc 1991; 265(21):2810].
387. Bezabeh S, Engel A, Morris CB, Lamm SH. Does benzene cause multiple myeloma? An analysis of the published case-control literature. Environ Health Perspect 1996; 104(suppl 6):1393–1398.
388. Bergsagel DE, Wong O, Bergsagel PL, Alexanian R, Anderson K, Kyle RA, et al. Benzene and multiple myeloma: appraisal of the scientific evidence. Blood 1999; 94:1174–1182.
389. Goldstein BD, Shalat SL. The causal relation between benzene exposure and multiple myeloma. Blood 2000; 95: 1512–1514.

390. Fu H, Demers PA, Costantini AS, Winter P, Colin D, Kogevinas M, et al. Cancer mortality among shoe manufacturing workers: an analysis of two cohorts. Occup Environ Med 1996; 53:394–398.

391. Dement JM, Hensley L, Kieding S, Lipscomb H. Proportionate mortality among union members employed at three Texas refineries. Am J Ind Med 1998; 33:327–340.

392. Raabe GK, Collingwood KW, Wong O. An updated mortality study of workers at a petroleum refinery in Beaumont, Texas. Am J Ind Med 1998; 33:61–81.

393. Wong O, Raabe GK. Multiple myeloma and benzene exposure in a multinational cohort of more than 250,000 petroleum workers. Regul Toxicol Pharmacol 1997; 26:188–199.

394. Gramenzi A, Buttino I, D'Avanzo B, Negri E, Franceschi S, La Vecchia C. Medical history and the risk of multiple myeloma. Br J Cancer 1991; 63:769–772.

395. Brown LM, Gibson R, Burmeister LF, Schuman LM, Everett GD, Blair A. Alcohol consumption and risk of leukemia, non-Hodgkin's lymphoma, and multiple myeloma. Leuk Res 1992; 16:979–984.

396. Heineman EF, Zahm SH, McLaughlin JK, Vaught JB, Hrubec Z. A prospective study of tobacco use and multiple myeloma: evidence against an association. Cancer Causes Control 1992; 3:31–36.

397. Brown LM, Pottern LM, Silverman DT, Schoenberg JB, Schwartz AG, Greenberg RS, et al. Multiple myeloma among Blacks and Whites in the United States: role of cigarettes and alcoholic beverages. Cancer Causes Control 1997; 8:610–614.

397a. Mills PK, Newell GR, Beeson WL, Fraser GE, Phillips RL. History of cigarette smoking and risk of leukemia and myeloma: results from the Adventist health study. J Natl Cancer Inst 1990; 82:1832–1836.

397b. Brown LM, Everett GED, Burmeister LF, Blair A. Hair dye use and multiple myeloma in white men. Am J Publ Health 1992; 82:1673–1674.

398. Fernandez E, Chatenoud L, La Vecchia C, Negri E, Franceschi S. Fish consumption and cancer risk. Am J Clin Nutr 1999; 70:85–90.

399. Chatenoud L, Tavani A, La Vecchia C, Jacobs DR Jr, Negri E, Levi F, et al. Whole grain food intake and cancer risk. Int J Cancer 1998; 77:24–28.

400. Friedman GD, Herrinton LJ. Obesity and multiple myeloma. Cancer Causes Control 1994; 5:479–483.

401. Thun MJ, Altekruse SF, Namboodiri MM, Calle EE, Myers DG, Heath CW Jr. Hair dye use and risk of fatal cancers in U.S. women. J Natl Cancer Inst 1994; 86:210–215.

402. Herrinton LJ, Weiss NS, Koepsell TD, Daling JR, Taylor JW, Lyon JL, et al. Exposure to hair-coloring products and the risk of multiple myeloma. Am J Public Health 1994; 84:1142–1144.

403. Bourguet CC, Grufferman S, Delzell E, DeLong ER, Cohen HJ. Multiple myeloma and family history of cancer. A case–control study. Cancer 1985; 56:2133–2139.

404. Brown LM, Linet MS, Greenberg RS, Silverman DT, Hayes RB, Swanson GM, et al. Multiple myeloma and family history of cancer among blacks and whites in the U.S. Cancer 1999; 85:2385–2390.

27

Bladder Cancers

Paolo Vineis

Unit of Cancer Epidemiology and Chair of Biostatistics, Dipartimento di Scienze Biomediche e Oncologia Umana, University of Turim, Turim, Italy

1. INTRODUCTION

In this chapter we review the most relevant data that permit the risk assessment of bladder cancer, based on the measurement of biomarkers. We consider separately biomarkers relevant to the etiology, and biomarkers relevant to the clinical assessment of such cancers. Many biomarkers have been suggested for use, particularly for clinical purposes, and our review cannot be exhaustive. Therefore, we have selected *p53* as a particularly representative clinical marker.

2. POPULATION RISK ASSESSMENT
2.1. Molecular Epidemiology of Bladder Cancer
2.1.1. Tobacco and Occupational Exposures

Bladder cancer is a relatively prevalent cancer, with age-adjusted incidence rates in Western population of about 30/100,000 men per year and 7–10/100,000 women (1).

The most important, single class of bladder carcinogens consists of aromatic amines. Aromatic amines are present in tobacco smoke and contaminate the ambient air where smokers are present (2). Exposure to aromatic amines occurs in different industrial and agricultural activities. Aromatic amines have been used as antioxidants in the production of rubber and in cutting oils, as intermediates in azo dye manufacturing, and as pesticides.

They are a common contaminant in several working environments, including the chemical and mechanical industries and aluminum transformation. Aromatic amine-based dyes are widely used, particularly in the textile industry.

The strongest evidence on the carcinogenicity of arylamines (benzidine, 2-naphthylamine) comes from large cohort investigations conducted in the 1950s in the British chemical industry. Carcinogenic arylamines such as 2-naphthylamine have been banned in the U.K. since 1967 (Carcinogenic Substances Regulation) (3) and in other Western countries subsequently (4). The International Labour Office had already concluded in 1921, based on early observations in humans, that 2-naphthylamine and benzidine were carcinogenic (5).

Occupational exposures to aromatic amines account for 5%–25% of bladder cancers occurring in some areas of Western countries. Estimates of the attributable fraction are strictly space- and time-specific, and might be higher in limited areas of developing countries.

According to the Working Groups of the International Agency for Research on Cancer Monographs Programme, seven arylamines have been classified as carcinogenic to humans (Group 1) or "probably" carcinogenic to humans (Group 2A). Categorized as such are three specific occupational chemicals (2-naphthylamine, benzidine, and MOCA), one medication (Chlornaphazine), one group of industrial compounds (benzidine-based dyes, i.e., Direct Black 38, Direct Blue 6, and Direct Brown 95), and two manufacturing processes (manufacture of auramine and magenta). Whereas for the other chemicals or industrial processes, the evidence of carcinogenicity in humans was sufficient, benzidine-based dyes and MOCA were considered "probably" carcinogenic because of a high level of evidence in experimental animals.

Tobacco smoking is a well-known cause of bladder cancer—accounting for more than 50% bladder cancers in men and 20% in women, in Western societies—and is a source of arylamines (6). Air-cured (black) tobacco, is particularly rich in arylamines such as 4-aminobiphenyl; smokers of black tobacco have a risk of bladder cancer that is about 2.5-fold in comparison with smokers of flue-cured blond tobacco (7). Studies of "molecular epidemiology" have suggested that smokers of air-cured black tobacco have higher levels of 4-aminobiphenyl–hemoglobin adducts (a marker of internal dose) in their blood, compared to smokers of flue-cured tobacco (8). Biopsies of bladder cancer from smokers contain a DNA adduct identified as a derivative of 4-aminobiphenyl (9). This same DNA adduct was present in exfoliated bladder cells of smokers (10); the presence and concentration of the DNA adducts was strongly correlated with 4-amino biphenyl–hemoglobin adducts but not with urinary 1-hydroxypyrene-glucuronide, a metabolite of benzopyrene (11) (Table 1; the derivative of 4-aminobiphenyl is adduct 4). The latter observation suggests that arylamines and not polycyclic aromatic hydrocarbons in tobacco smoke may be responsible of bladder cancer in smokers.

Table 1 Correlation Coefficients (Pearson) and *p*-Values (in Parentheses): Urinary Cotinine–Nicotine, Urinary 1-Hydroxyprene, Levels of 4-Aminobiphenyl-Hemoglobin Adducts (4-ABP), and Log DNA Adducts in Exfoliated Ladder Cells (39 Healthy Men)

	All subjects		Smokers ($N=18$)	
Adduct no.	1-Hydroxypyrene	4-ABP	1-Hydroxypyrene	4-ABP
1	−0.01	0.06	0.02	0.09
	(0.95)	(0.70)	(0.92)	(0.72)
2	0.44	0.42	0.37	0.52
	(0.005)	(0.007)	(0.12)	(0.03)
3	−0.22	−0.03	−0.19	0.37
	(0.17)	(0.84)	(0.44)	(0.13)
4	0.02	0.33	0.01	0.54
	(0.90)	(0.04)	(0.97)	(0.02)
5	0.08	0.07	0.16	0.28
	(0.62)	(0.67)	(0.53)	(0.26)
6	−0.01	0.01	−0.08	0.09
	(0.93)	(0.96)	(0.74)	(0.09)
7	−0.10	−0.02	−0.17	−0.28
	(0.52)	(0.88)	(0.49)	(0.27)
8	−0.04	−0.10	–	–
	(0.77)	(0.53)		
9	−0.14	0.05	−0.22	−0.35
	(0.39)	(0.75)	(0.36)	(0.14)
10	−0.09	0.37	−0.15	0.34
	(0.58)	(0.02)	(0.55)	(0.16)
11	−0.03	−0.14	0.09	0.06
	(0.87)	(0.40)	(0.71)	(0.82)
12	0.14	−0.13	0.05	−0.17
	(0.38)	(0.42)	(0.84)	(0.48)
Total diagonal zone	0.09	0.17	0.13	0.45
	(0.57)	(0.29)	(0.61)	(0.06)

Source: From Ref. 11.

The concentration of 4-aminobiphenyl–hemoglobin adducts in both smokers and non-smokers is modulated by the N-acetylation phenotype; irrespective of the smoking status of the subjects, the genetically based slow acetylator phenotype was associated with higher concentrations of the adduct (12). *N*-Acetyltransferase deactivates carcinogenic arylamines and has a genetically based polymorphic distribution in the population, with about 50% of Caucasians being slow acetylators. Slow acetylators have been shown to be at high risk of bladder cancer in epidemiological investigations (13). The consistency among the results obtained in different Caucasian populations and with different study designs seems to suggest that *N*-acetyl-transferase exerts a causal role in modulating the risk of bladder cancer in arylamine-exposed subjects (13). An exception is represented by studies in Asians, which show low relative risks in slow acetylators. In a meta-analysis of bladder cancer and the NAT-2 phenotype, the overall odds ratio (OR) was 1.37, while for GSTM1 the estimate was 1.57. However, such estimates tend to be higher in subjects exposed to specific carcinogens (13).

In conclusion, the risk of bladder cancer in Western countries is mainly explained by exposure to tobacco smoke and some occupational agents, and it is modulated by polymorphic genetic traits. Our knowledge, however, is insufficient as to allow individual risk assessment.

2.1.2. Dietary Factors

Several studies have suggested that "Mediterranean diet," and, more generally, a high consumption of cereals, fruits and vegetables decrease the risk of cancers at different sites, including colon, breast, bladder, and prostate cancers (14,15). In the case of bladder cancer, Table 2 shows the results of some epidemiological investigations suggesting a protective effect for this site. Different components of Mediterranean diet have attracted attention, particularly olive oil and tomatoes. A recent cohort study on American health professionals (15) has found a consistently decreased risk of prostatic cancer among heavy consumers of tomatoes and tomato sauce. It is not known which specific micronutrients are responsible for the protective effect of tomatoes, olive oil and other components of Mediterranean diet, although it is likely that different antioxidants including vitamins play a role (16). In vitro studies have shown that polyphenolic components of mediterranean diet, in particular oleuropein (responsible for the bitter taste of olives), interfere with biochemical events which are involved in atherogenic disease (17). In addition, in vivo studies have suggested that phenolics in red wine increase plasmatic antioxidant capacity and reduce the propensity of low density lipoprotein (LDL) to undergo peroxidation (18).

The consumption of phenolics has been shown to decrease the level of DNA adducts in experimental studies in humans and animals. Moderate wine consumption (a source of phenolics) inhibited peroxide-induced micronucleated cells (19), while the consumption of flavonoids inhibited DNA damage related to lipid peroxidation (20).The relationship of fruit and vegetable consumption to DNA adduct formation has been examined in a case–control study on bladder cancer (21). The level of aromatic DNA adducts in white blood cells (measured by ^{32}P-postlabeling) decreased with increasing levels of fruit and vegetable consumption; in addition, the association between the case/control status and the level of adducts (below or above the median value) was stronger in the subjects who consumed less than two portions of vegetables per day (OR 7.80; 95% confidence interval

Table 2 Results of Selected Epidemiological Studies on the Intake of Fruit and Vegetables and the Risk of Bladder Cancer (Odds Ratio for Highest vs. Lowest Intake)

Authors and year	Country	Design	No. of cases	Food	Odds ratio (a)
Mettlin and Graham, 1979	U.S.A.	Case–control	569	Carrots	0.6
				cruciferous	0.7
Claude et al., 1986	Germany	Case–control	431	Fresh fruit and vegetables	0.7
La Vecchia et al., 1989	Italy	Case–control	163	Carrots	0.6
				Green-leaf vegetables	0.5
Riboli et al., 1991	Spain	Case–control	432	Vegetables	1.0
Mills et al., 1991	USA	Cohort	52	Fruit juice	0.3
				Cooked green-leaf, vegetables	0.5
Nomura et al., 1991	USA	Case–control	261	Green-leaf vegetables	0.7
Chyou et al., 1993	USA	Cohort	96	Fruit	0.6
Momas et al., 1994	France	Case–control	219	Carrots, spinach, pumpkins	0.6

Source: Modified from Ref. 39.

CI 3.0–20.3) than in heavy consumers (OR = 4.98 for consumers of two portions per day; OR = 2.0 for consumers of three or more portions) (Table 3).

3. CLINICAL RISK ASSESSMENT

3.1. Oncogenes

Several genetic alterations have been detected in bladder cancer, and these have been proposed as biomarkers for the clinical follow-up of the patients. Recent reviews are available (see, e.g., 22–25). They suggest that currently no single marker is able to accurately predict the clinical course of bladder tumors and would serve as a reliable prognosticator. A combination of prognostic markers could predict which tumors need an aggressive form of therapy and/or adjuvant therapy.

Table 3 Case–Control Study on Bladder Cancer (162 Cases, 104 Controls): Distribution by WBC–DNA Adducts (^{32}P-postlabeling)[a]

Quartiles of DNA adducts	Cases	Controls	OR	95% CI
0.1 (detection limit)	32	50	1.0	–
>0.1	130	54	3.7	(2.2–6.3)
Below median [0.23]	64	72	1.0	–
Above median	98	32	3.6	(2.1–6.1)
0.1 (detection limit)	32	50	1.0	–
Tertiles above 0.1:				
0.11–0.23	33	24	2.1	(1.1–4.2)
0.23–0.51	44	19	3.5	(1.7–7.1)
>0.51	54	11	7.6	(3.6–16.1)

ORs are adjusted by age. Adducts are expressed as RAL $\times$ 10^{-8} (21).
[a]Missing data for seven cases and one control.
OR, odds ratio; CI, confidence interval.

The *ras* family was first discovered by studies of bladder cancer. Specifically a point mutation of codon 12 of the H-*ras* gene, in the bladder cancer cell line T24 (26). polymerase chain reation (PCR)-based methods suggest that the prevalence of *ras* mutations is around 40% in bladder tumors. Other oncogenes have been studied. p21 expression (waf1/cip1) was predictive of the outcome, but no relationship was found with survival (27).

Overexpression of the epidermal growth factor receptor (EGFR) has been reported in bladder cancer. Neal et al. observed increased expression in invasive vs. superficial bladder tumours, and suggested that overexpression was associated with high-grade, high-stage cancer and was an independent prognostic factor (28). However, in another study Nguyen et al. (29) reported that overexpression of EGFR was not an independent prognostic marker in advanced bladder cancer.

Promising data on oncogenes concern overexpression of ErbB2. Underwood et al.(30) studied 236 bladder patients and found that 16 out of 89 patients with recurrent disease had ErbB2 amplification, while amplification was not observed in nonrecurrent tumors. Although ErbB2 amplification was predictive of survival in multivariate analysis, stage and grade remained the most significant independent prognostic parameters. In another study (31) ErbB2 was a prognostic indicator in association with the combined EGRF and ErbB3 expression profile (31). Other markers have been reviewed elsewhere, including cell cycle markers like p27, and potential targets for novel therapies, such as cyclooxygenase 2 (COX 2) and factors of angiogenesis (32).

3.2. Tumor Suppressor Genes

Deletions of 3p and 17p have been correlated with tumor grade and stage. It has been suggested that different patterns of deletions or loss of heterozygosity (LOH), including 5q, 9q, 13q, and 19q, can be associated with different clinical behaviors (33,34). Loss of heterozygosity of 19q was particularly informative, since this chromosome includes the retinoblastoma (RB) locus, while 17p includes the *p53* gene. Both tumor suppressor genes exert a key role in carcinogenesis, and have collaborative roles. In two studies, survival was significantly decreased in patients with altered RB expression (35,36). Altered expression was more frequent in muscle invasive tumors.

Mutations of the *p53* gene were identified as common events in bladder cancer. *p53* nuclear overexpression correlated with both 17p LOH and gene mutations as identified by SSCP and sequencing (37). A series of studies have shown that *p53* overexpression is associated with tumour invasiveness and survival. However, it is not clear whether overexpression is a really independent predictive factor.

The relationship between *p53* mutations/overexpression, lymphnode invasion, covariates, and prognosis for bladder cancer has been considered in several investigations (Table 4). The most striking observation is the inconsistency of the findings: some studies show an association with prognostic factors or survival, while others do not. Overall, there seems to be an agreement on the fact that *p53* mutations are associated wih higher stage/grade and poorer prognosis. However, it is premature to develop guidelines for clinical practice on this basis. Issues that are still open, in particular, are (a) whether *p53* is predictive of the outcome as such, or its effect is mediated or confounded by lymphnode invasion; and (b) the degree of correspondence between immunohistochemistry and gene mutations. Additional methodological problems are related to the different antibodies and different thresholds (0, 5 or 20%) used in the investigations based on immunohistochemistry. In conclusion, it is not clear (a) whether the measurement of *p53* is worthwhile, in addition to the more traditional clinical markers in order to modify therapeutic choices; (b) whether immunohistochemistry can be reliably used as a surrogate of the search for mutations. This picture is confirmed by recent reviews. Schmitz-Drager et al. (38) have reviewed 43 trials on urothelial cancer and *p53* immunohistochemistry, including 3764 patients. They have concluded that the comparison between the trials yielded considerable differences due to technical aspects (selection of the antibody and the use of different cut-off values, study design and patient selection), and that there is an obvious need for standardization of the assay.

In conclusion, like for other cancer sites, it is premature to develop guidelines for the routinary use of *p53* mutation search or immunohistochemistry to make therapeutic decisions in bladder cancer patients (38).

Table 4 *p53* Immunohistochemistry as Prognostic Factor in Bladder Cancer (Grade, Stage, or Survival): Studies Published in 1997–1998

Authors	No. of cases	Biomarker	Results	Covariates
Caliskan et al., 1997 (40)	30 TCC *p*Ta/pT1	Nuclear accumulation of *p53* (Pab1801)	6/30 (20%) had nuclear accumul.: invasion or MTS 5/6 in: *p53*+ 6/24 *p53* neg.	Grade, stage, treatment (Cox model)
Casetta et al., 1997 (41)	31 pTa grade I without recurrence vs. 28 with recurrence	*p53* immunohistochemistry (threshold >0%)	16.1% *p53* positive in non-recurrent vs 53.6% in recurrent (chi-square*p* = 0.02)	Multivariate analysis: *p53* predicted progression (OR = 10) and recurrence (OR = 54)
Vollmer et al., 1998 (42)	229 TCC	*p53* immunohistochemistry	In grade II *p53* was predictive of invasion Interaction with MIB-1	Grade, stage, MIB-1, bcl-2, C-erbB-2
Al Abadi et al., 1998 (43)	147 TCC, 76 pTa/pT1, 35 pT2, 25 pT3, 11 pT4	Monoclonal antibody DO-7 (DAKO) threshold >7%	Association of *p53* with grade and stage: pTa=28% positive; pT1–2 73%; pT3–4 68%	Ploidy
Korkolopoulou et al., 1997 (44)	106 TCC	*p53* immunohistochemistry	*p53* was associated with grade, stage and papillary status. No significant impact on survival	Simultaneous expression of MDM2 and *p53* greatly shortened survival

Siu et al., 1998 (45)	118 TCC treated with cisplatin	p53 immunohistochemistry	p53 did not predict for survival	MIB-1 metallo-thionein, performance status, grade
Raitanen et al., 1997 (46)	51 TCC group 1: Ta/T1 with group 2: progressive group 3: metastatic	p53 immunohistochemistry	p53 positive: group 1 3/12 (25%) group 2:5/17 (29%) group 3:14/22 (64%) progression was associated with p53 positivity	—
Liukkonen et al., 1997 (47)	185 TCC superficial	p53 immunohistochemistry	36% positive for p53 ($>20\%$ threshold) p53 significantly related to stage and grade	—
Popov et al., 1997 (48)	114 TCC + 13 normal bladders	Monoclonal antibody Pab1801 (median value used as threshold)	Strong association between proliferation (MIB-1) and p53 expression ($p < 0.0001$)	In multivariate analysis p53, MIB-1 and stage were independently predictive of survival
Lebret et al., 1998 (49)	35 T1 G3	p53 immunomarking in 25 cases	Patients responding to BCG did not differ from nonresponding patients, using different p53 thresholds	—

(Continued)

Table 4 p53 Immunohistochemistry as Prognostic Factor in Bladder Cancer (Grade, Stage, or Survival): Studies Published in 1997–1998 (*Continued*)

Authors	No. of cases	Biomarker	Results	Covariates
Abdel Fattah et al., 1998 (50)	54 TCC	p53 immunohistochemistry and PCR direct sequencing	Association between p53 and grade and stage ($p = 0.01$); p53 positivity in $> 50\%$ nuclei was associated with lower survival ($p = 0.03$)	—
Sengelov et al., 1997 (51)	50 bladder cancers with MTS	Monoclonal antibody PAb1801	No relationship of p53 with response to cisplatin ($p = 0.14$) or with survival ($p = 0.38$)	Performance status
Hermann et al., 1998 (52)	143 TCC: 31 T1a, 60 T1b, 52 T1c	Monoclonal antibody Pab1801	p53 correlated with grade ($p < 0.05$) survival higher in p53 negative (73%) than in positive (61%) tumors ($p < 0.05$)	Multivariate analysis with age, grade and p53: only histology predicted survival
Ogura et al., 1998 (53)	111 TCC	p53 immunohistochemistry	No correlation of p53 with nuclear roundness factor; p53 associated with mean nuclear volume ($p = 0.008$)	—

Pfister et al., 1998 (54)	83 TCC	*p53* immunohistochemistry	*p53* correlated with stage and grade but was independent of MIB-1 in predicting progression	More marked progression if *p53* and pRB were both altered; stage and grade-adjustment
Tsuji et al., 1997 (55)	31 TCC with radical cystectomy	*p53* immunohistochemistry	Correlation between *p53* and Ki67 (MIB-1); expression of *p53* correlated with survival ($p < 0.05$)	
Schmitz et al., 1997 (56)	200 archival specimens from 92 patients	Monoclonal antibody DO-1 against *p53*	In 61 patients followed for >2 years, *p53* analysis with correlated with progression ($p = 0.01$)	Multivariate MDM2 and multifocality: both *p53* ($p = 0.01$) and MDM2 ($p = 0.009$) were associated with progression
Tsutsumi et al., 1997 (57)	47 patients	LOH of *p53* gene (SSCP analysis)	LOH: 0/10 grade 1; 9/23 grade 2 4/7 grade 3 LOH was associated with progression	—
Grossman et al., 1998 (58)	45 pT1 TCC	*p53* immunostaining	Association of *p53* with progression ($p = 0.04$)	Interaction with RB expression

(Continued)

Table 4 p53 Immunohistochemistry as Prognostic Factor in Bladder Cancer (Grade, Stage, or Survival): Studies Published in 1997–1998 (*Continued*)

Authors	No. of cases	Biomarker	Results	Covariates
Lianes et al., 1998 (59)	109 TCC T2-T3 and grade 2 or higher 57 lymphnode MTS 52 no MTS	Monoclonal antibody Pab1801 (>20%)	No significant association of *p53* with node invasion (*p* > 0.05)	MIB-1, DNA ploidy, microvascular counts
Jahnson et al., 1998 (60)	173 advanced bladder cancers	Antibody DO-7	Proportional hazards model: no association of *p53* with survival (*p* > 0.05)	PMG3-245 for RB

REFERENCES

1. Schottenfeld D, Fraumeni JF Jr. Cancer Epidemiology and Prevention. New York: Oxford University Press, 1996.
2. Maclure M, Ben-Abraham R, Bryant MS, Skipper PL, Tannenbaum ST. Elevated blood levels of carcinogens in passive smokers. Am J Public Health 1989; 79:1381–1384.
3. IARC Monographs on the Evaluation of Carcinogenic Risks to Humans. Vol. 4. Some Aromatic Amines, Hydrazine and Related Substances, N-Nitrosocompounds and Miscellaneous Alkykating Agents. Lyon: IARC, 1974.
4. US Government. Occupational safety and health standards. US Fed Reg 1973; 38(85):10929.
5. International Labour Office. Cancer of the Bladder among Workers in Aniline Factories. Studies and Reports, Series F, No. 1. Geneva: Internatinal Labour Office, 1921.
6. IARC Monographs on the Evaluation of Carcinogenic Risks to Humans. Vol. 38, Tobacco Smoking. Lyon: IARC, 1986.
7. Vineis P. Epidemiological models of carcinogenesis: the example of bladder cancer. Cancer Epidemiol Biomarkers Prev 1992; 1:149–153.
8. Bartsch H, Malaveille C, Friesen M, Kadlubar FF, Vineis P. Black (air cured) and blond (flue cured) tobacco—Cancer risk IV: molecular dosimetry studies implicate aromatic amines as bladder carcinogens. Eur J Cancer 1993; 29A:1199–1207.
9. Talaska G, Al-Juburi AZSS, Kadlubar FF. Smoking-related carcinogen–DNA adducts in biopsy samples of human urinary bladder: identification of N-(deoxyguanosin-8-yl)-4-aminobiphenyl as a major adduct. Proc Natl Acad Sci USA 1991; 88:5350–5454.
10. Talaska G, Schamer M, Skipper P, Tannenbaum SR, Caporaso N, Unruh L, Kadlubar FF, Bartsch H, Malaveille C, Vineis P. Detection of carcinogen–DNA adducts in exfoliated urothelial cells of cigarette smokers: association with smoking, hemoglobin adducts, and urinary mutagenicity. Cancer Epidemiol Biomarkers Prev 1991; 1:61–66.
11. Vineis P, Talaska G, Malaveille C, Bartsch H, Martone T, Sithisarankul P, Strickland P. DNA adducts in urothelial cells: relationship with biomarkers of exposure to arylamines and polycyclic aromatic hydrocarbons from tobacco smoke. Int J Cancer 1996; 65:314–316.
12. Vineis P, Bartsch H, Caporaso N, Harrington AM, Kadlubar FF, Landi MT, Malaveille C, Shields PG, Skipper PL, Talaska G, Tannenbaum SR. Genetically-based N-acetyltransferase metabolic polymorphism and low-level environmental exposure to carcinogens. Nature 1994; 369:154–156.
13. Vineis P, Malats N, Lang M, d'Errico A, Caporaso N, Cuzick J, Boffetta P. Metabolic Polymorphisms and Susceptibility to Cancer. IARC Scientific Publication No. 148. Lyon: IARC, 1999.
14. Miller AB, Berrino F, Hill M, Pietinen P, Riboli E, Wahrendorf J. Diet in the etiology of cancer: a review. Eur J Cancer 1994; 30A:207–220.
15. Giovannucci E, Ascherio A, Rimm EB, Stampfer MJ, Colditz GC, Willett WC. Intake of carotenoids and retinol in relation to risk of prostate cancer. J Natl Cancer Inst 1995; 87:1767–1776.

16. Block G, Patterson B, Subar A. Fruit, vegetables and cancer prevention: a review of the epidemiological evidence. Nutr Cancer 1992; 18:1–30.

17. Visioli F, Galli C. Oleuropein protects low density lipoprotein from oxidation. Life Sci 1994; 55(24):1965–1971.

18. Furman B, Lavy A, Aviram M. Consumption of red wine with meals reduces the susceptibility of human plasma and low-density lipoprotein to lipid peroxidation. Am J Clin Nutr 1995; 61:549–554.

19. Fenech M, Stockley C, Aitken C. Moderate wine consumpption protects against hydrogen-peroxide-induced DNA damage. Mutat Res 1997; 379(suupl 1): S173.

20. Cai Q, Rahan RO, Zhang R. Dietary flavonoids, quercetin, luteolin and genistein, reduce DNA damage and lipid peroxidation and quench free radicals. Cancer Lett 1997; 119:99–108.

21. Peluso M, Airoldi L, Magagnotti C, Fiorini L, Munnia A, Hautefeuille A, Malaveille C, Vineis P. White blood cell DNA adducts and fruit and vegetable consumption in bladder cancer. Carcinogenesis 2000; 21:183–187.

22. Halachmi S, Linn JF, Amiel GE, Moskovitz B, Nativ O. Urine cytology, tumours markers and bladder cancer. Br J Urol 1998; 82:647–654.

23. Harding M, Theodorescu D. Molecular markers: their role as prognostic indicators for bladder cancer. Curr Opin Urol 1997; 7:2822–2886.

24. Adshead JM, Kessling AM, Ogden CW. Genetic initiation, progression and prognostic markers in transitional cell carcinoma of the bladder: a summary of the structural and transcriptional change, and the role of developmental genes. Br J Urol 1998; 82:503–512.

25. Kausch I, Bohle A. Molecular aspects of bladder cancer III. Prognostic markers of bladder cancer. Eur Urol 2002; 41(1):15–29.

26. Reddy EP, Reynolds RK, Santos EM, Barbacid M. A point mutation is responsible for the acquisition of transforming properties by the T24 bladder carcinoma oncogene. Nature 1982; 300:149–152.

27. Lipponen P, Aaltomaa S, Eskelinen M, Ala-Opas M, Kosma M. Expression of p21 (waf1/cip1) protein in transitional cell bladder tumours and its prognostic value. Eur Urol 1998; 34:237–243.

28. Neal DE, Sharples L, Smith K, Fennelly J, Hall RR, Harris AL. The epidermal growth factor receptor and the prognosis of bladder cancer. Cancer 1990; 65:1619–1625.

29. Nguyen PL, Swanson PE, Jaszcz W, et al. Expression of epidermal growth factor receptor in invasive transitional cell carcinoma of the urinary bladder: a multivariate survival analysis. Am J Clin Pathol 1994; 101:166–176.

30. Underwood M, Bartlett J, Reeves J, Gardiner DS, Scott R, Cooke T. C-erb B-2 gene amplification: a molecular marker in recurrent bladder tumors? Cancer Res 1995; 55:2422–2426.

31. Chow NH, Chan SH, Tzai TS, Ho CL, Liu HS. Expression profiles of ErbB family receptors and prognosis in primary transitional cell carcinoma of the urinary bladder. Clin Cancer Res 2001; 7(7):1957–1962.

32. Tiguert R, Lessard A, So A, Fradet Y. Prognostic markers in muscle invasive bladder cancer. World J Urol 2002; 20(3):190–195.

33. Dalbagni G, Presti J, Reuter V, Fair WR, Cordon-Cardo C. Genetic alterations in bladder cancer. Lancet 1993; 324:469–471.
34. Habuchi T, Ogawa O, Kakehi Y, et al. Accumulated allelic losses in the development of invasive urothelial cancer. Int J Cancer 1993; 53:579–584.
35. Cordon-Cardo C, Zhang ZF, Dalbagni G, Drobnjak M, Charytonowicz E, Hu SX, Xu HJ, Reuter VE, Benedict WF. Cooperativ effects of p53 and pRB alterations in primary superficial bladder tumors. Cancer Res 1997; 57: 1217–1221.
36. Logothetis.
37. Cordon-Carlo C, Dalbagni G, Saez GT, Oliva MR, Zhang ZF, Rosai J, Reuter VE, Pellicer A. p53 mutations in human bladder cancer: genotypic vs. phenotypic patterns. Int J Cancer 1994; 56:347–353.
38. Schmitz-Drager BJ, Goebell PJ, Ebert T, Fradet Y. p53 immunohistochemistry as a prognostic marker in bladder cancer. Playground for urology scientists? Eur Urol 2000; 38(6):691–699.
39. La Vecchia C, Negri E. Nutrition and bladder cancer. Cancer Causes Control 1996; 7(1):95–100.
40. Caliskan M, Türkeri LN, Mansuroglu B, Toktas G, Aksoy B, Unlüer E, Akdas A. Nuclear accumulation of mutant p53 protein: a possible predictor of failure of intravesical therapy in bladder cancer. Br J Urol 1997; 79(3):373–377.
41. Casetta G, Gontero P, Russo R, Pacchioni D, Tizzani A. p53 Expression compared with other prognostic factors in OMS grade-I stage-Ta transitional cell carcinoma of the bladder. Eur Urol 1997; 32(2):229–236.
42. Vollmer RT, Humphrey PA, Swanson PE, Wick MR, Hudson ML. Invasion of the bladder by transitional cell carcinoma: its relation to histologic grade and expression of p53, MIB-1, c-erb-B-2, epidermal growth factor receptor, and bcl-2. Cancer 1998; 82:715–723.
43. Al Abadi H, Nagel R, Nehaus P. Immunohistochemical detection of p53 protein in transitional cell carcinoma of the bladder in correlation with DNA ploidy and pathohistological stage and grade. Cancer Detect Pre 1998; 22: 43–50.
44. Korkolopoulou P, Christodoulou P, Kapralos P, Exarchakos M, Bisbiroula A, Hadjiannakis M, Georgountzos C, Thomas Tsagli E. The role of p53, MDM2 and c-erb B-2 oncoproteins, epidermal growth factor receptor and proliferation markers in the prognosis of urinary bladder cancer. Pathol Res Pract 1997; 193:767–775.
45. Siu LL, Banerjee D, Khurana RJ, Pan X, Pflueger R, Tannock IF, Moore MJ. The prognostic role of p53, metallothionein, P-glycoprotein, and MIB-1 in muscle-invasive urothelial transitional cell carcinoma. Clin Cancer Res 1998; 4:559–565.
46. Raitanen MP, Tammela TL, Kallioinen M, Isola J. P53 accumulation, deoxyribonucleic acid ploidy and progression of bladder cancer. J Urol 1997; 157(4):1250–1253.
47. Liukkonen TJ, Lipponen PK, Helle M, Jauhiainen KE. Immunoreactivity of bcl-2, p 53 and EGFr is associated with tumor stage, grade and cell proliferation in superficial bladder cancer. Finnbladder III Group. Urol Res 1997; 25(1):1–7.

48. Popov Z, Hoznek A, Colombel M, Bastuji S, Lefrere MA, Bellot J, Abboh Mazerolles c, Chopin DK. The prognostic value of p53 nuclear overexpression and MIB-1 as a proliferative marker in transitional cell carcinoma of the bladder. Cancer 1997; 80:1472–1481.

49. Lebret T, Becette V, Barbagelatta M, Hervè JM, Gaudez F, Barrè P, Lugagne PM, Botto H. Correlation between p53 over expression and response to bacillus Calmette-Guerin therapy in a high risk select population of patients with T1G3 bladder cancer. J Urol 1998; 159(3):788–791.

50. Abdel-Fattah R, Challen C, Griffiths TR, Robinson MC, Neal DE, Lunec J. Alterations of TP53 in microdissected transitional cell carcinoma of the human urinary bladder: high frequency of TP53 accumulation in the absence of detected mutations is associated with poor prognosis. Br J Cancer 1998; 77:2230–2238.

51. Sengelov L, Horn T, Steven K. p53 nuclear immunoreactivity as a predictor of response and outcome following chemotherapy for metastatic bladder cancer. J Cancer Res Clin Oncol 1997; 123:565–570.

52. Hermann GG, Horn T, Steven K. The influence of the level of lamina propria invasion and the prevalence of p53 nuclear accumulation on survival in stage T1 transitional cell bladder cancer. J Urol 1998; 159(1):91–94.

53. Ogura K, Fukuzawa S, Habuchi T, Ogawa O, Yoshida O. Correlation of nuclear morphometry and immunostaining for p53 and proliferating cell nuclear antigen in transitional cell carcinoma of the bladder. Int J Urol 1997; 4(6):561–566.

54. Pfister C, Buzelin F, Casse C, Bochereau G, Buzelin JM, Bouchot O. Comparative analysis of MiB1 and p53 expression in human bladder tumors and their correlation with cancer progression. Eur Urol 1998; 33(3):278–284.

55. Tsuji M, Kojima K, Murakami Y, Kanayama H, Kagawa S. Prognostic value of Ki-67 antigen and p53 protein in urinary bladder cancer: immunohistochemical analysis of radical cystectomy specimens. Br J Urol 1997; 79(3):367–372.

56. Schmitz Dräger BJ, Kushima M, Goebell P, Jax TW, Gerharz CD, Bültel H, Schulz WA, Ebert T, Ackermann R. p53 and MDM2 in the development progression of bladder cancer. Eur Urol 1997; 32(4):487–493.

57. Tsutsumi M, Sugano K, Yamaguchi K, Kakizoe T, Akaza H. Correlation of allelic loss of the P53 gene and tumor grade, stage, and malignant progression in bladder cancer. Int J Urol 1997; 4(1):74–78.

58. Grossman HB, Liebert M, Antelo M, Dinney CP, Hu SX, Palmer JL, Benedict WF. p53 and RB expression predict progression in T1 bladder cancer. Clin Cancer Res 1998; 4:829–834.

59. Lianes P, Charytonowicz E, Cordon-Cardo C, Fradet Y, Grossman HB, Hemstreet GP, Waldman FM, Chew K, Wheedeless LL, Faraggi D. Biomarker study of primary nonmetastatic versus metastatic invasive bladder cancer. National Cancer Institute Bladder Tumor Marker Network. Clin Cancer Res 1998; 4:1267–1271.

60. Jahnson S, Karlsson MG. Predictive value of p53 and pRb immunostaining in locally advanced bladder cancer treated with cystectomy. J Urol 1998; 160(4):1291–1296.

61. Ross RK, Schottenfeld D. Prostate cancer. In: Schottenfeld D, Fraumeni JF Jr. Cancer Epidemiology and Prevention. New York: Oxford University Press, 1996.

62. Coley CM, Barry MJ, Flemng C, Mulley AG. Early detection of prostate cancer, part I: prior probability and effectiveness of tests. Ann Intern Med 1997; 126:394–406.

63. Stamey TA, Freiha FS, McNeal JE, Redwine EA, Whittemore AS, Schmid HP. Localized prostate cancer: relationship of tumor volume to clinical significance for treatment of prostate cancer. Cancer (suppl) 1993; 71:933–938.

64. Seidman H, Mushinki MH, Gelb SK, Silverberg E. Probabilities of eventually developing or dying of cancer. CA Cancer J Clin 1985; 35:36–56.

65. Meigs JB, Barry MJ, Giovannucci E, et al. High rates of prostate-specific antigen testing in men with evidence of benign prostatic hyperplasia Am J Med 1998; 104 517–525.

66. Catalona WJ, Richie JP, Ahmann FR, Hudson MA, Scardino PT, Flanigan RC, deKernion JB, Ratliff TL, Kavoussi LR, Dalkin BL, et al. Comparison of digital rectal examination and serum prostate specific antigen in the early detection of prostate cancer: results of a multicenter clinical trial of 6,630 men. J Urol 1994; 151(5) 1283–1290.

67. Catalona WJ, Partin AW, Slawin KM, Brawer MK, Flanigan RC, Patel A, Richie JP, deKernion JB, Walsh PC, Scardino PT, Lange PH, Subong EN, Parson RE, Gasior GH, Loveland KG, Southwick PC. Use of the percentage of free prostate-specific antigen to enhance differentiation of prostate cancer from benign prostatic disease: a prospective multicenter clinical trial. J Am Med Assoc 1998; 279(19):1542–1547.

68. Conseil d'Evaluation des Technologies de la Santè du Québec. Screening for cancer of the prostate: an evaluation of benefits, unwanted health effects, and costs Montréal, 1995.

69. Cote RJ, Shi Y, Groshen S, Feng AC, Cordon-Cardo C, Skinner D, Lieskovosky G. Association of p27^{Kip1} levels with recurrence and survival in patients with stage C prostate carcinoma. J Natl Cancer Inst 1998; 90:916–920.

70. Liu MC, Gelmann EP. P53 gene mutations: case study of a clinical marker for solid tumours. Semin Oncol 2002; 29:246–257.

28

Molecular and Biochemical Approaches to the Etiology of Prostate Cancer

Richard B. Hayes

Division of Cancer Epidemiology and Genetics, National Cancer Institute, DHHS, Bethesda, Maryland, U.S.A.

1. INTRODUCTION

Prostate cancer is the most commonly diagnosed form of cancer in men in the United States and, following lung cancer, is the second most common cause of cancer-related death, with 189,000 cases and 30,200 deaths in 2002. There is marked ethnic variation in prostate cancer incidence and mortality; the disease is most common among African-Americans. Internationally, prostate cancer rates also vary widely, with greater than a 25-fold difference in cancer incidence between low-risk countries, such as China, and high-risk countries, such as the United States.

Incidence of prostate cancer increases dramatically with age; about 80% of new cases occur among men 65 years of age or older. With advances in human longevity, the burden of prostate cancer will only increase. Reduction of the prostate cancer burden requires an understanding of the factors that cause the disease. Here, the current state of knowledge regarding risk factors for prostate cancer is reviewed, with particular attention to molecular and biochemical approaches to understanding the causes of this disease.

2. FAMILIAL RISK AND MAJOR CANCER GENES

Risks for prostate cancer are approximately doubled among men who have
a family history of this disease (1–9) (Table 1). Risks tend to be greater for
men who report prostate cancer in their brothers than in their fathers, consistent with recessive or X-linked transmission (4), however, segregation
analyses tend to show an autosomal dominant pattern (8,10).

Three loci on chromosome 1 (HPC1, PCAP, CAPB) (11–13), a locus
on chromosome X (HPCX) (14), a locus on chromosome 20 (HPC20)
(15), and a locus on chromosome 17 (HPC2/ELAC)(16) have been identified by linkage analysis in high-risk families as potential sites for high-pene-
trance prostate cancer genes, however, confirmation in other familiy series
has failed, suggesting that familial prostate cancer is hetreogeneous. Several
loci have also been suggested for prostate tumor aggressiveness (17), but the
search to determine specific prostate cancer genes at these and other loci is
still underway.

3. STEROIDAL HORMONES

Testosterone is required at puberty for prostate gland maturation and is
essential in adulthood for normal prostate function. Testosterone (T) is converted in the prostate to the more strongly androgenic dihydrotestosterone
(DHT) by 5-α-reductase. Dihydrotestosterone and, to a lesser extent, T bind
to cytosolic androgen receptors (ARs). These complexes translocate to the
nucleus to bind with DNA at androgen response elements, activating target
genes, including genes involved in the control of cell division.

Table 1   Family History and Risk for Prostate Cancer

	Brother		Father	
	n	Risk	*n*	Risk
Woolf, 1960 (1)	3	1.5	12	4.0
Whittemore et al., 1995 (2)	n.r.	2.0	n.r.	2.9[a]
Hayes et al., 1995 (3)	42	2.5	28	5.3
Monroe et al., 1995 (4)	138	1.0[b]	173	2.1
Keetch et al., 1995 (5)	136	3.5	133	4.7
Narod et al., 1995 (6)	18	1.2	19	2.6
Lesko et al., 1996 (7)	47	1.9	45	3.0
Schaid et al., 1998 (8)	n.r.	1.0[b]	n.r.	1.5
Bratt et al., 1999 (9)	24	2.2	23	3.6

[a]Father or son.
[b]Father's risk as referent.
n.r., not reported.

Interethnic comparisons provide evidence that serum androgen profiles may parallel population risks for prostate cancer. In one series of studies, T and T unbound to serum-binding proteins were higher in young African-American than white men (18), T was increased in pregnant African-American women, compared to whites (19), and androstanediol glucuronide (A-diol-g), a possible marker for DHT, was reduced in Japanese men (20). Another investigation did not find ethnic associations for T or unbound T, yet showed that the DHT:T ratio, a measure of 5-α-reductase enzyme activity, was highest in African-Americans, intermediate in whites, and lowest in Asian-Americans, corresponding to the respective incidence rates in these groups (21).

Although many epidemiologic investigations have been carried out, prostate cancer does not systematically show differences in serum levels of T and related compounds (22). Large studies that take into account more complex hormone interrelationships may be needed, as shown in a report that T is related to prostate cancer risk, after adjustment for SHBG, its major binding protein in blood (23).

The blood-based observational studies of androgenic hormones and prostate cancer risk may be limited for several reasons. Serum levels are only an indirect indicator of intraprostatic levels. All studies of prostate cancer cases have evaluated hormone levels at only one point in time; multiple measures may be needed to account for intraindividual variation. These studies have considered hormone levels in later adult life, while exposures at a younger age may also be important. An ongoing randomized trial of the 5-α-reductase inhibitor, finasteride, which blocks the intraprostatic conversion of T to DHT should provide insight about the role in prostate carcinogenesis of this key enzyme in androgen metabolism (24).

With increased understanding of the human genome, investigations have begun to explore the relationship to prostate cancer risk of genetic polymorphisms in the human prostatic (type II) steroid 5-α-reductase gene (*SRD5A2*, located at chromosome 2p23 and associated with prostatic metabolism of T to DHT), with polymorphisms in the androgen receptor gene (*AR*, located at chromosome Xq11–q12), and with *CYP17* (located on chromosome 10 and involved in testosterone biosynthesis in the gonads and adrenals).

Boys with selected germline mutations in *SRD5A2* are phenotypically female (25). A common polymorphic missense substitution (A49T) in *SRD5A2* was associated with increased risk for prostate cancer in African-American and Hispanic men (26). Longer TA dinucleotide repeats in the 3′ untranslated region of *SRD5A2* are more common in African-Americans, however, in one study longer TA repeats tended to be underrepresented among prostate cancer cases (27). Another missense substitution (V89L) in *SRD5A2*, resulting in decreased 5-α-reductase activity tended to be associated with increased risk for prostate cancer (28).

The N-terminal transactivation domain of *AR* is encoded by one large exon that contains two highly polymorphic trinucleotide repeats, coding, respectively, for glutamine (CAG) and glycine (GGN, where N is any one of the four nucleotides). A more than twofold expansion in the number of glutamine repeats causes Kennedy's disease, an androgen insensitivity syndrome (29), possibly through defective binding to an *AR* coactivator (30). Relatively long CAG repeats are also associated with infertility in otherwise healthy men (31) and have been related to decreased levels of T, free T, and albumin-bound T (32) and to decreased transcriptional activation by *AR* (33).

The length of CAG repeat sequences tend to be shorter in African-American than white and Asian men [34]. Several, but not all, studies show shorter CAG repeat sequences among prostate cancer cases, particulary for advanced disease (9,35–40) (Table 2). Evidence of gene–gene interrelationships has been found in two studies. In one, subjects with short CAG and short CGN repeats had the greatest risk (38), while in another investigation an interrelationship of risk was noted with short CAG repeat sequences and a polymorphism in the prostate-specific antigen (PSA) gene (41).

The *CYP17* A2 allele contains a T → C transition in the 5' promoter region that creates an additional (CCACC box) promoter site, which may increase the rate of transcription. The A2 allele has been associated with male pattern baldness in men and polycystic ovarian cancer in women, both of which are related to androgen metabolism and this allele has been associated with increased risk for prostate cancer in some studies (28,42).

4. GROWTH FACTORS

Greater serum levels of insulin-like growth factor 1 (IGF-1) and its major binding protein (IGFBP-3) have been related to prostate cancer in several

Table 2 CAG Repeat Polymorphisms in the Androgen Receptor (AR) and Risk for Prostate Cancer

	All cancer		Advanced cancer	
	n	Risk	*n*	Risk
Ingles et al., 1997 (35)	57	1.9	26	2.4[a]
Giovannucci et al., 1997 (36)	587	1.5[a]	269	2.1[a]
Hakimi et al., 1997 (37)	59	3.7[a]	25	8.2[a]
Stanford et al., 1997 (38)	281	1.2	129	1.2
Correa-Cerro et al., 1999 (39)	132	1.0	35	1.9
Bratt et al., 1999 (9)	160	n.s.		n.s
Hsing et al., 2000 (40)	190	1.6*		

[a]$p < 0.05$
n.s., not significant, risk estimates not specified.

studies (43) In a multivariate analysis, decreased levels of the serum IGF-1 binding protein, IGFBP-3, were also associated with increased risk, suggesting that the interrelationship of IGF-1 and its major binding protein are the important determinants of risk (44). Increased serum levels of IGFBP-1, which is involved in transvascular transport of IGF-1, has also been associated with increased risk for prostate cancer (45).

Other data support a role for insulin-like growth factors and related binding proteins in prostate cancer development. In some studies, risks for prostate cancer were greater for taller men (46–48), which may indirectly indicate the influence of the IGF axis on prostate cancer. IGFBP-3 is also lower in African-American men (49,50), consistent with their excess risk for this disease. Dietary factors (51,52) and tobacco use (53) influence the IGF axis and physiological control is exerted by vitamin D (54), androgens (55,56), and PSA (57). IGF-1 is a potent mitogen and antiapoptotic agent. IGFBP-3 inhibits cell growth by inhibiting access of IGF-1 to the IGF receptor. IGFBP-3 also stimulates apoptosis, independent of IGF-1 (58).

5. DIETARY FACTORS

Diet likely has a great impact on prostate cancer risk, however, the precise interrelationships of energy intake, dietary macronutrients, micronutrients, and other constituents are still not well understood. Dietary fat, particularly from animal sources, has been implicated as a risk factor for prostate cancer in many epidemiological studies; however, other studies have not shown an effect (59). Evidence that vegetarians have a lower risk of prostate cancer is also mixed (60,61). Total caloric intake (62) and energy imbalance (63), mutagens produced in cooking meats at high temperatures (64), and increased calcium intake (65,66) may increase risk for this disease, while intake of fish oils (67), micronutrients in fruits and vegetables (68,69), phytoestrogens (70), selenium (71), and vitamin E (72) may reduce risk.

5.1. Dietary Supplementation

A 32% decrease in the incidence of prostate cancer was found in the α-tocopherol (a form of vitamin E) treatment arm of a randomized control trial of α-tocopherol and β-carotene supplementation among 29,000 smokers in Finland (72). Vitamin E supplement users also had reduced risks for prostate cancer in some (73,74) but not all observational studies (75). Supplemental dietary selenium (Se) was associated with a 63% reduction in prostate cancer incidence among 974 men with a history of nonmelanoma skin cancer who were randomized to a daily supplement of Se (71). Observational studies tend also to support this finding (76,77).

Other dietary supplements, including β-carotene (78,79) and vitamins A and C have shown little association with prostate cancer (75), but interest in lycopene as a preventive is strong, based primarily on results from a number of observational epidemiological studies (80). The reductions in risk for prostate cancer identified in randomized control trials of α-tocopherol and Se are important because this study design eliminates many sources of bias found in observational studies. Prostate cancer was, however, not an a priori endpoint for the trials. Because of the earlier results, new randomized trials are beginning, to evaluate the effects on prostate cancer of supplementation, in one trial, with α-tocopherol and Se (SELECT Trial, D. Albanes, personal communication) and, in another trial, with α-tocopherol and β-carotene (81).

5.2. Calcium and Vitamin D

The interplay with prostate cancer of dietary calcium, dietary vitamin D and its metabolites, and polymorphisms in the vitamin D receptor are areas of current research. Vitamin D, derived from dietary sources and endogenous conversion in the skin via ultraviolet light, is metabolized by sequential hydroxylations, first in the liver to 25(OH)D, and subsequently in the kidney, mediated by 1-α-OH-ase, to 1,25(OH)$_2$D. Renal 1-α-OH-ase activity is enhanced by hypocalcemia, probably through stimulation of parathyroid hormone. The biologically active 1,25(OH)$_2$D binds to and activates the nuclear vitamin D receptor (VDR), promoting cellular differentiation and inhibiting cellular proliferation. The mechanism for this is unknown, although inter-relationships with IGF binding proteins (54) and the androgen receptor (82) may be involved.

Vitamin D levels decrease with age and can be reduced in the winter months in northern lattitudes, even when dietary supplementation is in effect. High prostate cancer death rates are found among whites in northern lattitudes of the United States, giving rise to the hypothesis that low UV exposure may be a risk factor for prostate cancer (83). Animal studies also show that 1,25(OH)$_2$D inhibits prostate tumors in experimental animals (84). However, serum 1,25(OH)$_2$D levels in humans have been inconsistently associated with prostate cancer, with one positive (85) and two negative studies (86,87). High calcium intake, which supresses conversion of 25(OH)D to 1,25(OH)$_2$D (88), has also been linked to increased risk for prostate cancer in some (65,66) but not all studies (66,89).

Genetic approaches have also been used to study interrelationships of the vitamin D axis with prostate cancer. Three polymorphisms in the vitamin D receptor (*VDR*), *BsmI*, and *TaqI* restriction site polymorphisms and a *poly(A)* length polymorphism, are in strong linkage disequilibrium in whites, such that only two *BsmI/TaqI/poly(A)* haplotypes, *BtS* and *bTL*, are commonly observed (90,91). These variants are not thought to be functional, but to possibly serve, through linkage disequilibrium, as markers for another as yet unidentified functional polymorphism, related to

Table 3 Vitamin D Receptor Polymorphic Variants and Prostate Cancer Risk Among Whites

	Relative risk		
	TaqI		
	TT	Tt	tt
Taylor et al., 1996 (94)	–	1.0	0.3[a]
Kibel et al., 1998 (95)	–	1.0	1.4
Correa-Cerro et al., 1999 (96)	1.0	0.5	1.2
Blazer et al., 2000[b] (97)	1.0	0.8	1.1
Ma et al., 1998 (93)	1.0	1.0	0.9
	Poly-A		
	LL	Ls	ss
Ingles et al., 1997[c] (90)	1.0	0.2[a]	0.2[a]

[a]$p < 0.05$.
[b]Relative risks recalculated for TT as the referent.
[c]Relative risks recalculated for LL as the referent.

bone density, osteoporosis, and serum vitamin D levels (92,93). In whites, the (*BsmI*) B, (*TaqI*) t, and [*poly(A)*] short allelic variants have been associated with reduced risk for prostate cancer in some studies (35,94). Others have not confirmed these findings, although effects have been noted in some subgroups (93,95–97) (Table 3).

In Asians and African-Americans, the linkage between the identified variants is weaker (90) and, consequently, the strength or direction of associations observed for these markers with prostate cancer risk may be different than those observed in whites. A Japanese study found no association with *TaqI* variants (98) and a Chinese study found no association with the BsmI polymorphism or with variants in an unrelated 5′ FokI polymorphic site (99), except for a subgroup of subjects in the highest tertile of IGFBP-3. In a study of African-Americans (91), risk for advanced cancer (but not localized cancer) was associated with the *BsmI/poly(A)* BL haplotype. It remains unclear whether VDR variants play a substantial role in prostate carcinogenesis.

6. METABOLIC POLYMORPHISMS

Meat cooked at high temperatures produces heterocyclic amines including PhIP (2-amino-1-methyl-6-phenylimidazol[4,5-b]pyridine). PhIp causes prostate cancer in rats; the cancers showing invasive characteristics in the presence of testosterone proprionate (64).

Polymorphisms in the N-acetyltransferases (*NAT1* and *NAT2*) result in differential metabolism of PhIP to carcinogenic metabolites and the homozygous *10 polymorphism in *NAT1*, which is related to rapid metabolism, tends to be associated with prostate cancer (100,101).

Prostate cancer was associated with the *CYP2D6 B* allele in one study ($p = 0.07$) (102) and, in another study, with the nondeleted (functional) genotype of *GSTT1* (odds ratio, 1.83; 95% confidence interval, 1.19–2.80) but not GSTM1 (odds ratio, 1.07; 95% confidence interval, 0.73–1.55) (103). No differences were found in a small case–control study of prostate cancer assessing the 609 $C \rightarrow T$ polymorphism in *NQO1* (the NAD(P)H: quinone oxidoreductase gene) (104). These results need to be evaluated in larger studies examining the inter-relationship of series of metabolic enzymes and prostate cancer risk.

7. SEXUALLY TRANSMITTED DISEASES

A history of syphilis and gonorrhea has been associated with risk for prostate cancer in a series of epidemiological studies (Table 4) (105–114). In the largest study, risks were shown to increase with increasing occurrences of gonorrhea and to be related to characteristics of sexual behavior. Also, serological investigations showed that risks were significantly greater for men exposed to *Treponema pallidum* (the causative agent of syphilis) (114).

Table 4   Sexually Transmitted Disease and Risk for Prostate Cancer

	Exposed cases	Risk
Wynder et al., 1971 (106)		
Whites	25	1.2
Blacks	12	0.7
Krain, 1974 (107)	28	5.6[a]
Heshmat et al., 1975 (108)	42	2.1[a]
Lees et al., 1985 (109)	29	1.5
Mishina et al., 1985 (110)	34	1.5
Mandel and Schuman, 1987, (111)	23	2.1[a]
Ross et al., 1987 (112)		
Whites	16	2.3
Blacks	70	1.7[a]
Honda et al., 1988 (113)	32	1.5
Hayes et al., 2000 (114)	142	1.6[a]
Rosenblatt et al., 2000 (105)	85	1.5[a]

[a]$p < 0.05$.

Since gonorrhea and syphilis could be sentinels for another sexually transmitted infectious agent, the risks observed may only partially reflect the true risks associated with the putative agent. For example, only after sensitive and specific assays were developed for human papilloma virus (HPV) did the relatively modest risks for cervical intraepithelial neoplasia associated with sexual activity (two- to four fold) translate to the substantial (50-fold) risks now established for cervical disease due to specific HPV subtypes (115).

Human papilloma virus, which occurs in human prostate cancer and benign prostatic tissue (116), transforms human prostate cells in vitro. Seropositivity for HPV-18 and HPV-16 has been associated with subsequent prostate cancer in a Finnish cohort study (117). Other studies (114,118), but not all (119) tend to support this. While an excess of prostate cancer has been observed in men with anal cancer, which is linked to HPV infection, the epidemiological patterns of HPV-related cervical cancer are not closely correlated with prostate cancer, although one study reported increased occurrence of cervical cancer in spouses of prostate cancer patients (120). No case–control differences have been found for prostate cancer with serologic responses to herpes simplex, cytomegalovirus, and Epstein–Barr virus (111,121,122). HHV8 RNA transcripts were reported in prostate cancers (123) but serologic studies for antibody have been negative (124).

8. SUMMARY

Age, race, and family history of prostate cancer are the three established risk factors for prostate cancer. Steroidal hormones are likely important in the pathogenesis of this disease, although the precise hormonal interrelationships and associated metabolic pathways are not yet defined.

Expanded molecular studies and an intervention trial with finasteride will provide insight about the role of hormones in prostate cancer. There is substantial evidence that some dietary factors, such as animal fat, increase risk for this disease and that other dietary factors, including selected micronutrients, are protective. Randomized trials have been initiated to assess the preventive impact on prostate cancer of selenium, α-tocopherol, and β-carotene. The association in epidemiologic studies of prostate cancer with sexually transmitted diseases suggests that sexually transmitted agents may also contribute to the occurrence of these tumors.

REFERENCES

1. Woolf CM. An investigation of the familial aspects of carcinoma of the prostate. Cancer 1960; 13:739–744.
2. Whittemore AS, Wu AH, Kolonel LN, John EM, Gallagher RP, Howe GR, West DW, Teh CZ, Stamey T. Family history and prostate cancer risk in

Black, White, and Asian men in the United States and Canada. Am J Epidemiol 1995; 141:732–740.

3. Hayes RB, Liff JM, Pottern LM, Greenberg RS, Schoenberg JB, Schwartz AG, Swanson GM, Silverman DT, Brown LM, Hoover RN, Fraumeni JF. Prostate cancer risk in US Blacks and Whites with a family history of cancer. Int J Cancer 1995; 60:361–364.

4. Monroe KR, Yu MC, Kolonel LN, Coetzee GA, Wilkins LR, Ross RK, Henderson BE. Evidence of an X-linked or recessive genetic component to prostate cancer risk. Nat Med 1995; 1:827–829.

5. Keetch DW, Rice JP, Suarez BK, Catalona WJ. Familial aspects of prostate cancer: a case–control study. J Urol 1995; 154:2100–2102.

6. Narod SA, Dupont A, Cusan L, Diamond P, Gomez JL, Subutu R, Labrie F. The impact of family history on early detection of prostate cancer. Nat Med 1995; 1:99–101.

7. Lesko SM, Rosenberg L, Shapiro S. Family history and prostate cancer risk. Am J Epidemiol 1996; 144:1041–1047.

8. Schaid DJ, McDonnell SK, Blute MI, Thibodeau SN. Evidence for autosomal dominant inheritance of prostate cancer. Am J Hum Genet 1998; 62: 1425–1438.

9. Bratt O, Borg A, Kristoffersson U, Lundgren R, Zhang QX, Olsson H. CAG repeat length in the androgen receptor gene is related to age at diagnosis of prostate cancer and response to endocrine therapy, but not to prostate cancer risk. Br J Cancer 1999; 81:672–676.

10. Carter BS, Beaty TH, Steinberg GD, Childs B, Walsh PC. Mendelian inheritance of familial prostate cancer. Proc Nat Acad Sci USA 1992; 89:3367–3371.

11. Smith JR, Freije D, Carpten JD, Gronberg H, Xu JF, Isaacs SD, Brownstein MJ, Bova GS, Guo H, Bujnovszky P, Nusskern DR, Damber JE, Bergh A, Emanuelsson M, Kallioniemi OP, WalkerDaniels J, BaileyWilson JE, Beaty TH, Meyers DA, Walsh PC, Collins FS, Trent JM, Isaacs WB. Major susceptibility locus for prostate cancer on chromosome 1 suggested by a genome-wide search. Science 1996; 274:1371–1374.

12. Berthon P, Valeri A, Cohen-Akenine A, Drelon E, Paiss T, Wohr G, Latil A, Millasseau P, Mellah I, Cohen N, Blanche H, Bellane-Chantelot C, Demenais F, Teillac P, Le Duc A, de Petriconi R, Hautmann R, Chumakov I, Bachner L, Maitland NJ, Lidereau R, Vogel W, Fournier G, Mangin P, Cohen D, Cussenot O. Predisposing gene for early-onset prostate cancer, localized on chromosome 1q42.2–43. Am J Hum Genet 1998; 62:1416–1424.

13. Gibbs M, Stanford JL, McIndoe RA, Jarvik GP, Kolb S, Goode EL, Chakrabarti L, Schuster EF, Buckley VA, Miller EL, Brandzel S, Li S, Hood L, Ostrander EA. Evidence for a rare prostate cancer-susceptibility locus at chromosome 1p36. Am J Hum Genet 1999; 64:776–787.

14. Xu JF, Meyers D, Freije D, Isaacs S, Wiley K, Nusskern D, Ewing C, Wilkens E, Bujnovszky P, Bova GS, Walsh P, Isaacs W, Schleutker J, Matikainen M, Tammela T, Visakorpi T, Kallioniemi OP, Berry R, Schaid D, French A, McDonnell S, Schroeder J, Blute M, Thibodeau S, Gronberg H, Emanuelsson M, Damber JE, Bergh A, Jonsson BA, Smith J, Bailey-Wilson J, Carpten J, Stephan D, Gillanders E, Amundson I, Kainu T, Freas-Lutz D, Baffoe-

Bonnie A, Van Aucken A, Sood R, Collins F, Brownstein M, Trent J. Evidence for a prostate cancer susceptibility locus on the X chromosome. Nat Genet 1998; 20:175–179.

15. Berry R, Schroeder JJ, French AJ, McDonald SK, Peterson BJ, Cunningham JM, Thibodeau SN, Schaid DJ. Evidence for a prostate cancer susceptibility locus on chromosome 20. Am J Hum Genet 2000; 67:82–91.

16. Tavtigian SV, Simard J, Teng DH, Abtin V, Baumgard M, Beck A, et al. A candidate prostate cancer susceptibility gene at chromosome 17p. Nat Genet 2001; 27:172–180.

17. Witte JS, Goddard KA, Conti DV, Elston RC, Lin J, Suarez BK, et al. Genome wide scan for prostate cancer aggressiveness gene loci. Am J Hum Genet 2000; 67:92–99.

18. Ross RK, Bernstein L, Judd H, Hanisch R, Pike MC. Serum testosterone levels in young black and white men. J Natl Cancer Inst 1986; 76:45–48.

19. Henderson BE, Bernstein L, Ross RK, Depue H, Judd H. The early in utero oestrogen and testosterone environment of blacks and whites: potential effects on male offspring. Br J Cancer 1988; 57:216–218.

20. Ross RK, Bernstein L, Lobo RA, Shimizu H, Stanczyk FZ, Pike MC. 5-alpha reductase activity and risk of prostate cancer among Japanese and U.S. white and black males. Lancet 1992; 339:887–890.

21. Wu A, Whittemore A, Kolonel LN, John E, Gallagher RP, West D, Hankin J, Teh C, Dreon D, Paffenbarger R. Serum androgens and sex hormone-binding globulins in relation to lifestyle factors in older African-American, white, and Asian men in the United States and Canada. Cancer Epidemiol Biomarkers Prev 1995; 4:735–741.

22. Eaton NE, Reeves GK, Appleby PN, Key TJ. Endogenous sex hormones and prostate cancer: a quantitative review of prospective studies. Br J Cancer 1999; 80:930–934.

23. Gann PH, Hennekens CH, Ma J, Longcope C, Stampfer HJ. Prospective study of sex hormone levels and risk of prostate cancer. J Natl Cancer Inst 1996; 88:1118–1126.

24. Thompson IM, Coltman CA Jr, Crowley J. Chemoprevention of prostate cancer: the Prostate Cancer Prevention Trial. Prostate 1997; 33:217–221.

25. Thigpen AE, Davis DL, Gautier T, Imperato-McGinley J, Russell DW. The molecular basis of 5-alpha-reductase deficiency in a large Dominican kindred. N Eng J Med 1992; 327:1216–1219.

26. Makridakis NM, Ross RK, Pike MC, Crocitto LE, Kolonel LN, Pearce CL, Henderson BE, Reichardt JKV. Association of mis-sense substitution in SRD5A2 gene with prostate cancer in African-American and Hispanic men in Los Angeles, USA. Lancet 1999; 354:975–978.

27. Kantoff PW, Febbo PG, Giovannucci E, Krithivas K, Dahl DM, Chang G, Hennekens CH, Brown M, Stampfer MJ. A polymorphism of the 5 alpha-reductase gene and its association with prostate cancer: a case–control analysis. Cancer Epidemiol Biomarkers Prev 1997; 6:189–192.

28. Lunn RM, Bell DA, Mohler JL, Taylor JA. Prostate cancer risk and polymorphism in 17 hydroxylase (CYP17) and steroid reductase (SRD5A2). Carcinogenesis 1999; 20:1727–1731.

29. La Spada AR, Wilson EM, Lubahn DB, Harding AE, Fischbeck KH. Androgen receptor gene mutations in X-linked spinal and bulbar muscular atrophy. Nature 1991; 352:77–79.
30. Hsiao PW, Lin DL, Nakao R, Chang C. The linkage of Kennedy's neuron disease to ARA24, the first identified androgen receptor polyglutamine region-associated coactivator. J Biol Chem 1999; 274:20229–20234.
31. Tut TG, Ghadesey FJ, Trifiro MA, Pinsky L, Yong EL. Long polyglutamine tracts in the androgen receptor are associated with reduced trans-activation, impaired sperm function, and male infertiltiy. J Clin Endocrinol Metab 1997; 82:3777–3782.
32. Krithivas K, Yurgalevitch SM, Mohr BA, Wilcox CJ, Batter SJ, Brown M, Longcope C, McKinlay JB, Kantoff PW. Evidence that the CAG repeat in the androgen receptor gene is associated with the age-related decline in serum androgen levels in men. J Endocrinol 1999; 162:137–142.
33. Chamberlain NC, Driver ED, Miesfeld RL. The length and location of CAG trinucleotide repeats in the androgen receptor N-terminal domain affect trans-activation function. Nucleic Acid Res 1994; 22:3181–3186.
34. Irvine RA, Yu MC, Ross RK, Coetzee GA. The CAG and GGC microsatellites of the androgen receptor gene are in linkage disequilibrium in men with prostate cancer. Cancer Res 1995; 55:1937–1940.
35. Ingles SA, Ross RK, Yu MC, Irvine RA, LaPera G, Haile RW, Coetzee GA. Association of prostate cancer risk with genetic polymorphisms in vitamin D receptor and androgen receptor. J Natl Cancer Inst 1997; 89:166–170.
36. Giovannucci E, Stampfer MJ, Krithivas K, Brown M, Brufsky A, Talcott J, Hennekens CH, Kantoff PW. The CAG repeat within the androgen receptor gene and its relationship to prostate cancer. Proc Natl Acad Sci U S A 1997; 94:3320–3323.
37. Hakimi JM, Schoenberg MP, Rondinelli RH, Piantadosi S, Barrack ER. Androgen receptor variants with short glutamine or glycine repeats may identify unique subpopulations of men with prostate cancer. Clin Cancer Res 1997; 3:1599–1608.
38. Stanford JL, Just JJ, Gibbs M, Wicklund KG, Neal CL, Blumenstein BA, Ostrander EA. Polymorphic repeats in the androgen receptor gene: molecular markers of prostate cancer risk. Cancer Res 1997; 57:1194–1198.
39. Correa-Cerro L, Wohr G, Haussler J, Berthon P, Drelon E, Mangin P, Fournier G, Cussenot O, Kraus P, Just W, Paiss T, Cantu JM, Vogel W. (CAG)n-CAA and GGN repeats in the human androgen receptor gene are not associated with prostate cancer in a French-German population. Eur J Hum Genet 1999; 7:357–362.
40. Hsing AW, Gao YT, Wu G, Wang X, Deng J, Chen YL, Sesterhenn IA, Mostofi FK, Benichou J, Chang C. Polymorphic CAG and GGN repeat lengths in the androgen receptor gene and prostate cancer risk: a population-based case–control study in China. Can Res 2000; 60:5111–5116.
41. Xue WM, Irvine RA, Yu MC, Ross RK, Coetzee GA, Ingles SA. Susceptibility to prostate cancer: interaction between genotypes at the androgen receptor and prostate-specific antigen loci. Cancer Res 2000; 60:839–841.

42. Wadelius M, Anderson AO, Johansson JE, Wadelius C, Rane E. Prostate cancer associated CYP17 genotype. Pharmacogenetics 1999; 9:635–639.
43. Insulin-like growth factor-1 and prostate cancer: a meta-analysis. Br J Cancer 2001; 85:991–996.
44. Chan JM, Stampfer MJ, Giovannucci E, Gann PH, Ma J, Wilkinson P, Hennekens CH, Pollack M. Plasma insulin-like growth factor I and prostate cancer risk: a prospective study. Science 1998; 279:563–566.
45. Signorello LB, Brismar K, Bergstrom R, Andersson SO, Wolk A, Trichopoulos D, Adami HO. Insulin-like growth factor-binding protein-1 and prostate cancer. J Natl Cancer Inst 1999; 91:1965–1967.
46. Giovannucci E, Rimm EB, Stampfer MJ, Colditz GA, Willett WC. Height, body weight, and risk of prostate cancer. Cancer Epidemiol Biomarkers Prev 1997; 6:557–563.
47. Hayes RB, Ziegler RG, Gridley G, Swanson C, Greenberg RS, Swanson GM, Schoenberg JB, Silverman DT, Brown LM, Pottern LM, Liff J, Schwartz AG, Fraumeni JF, Hoover RN. Dietary factors and risks for prostate cancer among blacks and whites in the United States. Cancer Epidemiol Biomarkers Prev 1999; 8:25–34.
48. Norrish AE, McRae CU, Holdaway IM, Jackson RT. Height-related risk factors for prostate cancer. Br J Cancer 2000; 82:241–245.
49. Platz EA, Pollak MN, Rimm EB, Majeed N, Tao YZ, Willett WC, Giovannucci E. Racial variation in insulin-like growth factor-1 and binding protein-3 concentrations in middle-aged men. Cancer Epidemiol Biomarkers Prev 1999; 8:1107–1110.
50. Tricoli JV, Winter DL, Hanlon AL, Raysor SL, Watkins-Bruner D, Pinover WH, Hanks GE. Racial differences in insulin-like growth factor binding protein-3 in men at increased risk of prostate cancer. Urology 1999; 54:178–182.
51. Thissen J-P, Ketelslegers J-M, Underwood LE. Nutritional regulation of the insulin-like growth factors. Endocr Rev 1994; 15:80–101.
52. Kaklamani VG, Linos A, Kaklamani E, Markaki I, Koumantaki Y, Mantzoros CS. Dietary fat and carbohydrates are independently associated with circulating insulin-like growth factor 1 and insulin-like growth factor-binding protein 3 concentrations in healthy adults. J Clin Oncol 1999; 17:3291–3298.
53. Kaklamani VG, Linos A, Kaklamani E, Markaki I, Mantzoros C. Age, sex, and smoking are predictors of circulating insulin- like growth factor 1 and insulin-like growth factor-binding protein 3. J Clin Oncol 1999; 17:813–817.
54. Nickerson T, Huynh H. Vitamin D analogue EB1089-induced prostate regression is associated with increased gene expression of insulin-like growth factor binding proteins. J Endocrinol 1999; 160:223–229.
55. Gregory CW, Kim D, Ye P, D'Ercole AJ, Pretlow TG, Mohler JL, French FS. Androgen receptor up-regulates insulin-like growth factor binding protein-5 (IGFBP-5) expression in a human prostate cancer xenograft. Endocrinology 1999; 140:2372–2381.
56. Huynh H, Seyam RM, Brock GB. Reduction of ventral prostate weight by finasteride is associated with suppression of insulin-like growth factor I (IGF-I) and IGF-I receptor genes and with an increase in IGF binding protein 3. Cancer Res 1998; 58:215–218.

57. Cohen P, Graves HCB, Peehl DM, Kamarei M, Giudice LC, Rosenfeld RG. Prostate-specific antigen (PSA) is an insulin-like growth factor binding protein-3 protease found in seminal plasma. J Clin Endocrinol Metabol 1992; 75:1046–1053.

58. Pollak M, Beamer W, Zhang JC. Insulin-like growth factors and prostate cancer. Cancer Metastasis Rev 1998; 17:383–390.

59. Kolonel LN, Nomura AMY, Cooney RV. Dietary fat and prostate cancer: current status. J Natl Cancer Inst 1999; 91:414–428.

60. Key TJ, Fraser GE, Thorogood M, Appleby PN, Beral V, Reeves G, Burr ML, Chang-Claude J, Frentzel-Beyme R, Kuzma JW, Mann J, McPherson K. Mortality in vegetarians and nonvegetarians: detailed findings from a collaborative analysis of 5 prospective studies. Am J Clin Nutr 1999; 70: 516S–524S.

61. Fraser GE. Associations between diet and cancer, ischemic heart disease, and all-cause mortality in non-Hispanic white California Seventh-day Adventists. Am J Clin Nutr 1999; 70:532S–538S.

62. Bosland MC. Dietary fat, calories, and prostate cancer risk—response. J Natl Cancer Inst 1999; 91:1692–1693.

63. Platz EA. Energy imbalance and prostate cancer. J Nutr 2002; 132:3471–3481.

64. Shirai T, Cui L, Takahashi S, Futakuchi M, Asamoto M, Kato K, Ito N. Carcinogenicity of 2-amino-1-methyl-6-phenylimidazo [4,5-b]pyridine (PhIP) in the rat prostate and induction of invasive carcinomas by subsequent treatment with testosterone propionate. Cancer Lett 1999; 143:217–221.

65. Giovannucci E, Rimm EB, Wolk A, Ascherio A, Stampfer MJ, Colditz GA, Willett WC. Calcium and fructose intake in relation to risk of prostate cancer. Cancer Res 1998; 58:442–447.

66. Berndt SI, Carter HB, Landis PK, Tucker KL, Hsieh LJ, Metter EJ, Platz EA. Calcium intake and prostate cancer risk in a long-term aging study: the Baltimore Longitudinal Study of Aging. Urology 2002; 60:1118–1123.

67. Norrish AE, Skeaff CM, Arribas GLB, Sharpe SJ, Jackson RT. Prostate cancer risk and consumption of fish oils: a dietary biomarker-based case–control study. Br J Cancer 1999; 81:1238–1242.

68. Cohen JH, Kristal AR, Stanford JL. Fruit and vegetable intakes and prostate cancer risk. J Natl Cancer Inst 2000; 92:61–68.

69. Gann PH, Ma J, Giovannucci E, Willett W, Sacks FM, Hennekens CH, Stampfer MJ. Lower prostate cancer risk in men with elevated plasma lycopene levels: results of a prospective analysis. Cancer Res 1999; 59:1225–1230.

70. Adlercreutz M. Epidemiology of phytoestrogens. Baillieres Clin Endocrinol Metab 1998; 12:605–623.

71. Clark LC, Dalkin B, Krongrad A, Combs GF, Turnbull BW, Slate EH, Witherington R, Herlong JH, Janosko E, Carpenter D, Borosso C, Falk S, Rounder J. Decreased incidence of prostate cancer with selenium supplementation: results of a double-blind cancer prevention trial. Br J Urol 1998; 81:730–734.

72. Heinonen OP, Albanes D, Virtamo J, Taylor PR, Huttunen JK, Hartman AM, Haapakoski J, Malila N, Rautalahti M, Ripatti S, Maenpaa H, Teerenhovi L, Koss L, Virolainen M, Edwards BK. Prostate cancer and

supplementation with alpha-tocopherol and beta-carotene: incidence and mortality in a controlled trial. J Natl Cancer Inst 1998; 90:440–446.

73. Chan JM, Stampfer MJ, Ma J, Rimm EB, Willett WC, Giovannucci EL. Supplemental vitamin E intake and prostate cancer risk in a large cohort of men in the United States. Cancer Epidemiol Biomarkers Prev 1999; 8:893–899.

74. Kristal AR, Stanford JL, Cohen JH, Wicklund K, Patterson RE. Vitamin and mineral supplement use is associated with reduced risk of prostate cancer. Cancer Epidemiol Biomarkers Prev 1999; 8:887–892.

75. Shibata A, Paganini-Hill A, Ross RK, Henderson BE. Intake of vegetables, fruits, B-carotene, vitamin C and vitamin supplements and cancer incidence in the elderly: a prospective study. Br J Cancer 1992; 66:673–679.

76. Yoshizawa K, Willett WC, Morris SJ, Stampfer MJ, Spiegelman D, Rimm EB, Giovannucci E. Study of prediagnostic selenium level in toenails and the risk of advanced prostate cancer. J Natl Cancer Inst 1998; 90:1219–1224.

77. Hardekk L, Degerman A, Tomic R, Marklund SL, Bergfors M. Levels of selenium in plasma and glutathione-peroxidase in erythrocytes in patients with prostate cancer or benign hyperplasia. Eur J Cancer Prev 1995; 4:91–95.

78. The α-Tocopherol and B-Carotene Cancer Prevention Study Group. The effect of vitamin E and B-carotene on the incidence of lung cancer and other cancers in male smokers. N Engl J Med 1994; 330:1029–1035.

79. Omenn GS, Goodman GE, Thornquist MD, Balmes J, Cullen MR, Glass A, Keogh JP, Meyskens FL, Valanis B, Williams JH, Barnhart S, Hammar S. Effects of a combination of beta carotene and vitamin A on lung cancer and cardiovascular disease. N Engl J Med 1996; 334:1150–1155.

80. Giovannucci E. A review of epidemiologic studies of tomatoes, lycopene, and prostate cancer. Exp Biol Med 2002; 227:852–859.

81. Christen WG, Gaziano JM, Hennekens CH. Design of physicians' health study II—A randomized trial of beta-carotene, vitamins E and C, and multivitamins, in prevention of cancer, cardiovascular disease, and eye disease, and review of results of completed trials. Ann Epidemiol 2000; 10:125–134.

82. Zhao XY, Ly LH, Peehl DM, Feldman D. Induction of androgen receptor by 1 alpha,25-dihydroxyvitamin D-3 and 9-cis retinoic acid in LNCaP human prostate cancer cells. Endocrinology 1999; 140:1205–1212.

83. Hanchette CL, Schwartz GG. Geographic patterns of prostate cancer mortality: evidence for a protective effect of ultraviolet radiation. Cancer 1999; 70:2861–2869.

84. Getzenberg RH, Light BW, Lapco PE, Konety BR, Nangia AK, Acierno JS, Dhir R, Shurin Z, Day RS, Trump DL, Johnson CS. Vitamin D inhibition of prostate adenocarcinoma growth and metastasis in the Dunning rat prostate model system. Urology 1997; 50:999–1006.

85. Corder EH, Guess HA, Huka BS, Friedman GD, Sadler M, Vollmer RT, Lobaugh B, Drezner MK, Vogelman JH, Orentreich N. Vitamin D and prostate cancer: a prediagnostic study with stored sera. Cancer Epidemiol Biomarkers Prev 1993; 2:467–472.

86. Braun MM, Helzlsouer KJ, Hollis BW, Comstock GW. Prostate cancer and prediagnostic levels of serum vitamin D metabolites. Cancer Causes Control 1995; 6:235–239.

87. Nomura AMY, Stemmermann GN, Lee J, Kolonel LN, Chen TC, Turner A, Holick MF. Serum vitamin D metabolite levels and the subsequent development of prostate cancer (Hawaii, United States). Cancer Causes Control 1998; 9:425–432.

88. Giovannucci E. Dietary influences of 1,25(OH)(2) vitamin D in relation to prostate cancer: a hypothesis. Cancer Causes Control 1998; 9:567–582.

89. Schuurman AG, van den Brant PA, Dorant E, Goldbohm RA. Animal products, calcium and protein and prostate cancer risk in the Netherlands Cohort Study. Br J Cancer 1999; 80:1107–1113.

90. Ingles SA, Haile RW, Henderson BE, Kolonel LN, Nakaichi G, Shi CY, Yu MC, Ross RK, Coetzee GA. Strength of linkage disequilibrium between two vitamin D receptor markers in five ethnic groups: implications for association studies. Cancer Epidemiol Biomarkers Prev 1997; 6:93–98.

91. Ingles SA, Coetzee GA, Ross RK, Henderson BE, Kolonel LN, Crocitto L, Wang W, Haile RW. Association of prostate cancer with vitamin D receptor haplotypes in African-Americans. Cancer Res 1998; 58:1620–1623.

92. Morrison NA, Qi JC, Tokita A, Kelly PJ, Crofts L, Nguyen TV, Sambrook PN, Eisman JA. Prediction of bone density from vitamin D receptor alleles. Nature 1994; 367:284–287.

93. Ma J, Stampfer MJ, Gann PH, Hough HL, Giovannucci E, Kelsey KT, Hennekens CH, Hunter DJ. Vitamin D receptor polymorphisms, circulating vitamin D metabolites, and risk of prostate cancer in united states physicians. Cancer Epidemiol Biomarkers Prev 1998; 7:385–390.

94. Taylor JA, Hirvonen A, Watson M, Pittman G, Mohler JL, Bell DA. Association of prostate cancer with vitamin D receptor gene polymorphism. Cancer Res 1996; 56:4108–4110.

95. Kibel AS, Isaacs SD, Isaacs MB, Bova GS. Vitamin D receptor polymorphisms and lethal prostate cancer. J Urol 1998; 160:1405–1409.

96. Correa-Cerro L, Berthon P, Haussler J, Bochum S, Drelon E, Mangin P, Fournier G, Paiss T, Cussenot O, Vogel W. Vitamin D receptor polymorphisms as markers in prostate cancer. Hum Gene 1999; 105:281–287.

97. Blazer DG, Umbach DM, Bostick RM, Taylor JA. Vitamin D receptor polymorphisms and prostate cancer. Mol Carcinog 2000; 27:18–23.

98. Furuya Y, Akakura K, Masai M, Ito H. Vitamin D receptor gene polymorphism in Japanese patients with prostate cancer. Endocr J 1999; 46:467–470.

99. Chokkalingam AP, McGlynn KA, Gao YT, Pollack M, Deng J, Sesterhenn IA, Mostofi FK, Fraumeni JF Jr, Hsing AW. Vitamin D receptor gene polymorphisms, insulin-like growth factors, and prostate cancer risk: a population-based case–control study in China. Cancer Res 2001; 61:4333–4336.

100. Fukutome K, Watanabe M, Shiraishi T, Murata M, Uemura H, Kubota Y, Kawamura J, Ito H, Yatani R. N-acetyltransferase 1 genetic polymorphism influences the risk of prostate cancer development. Cancer Lett 1999; 136:83–87.

101. Hein DW, Leff MA, Ishibe N, Sinha R, Frazier HA, Doll MA, Xiao GH, Weinrich MC, Caporaso NE. Association of prostate cancer with rapid N-acetyltransferase 1 (NAT1*10) in combination with slow N-acetyltransferase

2 acetylator genotypes in a pilot case–control study. Environ Mol Mutagen 2002; 40:161–167.

102. Febbo PG, Kantoff PW, Giovannucci E, Brown M, Chang G, Hennekens CH, Stampfer M. Debrisoquine hydroxylase (CYP2D6) and prostate cancer. Cancer Epidemiol Biomarkers Prev 1998; 7:1075–1078.

103. Rebbeck TR, Walker AH, Jaffe JM, White DL, Wein AJ, Malkowicz SB. Glutathione S-transferase-mu (GSTM1) and -theta (GSTT1) genotypes in the etiology of prostate cancer. Cancer Epidemiol Biomarkers Prev 1999; 8:283–287.

104. Steiner M, Hillenbrand M, Borkowsi M, Seiter H, Schuff-Werner P. 609 C →T polymorphism in NAD(P)H: quinone oxidoreductase gene in patients with prostatic adenocarcinoma or benign prostatic hyperplasia. Cancer Lett 1999; 135:67–71.

105. Rosenblatt KA, Wicklund KG, Stanford JL. Sexual factors and the risk of prostate cancer. Amer J Epidemiol 2000; 152:1152–1158.

106. Wynder EL, Mabuchi K, Whitmore WF. Epidemiology of cancer of the prostate. Cancer 1971; 28:344–360.

107. Krain LS. Some epidemiologic variables in prostatic carcinoma in California. Prev Med 1974; 3:154–159.

108. Heshmat MY, Kovi J, Herson J, Jones GW, Jackson MA. Epidemiologic association between gonorrhea and prostatic carcinoma. Urology 1975; 6:457–460.

109. Lees REM, Steele R, Wardle D. Arsenic, syphilis, and cancer of the prostate. J Epidemiol Community Health 1985; 39:227–230.

110. Mishina T, Watanabe H, Araki H, Nakao M. Epidemiologic study of prostate cancer by matched-pair analysis. Prostate 1985; 6:423–436.

111. Mandel JS, Schuman LM. Sexual factors and prostatic cancer: results from a case–control study. J Gerontol 1987; 42:259–264.

112. Ross RK, Shimzu H, Paganini-Hill A, Honda G, Henderson BE. Case–control studies of prostate cancer in Blacks and Whites in southern California. J Natl Cancer Inst 1987; 78:869–874.

113. Honda GD, Bernstein L, Ross RK, Greenland S, Gerkins V, Henderson BE. Vasectomy, cigarette smoking, and age at 1st sexual intercourse as risk factors for prostate cancer in middle-aged men. Br J Cancer 1988; 57:326–331.

114. Hayes RB, Pottern LM, Strickler H, Rabkin C, Pope V, Swanson GM, Greenberg RS, Schoenberg JB, Liff J, Schwartz AG, Hoover RN, Fraumeni JF. Sexual behaviour, STDs and risks for prostate cancer. Br J Cancer 2000; 82:718–725.

115. Schiffman MH, Bauer HM, Hoover RN, Glass AG, Cadell DM, Rush BB, Scott DR, Sherman ME, Kurman RJ, Wacholder S, Stanton CK, Manos MM. Epidemiologic evidence showing that human papilloma virus infection causes most cervical intraepithelial neoplasia. J Natl Cancer Inst 1993; 85:958–964.

116. Serth J, Panitz F, Paeslack U, Kuczyk MA, Jonas U. Increased levels of human papillomavirus type 16 DNA in a subset of prostate cancers. Cancer Res 1999; 59:823–825.

117. Dillner J, Knekt P, Boman J, Lehtinen M, Af G, Sapp M, Schiller J, Maatela J, Aromaa A. Sero-epidemiological association between human-papillomavirus infection and risk of prostate cancer. Int J Cancer 1998; 75:564–567.

118. Hisada M, Rabkin CS, Strickler HD, Wright WE, Christianson RE, van den Berg BJ. Human papillomavirus antibody and risk of prostate cancer. J Am Med Assoc 2000; 283:340–341.

119. Strickler HD, Burk R, Shah K, Viscidi R, Jackson A, Pizza G, Bertoni F, Schiller JT, Manns A, Metcalf R, Qu WM, Goedert JJ. A multifaceted study of human papillomavirus and prostate carcinoma. Cancer 1998; 82: 1118–1125.

120. Feminella JJ, Lattimer JR. An apparent increase in genital carcinoma among wives of men with prostatic cancer: an epidemiologic survey. Pirquet Bull Clin Med 1974; 20:3–9.

121. Baker LH, Mebust WK, Chin TDY, Chapman AL, Hinthorn D, Towle D. The relationship of herpesvirus to carcinoma of the prostate. J Urol 1981; 125:370–374.

122. Andersson SO, Baron J, Bergstrom R, Lindgren C, Wolk A, Adami HO. Lifestyle factors and prostate cancer risk: a case–control study in Sweden. Cancer Epidemiol Biomarkers Prev 1996; 5:509–513.

123. Staskus KA, Zhong WD, Gebhard K, Herndier B, Wang H, Renne R, Beneke J, Pudney J, Anderson DJ, Ganem D, Hasse AT. Kaposi's sarcoma-associated herpesvirus gene expression in endothelial (Spindle) tumor cells. J Virol 1997; 71:715–719.

124. Sitas F, Carrara H, Beral V, Newton R, Reeves G, Bull D, Jentsch U, Pacella-Norman R, Bourboulia D, Whitby D, Boshoff C, Weiss R. Antibodies against human herpesvirus 8 in black South African patients with cancer. N Engl J Med 1999; 340:1863–1871.

Index